25 Update in Intensive Care and Emergency Medicine

Edited by J.-L. Vincent

Springer
Berlin
Heidelberg
New York
Barcelona
Budapest
Hong Kong
London
Milan
Paris
Santa Clara
Singapore
Tokyo

D. Tibboel E. van der Voort (Eds.)

Intensive Care in Childhood

A Challenge to the Future

With 50 Figures and 62 Tables

Springer

Series Editor

Prof. Jean-Louis Vincent
Clinical Director, Department of Intensive Care
Erasme University Hospital
Route de Lennik 808, B-1070 Brussels, Belgium

Volume Editors

Prof. Dr. Dick Tibboel
University Hospital Rotterdam, Dept. of Pediatric Surgery
Pediatric Surgical Intensive Care Unit
Sophia Children's Hospital
Dr. Molewaterplein 60, NL-3015 GJ Rotterdam, The Netherlands

Prof. Dr. Edwin van der Voort
University Hospital Rotterdam, Dept. of Pediatrics
Subdivision of Pediatric Intensive Care
Sophia Children's Hospital
Dr. Molewaterplein 60, NL-3015 GJ Rotterdam, The Netherlands

ISBN-13: 978-3-642-80229-4 e-ISBN-13: 978-3-642-80227-0
DOI: 10.1007/978-3-642-80227-0

Die Deutsche Bibliothek – CIP-Einheitsaufnahme
Intensive care in childhood : a challenge to the future / D. Tibboel ; E. v. d. Voort (ed.). – Berlin ; Heidelberg ; New York ; Barcelona ; Budapest ; Hong Kong ; London ; Milan ; Paris ; Santa Clara ; Singapore ; Tokyo : Springer, 1996
(Update in intensive care and emergency medicine ; 25)
ISBN-13: 978-3-642-80229-4
NE: Tibboel, Dick [Hrsg.]; GT

Softcover reprint of the hardcover 1st edition 1996

Typesetting and printing: Zechnersche Buchdruckerei, Speyer
Bookbinding: J. Schäffer, Grünstadt

SPIN: 10537180 19/3133-5 4 3 2 1 0 – Printed on acid-free paper

Preface

Specialized intensive care units for treatment of critically ill children have been instituted all over the world during the past 25 years, either within the framework of hospital organisations or through personal initiatives of pediatricians, pediatric surgeons, pediatric anesthesiologists etc. As a consequence the supervisors of these units have different backgrounds, which proves that a high standard of intensive care in childhood is not the unique ability of one kind of physicians. The question is whether ongoing specialization and sometimes super-specialization will automatically yield better treatment results. The intrinsic hazard of this development is losing the holistic view and broad knowledge essential for optimal care of critically ill children. For this reason we are very proud of the subtitle of the 2nd World Congress on Pediatric Intensive Care: 'From Differentiation to Integration'. An integrated approach is necessary, not only to obtain optimal treatment results in the acute phase of critical illness, but also, and maybe even more important, to evaluate treatment results and long-term morbidity. We have to realize that morbidity is not always caused by the underlying disease: in a number of children it is directly related to the treatment modalities.

We are convinced that the 44 chapters in this book represent expert views from leading authorities in the different specialties involved in care of the critically ill child. Importantly, not only physicians but specialized nurses as well have contributed to this update in intensive care and emergency medicine. The fact that Prof.Dr.J.L.Vincent as chief editor of the series has recognized the increasing importance of intensive care in childhood proves that this area of medicine has reached adulthood.

The enormous success of the 1st World Congress on Pediatric Intensive Care, held in Baltimore, U.S.A. in 1992, strengthens our hope that his kind of meeting will serve as an international forum contributing to the development of the field of intensive care in childhood, now and in the future.

In this book our faculty members provide the reader with 'state-of-the-art' chapters on a variety of subjects, for which we are very grateful. We also like to thank Annemarie Illsley-de Jonge for her enthusiastic and energetic secretarial support which made our work so much easier than it seemed at the beginning.

Dick-Tibboel, Chairman	Edwin van der Voort, Chairman
Scientific Committee 2nd World Congress on Pediatric Intensive Care	Organing Committee 2nd World Congress on Pediatric Intensive Care

Contents

The Fragile Balance Between Cells, Organisms and Environment
(D. Tibboel and E.v.d. Voort) 1

Neonatology/Pediatric Surgery

Persistent Pulmonary Hypertension of the Newborn
(K.R. Stenmark, M.G. Frid and E.C. Dempsey) 11

Free Radicals in Neonatal Intensive Care
(O.D. Saugstad) 36

Bronchopulmonary Dysplasia: Strategies for Therapeutic Intervention
(A.K. Tanswell, M. Liu and M. Post) 53

Adverse Effects of Dexamethasone Treatment in Preterm Neonates
(A.F. Bos and S. Bambang Oetomo) 66

Neonatal Metabolism of Surfactant Phosphatidylcholine: Therapeutic Implications
(L.J.I. Zimmermann) 75

The Lung in Congenital Diaphragmatic Hernia (CDH)
(D. Tibboel, T. Okazaki and T. Miyano) 90

Congenital Diaphragmatic Hernia, a Defect beyond Surgical Repair
(J.C. Molenaar) 100

Neonatal Intensive Care and Neurodevelopmental Outcome
(N. Weisglas-Kuperus) 104

Organization

Outcome Assessment and Quality Assurance
in Pediatric Intensive Care
(R.J.B.J. Gemke, G.J. Bonsel and A.J. van Vught) 117

Effectiveness and Efficiency in Pediatric Intensive Care
(F. Shann) 133

Specialized Pediatric Interhospital Transfer
(J. Britto, C. DeMunter and P. Habibi) 146

The Nursing Mutual Participation Model of Care
(M.A.Q. Curley) 159

Neuroscience

The Role of Leukocytes in Global and Focal Brain Ischemia
(C.L. Schleien and J.W. Kuluz) 175

Hypoxia and Acute Brain Insult
(R.C. Tasker) 187

Current Management of Seizures and Status Epilepticus
in Children
(R. Rivera Brenes and A. Baltodano Agüero) 193

Nursing Aspect of Head-Injured Children
(P.A. Moloney-Harmon) 206

Sepsis

Neonatal Sepsis
(H. Stopfkuchen) 219

Definitions, Risk Factors, and Outcome of Sepsis in Children
(F. Leclerc, A. Martinot and C. Fourier) 229

Systemic Inflammatory Response Syndrome (SIRS)
in Pediatric Patients
(J. Fischer and S. Fanconi) 239

Septic Shock: Cardiovascular Function and Management
(M.M. Parker) 255

Plasma Concentrations of Fibronectin
in Critically Ill Children
(L. Shao, D. Guo and J. Huang) 263

Pulmonary

Mechanisms of Respiratory Failure
and New Management Strategies
(B. Lachmann, D. Gommers and S. Böhm) 271

High-Frequency Jet Ventilation or Oscillation?
(A.J. van Vught, D.G. Markhorst and R.J.B.J. Gemke) 284

The Changing Pattern of Neonatal ECMO:
Do we Really Need it ?
(J.D. Cornish) 294

Pediatric ECMO: Is there a Problem?
(P.P. O'Rourke) 312

Inhaled Nitric Oxide Therapy
in Neonatal and Pediatric Cardiorespiratory Disease
(S.H. Abman) 322

Airflow Obstruction in Asthma:
There is More than Smooth Muscle
(H.A.W.M. Tiddens and J.C. de Jongste) 337

Treatment of Severe Acute Asthma in the Child
(J.P. Piva, S. Amantéa and P.C.R. Ramos Garcia) 344

Treatment of Respiratory Syncytial Virus Bronchiolitis:
Hope and Despair
(J.L.L. Kimpen) 354

Pharmacology

Fetal Pharmacology and Therapy
(E. Jacqz Aigrain) 365

Principles of Neonatal Pharmacology
(C.M.A. Rademaker, A. Fleer and J.N. van den Anker) 375

Drug Metabolism in the Neonate and Young Infant
(G.L. Kearns and J.N. van den Anker) 385

Pharmacology of Antimicrobial Agents in Preterm Infants
(J.N. van den Anker, G.L. Kearns and R. de Groot) 400

Pulmonary Function

Monitoring and Assessment of the Pulmonary Function in Ventilated Infants and Children
(Y. Sivan and Chr.J.L. Newth) 413

Pulmonary Function Testing in Sick, Preterm Infants
(K.E. Edberg) 439

Cardiac Surgery

Long-Term Outcome After Surgery for Congenital Heart Disease
(F.J. Meijboom, A.J.J.C. Bogers, E.M.W.J. Utens and J. Hess) . 449

Curative Repair in Pediatric Cardiac Surgery is Increasingly Feasible
(A.J.J.C. Bogers and F.J. Meijboom) 458

Ethics

Ethics
(R. Truog, J. Burns and M.C. Rogers) 467

"Good" Medicine: Ethics and Pediatric Critical Care
(F.A. Carnevale) 491

Pain

Developmental Neurobiology of Pain in Neonatal and Pediatric I.C.U. Patients
(K.J.S. Anand) 507

Pain in Children: A State of the Art
(H. Huijer Abu-Saad) 517

Perspectives on Pediatric Pain Control
(A.R. Lloyd-Thomas) 527

Emergency

Management of Liver Failure
Secondary to Mushroom Poisoning in Children
(S. Clément de Cléty and D. Moulin) 539

Subject Index 549

List of Contributors

Abman, S.H.
Pulmonary and Critical Care
Medicine, B-395,
The Children's Hospital,
1056 E. Nineteenth Ave.,
Denver, CO 80218-1088
USA

Amantéa, S.
Dept of Intensive Care
Hospital da Criançia Santo Antônio
Sociedade de Pediatra do Rio Grande do Sul
Rua Eleutério de Araujo 14, Sala 501,
CEP 90680–410, Bairro Partenon,
Porto Alegre - RS
Brazil

Anand, K.J.S.
Dept of Pediatrics
Egleston Children's Hospital
at Emory University
1405 Clifton Road, NE,
Atlanta, Georgia 30322
USA

Anker van den, J.N.
Dept of Pediatrics
Sophia Children's Hospital,
Dr. Molewaterplein 60,
3015 GJ Rotterdam,
The Netherlands

Baltodano Agüero, A.
Dept of Intensive Care
National Children's Hospital
PO Box 1654–1000, San José,
Costa Rica

Bambang Oetomo, S.
Dept of Pediatrics, Division
of Neonatology
Beatrix Children's Hospital,
University Hospital
Hanzeplein 1, 9713 GZ Groningen
The Netherlands

Bogers, A.J.J.C.
Dept of Thoracic Surgery,
Thoraxcentre, BD 156,
University Hospital Sophia/Dijkzigt,
Dr. Molewaterplein 40,
3015 GD Rotterdam,
The Netherlands

Böhm, S.
Dept of Anesthesiology
Erasmus University Rotterdam
Post Box 1738
3000 DR Rotterdam
The Netherlands

Bonsel, G.J.
Dept of Clinical Epidemiology,
Academic Medical Center,
Amsterdam
Meibergdreef 9
1105 AZ Amsterdam
The Netherlands

Bos, A.F.
Dept of Pediatrics, Division
of Neonatology
Beatrix Children's Hospital,
University Hospital
Hanzeplein 1, 9713 GZ Groningen
The Netherlands

Britto, J.
Dept of Pediatrics, St. Mary's
Hospital Medical School,
South Wharf Road,
Praed Street, London W2 1NY.
United Kingdom

Burns, J.
Children's Hospital
MICU Office/Farley 517
300 Longwood Avenue
Boston, MA 02115
USA

Carnevale, F.A.
Dept of Pediatric Intensive Care
Montreal Children's Hospital
McGill University
2300 Tupper
Montreal, Quebec, Canada, H3H 1P3

Clément de Cléty, S.
Dept of Pediatric Intensive Care
Saint-Luc University Hospital
Avenue Hippocrate 10
B-1200 Brussels
Belgium

Cornish, J.D.
Dept of Pediatrics
Emory School of Medicine
2040 Ridgewood Dr., N.E.,
Atlanta, Georgia 30322, USA

Curley, M.A.Q.
Multidisciplinary ICU
Children's Hospital, Boston
46 Ripley St
Newton Centre, MA 02159-2297
USA

Dempsey, E.C.
Dept of Pediatric Critical Care
Developmental Lung Biology
and Pulmonary Medicine
University of Colorado Health
Sciences Center
4200 E. 9th Ave.
Denver, CO 80262
USA

DeMunter, C.
Dept of Pediatrics,
St. Mary's Hospital,
South Wharf Road,
Praed Street
London W2 1NY
United Kingdom

Edberg, K.E.
Dept of Pediatric Anaesthesia
& Intensive Care,
Children's Hospital, University
of Göteborg
Smorslottsgatan, 1
S-416 85 Göteborg
Sweden

Fanconi, S.
Dept of Intensive Care
University Children's Hospital
Steinwiesstrasse 75
CH-8032 Zurich
Switzerland

Fischer, J.
Dept of Intensive Care
University Children's Hospital
Steinwiesstrasse 75
CH-8032 Zurich
Switzerland

Fleer, A.
Dept of Medical Microbiology
Wilhelmina Children's Hospital
PO Box 18009
3501 CA Utrecht
The Netherlands

Fourier, C.
Dept of Pediatric Intensive Care
Hopital Jeanne de Flandre
59037 Lille
France

Frid, M.G.
Dept of Pediatric Critical Care
Developmental Lung Biology
and Pulmonary Medicine
University of Colorado Health
Sciences Center
4200 E. 9th Ave.
Denver, CO 80262
USA

Gemke, R.J.B.J.
Wilhelmina Children's Hospital and
Utrecht University Medical School
Dept of Pediatrics, P.O. Box 18009
3501 CA Utrecht
The Netherlands

Gommers, D.
Dept of Anesthesiology
Erasmus University Rotterdam
Post Box 1738
3000 DR Rotterdam
The Netherlands

Groot de, R.
Dept of Pediatrics, Division
of Pediatric Infectious Diseases,
Sophia Children's Hospital,
Dr. Molewaterplein 60, 3015 GJ
Rotterdam,
The Netherlands

Guo, D.
Tianjin Children's Hospital
Tianjin 300074
China

Habibi, P.
Dept of Pediatrics,
St. Mary's Hospital,
South Wharf Road,
Praed Street, London W2 1NY
United Kingdom

Hess, J.
Dept of Pediatrics,
Division of Cardiology
Sophia Children's Hospital
Dr Molewaterplein 60, 3015 GJ
Rotterdam
The Netherlands

Huang, J.
Tianjin Children's Hospital
Tianjin 300074
China

Huijer Abu-Saad, H.
Dept of Nursing Science
University of Limburg
Post Box 616
6200 MD Maastricht
The Netherlands

Jacqz Aigrain E.
Unité de Pharmacologie
Clinique Hopital Robert Debré
48 Boulevard Sérurier 75019 Paris,
France

Jongste de, J.C.
Dept of Pediatrics
Sophia Children's Hospital
Dr. Molewaterplein 60
3015 GJ Rotterdam
The Netherlands

Kearns, G.L.
Dept of Pediatric Clinical
Pharmacology
and Experimental Therapeutics,
The Children's Mercy Hospital,
2401 Gillham Road
Kansas City, Missouri 64108
USA

Kimpen, J.L.L.
Beatrix Children's Hospital -
University Hospital Groningen
Hanzeplein 1, POB 30.001,
9700 RB Groningen
The Netherlands

Kuluz, J.W.
Dept of Pediatrics
University of Miama School
of Medicine
Pediatric Clinical Care Medicine
PO Box 016960
Miami, Florida
USA

Lachmann, B.
Dept of Anesthesiology
Erasmus University Rotterdam
Post Box 1738
3000 DR Rotterdam
The Netherlands

Leclerc, F.
Dept of Pediatric Intensive Care
Hopital Jeanne de Flandre
59037 Lille
France

Liu, M.
Dept of Neonatology
Hospital for Sick Children
555 University Avenue
Toronto Ontario,
Canada M5G 1X8

Lloyd-Thomas, A.R.
Dept of Pediatric Anesthesia
Great Ormond Street Hospital
for Children NHS Trust
and the Institute of Child Health
Great Ormond Street
London WC1N 3JH
England

Markhorst, D.G.
Dept of Pediatrics,
Pediatric Intensive Care Unit,
Academic Hospital Vrije Universiteit,
De Boelelaan 1117
1081 HV Amsterdam
The Netherlands

Martinot, A.
Dept of Pediatric Intensive Care
Hopital Jeanne de Flandre
59037 Lille
France

Meijboom, F.J.
Dept of Pediatrics, Division
of Pediatric Cardiology
Sophia Children's Hospital
Dr Molewaterplein 60
3015 GJ Rotterdam
The Netherlands

Miyano, T.
Juntendo University School
of Medicine
2-1-1 Hongo, Bunkyo-ku
Tokyo 113
Japan

Molenaar, J.C.
Dept of Pediatric Surgery
Sophia Children's Hospital
Dr. Molewaterplein 60
3015 GJ Rotterdam
The Netherlands

Moloney-Harmon, P.A.
Children's Services
Sinai Hospital of Baltimore
125 W. Lafayette Avenue
Baltimore, MD 21217
USA

Moulin, D.
Dept of Pediatric Intensive Care
Saint-Luc University Hospital
Avenue Hippocrate 10
B-1200 Brussels
Belgium

Newth, Chr.J.L.
Dept of Pediatric Critical Care
Children's Hospital of Los Angeles,
University of Southern California
School of Medicine
4650 Sunset Blvd, Mail Stop 12
Post Office Box 54700
Los Angeles, CA 90054-0700
USA

Okazaki, T.
Juntendo University School
of Medicine, Tokyo, Japan
and Sophia Children's Hospital
Dept. of Pediatric Surgical
Intensive Care
Dr. Molewaterplein 60
3015 GJ Rotterdam
The Netherlands

O'Rourke, P.P.
Children's Hospital and Medical
Center
4800 Centpointway NE,
PO Box C5371
Seattle BA 98105
Washington
USA

Parker, M.M.
Dept of Pediatrics
HSC, T-11, SUNY at Stony Brook,
Stony Brook, NY 11794-8111
USA

Piva, J.P.
Dept of Intensive Care
Hospital da Criança Santo Antônio
Sociedade de Pediatra do Rio Grande
do Sul
Rua Eleutério de Araujo 14, Sala 501,
CEP 90680-410, Bairro Partenon,
Porto Alegre - RS
Brazil

Post, M.
Dept of Neonatology
Hospital for Sick Children
555 University Avenue
Toronto, Ontario
Canada, M5G 1X8

Rademaker, C.M.A.
Dept of Clinical Pharmacy
Wilhelmina Children's Hospital
PO Box 18009
3501 CA Utrecht
The Netherlands

Ramos Garcia, P.C.R.
Dept of Intensive Care
Sao Lucas Hospital,
Pontificia Universidade Católica
do Rio Grande do Sul,
Brazil

Rivera Brenes, R.
Dept of Intensive Care
National Children's Hospital
PO Box 1654-1000
San José
Costa Rica

Rogers, M.C.
Duke University Medical Center
Box 3708, Erwin Road
Durham, NC 27710
USA

Saugstad, O.D.
Dept of Pediatrics
Rikshospitalet
0027 Oslo
Norway

Schleien, C.L.
Dept of Pediatrics
University of Miama School
of Medicine
Pediatric Clinical Care Medicine
PO Box 016960
Miami, Florida
USA

Shann, F.
Dept of Intensive Care
Royal Children's Hospital
Parkville, Victoria 3052,
Australia

Shao, L.
Tianjin Children's Hospital
Tianjin 300074
China

Sivan, Y.
Dept of Pediatric Intensive Care
Dana Children's Hospital
Tel-Aviv Sourasky Medical center
6 Weizman street
Tel-Aviv
Israel 64239

Stenmark, K.R.
Dept of Pediatric Critical Care
Developmental Lung Biology and
Pulmonary Medicine
University of Colorado Health
Sciences Center
4200 E. 9th Ave.
Denver, CO 80262
USA

Stopfkuchen, H.
Universitätskinderklinik
Langenbeckstrasse 1
55101 Mainz
Germany

Tanswell, A.K.
Dept of Neonatology
Hospital for Sick Children
555 University Avenue
Toronto, Ontario
Canada, M5G 1X8

Tasker, R.C.
Dept of Paediatric Intensive Care
Hospital for Sick Children
Great Ormond Street
London, WC1N 3JH
United Kingdom

Tibboel, D.
Dept of Pediatric Surgical
Intensive Care
Sophia Children's Hospital
Dr. Molewaterplein 60
3015 GJ Rotterdam
The Netherlands

Tiddens, H.A.W.M.
Dept of Pediatrics
Sophia Children's Hospital
Dr. Molewaterplein 60
3015 GJ Rotterdam
The Netherlands

Truog, R.
Director Multidisc. ICU
Children's Hospital
MICU Office/Farley 517
300 Longwood Avenue
Boston, MA 02115
USA

Utens, E.M.W.J.
Dept of Child Psychiatry
Sophia Children's Hospital
Dr Molewaterplein 60,
3015 GJ Rotterdam,
The Netherlands

Voort v.d., E.
Dept of Pediatrics, Division of
Pediatric Intensive Care,
Sophia Children's Hospital
Dr. Molewaterplein 60
3015 GJ Rotterdam
The Netherlands

Vught van, A.J.
Dept of Pediatric Intensive Care
University Children's Hospital
Het Wilhelmina Kinderziekenhuis
POB 18009
3501 CA Utrecht
The Netherlands

Weisglas-Kuperus, N.
Dept of Pediatrics
Sophia Children's Hospital
Dr. Molewaterplein 60,
3015 GJ Rotterdam,
The Netherlands

Zimmermann, L.J.I.
Dept of Pediatrics
Sophia Children's Hospital
Dr. Molewaterplein 60
3015 GJ Rotterdam
The Netherlands

Abbreviations

ALS	Air leak syndrome
ARDS	Acute respiratory distress syndrome
ARF	Acute respiratory failure
BPD	Bronchopulmonary dysplasia
C	Compliance
CAH	Congenital adrenal hyperplasia
CDH	Congenital diaphragmatic hernia
CLD	Chronic lung disease
$CMRO_2$	Cerebral metabolic rate for oxygen
CMV	Conventional mechanical ventilation
CPP	Cerebral perfusion pressure
CRIB	Clinical risk index for babies
CRP	C-Reactive protein
CT	Computerized tomography
DNR	Do-not resuscitate
DSPC	Desaturated phosphatidylcholine
EAA	Excitatory amino acid
$ECCO_2R$	Extracorporeal CO_2 removal
ECMO	Extracorporeal membrane oxygenation
EDRF;1	Endothelium-derived relaxing factor
E_TCO_2	End-tidal carbon dioxide
FEFV	Expiratory flow-volume
FHF	Fulminant hepatic failure
Fn	Fibronectin
FRC	Functional residual capacity
G-CSF	Granulocyte-colony stimulating factor
GFR	Glomerular filtration rate
GPx	Glutathione peroxidase
He	Helium

HFFI	High-frequency flow interruption
HFJV	High-frequency jet ventilation
HFO	High-frequency oscillation
HFPPV	High-frequency positive pressure ventilation
HIE	Hypoxic-ischemic encephalopathy
I	Inertia
ICP	Intracranial pressure
IL-6	Interleukin-6
IVIG	Intravenous immunoglobulins
MAS	Meconium aspiration syndrome
MOF	Multiple organ failure
MOSF	Multi-organ system failure
MRI	Magnetic resonance imaging
NMDA	N-methyl-D-aspartate
NMPMC	Nursing mutual participation model of care
NO	Nitric oxide
NTB	Necrotizing tracheobronchitis
OLT	Orthotopic liver transplantation
PAGE	Perfluorocarbon-associated gas exchange
PC	Phosphatidylcholine
PCA	Patient controlled analgesia
PDE5	Phosphodiesterase
PEEP	Positive end-expiratory pressure
PGI_2	Prostacyclin
PIVH	Periventricular-intraventricular hemorrhage
PKC	Protein kinase C
PLV	Partial liquid ventilation
PPH	Primary pulmonary hypertension
PPHN	Persistent pulmonary hypertension of the newborn
PVL	Periventricular leucomalacia
PVR	Pulmonary vascular resistance
PRISM	Pediatric risk of mortality
R	Resistance
RDS	Respiratory distress syndrome
RES	Reticuloendothelial system
ROP	Retinopathy of prematurity
ROS	Reactive oxygen species

RSIVIG	Respiratory syncytial virus specific intravenous immunoglobulins
RSV	Respiratory syncytial virus
SIRS	Systemic inflammatory response syndrome
SMC	Smooth muscle cell
SNAP	Score for neonatal acute physiology
SODs	Superoxide dismutases
SP-A	Surfactant protein A
SP-B	Surfactant protein B
SP-C	Surfactant protein C
SVR	Systemic vascular resistance
TGFβs	Transforming growth factor βs
THR	Thyroid hormone receptor
TISS	Therapeutic intervention scoring system
TLV	Total liquid ventilation
TNF	Tumor necrosis factor
TRH	Thyrotropin-releasing hormone

The Fragile Balance Between Cells, Organisms and Environment

D. Tibboel and E. v. d. Voort

Introduction

Along different lines specialized units have been instituted providing intensive care for children with a large variety of bodyweight, age and disease entities. Not only the diseases treated in these units are very diverse, the same is through for the medical background of the physicians who are primary responsible for the care of these critically ill children. Due to local differences in set up pediatricians, pediatric surgeons or anesthesiologists have been appointed chairman of a specialized intensive care unit. Although new modes of treatment are continuously developed, in many instances the treatment modalities are symptomatic and as such not always based on a profound scientific basis.

Besides developments in intensive care in the last 5 to 10 years, major changes have taken place through the effort of basic scientists, elucidating basic mechanisms of cell growth, cellular differentiation and the importance of growth factors. Moreover genes responsible for certain diseases such as Duchenne muscular dystrophy, cystic fibrosis have been identified.

Intensivists can not close their eyes for the fast developments in molecular biology and we have to realize that the gain of knowledge in the basic science laboratories will have implications for our daily clinical practice.

Molecules and Cells

Today billions of US dollars are spend to unravel the human genome. As a consequence of this international collaboration genes are identified which are responsible for devastating diseases such as multicystic kidney disease, cystic fibrosis, hemophilia etc. The identification of these genes will lead to the increasing use of prenatal diagnostic procedures and as such result in real prevention and hopefully disappearance of a disease. This will inevitably lead to changes in disease patterns in the pediatric and pediatric surgical ICU's.

In the field of developmental biology, researchers are encircling basic mechanisms of cell multiplication and cell death, both important processes for normal morphogenesis and organ differentiation. Important processes such as cell-cell signalling during development, the molecular mechanisms of morphogenesis and the control of tissue differentiation by transcription factors are nowadays studied. These studies take place in animal systems which at first sight are far away from the human, like the zebrafish, axolotl, tadpoles, fruit fly, and to some extent in mice [1–4]. We can not close our eyes for these tremendous developments because the application of newly developed technics such as transgenic mice, in which certain genes can be blocked or overexpressed, can provide new insight into the etiology and pathogenesis of a disease. As a consequence of these developments, so called suicide genes in retrovirus mediated vectors can be of additional help in the treatment of certain forms of cancer such as brain tumors. Another example is the treatment of the respiratory manifestations of CF through transfer of the CFTR cDNA using adenovirus or liposome vectors [5]. Today neither conceptual or technological limitation will limit the progress in molecular genetics. The greatest challenge we face is not the scientific question of how to do this research, but the question of what to do with its products. Once applied in human, the reaction of the critically ill child will be sometimes unpredictable. Intensivists have to be aware of the background and side effects but are they really able to understand?

Along these lines of research, specific chromosomal locations have been identified to contain the genes for tumors like retinoblastoma, neurofibromatosis and Wilms's tumor. Tumor suppressor genes are of great importance in the normal regulation of cellular proliferation and differentiation [6].

In conjunction with the increased understanding of the normal behavior of cells, progress is made in the cellular and subcellular mechanisms involved in cell damage as occurs in different organs and endothelial cells such as occur during shock (polytrauma, burn shock) or during massive intra-operative stress (prolonged ischemia, major soft tissue injury). These are examples of non-bacterial inflammation, triggered by activation of various mediators of both humoral and cellular systems. Besides knowledge of the intracellular mechanisms resulting in the release of cytotoxic agents as part of the (normal) inflammatory response, biochemistry has provided us with increased knowledge of the membrane associated oxidases. We have to understand that there is still a limitation in our understanding of supply of oxygen in disease states, mostly because of unavailability of methods to assess organ specific cellular metabolism [7–9].

From time to time new molecules are discovered of which nitric oxide is the most exciting one of the last decade. Nitric oxide activity and changes in nitric oxide synthase is suggested to be of importance in a variety of diseases ranging from pulmonary hypertension to organ damage such as acute respiratory distress syndrome (ARDS) [10–12]. Today it is nearly impossible to make a list of accepted indications for the use of inhaled nitric oxide because the full spectrum of effects has to be elucidated in more detail improperly designed perspective randomized control trials (PRCT's).

Organisms

Following an infectious or a non-infectious insult, the body will depending on age and preceding disease state react with an inflammatory response. This inflammatory response can be triggered by an infectious agent but the sequence of events which is nowadays known as the systemic inflammatory response syndrome (SIRS) can be present without sepsis. It may occur following uninfected trauma, part of this has long been known as the metabolic stress response. The identification of a number of humoral factors released by cells of the host or by the invading micro-organisms, can result in an overreaction of the host which is no longer controlled anymore by natural inhibitors [13, 14].

Although the principles of management of septic shock such as meningococcal disease are well determined, the very complicated response, from a cellular point of view, impairs the widespread use of specific inhibitors of the different pathways involved such as monoclonal antibodies raised against specific cytokines or factors [15, 16]. Although the interleukin number has reached already number 13, no clinical trial has proven significant reduction in mortality. Especially identification of the tumor necrosis factor and its gene on one hand and the use of corticosteroids on the other, has attracted investigators to search for the final solution for the high mortality in septic shock both in children and adults. Acute respiratory distress syndrome (ARDS), know to occur in newborns as well, is a good example of the difficulty there is to pinpoint the crucial step in the pathogenesis of the reaction of the body to an insult. Besides measurements to maintain tissue oxygenation and adequate blood pressure, the variety of treatment modalities proposed, clearly demonstrates the lack of real understanding of the complex pathophysiological sequence of events which occur in the symptom complex called ARDS [17].

In this context old questions are reconsidered such as whether the lung should be rested or recruited. For over 15 years barotrauma has been the key feature explaining ongoing lung damage in which the high inspiratory pressures were thought to be crucial. Today this acronym is replaced more and more through volutrauma [18, 19].

One of the most exciting developments in the application of new technologies in pediatric intensive care is extracorporeal membrane oxygenation (ECMO). Although originally practiced in neonates with different disease entities, considerable doubt exists to apply ECMO in congenital diaphragmatic hernia. Following an almost religious appreciation of ECMO for 10 years now [20, 21] ECMO is only one of the treatment modalities together with high frequency oscillation with or without nitric oxide and more recently partial liquid ventilation [22, 23] enabling us to treat respiratory insufficiency.

The application of high frequency oscillation has significantly decreased the use of ECMO in case of neonatal respiratory insufficiency. In contrast there seems to be a tendency to increase the use of ECMO in non-neonatal therapy refractory respiratory insufficiency. Today no clear indications are available when and how to apply ECMO in non-neonates because prospective randomized trials are lacking and entry criteria are not well established [24].

Due to the development of perinatology birth of a child is not anymore the natural boundary when neonatologists and pediatric surgeons start to face their patient. The continuous development of fetal surgery for a variety of congenital anomalies, such as cystic adenomatoid malformation of the lung (CCAML), aortic valve obstruction and urinary tract obstruction, resulted in survival of a number of fetuses who would otherwise be born with an endstage disease or therapy-refractory respiratory insufficiency. It is obvious that these procedures should only be performed in a limited number of centers [25, 26]. The same holds through for the transplantation of stem cells, taking advantage of the immature and therefore highly tolerant immune system of the fetus for treatment of hereditary or metabolic diseases.

Advances in understanding the specific immunology related to organ transplant, including the concept of chimerism, will result in altered treatment schemes for immunosuppression with hopefully less secondly malignancies following organ transplant [27]. Next to this development, transplants are being performed in young children now, such as liver transplant in babies under 1 year of age in which reduction hepatectomy has resulted in a significant change in treatment [28].

Identification of the genes for insulin, growth hormone and a number of different growth factors, like insulin like growth factors (IGFs), has opened the opportunity for recombinant human DNA hormone manufacturing [29]. As such these hormones are easy obtainable and will probably find their way therapeutic agents in the critically ill. Today IGF trials started in adults have been stopped in children. The application of growth hormone as adjuvant therapy in pediatric intensive care is dependent on the proper assessment of the metabolic rate and progress in nutritional assessment in small children.

This is mainly influenced by the lack of data describing
1) steady state following an operative procedure in the immediate postoperative period;
2) a clear description of disease specific changes in resting energy expenditure (REE) and
3) difficulty of interpretation of the obtained values by indirect calorimetry due to tube leakage.

Not only hormones but DNAse is used as well. The gene for DNA-ase has been cloned now which has resulted in human recombinant DNA-ase I used as aerosol inhalation in cystic fibrosis patients [30]. This kind of developments will probably influence the morbidity and length of stay in the ICU and should be evaluated in properly designed prospective randomized trials.

Environment

The child in the ICU is prone to encounter iatrogenic side effects due to the non-natural environment. This may have a major impact not only on the span of life but on the occurrence of long term morbidity as well. In this context should be mentioned: the immature brain in the premature born infant has a high susceptibility to develop intracranial hemorrhage, the child with the short gut syndrome developing end stage liver disease through a combination of total parenteral nutrition and recurrent periods of sepsis. Moreover following a difficult intubation a child may end up with a trachea canula and repeated ENT surgery for treatment of the laryngeal problems.

People working in the intensive care unit are starting to realize that mortality is not the only outcome parameter to compare treatment results of different ICU's [31]. Morbidity at predetermined intervals following admission to the intensive care is at least as important as publishing mortality rates [32–36]. A number of scoring systems is developed which objectively enables us to judge upon new treatment modalities, such as the use of monoclonal antibodies to endotoxin, tumor necrosis factor or interleukin 1 receptor antagonists. Most neonatal intensive care units have well organized follow-up programs and people specially trained in child development and psychological assessment. Follow–up of intensive care treatment in older children, including pediatric surgical diseases, is lacking behind in this respect. Other specialists, apart from doctors, have developed new ways of measuring outcome. Consequently in a number of countries technology assessment is an integral part of evaluating treatment children admitted to the ICU [37]. The problem remains however, whether application of validated scoring system has the same significant for the individual patient as for patient groups as a whole [38]. Although applied technology and treatment results are frequently the scope of publications of intensive care physicians, this is only one part of the spectrum. The humane part is at least as important as the application of technology. We are awaiting bereavement in the ICU and the circumstances surrounding a bereavement may influence future morbidity and even mortality in surviving family members. Fortunately, in most intensive care unit guidelines are available for both physicians and nurses to cope with this part of their everyday workload in the intensive care unit, being death and the dying process [39].

Concluding Remarks

Every decade trends of treatment are changing as shown in Table 1. Intensivists, both physician and nurse, are confronted with the new possibilities of molecular genetics and are part of the process to transfer basic laboratory science into clinical practice. Consequently the intensivist is facing unknown technologies

Table 1. Trends in treatment modalities during the last decade

- The use of high frequency ventilation and optimal mode of ventilation
- Steroids and septic shock
- The role and dosage of epinephrine in treatment of septic shock
- Emergency operation in congenital diaphragmatic hernia
- Hyperventilation, hypothermia and barbiturates in increased intracranial pressure
- Intra-osseal infusions
- Indications for sodium bicarbonate
- Hemodynamic monitoring with Swan-Ganz catheters

and consequences of new findings which are now ready to be used in humans. We have to be aware not to act only as servants to scientists trying to apply new technologies, operative procedures or just thoughts to the individual patient. On the other hand, the intensivist should not be the factor hampering progress in this respect. We have to protect the balance and be aware how new treatment modalities are evaluated. Therefore we need an open mind for new thoughts and ideas but have to be protective in an attempt to do what is in the best interest for the individual child and his parents. Making a career in intensive care in childhood may include knowledge of developmental biology, technology assessment and application of new technologies to go hand in hand with a common sense to guarantee dignity of the individual patient under all circumstances.

In this way the fragile balance between cells, (micro)organisms and environment can be maintained.

References

1. Editorial: Looking to Development's Future. Science 1994;266:561–614.
2. Paigen K (1995) A Miracle Enough: the Power of Mice. Nature Med 1:215–220.
3. Culliton BJ (1995) Molecular medicine in a changing world. Nature Med 1:1.
4. Kirschner MW, Marincola E, Olmsted Teisberg E (1994) The role of biomedical research in health care reform. Science 266:49–54.
5. Crystal RG (1995) The gene as the drug. Nature Med 1:15–17.
6. Skuse GR, Ludlow JW (1995) Tumour suppressor genes in disease and therapy. Lancet 345:902–906.
7. Schlag G, Redl H, Hallström S (1991) The cell in shock: the origin of multiple organ failure. Resuscitation 21:137–180.
8. Babcock GT, Wikström M (1992) Oxygen activation and the conservation of energy in cell respiration. Nature 356:301–309.
9. Wagner PD (1995) Limitations of oxygen transport to the cell. Intensive Care Med 21:391–398.
10. Giaid A, Saleh D (1995) Reduced expression of endothelial nitric oxide synthase in the lungs of patients with pulmonary hypertension. N Eng J Med 333:214–221.
11. Loscalzo J (1995) Editorial: Nitric Oxide and Vascular Disease. N Engl J Med 333:251–253.
12. Fink MP, Payen D (1996) The role of nitric oxide in sepsis and ARDS. Intensive Care Med 22:158–165.
13. Pittet D, Rangel-Frausto S, Li N et al. (1995) Systemic inflammatory response syndrome, sepsis, severe sepsis and septic shock: incidence, morbidities and outcomes in surgical ICU patients. Intensive Care Med 21:302–309.
14. Lamy M, Deby-Dupont G (1995) Is sepsis a mediator-inhibitor mismatch ? Intensive Care Med 21:S250-S257.
15. Parillo JE (1993) Pathogenetic mechanisms of septic shock. N Engl J Med 328:1471–1477.
16. Giroir BP (1993) Mediators of septic shock: New approaches for interrupting the endogenous inflammatory cascade. Crit Care Med 21:780–789.
17. Kollef MH, Schuster DP (1995) The acute respiratory distress syndrome. N Engl J Med 332:27–37.
18. Dreyfuss D, Saumon G (1992) Barotrauma is volutrauma, but which volume is the one responsible ? Intensive Care Med 18:139–141.

19. Dreyfuss D, Saumon G (1994) Should the lung be rested or recruited ? The Charybdis and Scylla of Ventilator Management. Am J Respir Care Med 149:1066–1068.
20. Kanto WP (1994) A decade of experience with neonatal extracorporeal membrane oxygenation. J Pediatr 124:335–347.
21. Walsh-Sukys M, Stork EK, Martin RJ (1994) Neonatal ECMO: Iron lung of the 1990's? J Pediatr 124:427–430.
22. Curtis S (1991) Perfluorocarbon-associated gas exchange: A hybrid approach to mechanical ventilation. Crit Care Med 19:600–601.
23. Shaffer TH, Wolfson MR, Clark LC (1992) Liquid Ventilation. Pediatr Pulm 14:102–109.
24. Moler FW, Palmisano J, Custer JR (1993) Extracorporeal life support for pediatric respiratory failure: Predictors of survival from 220 patients. Crit Care Med 21:1604–1611.
25. Adzick NS, Harrison MR (1994) Fetal surgical therapy. Lancet 343:897–901.
26. Luks FI (1995) Fetal surgery; New techniques have given surgeons a second chance. Br Med J 311:1449–1453.
27. Starlz TE, Todo S, Tzakis A et al. (1993) The transplantation of gastrointestinal organs. Gastroenterology 104:673–679.
28. Beath SV, Brook GD, Kelly DA et al. (1993) Successful liver transplantation in babies under 1 year. Br Med J 307:825–828.
29. Ross RJM, Rodrigues-Arnao J, Bentham J et al. (1993) The role of insulin, growth hormone and IGF-I as anabolic agents in the critically ill. Intensive Care Med 19:S54-S57.
30. Hodson ME, Shah PL (1995) DNase trials in cystic fibrosis. Eur Respir J 8:1786–1791.
31. Outcome Assessment of Pediatric Intensive Care; Principles and Applications. Gemke RJBJ, Thesis, Utrecht (1994).
32. Horbar JD, Onstad L, Wright E et al. (1993) Predicting mortality risk for infants weighing 501 to 1500 grams at birth: A national institutes of health neonatal research network report. Crit Care Med 21:12–18.
33. Bion J (1993) Outcomes in intensive care. Br Med J 307:953–954.
34. Sanderson C, Hall DMB (1995) The outcomes of neonatal intensive care. Br Med J 310:681–682.
35. Smit R (1995) Rationing: the debate we have to have. Br Med J 310:686.
36. Petros AJ, Marshall JC, van Saene HKF (1995) Should morbidity replace mortality as an endpoint for clinical trials in intensive care ? Lancet 345:369–371.
37. Franklin C (1993) Basic concepts and fundamental issues in technology assessment. Intensive Care Med 19:117–121.
38. Lemeshow S, Klar J, Teres D (1995) Outcome Prediction for Individual Intensive Care Patients: useful, misused, or abused ? Intensive Care Med 21:770–776.
39. Granger CE, George C, Shelly MP (1995) The management of bereavement on intensive care units. Intensive Care Med 21:429–436.

Neonatology/Pediatric Surgery

Persistent Pulmonary Hypertension of the Newborn

K. R. Stenmark, M. G. Frid, and E. C. Dempsey

Introduction

Pulmonary hypertension in humans is characterized by significant increases in cell proliferation and extracellular matrix protein production in pulmonary vascular wall cells [1]. The fibroproliferative response in neonatal pulmonary hypertension is particularly exuberant compared with changes observed in adults, yet the reasons for these age-related differences remain, for the most part, obscure (Fig. 1).

Observations in animal models suggest, however, that the proliferative and matrix producing potential of the neonatal pulmonary circulation in response to injury exceeds that of the adult [2, 3]. Pulmonary artery smooth muscle cell (SMC) and fibroblasts isolated from bovine fetuses and neonatal calves and humans have been found to have enhanced growth in vitro when compared with adult cells [4, 5]. A reversion to a more immature phenotype following

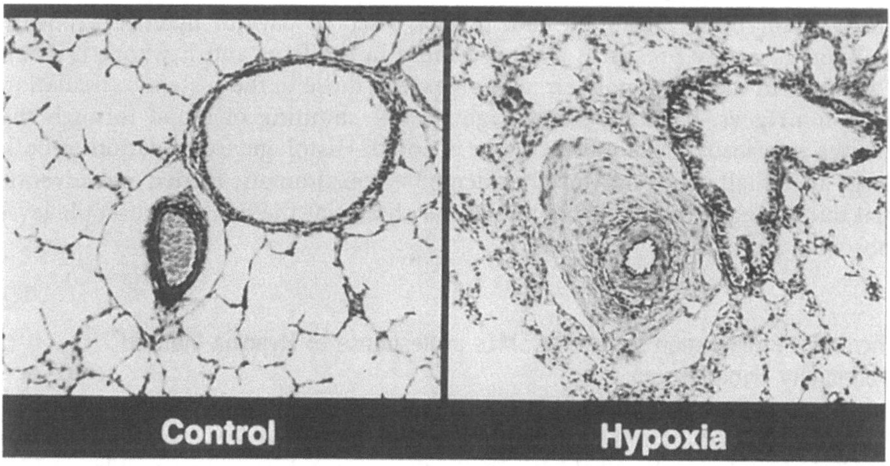

Fig. 1. Medial and adventitial thickening are observed in severe neonatal pulmonary hypertension. Shown on the left is a small pulmonary artery from a 15 day old control calf. Shown on the right is a small pulmonary artery from a 15 day old calf exposed for 14 days to hypobaric hypoxia (PB = 430 mm Hg).

exposure to mechanical injury has been described in the systemic circulation and in association with scar formation in the interstitial space of the lung [6, 7]. Tropoelastin production is also known to be developmentally regulated, and elastogenesis in arteries is limited to a brief period from mid-fetal to early neonatal life [2].

Developmental regulation of both cell proliferation and matrix protein production in the vasculature appears to be influenced to a large degree by hemodynamic forces [2, 8]. Because hemodynamic factors modulate arterial growth and protein synthesis and large and abrupt changes in hemodynamic function in the pulmonary vascular bed occur around the time of birth, we reasoned that major changes in cell proliferation and expression of tropoelastin mRNAs (taken as an example of matrix protein changes) should take place in the perinatal period. Thus, study of cell proliferation and matrix protein gene expression in the normal and hypertensive neonatal pulmonary circulation could provide clues as to the mechanisms contributing to the excessive thickening of the vessel wall observed in response to injury in the neonatal period.

In Vivo Changes in Smooth Muscle Cell and Fibroblast Proliferation in Neonatal Pulmonary Hypertension

Animal Model Used for Experimentation

We have shown that the normal decline in pulmonary artery pressure occurring after birth is inhibited by exposure of neonatal calves to hypobaric hypoxia (Fig. 2) [9, 10].

When calves, 1 day of age, are placed in a hypobaric (thus hypoxic) environment (PB = 430 mmHg) the steady decline in pulmonary artery pressure normally observed is prevented and, in fact, after 14 days of hypoxic exposure pulmonary artery pressures exceeded those in the fetus and newborn (Fig. 2). Pressures in the pulmonary circulation exceed those in the systemic circulation (110 mmHg vs. 85 mmHg) and right to left shunting of blood through the ductus arteriosus and foramen ovale is noted. Histologic examination of both large and small pulmonary arteries demonstrates dramatic medial and adventitial thickening with only minimal intimal change at the light microscopic level observed [9, 10].

Increased Proliferation in Arterial SMCs in Response to Hypoxia-Induced Pulmonary Hypertension

The contribution of cell proliferation and/or increased DNA synthesis in hypoxia-induced vessel wall thickening in the neonatal period was addressed by examining bromodeoxyuridine (BrdU; a thymidine analogue) incorporation in medial SMCs of main and intralobar pulmonary arteries of hypertensive and control calves at 2, 8, and 15 d of age [11]. In the arterial media of control

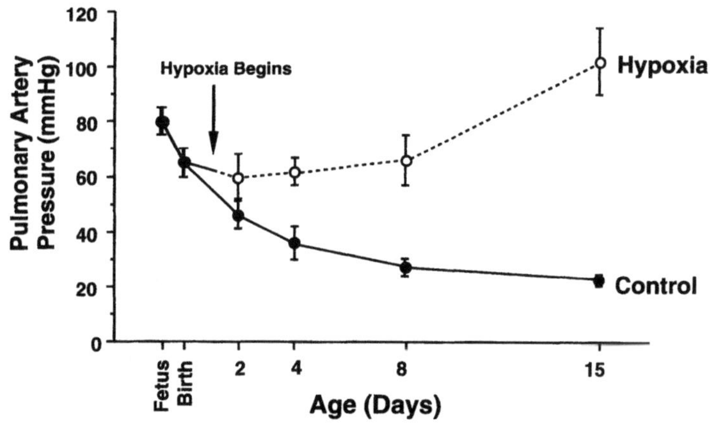

Fig. 2. Exposure to hypoxia prevents the normal decline in pulmonary artery pressure that takes place during early neonatal life. A rapid decline in pulmonary artery pressure is observed in animals born and residing at 1,500 m (•, control). When calves are made chronically hypoxic beginning on day 1 of life, (○, hypoxia), the normal decline in pressure is prevented, and by 2 wk of life, pulmonary artery pressures are greater than those observed in the fetus and even exceed those measured in the systemic circulation (mean aortic pressure. 85 + 5 mm Hg at 15 d of age).

animals the labeling index (percentage of nuclei incorporating BrdU versus total nuclei number) was highest on day 2 and progressively decreased over the first 2 wk of life (Fig. 3).

A similar pattern of decreasing cell replication was also noted in the arterial adventitia in all vessels along the longitudinal axis of the pulmonary artery. In contrast, in hypertensive animals, BrdU incorporation in the arterial media of large elastic vessels was increased on days 8 and 15, where it was 14- and 10-fold higher, respectively, than in age-matched controls (Fig. 3; [11]). Similar and even more dramatic changes were observed in small muscular pulmonary arteries. Increases in DNA synthesis in adventitial fibroblasts occurred earlier (day 2) and were even more dramatic than those observed in the arterial media. Previous studies in this model have demonstrated that the increased BrdU labeling index reflects actual cell proliferation and not simply increased DNA synthesis [12].

Heterogeneous Response of Phenotypically Distinct Pulmonary Artery SMC Subpopulations to Hypoxia-Induced Neonatal Pulmonary Hypertension

The possibility that not all medial SMCs participated equally in the proliferative responses observed, was raised by our recent observations demonstrating that the bovine arterial media is comprised of multiple phenotypically distinct SMC subpopulations [13]. Fig. 4 shows that the media of the neonatal bovine pulmonary artery is heterogeneous both with regard to structural organization

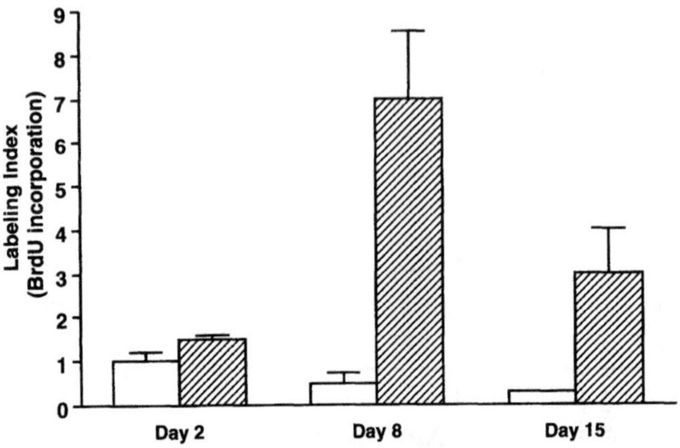

Fig. 3. BrdU labeling is increased in the pulmonary arterial media of neonatal calves with hypoxic pulmonary hypertension. The BrdU labeling index (nuclei incorporating BRDU/total nuclei × 100) in pulmonary arteries of control calves (open bars) decreased postnatally (**P < 0.05 compared with day 2). In neonatal calves with pulmonary hypertension (stippled bars), on the other hand, not only was this decline prevented, but significant increases in proliferation, compared to age-matched control animals, were observed (*P < 0.05). (n = 3 in each age group at each time point).

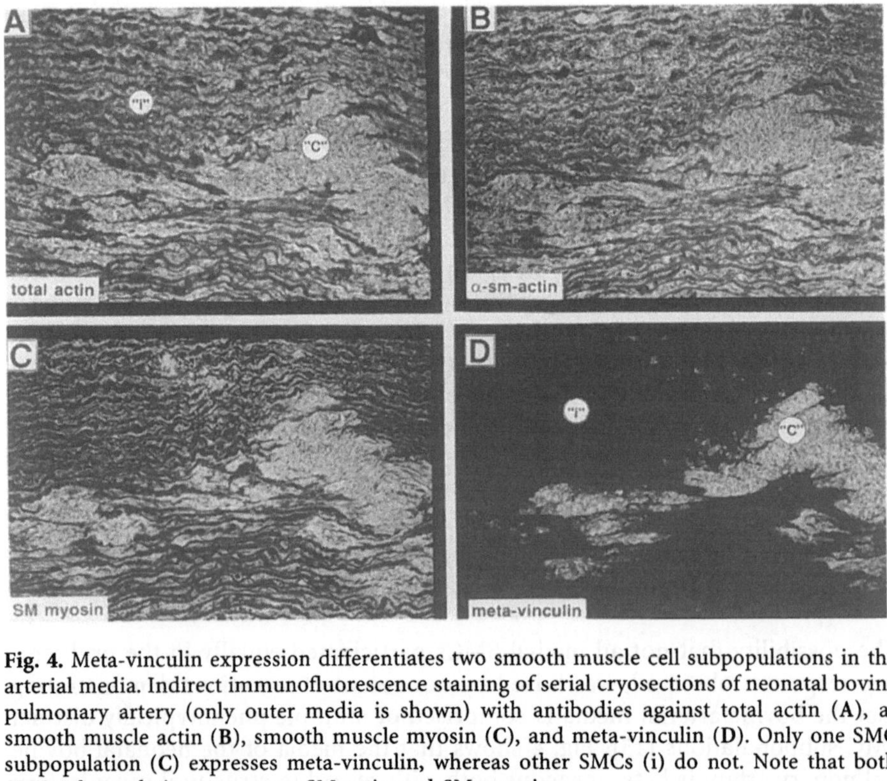

Fig. 4. Meta-vinculin expression differentiates two smooth muscle cell subpopulations in the arterial media. Indirect immunofluorescence staining of serial cryosections of neonatal bovine pulmonary artery (only outer media is shown) with antibodies against total actin (**A**), a-smooth muscle actin (**B**), smooth muscle myosin (**C**), and meta-vinculin (**D**). Only one SMC subpopulation (C) expresses meta-vinculin, whereas other SMCs (i) do not. Note that both SMC subpopulations express a-SM-actin and SM-myosin.

and SMC phenotype. Structural heterogeneity was revealed by gross microscopic examination of sections stained with antibodies against total actin which react with all cells in the vessel wall (Fig. 4A). Compact cell clusters ("C" in Fig. 4A) composed of longitudinally oriented cells, were identified within the outer media. These cell clusters were interspersed among more typical appearing thin, elongated and circumferentially oriented cells ("i" in Fig. 4A). Diversity in SMC phenotype was demonstrated by the differential expression of the high molecular weight variant of vinculin, meta-vinculin, by a specific subpopulation of SMCs in the outer media. Cells in compact clusters ("C" in Fig 4, A and D) expressed meta-vinculin, whereas other cells ("I" in Fig. 4, A and D) did not. Fig. 4 shows that in the outer media of the neonatal pulmonary artery all SMCs expressed a-smooth muscle actin (a-SM-actin), smooth muscle-myosin (SM-myosin) (Fig. 4, B and C), and as previously reported calponin and desmin [13].

To determine if hypoxic pulmonary hypertension stimulated proliferation equally in all SMC subpopulations, or if one subpopulation was preferentially effected, we used double-labeling immunofluorescence analysis. Ki-67, an antibody against a proliferation-associated nuclear antigen, was used to assess SMC proliferation. Concurrently, meta-vinculin expression was evaluated to distinguish the two SMC subpopulations within the neonatal pulmonary arterial media. Proliferation (Ki-67 positive nuclei) was seen to occur in cells throughout the entire media but rarely, if ever, within the subpopulation of SMCs expressing meta-vinculin [11]. Quantitative analysis of proliferation within the two SMC subpopulations (meta-vinculin-positive versus meta-vinculin-negative) in the arterial media of hypertensive neonatal calves showed that at all postnatal ages studied, in both the main and right pulmonary arteries, proliferation occurred almost exclusively in the meta-vinculin-negative SMC population (Fig. 5; [11]). In the pulmonary arteries of 8-d old hypertensive calves (where we had observed the highest labeling index), the percentage of replicating/meta-vinculin-positive SMCs relative to all replicating cells, was $< 5\%$ in the right pulmonary artery (right PA) and $< 2\%$ in the main pulmonary artery (main PA) (Fig. 5).

The concept that unique SMC subpopulations comprise the arterial media and respond selectively to pathologic stress is supported by previous in vivo and in vitro studies. Several laboratories have reported the existence of SMCs of different size, shape and differentiation state in the normal arterial media [13, 14]. Further, increased numbers of SMCs with an "immature" phenotype have been reported in the arterial intima and/or media in vascular diseases such as atherosclerosis, restenosis, and renovascular hypertension [15]. The presence of "less differentiated" cells in the vessel wall could be the result of either dedifferentiation/ "phenotypic modulation" of differentiated medial SMCs or the expansion of a preexisting subpopulation of "immature" SMCs during the pathogenesis of vascular disease. Further, although indirect, support for the concept that genetically distinct SMCs exist in the arterial media and exhibit differential proliferative responses to growth promoting stimuli is derived from recent in vitro studies. Several laboratories have demonstrated that

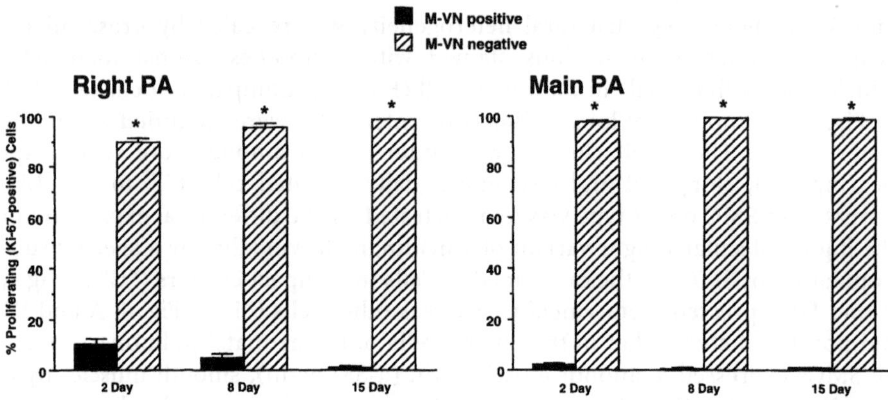

Fig. 5. Quantitative analysis demonstrates that proliferation occurs almost exclusively in the meta-vinculin-negative cell population in the pulmonary arteries of hypertensive neonatal calves. Double-label immunofluorescence staining of right and main pulmonary artery cryosections was utilized to quantitatively assess proliferation (as determined by a nuclear Ki-67 antigen expression) in two phenotypically distinct SMC subpopulations, meta-vinculin-positive (solid bars) and meta-vinculin-negative (hatched bars) (*$P < 0.001$). ($n = 3$ in each age group at each time point).

at least two SMC populations, which exhibit differential responses to the same stimulus, can be isolated from normal arteries. A subpopulation of SMCs has been isolated from the normal arterial media of neonatal and adult rats and monkeys which can grow in PDGF free media, whereas another simultaneously isolated SMC population requires PDGF for proliferation [16]. Other studies have shown that a subpopulation of SMCs less sensitive to the growth inhibitory effects of heparin could be selectively isolated from adult rat aortic media [17]. Two stable subtypes of SMCs were isolated from human adult carotid arteries based on markedly different growth characteristics [18]. Most recently, two morphologically distinct SMC populations isolated from the mature rat aortic media were shown to differ dramatically in their ionic responses to vasoactive agonists [19]. Thus, the in vivo data of our studies extend the in vivo and in vitro observations of other investigators and strongly support the idea that distinct SMC subpopulations exist in the arterial media which exhibit uniquely different responses to a given mitogenic stimulus. Specific subpopulations of medial SMCs with enhanced proliferative potential may thus contribute selectively to the process of vascular remodeling observed in neonatal pulmonary hypertension.

Homogeneous Pattern of Proliferation in Fetal Arteries

To determine if the remarkable differences in proliferative behavior of the distinct SMC subpopulations observed in the hypertensive neonate existed under other conditions associated with high rates of SMC replication, we examined the pattern of SMC proliferation in fetal pulmonary arteries, where pressure and wall stress are high (as in hypertensive neonatal animals) and where a high index of proliferation exists.

Two phenotypically distinct SMC subpopulations (meta-vinculin-positive and meta-vinculin-negative), identical to those in the neonatal arterial media, were also identified in the fetal arteries (140–270 d of gestation). The proliferative behavior of these two SMC populations was analyzed by double-labeling immunofluorescence utilizing Ki-67 and meta-vinculin antibodies. In contrast to the hypertensive neonatal arteries (Fig. 5), coexpression of Ki-67 antigen and meta-vinculin within the same cell was frequently observed in the fetal arteries of all gestation ages analyzed. To quantitatively analyze the relative rates of proliferation within each of the two arterial SMC populations at different gestational ages, we performed triple-labeling immunofluorescence staining utilizing Ki-67 and meta-vinculin antibodies, as well as the nuclear stain Hoechst-33342 on main pulmonary arteries of fetuses at different gestational ages (from 135 to 265 days). We found that the meta-vinculin-positive and meta-vinculin-negative SMC subpopulations had equal proliferative rates at each gestational age (Fig 6; [11]). Thus, in the fetal arterial media both SMC subpopulations had similar proliferative capabilities.

These observations demonstrate that significant changes in the proliferative behavior and/or potential of different SMC subpopulations appear to take place over a very short period of time between late gestation and early neonatal life.

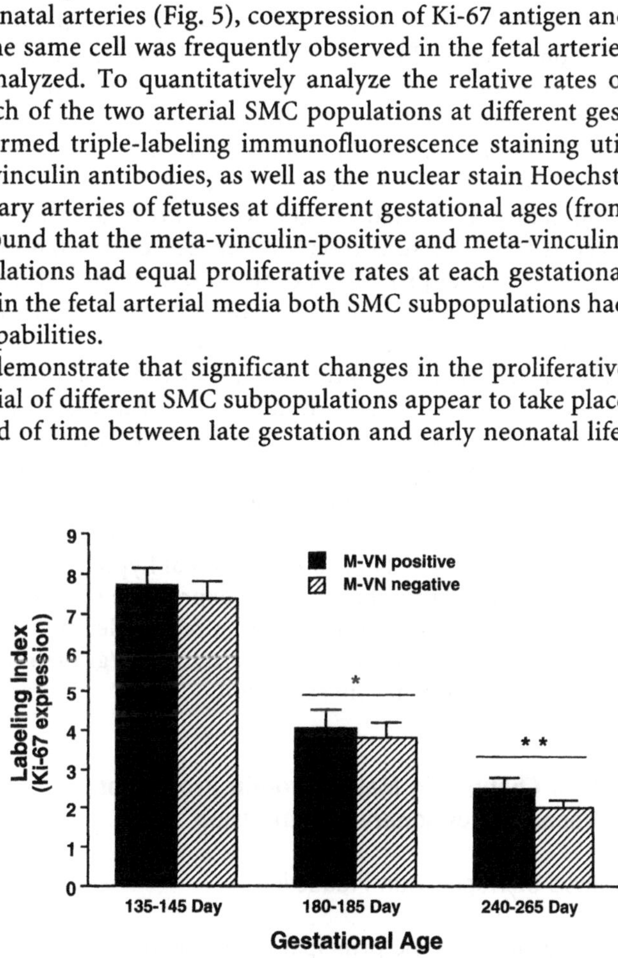

Fig. 6. Labeling index for meta-vinculin-positive and -negative SMC subpopulations in the outer media is equal in the fetus. The Ki-67 labeling index (nuclei expressing Ki-67 antigen/total number of nuclei within each SMC subpopulation [i. e., meta-vinculin-positive or meta-vinculin-negative] × 100) was calculated for the two distinct SMC subpopulations in the outer media of early (135-140-d-old), middle (180-185-d-old), and late (240-265-d-old) gestation fetal main pulmonary arteries (n = 3 at each gestational age). Relative rates of proliferation within both SMC subpopulations is equal at all gestational ages studied. Note that proliferation in both cell subpopulations declines with advancing gestational age (*$P < 0.05$ compared to 140-d-old fetus, **$P < 0.05$ compared with 180-d-old fetus.)

In fetal arteries, relatively high rates of proliferation were observed in all SMC subpopulations. After birth, a decline in the replication rate of both pulmonary arterial SMC subpopulations examined was observed under normal conditions. In the setting of severe pulmonary hypertension, overall SMC replication remained equal to or even greater than that observed in the late gestation fetus. However, one subset of SMCs (meta-vinculin-positive) which had simultaneously expressed meta-vinculin and the replication-associated marker Ki-67 in the late gestation fetus, did not proliferate under hypertensive conditions. Thus, it appears that dramatic changes in the mechanisms controlling cell proliferation occur at the time of birth in some but not all SMC populations. The factors regulating such dramatic changes in the proliferative potential of arterial SMCs before and after birth are not known.

We also observed that in fetal arteries meta-vinculin, which is believed to be a cytodifferentiation related marker, was simultaneously expressed with the proliferation-associated antigen Ki-67. Previous studies, mostly in vitro, have suggested an inverse correlation between expression of cytodifferentiation-related cytoskeletal proteins and proliferation [20, 21]. Our observations in fetal arteries do not support this idea. Moreover, we observed that cells not expressing meta-vinculin in the outer media of fetal and neonatal arteries did express other muscle specific contractile and cytoskeletal proteins such as a-SM-actin, SM-myosin, calponin and desmin and coexpression of these proteins with a proliferation associated nuclear marker Ki-67 was routinely observed (authors' unpublished observation). These results are consistent with recent studies by other investigators demonstrating that proliferation of SMCs can occur without downregulation of muscle specific proteins traditionally associated with SMC differentiation state. Thus, the traditional hypothesis regarding the existence of an inverse correlation between the expression of cytodifferentiation-associated markers and proliferation should be reconsidered. The mechanisms responsible for differential effect of various mitogens/growth factors on SMC differentiation warrant further investigation.

In Vivo Changes in Matrix Protein Production in Neonatal Pulmonary Hypertension

Analysis of Tropoelastin Production

Because elastin is the principal matrix component of large conducting arteries, tropoelastin mRNA expression provides a reliable marker of vascular SMC phenotype during normal and abnormal growth and development. Therefore, using in situ hybridization techniques we evaluated the distribution of tropoelastin mRNA in intralobar pulmonary arteries from late gestation fetuses and in animals exposed to hypobaric hypoxia from birth for 1, 3, 7, or 14d as well as in age-matched and adult room-air breathing controls [8]. We found, in the late gestation fetus (240–270 d), that tropoelastin mRNA was expressed by cells throughout the media of the lobar pulmonary artery, but, the relative signal strength varied within the vessel wall. The strongest signal was detected in the outer media where tropoelastin mRNA-positive SMC were found interspersed among dense foci of tropoelastin mRNA-negative cells (Fig. 7A). Consistent with a lack of detectable tropoelastin mRNA, these outer medial cell foci were also devoid of well-developed elastic laminae. Inner medial cells, as well as some endothelial cells, of the fetal lobar pulmonary arteries were consistently positive for tropoelastin mRNA. The signal per cell, however, appeared less in areas closer towards the vessel lumen, indicating a radial gradient of tropoelastin mRNA expression. In addition, the hybridization pattern in the innermost part of the arterial wall was random and punctate rather than arranged in a lamellar pattern as in the outer media. Arteries from 4–5 hour old newborn calves had essentially the same morphology and pattern of tropoelastin expression as that seen in the fetal vessel (Fig. 7A). After birth, the wall of the lobar pulmonary artery gradually thinned, and the pattern of tropoelastin expression was markedly altered in normal animals. At 2 d postpartum, arteries from normoxic calves demonstrated some thinning but continued to resemble fetal vessels both in the pattern and level of tropoelastin expression. By 4 d postpartum, the vessel had thinned significantly, and the signal intensity for tropoelastin mRNA was diminished. In addition, tropoelastin expression was seen mostly in middle medial cells. At 8 d after birth, no additional thinning of the artery or reduction in tropoelastin mRNA expression was evident. In 15-d-old normal neonatal calves, however, a marked change in the distribution of tropoelastin expression was seen (Fig. 7A). Unlike earlier ages, little to no signal was typically seen in outer medial wall cells but was consistently seen within cells in the first few layers of the inner media. By maturity, no consistent hybridization signal was observed in the lobar pulmonary artery [8].

In the calves subjected to hypoxia from day 1 of life, however, these age-dependent changes in pulmonary vessel morphology and tropoelastin expression did not occur. Instead, the fetal and early neonatal pattern of tropoelastin expression and wall thickness persisted after 1, 3, 7, and 14d of hypoxia exposure (Fig. 7B). Consistent among fetal, early neonatal, and all hypertensive arteries was the relative wall thickness, the increasing signal of tropoelastin mRNA expression from the inner to outer media, and the presence of foci of tropoelastin mRNA-negative cells with no intervening elastic lamellae. Very consistent was the fact that tropoelastin mRNA expression was greatest in the outer media [8].

To assess if the changing distribution of tropoelastin mRNA expression was specific to the pulmonary vasculature, we also examined sections of thoracic aorta from these same control and hypertensive calves. Strong hybridization signal was observed throughout the vessel wall, with the exception of tropoelastin mRNA-negative cell foci similar to those observed in the pulmonary artery. No changes were observed in the distribution pattern of tropoelastin mRNA in the aorta of control or hypertensive calves over the time period during which dramatic changes were observed in the pulmonary artery.

Northern blot hybridizations were done to confirm that in situ hybridization findings predicted steady state mRNA levels. High steady state tropoelas-

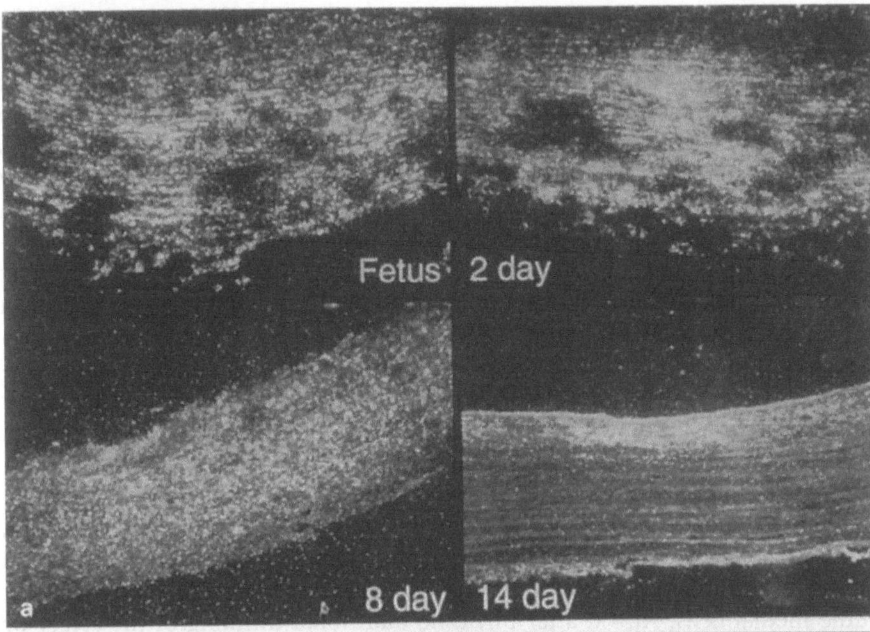

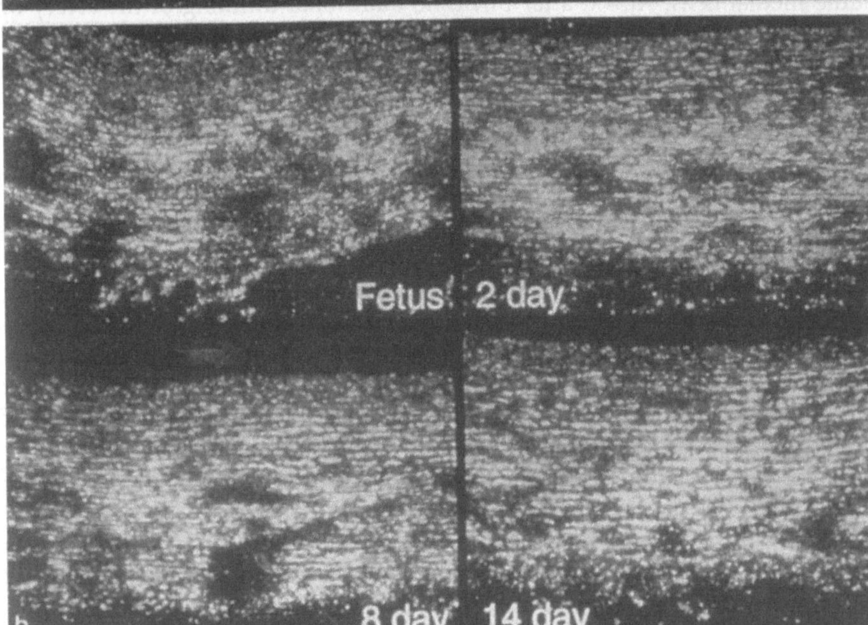

Fig. 7. Persistence of the fetal pattern of tropoelastin mRNA expression and lobar pulmonary arteries of calves with neonatal pulmonary hypertension. **a** In situ hybridization demonstrating a radial decline in tropoelastin mRNA expression over the first 14 days of normal postnatal life. In the fetus, tropoelastin mRNA is observed throughout the vessel wall (hybridization signal demonstrated by the white dots). By 8 days of life a decrease in the overall hybridization signal is observed with the greatest decrease observed in the outer wall. By 14 days tropoelastin mRNA signal is observed only in the inner third of the vessel wall. By 2 months of age, no tropoelastin mRNA signal was seen in the vessel wall (data not shown). **b** No decrease in tropoelastin mRNA hybridization signal was observed at any time point in animals made hypoxic at birth. A persistence of the fetal pattern of tropoelastin mRNA expression was observed at all time points [8].

tin mRNA levels were observed in the lobar pulmonary arteries of the fetus, a time when pulmonary artery pressure is high and when there is presumably a high degree of wall stress in the pulmonary artery. Consistent with the in situ hybridization findings, tropoelastin mRNA levels progressively declined over the first 15d of life in the lobar pulmonary artery of control animals (Fig. 8). This decline was concomitant with the progressive decrease in pulmonary artery pressure and pulmonary vascular resistance over this period of time (Fig. 2). On the other hand, tropoelastin mRNA levels remained elevated in animals exposed to hypoxia in whom pulmonary artery pressure did not decline and, in fact, were slightly elevated compared with control neonatal calves (Fig. 8). To better evaluate the relationship between tropoelastin mRNA expression and pulmonary artery pressure, we plotted relative tropoelastin levels against pressure (Fig. 9) and demonstrated a highly significant correlation (r=0.89) between pressure and tropoelastin mRNA levels.

Our studies are consistent with and extend previous studies demonstrating that expression of structural matrix proteins are apparently at least partially coupled to the hemodynamic stresses accompanying the development of the circulatory system. For instance, elastin and collagen deposition were shown to be similar in the pulmonary arterial trunk and the ascending aorta of the newborn rabbit, but by 2 mo of age, when the aortic pressure greatly exceeded that in the pulmonary artery, the contents of elastin and collagen in the aorta were also greater [22]. Increases in wall tension in both the systemic and pulmonary arterial wall have been shown to stimulate an increase in matrix protein production both in vivo and in vitro [23]. These changes occur within hours, well before an increase in many other proteins, suggesting that the matrix proteins

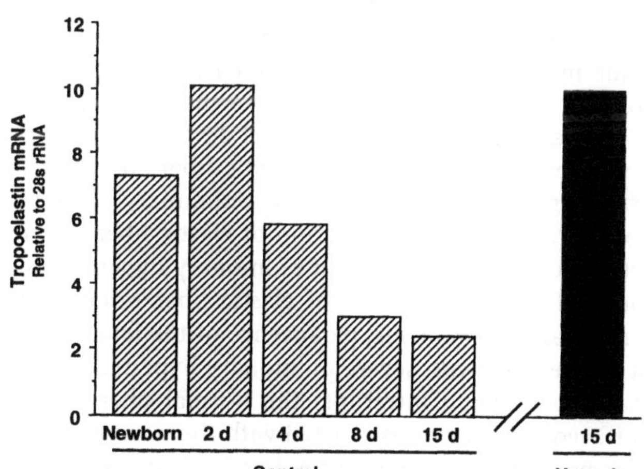

Fig. 8. Steady state tropoelastin mRNA levels decrease rapidly during normal development in lobar pulmonary arteries. Densito-metric scanning demonstrated that tropoelastin mRNA levels (relative to 28s rRNA) declined steadily over the first 15 d of life. This decline in steady state tropoelastin levels was not observed in animals exposed to hypobaric hypoxia with resultant pulmonary hypertension (15 d hypoxia).

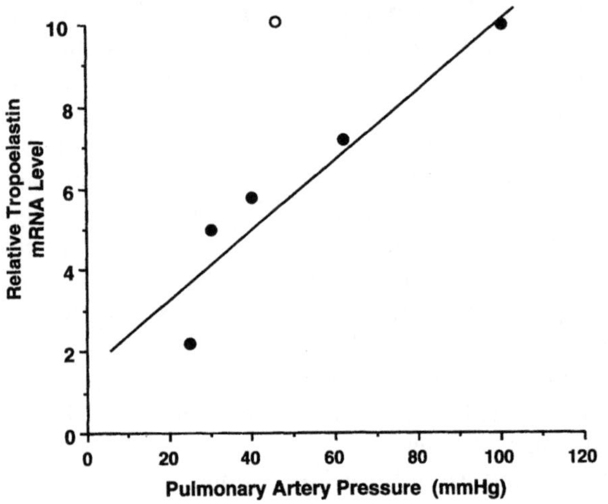

Fig. 9. Correlation of pulmonary artery pressure to relative tropoelastin mRNA levels in the pulmonary artery. When relative tropoelastin mRNA levels (to 28s rRNA) were plotted against pulmonary artery pressure, a strong correlation ($r = 0.89$) was observed. One point (o) from the 2-d-old control animals fell significantly outside this line.

quickly adapt to assist in maintenance of vessel geometry depending on the stresses that are imposed. However changes in pressure and wall stress are not the only factors controlling tropoelastin expression in the perinatal period. Recent studies have shown that increases in elastin accumulation in the aorta occur just before birth in the absence of significant changes in arterial pressure [24]. The mechanism of this increase is not known but is felt to be an adaptive response in preparation of subsequent increases in pressure. Nonetheless, the current and previous observations are consistent with the concept that pressure and wall stress likely play an important role in the pulmonary vascular pattern of elastin expression.

The current findings explain and confirm at the molecular level observations made many years ago from histologic/pathologic specimens. In the fetus, the configuration of the elastic fibers in the pulmonary trunk is similar to that of the aorta. During normal postnatal development marked differences in the arrangement of the network of elastic fibers between the aorta and pulmonary artery are observed [25]. When pulmonary hypertension exists from birth, however, the fetal configuration of elastic fiber distribution in the pulmonary artery persists. In contrast, if pulmonary hypertension is acquired later in life, the fetal or aortic pattern of elastic fiber orientation is not observed in the pulmonary artery. Thus, persistence of the fetal pattern of tropoelastin mRNA in the neonate with severe pulmonary hypertension is consistent with the idea that hypertension interrupts the normal phenotypic adaptations in vascular SMC required for or associated with the normal transition to extrauterine life. It is possible that other genes involved in the regulation of structure and/or function of the pulmonary circulation are similarly affected in the setting of neonatal pulmonary hypertension.

In Vitro Analysis of Fetal and Neonatal SMC Proliferation

Our in vivo observations suggested that isolated PA SMC would likely display developmental and injury-induced changes in proliferative phenotype and that injury (i. e. hypoxia) applied during the neonatal period might cause a persistence of a more immature, fetal-like growth phenotype. We therefore hypothesized that isolated fetal PA SMC would demonstrate increased growth properties compared to neonatal and adult cells and that PA SMC from calves exposed to chronic hypoxia would retain and/or re-express fetal-like growth characteristics. To test this hypothesis, PA SMC were isolated at three developmental stages (100–120 day fetal, 15 day neonatal, and adult), and compared to those from 15 day old calves exposed to hypoxia since the day after birth [26]. Growth responses to maximal serum stimulation (10% serum), serum withdrawal, peptide mitogens, and one physiologically relevant antiproliferative agent - heparin, were then compared. In addition, responsiveness to selective activation of the protein kinase C (PKC) pathway (using the cell-permeable phorbol ester, phorbol 12-myristate 13-acetate [PMA]) and to hypoxia were assessed. These comparative studies were designed to also detect any new and unique growth properties that neonatal PA SMC might acquire following exposure to hypoxia although there is little precedent for this in the literature.

Following these comparisons, the contribution of the PKC pathway to the differences in cell growth potential observed was then assessed. This pathway is developmentally regulated [27] and has been found to contribute to the enhanced growth of neonatal PA SMC as well as fetal and neonatal PA adventitial fibroblasts in vitro [4, 5]. Activation of PKC also increases responsiveness to developmentally-regulated mitogens and is a requisite step for PA SMC to respond directly to hypoxia [28, 29]. Many isozymes of PKC have been described [30]. Both calcium-dependent and calcium-independent PKC isozymes have been detected in PA SMC. However, their role in developmental and hypoxia-induced changes in growth of vascular cells remains unknown. The approach we used here was to examine the effects of complimentary PKC antagonist strategies - dihydrosphingosine, light-activated calphostin C, and phorbol-ester-induced PKC downregulation - on serum-stimulated growth of the different groups of PA SMC (fetal, control and hypertensive neonatal, and adult). Results with these inhibitors were then compared with those obtained with the PKC-dependent antagonist, heparin. Because these studies suggested a key role for PKC, we attempted to determine if the calcium-dependent family of PKC isozymes contributed to the growth differences. For this purpose we compared the antagonistic effects of the specific, but isozyme non-selective, PKC inhibitor, RO31-8220, with GF109203X, a structural analogue with relative specificity for the calcium-dependent isoforms of PKC (a and b in PA SMC). Finally, we compared whole cellular PKC catalytic activity in the four different groups of PA SMC(fetal, control and hypertensive neonatal, and adult).

Persistence of Fetal-like Growth Properties Following Hypoxia Exposure

To determine if there were developmental and/or injury (i. e. hypoxia)-induced differences in cell growth in response to a maximal serum stimulus, we measured the rate of SMC proliferation of fetal, control neonatal, and adult PA SMC in media supplemented with 10% serum and compared the results with those obtained with SMC harvested from hypoxic calves. These studies are useful because they tend to obscure mitogen-specific differences in growth capacity. Persistent abnormalities in growth under these conditions are likely due to more global derangements in signalling mechanisms. Fetal and neonatal hypoxic PA SMC had increased DNA synthesis and proliferative rate compared to control neonatal or adult cells (data not shown). Similar results were obtained under conditions of submaximal (1 to 5%) serum stimulation. Under serum-deprived conditions (0.1% serum) PA SMC from fetuses and hypoxic calves also exhibited persistent growth that greatly exceeded that observed for control neonatal or adult cells.

To determine if the growth pattern observed with serum stimulation would also be seen in response to purified peptide mitogens, DNA synthesis was measured in each cell culture following stimulation with 100 ng/ml IGF-I and 30 ng/ml PDGF-BB. We found that PA SMC from fetuses and hypoxia-exposed calves were more responsive to both IGF-1 and PDGF-BB than neonatal control or adult cells.

These observations demonstrated that fetal PA SMC had enhanced growth capacity compared to cells isolated at later stages of normal development, and that PA SMC from calves exposed to chronic hypoxia since day one of life retained and/or re-expressed these enhanced fetal-like growth properties. To our knowledge this is the first in vitro demonstration of a phenotypic change in growth properties of isolated PA SMC following whole animal exposure to hypoxia. The observation that hypoxic cells retain fetal-like growth properties is consistent with in vivo observations in this same animal model demonstrating persistent fetal-like growth and matrix protein synthesis in response to chronic hypoxia [8]. It is also consistent with our in vivo observations that a subpopulation of SMC in the neonatal pulmonary arterial media, that is actively proliferating during fetal life, persists in a state of rapid cell division under exposure to chronic hypoxia shortly after birth [11]. SMC from the systemic circulation have also been shown to manifest similar changes in their growth properties in response to injury. For example, human SMC harvested from restenotic lesions displayed enhanced response to PDGF compared with SMC isolated from primary stenotic lesions. During repair of arterial injury rat carotid neointimal SMC have also been shown to reexpress a developmentally regulated mRNA phenotype characteristic of earlier stages of artery wall development [6].

Hypoxia-Induced Acquisition of a More Heparin-Sensitive Growth Phenotype

We have also compared PA SMC isolated at different stages of normal development to those isolated from hypoxia-exposed neonatal calves in terms of their susceptibility to the growth-inhibitory effects of heparin. The more immature the SMC tested, the greater the susceptibility to the anti-proliferative effects of heparin observed (fetal > neonatal > adult; data not shown). PA SMC from hypoxia-exposed calves also retained and/or re-expressed a "fetal-like" pattern of enhanced sensitivity to heparin (data not shown). To our knowledge this is the first report of vascular cells acquiring a more heparin-sensitive phenotype. A phenotypic switch to a more heparin-resistant phenotype has been observed, but only after a non-physiological stimulus (i. e. chronic exposure to heparin).

Acquisition of New and Unique Growth Properties Following Exposure to Hypoxia

We then determined if the time course of developmental and hypoxia-induced changes in response to peptide mitogens were the same for a non-peptide, cell-permeable mitogen, phorbol 12-myristate 13-acetate (PMA) that directly activates the PKC pathway. DNA synthesis was measured in each cell group following stimulation with 10 nM PMA. PA SMC from hypoxia-exposed calves again had enhanced responsiveness compared to neonatal control and adult cells. Unlike for the peptide mitogens tested, fetal PA SMC did not exhibit enhanced responsiveness to PMA (and in fact were even less responsive) compared to neonatal control cells. The mitogenic response of each group of PA SMC to hypoxia following selective activation of PKC by PMA was also tested. This "priming" has been demonstrated to be necessary for a hypoxia-induced proliferative response in PA SMC. The growth response to hypoxia (3% O2) following PMA stimulation was detected in control neonatal and adult, but not fetal, PA SMC. Cells from calves exposed to chronic hypoxia had an enhanced response compared to control neonatal PA SMC.

These studies demonstrate that PA SMC from hypoxia-exposed neonatal calves have also acquired a new and unique proliferative phenotype compared to fetal cells. SMC from hypoxic calves exhibited increased responsiveness to a non-peptide cell permeable mitogen, PMA, and to hypoxia compared with neonatal control and adult cells. Fetal cells were found to be less responsive to PMA than control or hypertensive cells and unresponsive to hypoxia. This observation suggests that the developmentally regulated changes in responsiveness to growth factors may be mitogen-specific. These changes may also be cell-type specific because fetal PA adventitial fibroblasts (unlike SMC) were actually found to be more responsive to PMA than neonatal or adult fibroblasts [5]. Further, we found that responsiveness to peptide mitogens important in normal lung development are enhanced in the most immature cells while the response to a phorbol PKC activator and to hypoxia are blunted. The reasons for this phenomenon are unclear. One possible explanation is that a part of the PKC signaling cascade required for fetal PA SMC to proliferate in response to PMA and hypoxia does not mature until after birth.

Developmental and Hypoxia-Induced Changes in SMC Growth are Dependent on PKC

To determine if the enhanced growth of fetal PA SMC and cells from hypoxia-exposed calves was dependent of PKC, we compared the susceptibility of each cell group (fetal, neonatal control, adult and neonatal hypoxic) to several different PKC inhibitor strategies. We found that dihydrosphingosine (DS, 3mM), light activated calphostin C (30 nM, 1 hr each day), and PMA-induced PKC downregulation (1 mM PMA pretreatment × 24 hr), each inhibited growth of PA SMC from hypoxic calves, as well as fetal cells, to a greater extent than neonatal control or adult cells (data not shown). They each mimicked the antiproliferative effect of heparin.

Because of these findings we tested whether the calcium-dependent family of PKC isozymes contributed to the developmental and hypoxia induced changes in serum-stimulated growth observed. The inhibitory effects of the specific, but isoform non-selective, PKC antagonist, RO31-8220, were contrasted with GF109203X, a structural analogue with relative specificity for the calcium-dependent isoforms of PKC. The antiproliferative effects of the two related bisindolamide compounds on PA SMC from hypoxia-exposed calves were initially compared. Both compounds exerted the same antagonistic effects on DNA synthesis and late cell counts and thus were equipotent. We then compared the effects of 5 mM RO31-8220 and GF109203X on the developmental and hypoxia-induced changes in growth previously observed. Like for the other PKC inhibitors, fetal and hypoxic neonatal PA SMC were more susceptible to the growth inhibitory effects of both RO31-8220 and GF109203X than neonatal control and adult cells. The bisindolamide compounds were again equipotent. A lower concentration (1 mM) of these antiproliferative agents yielded similar results. To test whether developmental and/or hypoxia-induced differences in cell growth responses and susceptibility to PKC antagonists were associated with differences in PKC catalytic activity, enzyme activity was also measured in the four cell groups. The measurements paralleled the pattern of cell growth and susceptibility to PKC inhibition observed. PA SMC from fetuses and hypoxia-exposed calves had increased total catalytic activity compared with control neonatal or adult cells (data not shown). These findings suggest that the developmental and hypoxia-induced changes in PA SMC growth capacity observed here are dependent on the calcium-dependent family of PKC isozymes.

In these recently completed in vitro studies, we have found that PA SMC from hypoxia-exposed calves, like fetal cells, have enhanced growth properties compared to neonatal control and adult cells which are dependent on the PKC pathway. The family of calcium-dependent PKC isozymes appear to be particularly important here. PA SMC from hypoxia-exposed calves also acquire new and unique growth characteristics that are not detectable in fetal cells (i. e. increased responsiveness to PMA and hypoxia). These persistent and newly acquired growth properties detected in vitro likely contribute to the enhanced proliferation of neonatal PA SMC following exposure to hypoxia found in vivo.

In Vitro Analysis of Fetal and Neonatal Fibroblast Proliferation

The earliest and most striking proliferative changes in vivo in response to chronic hypoxia occur in the pulmonary artery adventitia where the fibroblast resides [31]. These adventitial changes are more impressive in the neonatal than in the adult pulmonary circulation [10]. This finding is compatible with observations showing that the proliferative and matrix producing potential of the neonatal pulmonary circulation in response to injury exceeds that of the adult [2,3, 32]. The mechanisms responsible for the increased growth of neonatal vascular wall cells in general or the adventitial fibroblast in particular are poorly understood.

Distinct morphological, structural, and functional characteristics have been described for fibroblasts isolated from different nonvascular sites [33]. However, little is known about the growth properties of fibroblasts isolated from the PA adventitia. Age-related differences in growth of skin and whole lung fibroblasts have also been described [33, 34]. Similar developmental differences in PA adventitial fibroblasts likely exist but had not been reported. Mechanisms responsible for the heterogeneity of and developmental differences in fibroblast growth responses were not known. For these reasons, a developmental comparison of pulmonary artery adventitial fibroblast growth was needed. Because persistent fetal-like growth characteristics of vascular cells in the hypertensive neonatal pulmonary arterial wall had been described in vivo [8, 11], we wanted to study cells isolated from the fetal as well as neonatal period.

We addressed the hypothesis that PA adventitial fibroblasts from neonatal and fetal animals would demonstrate enhanced growth characteristics in vitro compared with adult cells and that, similar to our observations in SMC, at least some of these properties would be dependent on PKC. To test this hypothesis, PA adventitial fibroblasts were isolated from 70- to 180-day-old bovine fetuses, 12- to 14-day-old neonatal calves, and adult cows and their growth responses to maximal serum stimulation, serum withdrawal, and stimulation with a select group of mitogens after induction of a quiescent state were first compared. Then we examined the effects of three different PKC antagonist strategies on serum-stimulated growth of fibroblasts from each developmental stage: dihydrosphingosine (also called sphinganine), phorbol-ester-induced PKC downregulation, and heparin. Finally , we compared PKC catalytic activity in lysates of fetal, neonatal, and adult fibroblasts [5].

Developmental Differences in Proliferation of Pulmonary Artery Fibroblasts

To determine whether there were developmental differences in growth in response to a maximal serum stimulus, we measured the rate of fetal, neonatal, and adult fibroblast proliferation in 10% serum-containing media. Fetal and neonatal fibroblasts grew more rapidly than adult cells (Fig. 10).

Differences became most striking after the cells reached their respective plateau densities at days 7–10. By day 10, there were 41.7 + 2.0 (fetal), 29.1 + 0.8

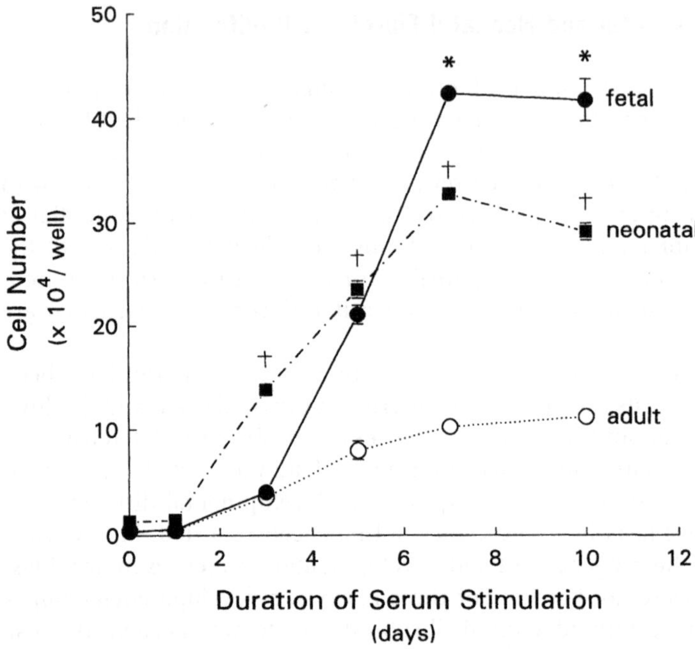

Fig. 10. Serum-stimulated fetal and neonatal pulmonary artery adventitial fibroblasts grow faster and reach higher plateau densities than adult cells. Values are means + SE for this and all subsequent figures; n = 4 replicate wells. Cells were seeded at low density (0.5 × 104 cells/cm^2) and grown in MEM/10% serum. Fetal fibroblasts used here were isolated at day 70 of gestation.. *$P < 0.05$ compared with day 0 result and matched neonatal and adult result at same time. † $P < 0.05$ compared with day 0 result and matched adult result at same time. Similar results both in direction and degree were obtained with different cell populations in 2 other independent experiments.

(neonatal), and 11.3 + 0.6 (adult) × 104 fibroblasts/well, respectively. Similar developmental differences in growth were detected by measuring DNA synthesis during log growth. Fetal and neonatal cells had increased [3H]thymidine incorporation compared with adult fibroblasts.

To determine whether the increased growth of fetal fibroblasts was dependent on time of harvest during gestation, we compared the rate of proliferation for fibroblasts isolated from 120-, 140-, and 180-day-old fetuses and an adult cow (Fig. 11). Fibroblasts isolated from 120- and 140-day fetal tissue grew more rapidly than cells harvested later in gestation (180 days). All populations of fetal cells grew faster than adult fibroblasts.

To determine whether the enhanced growth of fetal and neonatal fibroblasts was associated with increased responsiveness to a cell-permeable activator o. the PKC pathway (PMA, 10 nM), two peptide mitogens important in the local control of vascular growth (IGF-I, 100 ng/ml, and PDGF-BB, 30 ng/ml), or to a synergistic combination of PMA (10 nM) and IGF-I (100 ng/ml), [3H]-thymidine incorporation was measured in each cell population after stimulation with

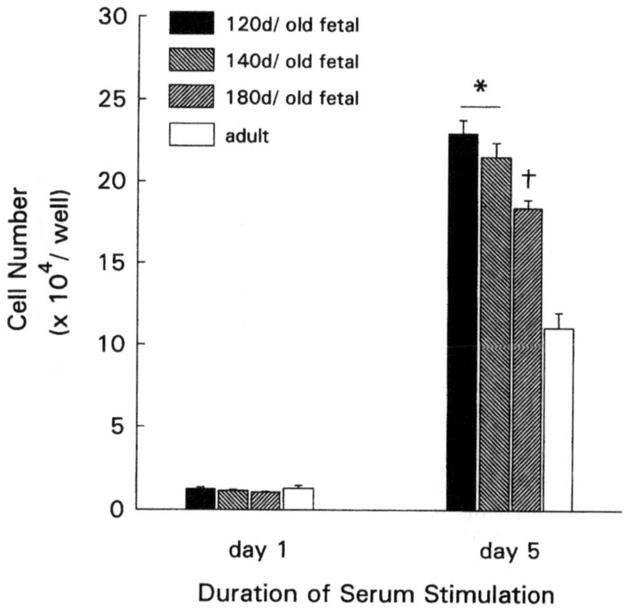

Fig. 11. Growth of fetal pulmonary artery adventitial fibroblasts is dependent on time of harvest during the fetal period; n = 4 replicate wells. Fetal (120-, 140-, and 180-day-old) and adult pulmonary artery adventitial fibroblasts were seeded at 0.5 × 104 cells/cm^2 and grown in MEM-10% serum. Medium was supplemented but not replaced on day 4. *P < 0.05 compared with 180-day-old fetal and adult values. † P < 0.05 compared with adult.

this panel of mitogens. For these experiments, the cells were growth arrested before addition of mitogens. Fetal fibroblasts had greater DNA synthesis than adult cells in response to each stimulus (Fig. 12). Neonatal cells also had increased [3H] thymidine incorporation in response to PMA alone and in combination with IGF-I compared with adult fibroblasts [5].

The increased proliferation of fetal and neonatal fibroblasts that we observed is compatible with previous growth-related studies of fetal cells. Fetal fibroblasts from other sites have been shown to have a number of unique features, including phenotypic instability, malignant growth characteristics, proliferative response to transforming growth factor-b, synthesis of certain isoforms of matrix molecules, and production of a growth factor with PDGF-like activity in comparison to adult cells [33, 34]. It is well known that there is heterogeneity in the proliferative responses of fibroblasts derived from the same anatomical site. Therefore the differences in growth capacity of fibroblasts that we have found may be due to variations in phenotype and/or differences in signaling mechanisms [2]. The increased growth capacity of fetal and neonatal PA fibroblasts in response to a maximal serum stimulus (i.e., 10%), a test condition that would likely obscure mitogen-specific differences, suggested however, that developmental differences in signal transduction mechanisms were present.

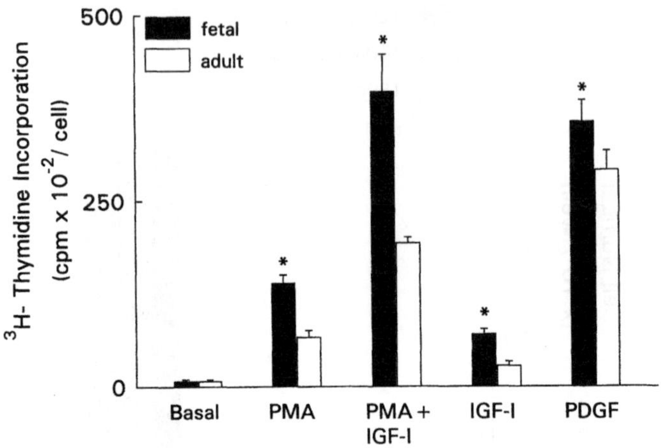

Fig. 12. Fetal pulmonary artery adventitial fibroblasts have greater DNA synthesis in response to growth factors than adult cells; n = 4 replicate wells. Cells were seeded at 0.75 × 104 cells/cm^2 in MEM-10% serum, grown for 2 days, and growth arrested for 2 days with 0.1% serum containing MEM. Fetal and adult cells were exposed to 10nM phorbol 12-myristate 13-acetate (PMA), 100 ng/ml insulin-like growth factor (IGF)-I, 30 ng/ml platelet-derived growth factor (PDGF)-BB, and the combination of 10nM PMA and 100 ng/ml IGF-I. In a separate experiment, neonatal cells also had increased responsiveness to PMA and PMA + IGF-I compared with adult cells. *$P < 0.05$ compared with matched adult. Similar results were obtained in a second independent experiment.

In response to the cell-permeable PKC activator PMA, alone or in combination with IGF-I, there was greater DNA synthesis in both fetal and neonatal fibroblasts than in adult cells. Interestingly, only fetal cells also had increased responsiveness to peptide growth factors alone (IGF-I or PDGF-BB). Others also have reported equal responses to PDGF in nonvascular neonatal and adult fibroblasts [34]. Betsholtz and Westermark [35] reported that an enhanced neonatal response to PDGF could be obtained in fibroblasts by manipulating the extracellular calcium concentration. However, we did not find that this maneuver unmasked developmental differences in PDGF responses in our neonatal and adult PA fibroblasts. We found only prestimulation with the direct PKC activator PMA allowed this to occur. These observations suggest that developmental changes in signal transduction mechanisms (like PKC) and mitogen receptors (such as receptors for PDGF and IGF-I) may be regulated by different time-dependent mechanisms. The enhanced response of fetal and neonatal fibroblasts to PMA and a combination of PMA and IGF-I is similar to our observation reported for PA SMC [4]. Collectively, these data also suggest that PKC likely contributes to the developmental differences in growth of PA adventitial fibroblasts.

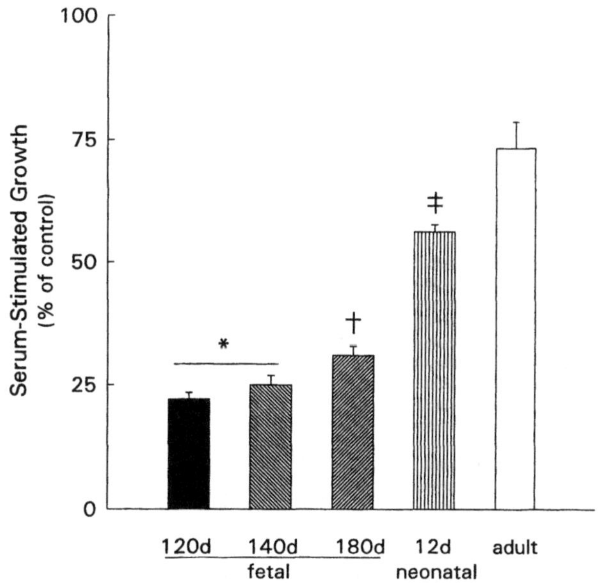

Fig. 13. Fetal and neonatal pulmonary artery adventitial fibroblasts are more sensitive than adult cells to the antiproliferative effects of the protein kinase C (PKC) inhibitor dihydrosphingosine (DS); n = 4 replicate wells. Cells were seeded at 0.5 × 104 cells/cm2 in 10% serum-containing media. On day 1 DS (3mM) or vehicle (EtOH and 2.5 mM bovine serum albumin) was added. Cells were counted on day 1 and day 5. Similar results were obtained is DS was re-added on day 3. *$P < 0.05$ compared with 180-day-old fetal, neonatal, and adult. † $P < 0.05$ compared with adult and neonatal. ‡ $P < 0.05$ compared with adult. Similar results were obtained with different cell populations in a second independent experiment.

Developmental Differences in Growth of Pulmonary Artery Fibroblasts are Dependent on PKC

To determine whether the enhanced serum-stimulated growth of fetal and neonatal fibroblasts was dependent on PKC, we compared the susceptibility of fetal, neonatal, and adult cells to three different PKC-inhibitor strategies. The PKC antagonist dihydrosphingosine inhibited growth of fetal and neonatal fibroblasts to a greater extent than adult cells (Fig. 13). Fibroblasts isolated earlier in gestation (120 and 140 days) were even more susceptible than the 180-day fetal cells to the growth-inhibiting effects of dihydrosphingosine. A complementary PKC-antagonist strategy, PMA-induced PKC downregulation, had a similar inhibitory effect on serum-stimulated growth of fibroblasts [5].

Heparin was the final PKC-inhibitor strategy analyzed (Fig. 14). It is important that this compound has been shown to exert PKC-dependent anti-proliferative effects on systemic vascular cells [36] and to attenuate the pulmonary vascular remodeling associated with adult forms of chronic hypoxic pulmonary hypertension [37]. Susceptibility to the inhibitory effects of heparin was found to parallel that observed with the other two PKC-antagonist strategies (fetal > neonatal > adult). Growth of fetal fibroblasts was antagonized by a lower con-

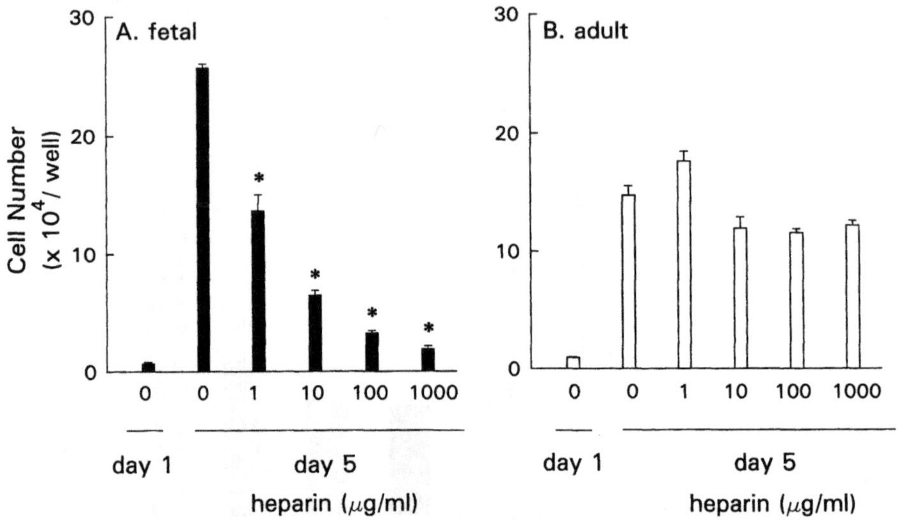

Fig. 14. Fetal pulmonary artery adventitial fibroblasts (A) are more sensitive than adult cells (B) to the PKC-dependent antiproliferative effects of heparin; n = 4 replicate wells. Cells were seeded at 0.5 × 104 cells/cm^2 in 10% serum-supplemented medium. Heparin (1-1,000 mg/ml) was added on day 1 and again on day 3. Cells were counted on days 1 and 5. *P < 0.05 compared with untreated day 5 control (heparin, 0 mg/ml). In a separate experiment, neonatal fibroblasts were also found to be more sensitive than adult cells to the antiproliferative effects of heparin (threshold, 10 mg/ml; maximum, 100 mg/ml heparin). Similar results were obtained with different cell populations in a second independent experiment.

centration (1 mg/ml) than neonatal or adult cells (10 mg/ml). Both fetal and neonatal cell proliferation were maximally inhibited to a greater extent (87 + 1 and 71 + 2%, respectively; n= 4; P < 0.05) than adult (17 + 3%) cells. The effect on adult fibroblasts was so modest that it did not reach statistical significance.

To test whether developmental differences in serum-stimulated growth and susceptibility to PKC antagonists were associated with differences in PKC catalytic activity, whole cellular enzyme activity was measured in matched fetal, neonatal, and adult pulmonary artery fibroblast. Fetal fibroblasts had higher catalytic activity than neonatal or adult cells [5].

Results with these three different PKC antagonists support the hypothesis that enhanced fetal and neonatal fibroblast growth is dependent on PKC. It has been suggested that PKC activity is an important signalling mechanism in maturing cells. As shown above, PKC is important in the enhanced growth of neonatal PA SMC compared with adult cells. Our direct measurements of PKC catalytic activity parallel the developmental differences found in growth and susceptibility to PKC inhibitors. Therefore, these results suggest a link between increased growth, increased susceptibility to PKC inhibitors, and increased whole cellular PKC activity.

The enhanced growth capacity of neonatal PA adventitial fibroblasts found in vitro is consistent with in vivo observations of dramatic adventitial thickening occurring in neonatal pulmonary hypertension. A variety of clinical and experimental studies have shown that developmentally regulated growth phenotypes may be reiterated in fibroblasts after injury and in the setting of abnormal fibrotic response. A persistent fetal phenotype may be expressed in adventitial fibroblasts during pulmonary hypertension in neonates. Therefore, the increased growth capacity of fetal and neonatal fibroblasts may contribute to the dramatic structural remodeling of the neonatal pulmonary circulation that occurs in vivo after hypoxic exposure. Furthermore, PKC-antagonist strategies like heparin may be particularly useful in attenuating pulmonary vascular remodeling in neonatal forms of pulmonary hypertension.

References

1. Morin FC, Stenmark KR (1995). Persistent pulmonary hypertension of the newborn: State-of-the-Art. Am J Respir Crit Care Med 151;2010–2032.
2. Stenmark KR, Dempsey EC, Badesch DB, Frid M, Mecham RP, Parks WC (1993). Regulation of pulmonary vascular wall cell growth: developmental and site-specific heterogeneity. Eur Respir Rev 16;629–637.
3. Rabinovitch M, Bamble WJ, Miettinen OS, Reid L (1981). Age and sex influence on pulmonary hypertension of chronic hypoxia and recovery. Am J Physiol 240;H62–H72.
4. Dempsey EC, Badesch DB, Dobyns EL, Stenmark KR (1994). Enhanced growth capacity of neonatal pulmonary artery smooth muscle cells in vitro: Dependence on cell size, time from birth, insulin-like growth factor 1, and auto-activation of protein kinase C. J Cell Physiol 160;469–481.
5. Das M, Stenmark KR, Dempsey EC (1995). Enhanced growth of fetal and neonatal pulmonary artery adventitial fibroblasts is dependent on protein kinas C. Am J Physiol 269;L660–L667.
6. Majesky MW, Giachelli CM, Reidy MA, Schwartz SM (1992). Rat carotid neointimal smooth muscle cells reexpress a developmentally regulated mRNA phenotype during repair of arterial injury. Circ Res 71;759–768.
7. Torrey DJ, Richards CD, Podor TJ, Gauldie J (1994). Anchorage-independent colony growth of pulmonary fibroblasts derived from fibrotic human lung tissue. J Clin Invest 93;1525–1532.
8. Stenmark KR, Mecham RP, Durmowicz AG, Parks WC (1994). Persistence of the fetal pattern of tropoelastin gene expression in severe neonatal pulmonary hypertension. J Clin Invest 93;1234–1242.
9. Durmowicz AG, Orton EC, Stenmark KR (1993) Progressive loss of vasodilator responsive component of pulmonary hypertension in neonatal calves exposed to 4,570m. Am J Physiol 265:H2175–H2183.
10. Stenmark KR, Fasules J, Voelkel NF, Henson J, Tucker A, Wilson H, Reeves JT (1987). Severe pulmonary hypertension and arterial adventitial changes in newborn calves at 4300m. J Appl Physiol 62;821–830.
11. Wohrley JD, Frid MG, Orton EC, Belknap JK, Stenmark KR (1995). Hypoxia selectively induces proliferation in a specific subpopulation of smooth muscle cells in the bovine neonatal pulmonary arterial media. J Clin Invest 96;273–281.
12. Orton EC, LaRue SM, Ensley B, Stenmark KR (1992). Bromodeoxyuridine labeling and DNA content of pulmonary arterial medial cells from normal and hypoxia exposed calves. Am J Vet Res 53;1925–2930.
13. Frid MG, Moiseeva EP, Stenmark KR (1994). Multiple phenotypically distinct smooth muscle cell populations exist in the adult and developing bovine pulmonary arterial media in vivo. Circ Res 75:669–681.

14. Zanellato AMC, Borrione AC, Giuriato L, Tonello M, Scannapieco G, Pauletto P, and Sartore S. (1990). Myosin isoforms and cell heterogeneity in vascular smooth muscle in developing and adult bovine aorta. Dev Biol 141:431–446.
15. Okamoto E, Imataka K, Fuji J, Kuro-o M, Nakahara K, Nishimura H, Yazaki Y, Nagai R (1992). Heterogeneity in smooth muscle cell population, accumulating in the neointima and the media of posterionotic dilation of rabbit carotid artery. Biochem Biophys Res Commun 185;459–464.
16. Lemire J, Covin CW, White S, Ciiachelli CM, Schwartz SM (1994) Characterization of cloned aortic smooth muscle cells from young rats. Am J Pathol 144:1068–1081.
17. Barzu T, Herbert JM, Deainouliere A, Carayon P, Pascal M (1994). Characterization of rat aortic smooth muscle cells resistant to the antiproliferative activity of heparin following long-term heparin treatment. J Cell Physiol 160;239–248.
18. Fujita H, Shimokado K, Yutani C, Takaichi S, Masada J, Ogata J (1993). Human neonatal and adult vascular smooth muscle cells in culture. Exp Mol Pathol 58;25–39.
19. Neylon CB, Avdonin PV, Dilley RJ, Larsen MA, Tkachuk VA, Bobik A (1994). Different electrical responses to vasoactive agonists in morphologically distinct smooth muscle cell types. Circ Res 75;733–741.
20. Fager G, Hansson GK, Gowa AM, Larson DM, Skalli O, and Bondjers G. (1989). Human arterial smooth muscle cells in culture: inverse relationship between proliferation and expression of contractile proteins. In Vitro Cell & Dev Biol 25:511–520.
21. Campbell JH, Kocher O, Skalli O, Gabbiani G, Campbell GR (1989). Cytodifferentiation and expression of a-smooth muscle actin mRNA and protein during primary culture of aortic smooth muscle cells. Atherosclerosis 9;633–643.
22. Leung DYM, Glagov S, Mathews MG (1977). Elastin and collagen accumulation in rabbit ascending aorta and pulmonary trunk during postnatal growth. Circ Res 41;316–323.
23. Tozzi CA, Poiani GJ, Harangozo AM, Boyd CD, Riley DJ (1989). Pressure-induced connective tissue synthesis in pulmonary artery segments is dependent on intact endothelium. J Clin Invest 84;1005–1012.
24. Bendeck MP, Langille RL (1991). Rapid accumulation of elastin and collagen in the aortas of sheep in the immediate perinatal period. Circ Res 69;1165–1169.
25. Heath D, Wood EH, DuShane JW, Edwards JE (1959). The structure of the pumonary trunk at different ages and in cases of pulmonary hypertension and pulmonary stenosis. J Pathol Bacteriol 77;443.
26. Xu Y, Stebnmark KR, Walchak SJ, Ruff LJ, Dempsey EC (1996). Pulmonary artery smooth muscle cells from hypoxia-exposed neonatal calves retain and/or re-express fetal-like growth properties. Submitted for presentation at 1996 annual meeting of the American Thoracic Society.
27. Otte AP, Moon RT (1992). Protein kinase C isozymes have distinct roles in neural induction and competence in Xenopus. Cell 68;1021–1029.
28. Dempsey EC, Stenmark KR, McMurtry IF, O'Brien RF, Voelkel NF, Badesch DB (1990). Insulin-like growth factor 1 and protein kinase C activation stimulate pulmonary artery smooth muscle cell proliferation through separate but synergistic pathways. J Cell Physiol 144;159–165.
29. Dempsey EC, McMurtry IF, O'Brien RF (1991). Protein kinase C activation allows pulmonary artery smooth muscle cells to proliferate to hypoxia. Am J Physiol 260;L136–L145.
30. Nishizuka Y (1992). Intracellular signaling by hydrolysis of phospholipids and activation of protein kinase C. Science 258:607–614.
31. Meyrick B, Reid L (1979). Hypoxia and incorporation of 3H-thymidine by cells of the rat pulmonary arteries and alveolar wall. Am J Pathol 96;51–70, 1979.
32. Haworth SG (1993). Pulmonary hypertension in childhood. Eur Respir J 6;1037–1043.
33. Jordana M, Kirpalaini H, Gauldie J (1992). Heterogeneity of human lung fibroblast proliferation in relation to disease expression. In: Phipps RP (ed) Pulmonary Fibroblast Heterogeneity, CRC, Boca Raton, FL, pp 229–249.
34. Karlsson C, Paulsson Y (1994). Age related reduction of platelet-derived growth factor A-chain mRNA in normal human fibroblasts. J Cell Physiol 158;256–262.

35. Betsholtrz C, Westermark B (1984). Growth factor-induced proliferation of human fibroblasts in serum-free culture depends on cell density and extracellular calcium concentration. J Cell Physiol 188;203–210.
36. Wright TC, Jr., Pukac LA, Castellot JJ, Jr., Karnovsky MJ, Levine RA, Kim-Park H-Y, Campisi J (1989). Heparin suppresses the induction of c-fos and c-myc mRNA in murine fibroblasts by selective inhibition of a protein kinase C dependent pathway. Proc Natl Acad Sci USA 86;3199–3203.
37. Thompson BT, Spence CR, Janssens SP, Joseph PM, Hales CA (1994) Inhibition of hypoxic pulmonary hypertension by heparins of differing in vitro antiproliferative potency. Am J Respir Crit Care Med 149;1512–1517.

Free Radicals in Neonatal Intensive Care

O. D. Saugstad

Introduction

The preterm baby is especially vulnerable to tissue injury. The eyes may be damaged by retinopathy of prematurity, the brain by intracranial hemorrhage and periventricular leukomalacia, the lungs by bronchopulmonary dysplasia, the ductus arteriosus may be persistent, and the intestine may suffer from necrotizing enterocolitis. Up to now most investigators have considered these conditions to be different diseases, but recently we have hypothesized that they are only different facets of the same disease, *"The oxygen radical disease in neonatology"* [1].

In fact, the field of medicine has lately experienced an explosive interest in the study of effects of free radicals. It has been suggested that free radicals are involved in a series of human diseases such as cancer, atherosclerosis, rheumatoid arthritis, and so forth. Which role do free radicals play in the perinatal period? When trying to answer this question we are moving into a field with many questions, but fewer facts.

Oxygen was discovered independently by Scheele in 1772 and Priestly in 1774. Priestly understood very early that oxygen produces toxic effects. Already in the nineteenth century such effects had been described scientifically. Further, it has recently become evident that hypoxic tissue injury is not only caused by lack of oxygen as was previously believed. Today it is clear that tissue injury associated with hypoxia occurs to a large extent in the post-hypoxic reoxygenation period. The irreversible damage to for instance the brain is not caused by complete exhaustion of substrates for energy supplies. Less than five minutes of complete ischemia is sufficient for the total exhaustion of intracellular adenosine triphosphate (ATP). Yet, in spite of this, the brain is capable of complete recovery of its adenylate pool [2, 3]. It is evident that factors other than lack of oxygen, or lack of substrates for the generation of energy, may be even more important. One such factor is oxygen radicals.

The Oxygen Paradox

When oxygen is administered after a significant period of lack of oxygen, an explosive tissue injury is found. This phenomenon which has been described in both clinical and experimental medicine, has been designated the *oxygen paradox* since it seems paradoxical that administration of oxygen to tissues lacking oxygen can be deleterious. According to Latham [4] this term was first introduced by Ruff and Strughold in 1939.

In 1980 we proposed an explanation for the oxygen paradox by introducing the hypothesis that oxygen radicals are formed in excess by the hypoxanthine-xanthine oxidase system in the post-hypoxic period [5]. I have called this phenomenon *hypoxia-reoxygenation injury*, and I believe it is of interest in a number of clinical conditions: when a patient is resuscitated with oxygen after hypoxia like the newborn baby who suffers from hypoxia during delivery and is resuscitated with high concentrations of oxygen; the preterm baby with pulmonary insufficiency who is ventilated with high concentrations of oxygen; patients resuscitated after cardiac arrest; resuscitation of organs after hypoxia or ischemia e.g. the myocard after cardiac surgery or myocardial infarction; and perfusion of organs like kidneys, liver, heart and lung in connection with transplantation.

Since we proposed this hypothesis we have developed it further in a series of publications [6, 7, 8, 9, 10] and it has been adopted by numerous other investigators. Many authors in the field mix this with the term "ischemia-reperfusion injury". I consider that hypoxia - reoxygenation injury is a more accurate term for the specific injury caused by oxygen radicals formed by hypoxanthine-xanthine oxidase and other systems in the reoxygenation period. Ischemia-reperfusion is much more complex and includes a series of additional, known and unknown, mechanisms contributing to tissue injury.

Clinical Effects Of Hyperoxia

Today we know that oxygen exerts acute and chronic toxic effects on a number of organs such as the lung and brain. It influences the circulation, endocrinological functions, enzyme systems and molecular organization. The acute clinical effects of hyperoxia on the brain are: vertigo, nausea, involuntary movements, convulsions, auditory hallucinations and paresthesia [11, 12, 13, 14].

Exposure of the lung to high oxygen concentrations produces dyspnea, tachypnea and respiratory inhibition [15]. The content of bacteria in the lung increases rapidly, partly because both the epithelium in the airways and the ciliae are affected. The blood-air barrier becomes thicker and after a while the type I alveolar cells disappear and the type II cells increase in thickness. Change in cell diameter may also be seen [16] and mitochondria increase in number and size, and eventually the cells may degenerate and die [17,18,19,20]. The interstitium also becomes thickened by increased edema and the influx and proliferation of fibroblasts. Reactive oxygen species activate human neutrophil collagenase [21] and alveolar macrophages have been shown to produce fibroblasts.

Oxygen exposed lungs have a decline in phospholipid and increase in protein levels in bronchopulmonary lavage fluid [16] surfactant protein A, B and C have been found in increased amounts in lavage fluid after oxygen exposure [22], this is associated with increased relative abundance of mRNA encoding each of these surfactant proteins in the lung tissues. Oxygen exposure also increases mRNA encoding for the tissue inhibitor of metalloproteinase a protein which seems to play a key role in regulating connective tissue turnover [23]. An oxygen injured lung therefore becomes stiff and fibrotic, with a reduced lung compliance.

Since oxygen treatment of newborn babies was introduced new effects of hyperoxia have been discovered, including retrolental fibroplasia (retinopathy of prematurity, ROP, is a more common term today). Lungs exposed to artificial ventilation and extra oxygen occasionally develop bronchopulmonary dysplasia (BPD) [24] (many authors today prefer to call this condition chronic lung disease). A series of other conditions affecting the sick newborn may partly be caused by hyperoxia as well.

Oxygen Radicals

Why is oxygen toxic? Rebecca Gerschman and coworkers [25] answered this question by postulating that oxygen generates oxygen radicals. Free radicals are highly reactive substances many of these having half life of only a fraction of a second. However, they might initiate chain reactions and thus an explosive production of free radicals can be generated if the process has been initiated. For instance if a molecule of polyunsaturated fatty acids reacts with a free radical a lipid radical is formed which can be oxidized to a hydroperoxide radical which can react with a new polyunsaturated fatty acid molecule to form a new lipid radical. Thus a chain reaction is initiated if it is not quenched by for instance vitamin E. Free radicals not only injure polyunsaturated fatty acids in membranes they may degrade structural proteins, inactivate enzymes and even destroy DNA.

Oxygen radicals of which a number of different species are known, as the superoxide and the hydroxyl radical, can be produced by different sources as in the normal energy metabolism, by hypoxanthine- xanthine oxidase [26], metabolism of catecholamine and arachidonic acids and so forth. Activated phagocytes produce high concentrations of oxygen radicals which are an important part of the antibacterial defense [27], and further phagocytes are attracted to ischemic organs and activated during reoxygenation [28]. The very low birth weight baby seems to have a higher capacity than the term one to produce oxygen radicals by the respiratory burst [29]. On the other hand, newborn rabbits treated with natural surfactant had an impairment of lung macrophage bactericidal activity, and therefore surfactant treatment may reduce the bactericidal activity of pulmonary alveolar macrophages [30]. Further, hyperoxia per se seems to damage phagocytic defenses by inducing a decrease in superoxide radical release in alveolar macrophages of neonatal rabbits [31]. From animal and cellular studies it might therefore be speculated that surfactant treatment and hyperoxia alone or in combination may alter the phagocytic defense and increase the susceptibility for infections also in the human.

Hypoxia – Reoxygenation Injury

About thirty years ago several investigators found improved results in shock and ischemia when animals were pretreated with allopurinol. The rationale at that time was that inhibition of xanthine oxidase protects against irreversible loss of purines catabolized from adenine nucleotides [32].

The first experimental evidence supporting the hypothesis that the hypoxanthine-xanthine oxidase system plays a role in hypoxia – reoxygenation injury was, however, published by Granger et al [33] when they showed that allopurinol protects the feline intestine during postischemic reperfusion. This was an important step forward in linking such damage to the hypoxanthine-xanthine oxidase system. They called this phenomenon ischemia–reperfusion injury.

The Hypoxanthine-Xanthine Oxidase System

The hypoxanthine-xanthine oxidase system probably plays an important role in clinical medicine especially because of its ability to generate free radicals [26]). The hypoxanthine and xanthine converting enzyme exists in two forms: xanthine dehydrogenase and xanthine oxidase. Only the latter form can produce oxygen radicals. The main bulk of the enzyme is present, however, in the dehydrogenase form. Ischemia and hypoxia seem to transform it to the oxidase form, although the degree and velocity of this reaction have been disputed [34].

In humans liver xanthine oxidase activities increase toward term while the opposite occurs in the intestine [35]. The clinical significance of this finding is difficult to understand. But since the intestine of the preterm contains more xanthine oxidase than at term, it is perhaps more susceptible than that of the term baby to hypoxanthine-xanthine oxidase derived injury? This may be of interest in understanding necrotizing enterocolitis.

After normal birth a washing out of hypoxanthine into the circulation has been found and after intrauterine hypoxia this is even more pronounced [36]. This wash out phenomenon was illustrated in an experimental model in which we induced endotoxic shock in dogs by infusion of *Escherichia coli* endotoxin. During the shock phase the plasma hypoxanthine concentration was low. When the animals were resuscitated with volume therapy and artificial ventilation, there was, however, an enormous washing out of hypoxanthine into the circulation with an increase from almost zero to approximately 100 umol/l in the course of 10 min [37]. It seems possible that these findings may reflect the clinical condition when hypotensive or hypoxic patients are resuscitated.

If oxygen is added during resuscitation, large amounts of oxygen radicals may thus be produced by the hypoxanthine-xanthine oxidase system. These oxygen radicals may attack several organs, and if the defense systems are overcome many organs may be injured simultaneously. To what extent xanthine oxidase is present in the different organs of the human body is not known (for overview see [34]), but we have hypothesized that the enzyme may be released from the liver during shock or severe hypoxia, and hence circulates in the body [7]. In fact, several groups including ourselves have shown that this is the case [38]), and recently Supnet and coworkers [39] could demonstrate that xanthine oxidase is present in umbilical cord blood after normal delivery and that infants with a poor outcome have significantly higher xanthine oxidase activity and lipid peroxidation production in blood four hours after birth.

The Defense Systems Against Oxygen Radicals

The body contains a complex system that form a defense against free radicals. Several vitamins have antioxidative properties like vitamin C and E and β-carotene. The superoxide dismutases (SOD), of which different types have been described, protect against the superoxide radical and catalyze the transformation from superoxide to hydrogen peroxide [40]. SOD is mainly found in the cytosol but can also be detected in the mitochrondria and extracellular fluid. Catalase and glutathione peroxidase are necessary for a quick conversion of hydrogen peroxide to molecular oxygen and water. Glutathione peroxidase is mainly selenium dependent and selenium therefore represents an important part of the natural defense against free radicals. A series of compounds and metabolites like mannitol, uric acid and bilirubin act as oxygen radical scavengers [41].

It has been speculated that aging depends on the levels of scavengers and antioxidants such as uric acid and vitamin C. A relationship has actually been found between potential life span in different mammals and the concentration of scavengers [42].

Role Of Iron. Is the Early Anemia of Prematurity Protective?

Iron speeds up the reaction between superoxide anion and hydrogen peroxide so that the toxic hydroxyl radical is formed. This is the so called Haber-Weiss reaction. Nutritional iron deficiency may therefore be protective in several types of oxygen radical-mediated injury. Birth is a point of transition for the neonate from a relatively iron-rich environment in utero to the iron-poor extrauterine environment. Sullivan [43] has recently speculated that iron plays an important part in pathogenesis of oxygen radical disease in neonatology and as he points out; maybe the early anemia of prematurity is advantageous? Perhaps one should therefore be careful in interfering by giving iron supplementation or even treatment with erythropoietin?

The plasma proteins, apotransferrin and ceruloplasmin, have strong antioxidant activities [44,45,46]. The antioxidative activity of apotransferrin depends on its ability to bind two ferric ions. Ceruloplasmin is a potent antioxidant by facilitating binding of iron to transferrin. The antioxidant potency of these two proteins in the brain homogenate assay has been estimated by Stocks et al [44] to be 200–500 times that of α-tocopherol. In premature infants apotransferrin and ceruloplasmin concentrations are low [47, 48]. Over 90% of the preventive antioxidant activity of plasma is associated with ceruloplasmin and apotransferrin.

Lactoferrin is a transferrin like iron binding protein present in breast milk and neutrophils. Both purified apolactoferrin and human milk have substantial antioxidant activity. Breast fed premature infants may therefore have an extra protection against oxygen radical injury.

Role Of Bilirubin. Does the Preterm Baby Need Hyperbilirubinemia?

Bilirubin is generally regarded as a toxic compound when it in unconjugated form accumulate at abnormally high concentrations in biological tissues and it is responsible for the development of kernicterus. However, it has also been demonstrated by Stocker et al [49] that the bile pigments bilirubin and biliverdin may protect linoleic acid from oxidative destruction. In the presence of 21% oxygen bilirubin was much less efficient than α-tocopherol, but about equal to β-carotene as an antioxidant. When the oxygen concentration was lowered to 2%, the same concentration as found in tissues, the antioxidant activity of bilirubin increased and it suppressed oxidation of linoleic acid even more efficiently than α-tocopherol. Stocker et al [50] have also found evidence that bilirubin, when bound to human albumin at concentrations present in normal adult human plasma, acts as an oxygen radical scavenger. Ascorbate was found to be a better antioxidant than bilirubin. The relative importance of albumin bound bilirubin as a plasma antioxidant is therefore expected to increase as its concentration increases or under conditions where plasma ascorbate is low. It is therefore interesting that the activity of heme oxygenase, which is the rate-limiting enzyme in bilirubin formation, has been shown to be increased in animals deprived of ascorbate. Further, albumin has been reported to leave the blood stream and to appear in inflammatory exudate thereby transporting bound substances, such as bilirubin, across the vascular wall into these sites of increased production of oxygen radicals by phagocytic cells. Stocker et al [49, 50] therefore believe that bilirubin serves a beneficial role as endogenous antioxidant. For this reason it might be advantageous for the preterm baby, with is lowered antioxidant defense, to have a higher bilirubin level in plasma and the extracellular space than term babies. Fortunately, phototherapy does not seem to inactivate the antioxidant effects of bilirubin.

Bracci et al [51] demonstrated lower erythrocyte concentrations of oxygen radical scavengers in babies who developed hyperbilirubinemia, and these authors speculate that a lowered antioxidant defense in the erythrocyte may contribute to hemolysis and hyperbilirubinemia. Since bilirubin itself is a free radical scavenger its presence may be a useful way to limit free oxygen radical damage in babies with an otherwise lowered antioxidant defense.

Lindeman et al [52] found in plasma of the preterm baby that the trapping capacity of free radicals was highest by uric acid and vitamin C, bilirubin having a trapping capacity of only 1/4 of vitamin C and 1/6 of uric acids.

Role of Vitamin E

Vitamin E, or tocopherol, is the body's principle lipid-soluble antioxidant. Plasma and tissue vitamin E levels are lower at birth than during adulthood. There is, however, no difference between plasma α-tocopherol levels in preterm and term babies. Hågå and Lunde [53]) found that the plasma α-tocopherol concentration correlated well with β-lipoprotein concentration which is the principle carrier of tocopherol in plasma. It therefore seems that differences in transport capacity rather than a relative impermeability of the plasma for tocopherol is the reason for the low levels in newborn infants. At birth there is a rapid increase of vitamin E level in the liver and a more slowly one in the blood and the lung.

In 1949 Owens and Owens [54] reported that oral tocopherol acetate prophylaxis was effective in preventing retinopathy of prematurity. Since then a series of randomized controlled vitamin E trials have been published with inconsistent results. In a randomized controlled trial by Phelps and coworkers [55] they where not able to find any positive effect on ROP incidence by intravenous (20 mg/kg within 24 hours of birth) vitamin E prophylaxis. By the contrary, grades III and IV intraventricular hemorrhage occurred more frequently in infants weighing less than 1 kg at birth who had received tocopherol. These authors concluded that the evidence for the efficacy of vitamin E in preventing ROP is not convincing. On the other hand, Chiswick and coworkers [56] reported that intramuscular vitamin E (25 mg/kg) at the first three days after birth reduced the incidence of intraventricular hemorrhage from 56% to 18% in preterm babies less than 32 weeks gestation. These authors believed that vitamin E protects endothelial cell membranes from oxidative damage and disruption, and therefore limits the magnitude of hemorrhage and its spread from the subependyma into the ventricles. Recently Inan et al [57] found that prenatal vitamin E injections to rats protect the fetus and newborn against hypoxic injury.

Tappel [58] and Packer et al [59] have found evidence demonstrating that vitamins E and C act synergistically. Vitamin E acting as the primary antioxidant and the resulting vitamin E radical then reacting with vitamin C to regenerate vitamin E. There is a high vitamin C concentration in umbilical cord blood with a marked decline after birth.

Development Of Antioxyenzymes in the Perinatal Period

The concentrations of most antioxyenzymes increase during pregnancy. This has been shown by Frank and coworkers [60] and several other investigators. The same pattern was found in the kidney [61]. In the heart there was an increase in glutathione peroxidase but not in SOD and catalase [61]. The antioxidant defense of guinea pig mitochondria was studied specifically. Superoxide dismutase activity increased from between 1.5 to 3 fold from the fetal to the adult period in kidney, liver and heart, while glutathione peroxidase activity was almost constant from birth until adult age [62]. Mishra and Delivoria-Papadopoulos [63] studied the development of antioxidant enzymes in the guinea pig brain. They found no change in superoxide dismutase during pregnancy. Catalase activity increased from day 45 (term at 60 days). The levels were not influenced by maternal hypoxemia.

The developing pattern of antioxidants in the tissues therefore seems to be rather complex in the perinatal period, with differences between species, organs and between the different enzymes as well. At present it is unclear whether the concentrations of these enzymes reach a peak at term followed by a gradual decrease toward adult levels, or whether the concentration continues to increase post partum.

What is the situation in humans? In studies in man the erythrocyte superoxide dismutase activity did not change significantly with gestational age and no significant differences were observed among preterm infants, term neonates and adults. By term catalase activity reached a level similar to the adult level, but glutathione peroxidase activity was markedly lower in preterm and term babies than in adults [64]. Very recently, however, with new techniques, Phylactos et al [65] actually have demonstrated that preterm babies have lower erythrocyte SOD activities than term babies, thus indicating that also in humans there is a development of antioxyenzyme activity toward term.

Frank and Sosenko [66] could further demonstrate that term by contrast to preterm rabbits have the capacity to induce antioxyenzymes in the lung when exposed to hyperoxia. If this is the case also for humans it means that preterm infants have lowered defence against oxygen radicals than term infants at birth, in addition they have not the capability to protect themselves against oxidative stress by enzyme induction as the term infants might do.

Adult mammals are known to be less resistant to hyperoxia than newborn ones. In one study, all the newborn rats which were exposed to 95% oxygen for 72 hours survived by contrast to 20% survival in 60-day-old rats [67]. One reason for this difference between the newborn and adult rat may be that only the newborn rat can adapt to hyperoxia by induction of antioxyenzymes. This adaptive mechanism seems to be present only during a short period post partum [68].

The antioxidant activity in plasma seems, however, by contrast to the situation in the tissues, to be at about the same level in the preterm, term and adult [69].

Bronchopulmonary Dysplasia

Since Northway et al [24] more than twenty years ago described bronchopulmonary dysplasia in newborn babies who were ventilated artificially because of the respiratory distress syndrome (RDS), this entity has become a dreaded complication in every neonatal intensive care unit. The list of etiological factors is long [70, 71]. In addition to prematurity itself, two particular factors have been discussed especially: the role of high pressure applied to the airways by the ventilator, and the consequence of a high concentration of oxygen in the inspired air [72]. I think the oxygen radical hypothesis can now explain the effects of both these two factors and how they are connected [10]. In fact, most of the etiological factors mentioned in the literature are related to an increased oxygen radical production or a lowered defense against them.

Experimental and Clinical Data

Instillation of xanthine oxidase into the trachea of rats [73] and guinea pigs [8, 9] produced edema and hemorrhage, and the lung compliance was reduced. This effect could to some extent be prevented by the addition of superoxide dismutase. Further, intravenous infusion of hypoxanthine in rats breathing 100% oxygen for 48 hours produced lung hemorrhage and edema. There was an increase in the protein concentration of bronchoalveolar lavage compared with controls, and the surfactant function was abolished [6]. Similar findings were done by Holm et al [17] in rats breathing 100% oxygen for 64 hours. In bronchoalveolar lavage fluid there was a three-fold increase in protein content and a 30% decline in the phospholipid levels. Twenty-four hours after exposure to oxygen the phospholipid concentration was reduced even more, down to half of values of controls. Furthermore, the protein level in lavage fluid was increased to eight time the control values. These lavages exhibited severely impaired dynamic surface activity [17].

Pitkanen and coworkers [74] measured pentane and ethane in expired air of premature babies. These gases are products from lipid peroxidation, and a high concentration indicates a high peroxidation activity due to presence of oxygen radicals. During the first days after birth babies who later developed BPD had higher pentane and ethane concentrations in expired air than babies who did not develop BPD. This study is important since it to my knowledge represents the first data indicating that an increased oxygen radical production finds place in babies who later develop BPD. Varsila et al [75] have further shown that preterm babies exhale higher concentrations of these gases than term infants indicating that preterm babies are prone to more lipid peroxidation than term infants may be because of the lowered oxidative defence?

Recently Gladstone and Levine [76] have shown that protein oxidation is enhanced in babies exposed to high oxygen concentrations compared with babies with low oxygen supplementation, and Varsila et al [77] found that babies developing BPD have higher concentration of protein oxidation products in the lung lavage than normal babies also indicating that these babies are exposed to higher oxygen stress than the controls. Clement et al [78] found that activated macrophages from bronchopulmonary dysplasia patients produce more oxygen radicals than those from normal subjects.

All these findings indicate that oxygen radicals, in one way or another, are involved in development of bronchopulmonary dysplasia, the oxygen radicals probably are generated by a number of systems. A low compliant lung for instance has probably a higher hypoxanthine concentration in the tissue than a normal lung. Especially during positive pressure ventilation with high inspiratory pressures there is reason to assume that the hypoxanthine concentration increases [10].

Retinopathy of Prematurity

Retinopathy of prematurity (ROP) was the first disease entity, at least in neonatology, which was referred to the effect of hyperoxia. When the relation between hyperoxia and ROP became known, fairly strict guidelines were laid down for oxygen treatment, and the use of more than 40% oxygen was to be avoided. Consequently the incidence of ROP decreased, however, mortality and the number of babies with cerebral palsy increased dramatically [79]. During the last decade or so a new rise in the number of ROP cases has been observed in most developed countries. This may be caused by a higher survival rate of very low birthweight preterm babies. Today it is clear that a series of etiological factors contribute to ROP [80, 81] including both hyperoxia and hypoxia, as well as low birthweight per se. Such a long list of etiological factors may indicate that the pathogenesis of this disease is still hidden. Most of these etiological factors are, however, in some respects related to free radicals either because they contribute to a higher oxygen radical production or a lowered defense against them. Transfused blood for instance, contains very high concentrations of both hypoxanthine and iron.

We have therefore proposed that the hypoxanthine - xanthine oxidase system also plays a role in development of ROP [1]. The free radical hypothesis contributes to explain why the incidence of ROP increases with decreasing gestational age since it is reasonable to suggest, although it has to my knowledge to date not been proven, that the defense against free radicals in the eye is lower early in gestation than at term.

To explore this hypothesis we measured the hypoxanthine concentration in the vitreous fluid post mortem in preterm babies who had died from RDS. In these babies we found significantly higher hypoxanthine concentration than in the controls [82]. These data do not prove that an increased production of oxygen radicals takes place in the eyes of babies at risk for developing ROP. They do, however, show that such babies have high concentration in the eye of one substrate for oxygen radical production, i.e. hypoxanthine. We do not know to what extent xanthine oxidase is present in the human eye for instance in the retinal vascular endothelium. We know that oxygen radicals have vasoactive properties, but nothing is known about the effects on the retinal vessels. It is, however, reasonable to speculate that oxygen radicals affect the retinal circulation. It seems clear that the etiology of ROP is multifactorial but the considerations above may elucidate important aspects of the pathogenesis of this condition.

Necrotizing Enterocolitis

Necrotizing enterocolitis in the newborn represents a severe clinical problem. The pathogenesis is, however, still unclear. There is a substantial body of experimental data supporting the hypothesis that reactive oxygen metabolites mediate the microvascular and mucosal permeability changes observed after reperfusion of the ischemic intestine in adult animals [28, 83]. Grøgård and coworkers [84] found increased mucosal albumin clearance in jejunal segments of dogs with arterial occlusion and intraluminal perfusion with hypoxanthine-xanthine oxidase. The effect of hypoxanthine-xanthine oxidase was prevented by superoxide dismutase.

Hernandez et al [85] have assessed the role of iron catalyzed oxidant production in ischemia-reperfusion injury. The intestinal vascular permeability is increased after one hour ischemia followed by 30 min reperfusion. Apotransferrin, an antioxidant, and deferoxamine, an iron chelator, were given intravenously as an infusion five minutes before reperfusion. Both apotransferrin and deferoxamine reduced ischemia-reperfusion induced vascular permeability when compared with untreated animals. Treatment with iron-loaded deferoxamine did not offer any protection against ischemic injury. These data support the hypothesis that iron plays an important role in the formation of hydroxyl radicals after reperfusion of the ischemic bowel.

Grisham and coworkers [28] found, that myeloperoxidase activity in the intestine increased during ischemia and a further augmentation was found during reperfusion. The myeloperoxidase activity reflects the amounts of leukocytes present. It seems therefore to be at least two major sources of oxygen radicals in the postischemic intestine: hypoxanthine-xanthine oxidase and activated phagocytes.

Brain Injury

Scheuch et al [86] have found that the hypoxanthine-xanthine oxidase system increases the release of dopamine from isolated rat brain synaptosomes. The effect was inhibited by catalase but not by superoxide dismutase. Oxygen radical induced release of dopamine, and possibly other neurotransmitters as well, may therefore play a role in development of hypoxic brain injury. Palmer et al [87] found that pretreatment with allopurinol (xanthine oxidase inhibitor) reduced perinatal hypoxic-ischemic brain damage in the developing brain of 7 day old rat pups. Does these data justify routine treatment with allopurinol of hypoxic newborn babies? I don't think so. Many questions concerning effects of allopurinol have not yet been solved [34]. The possible relation between oxygen radicals and brain injury in the preterm baby deserves still a thorough examination.

Oxygen Radicals and the Perinatal Circulation

Oxygen radicals have vasoactive properties, do they play a role in the normal regulation? Tate and coworkers [88] created an oxygen radical producing system in the isolated rabbit lung by infusing xanthine oxidase together with a purine. This gave an increase in the perfusion pressure. The effect could be inhibited by catalase but not by superoxide dismutase. The effect was therefore probably mediated by hydrogen peroxide or hydroxyl radicals.

Clyman et al [89] studied the effect of oxygen radicals on isolated ductal rings from lamb fetuses. Maximally constricted isolated ductal rings became dilated when exposed to a high concentration of hypoxanthine ($> 100\ \mu mol/l$). When xanthine oxidase was added as well, the dilatation occurred already at physiological concentrations of hypoxanthine (1–10 $\mu mol/l$). The effect was blocked by indomethacin, which inhibits prostaglandin synthesis. Simultaneously there was a marked increased production of PGE_2. It therefore seems evident that oxygen radicals are potent dilatators of the isolated ductus arteriosus of fetal lambs. This is probably due to free radical initiation of prostaglandin production in the ductal wall.

Recently Sanderud et al [90] have shown that the hypoxanthine-xanthine oxidase system constricts the intact pulmonary circulation of pigs. This effect was inhibited by indomethacin, allopurinol and catalase. The output of 6-keto-$PGF_1\alpha$, the stable metabolite of prostacyclin, and thromboxane B_2, the stable metabolite of thromboxane A_2, peaked 40–60 minutes after xanthine oxidase was given. The output of these prostanoids was inhibited not only by indomethacin but by catalase as well.

From these data we speculate that oxygen radicals may be of importance in regulating the perinatal circulation by constricting the pulmonary circulation and dilating the ductus arteriosus [10, 90]. This fits in with the knowledge that persistent fetal circulation may be precipitated by hypoxia.

Interrelation Between Oxygen Radicals, Excitatory Amino Acids and Nitric Oxide

Oxygen radicals may react with NO and generate the toxic peroxynitrite radical. In hypoxia-reoxygenation conditions excitatory aminoacids as glutamate are released from the presynaptic membrane and activate the NMDA and AMPA/kainate receptor at the postsynaptic membrane. Ca^{++} enters the neuron and induces synthesis of a number of enzymes as nitric oxide synthetase. In the reoxygenation period the concentration of both oxygen radicals and NO are high and as mentioned these may react and generate toxic products. In patients treated with NO it is possible that high concentrations of peroxynitrite are formed. Possible adverse effects of this has not been discussed thoroughly [91].

Prevention of Oxygen Radical Disease in Neonatology. Should Resuscitation be Performed with Room Air?

The presented hypothesis of both hypoxia-reoxygenation injury and an oxygen radical disease in neonatology may have a number of clinical implications. If it is correct, it opens for a completely new understanding of the pathogenesis of some of the most challenging problems in neonatology. This new understanding opens up for new treatment modalities, for example by administration of different oxygen radical scavengers or xanthine oxidase inhibitors to patients.

The present hypothesis clearly indicates that the alternation between hypoxia and hyperoxia may be harmful and such should be avoided. During the resuscitation of hypoxic newborns it could be beneficial to use as low supplementary oxygen concentration as possible since most of infants seem to be resuscitated satisfactory with room air [92]. Since we introduced the hypothesis that room air should be tested out during resuscitation a series of animal studies have supported the idea that it is at least equally efficient as 100% oxygen [93, 94]. Further, there are accumulating data documenting the adverse effects by using oxygen during resuscitation. A large international controlled multicenter resuscitation study enrolling up to 700 newborn infants is ended by may 1996. In this study, Resair 2, the room air hypothesis is tested out.

Conclusion

In recent years we have begun to understand far more of the pathogenesis of oxygen toxicity in neonatology, although I believe we are only at the very beginning of a new era that may completely change our understanding and treatment of the diseases discussed in this article. The pathogenesis of post-hypoxic reoxygenation injury is so complex that so far we have only scratched at the surface of an understanding of it.

Acknowledgements. This study has been supported by: The Norwegian Research Council, The Norwegian Cancer Society, The Norwegian Council for Cardiovascular Diseases, The Laerdal Foundation for Acute Medicine, Odd Fellow Medical Research Foundation, Anders Jahres Research Foundation, and Eckbo's legat.

References

1. Saugstad OD (1988) Hypoxanthine as an indicator of hypoxia: Its role in health and disease through free radical production. Pediatr Res 23:143–150.
2. Hossmann KA (1983) Neuronal survival and revival during and after cerebral ischemia. Am J Emerg Med 1:191–197.
3. Kjellmer I (1988) Prenatal and intrapartum asphyxia. In: Levene MI, Bennett MJ, Punt J (eds) Fetal and neonatal neurology and neurosurgery. Churchill Livingstone, Edinburgh, London, Melbourne, New York, pp 357–369.

4. Latham F (1951) The oxygen paradox. Experiments on the effects of oxygen in human anoxia. Lancet 1:77–81.
5. Saugstad OD, Aasen AO (1980) Plasma hypoxanthine levels as a prognostic aid of tissue hypoxia. Europ Surg Res 12:123–129.
6. Saugstad OD, Hallman M, Abraham J, Cochrane CG, Epstein B, Gluck L (1984) Hypoxanthine and oxygen induced lung injury: A basic mechanism of tissue damage? Pediatr Res 18:501–504.
7. Saugstad OD (1985) Oxygen radicals and pulmonary damage. Pediatr Pulmonol 1:167–175.
8. Saugstad OD, Becher G, Grossmann M, Oddoy A, Merker G, Lachmann B (1987) Acute and chronic lung damage in guinea pigs induced by xanthine oxidase. Intensive Care Med 13:30–32.
9. Saugstad OD, Hallman M, Becher G, Oddoy A, Lium B, Lachmann B (1988) Respiratory failure by intratracheal saline: Additive effect of xanthine oxidase. Biol Neonat 54:61–67.
10. Saugstad OD (1990) Oxygen toxicity in the neonatal period. Acta Paediatr Scand 79:881–892.
11. Gilbert DL (1985) Oxygen an overall biological view. In: Gilbert DL (ed) Oxygen and living processes. Springer Verlag, New York, pp 376–92.
12. Wolfe WG, DeVries WC (1975) Oxygen toxicity. Ann Rev Med 26:203–217
13. Kovachich GB, Haugaard N (1985) Biochemical aspects of oxygen toxicity in the metazoa. In: Gilbert DL (ed) Oxygen and living processes. Springer Verlag, New York, pp 210–34.
14. Schaefer KE (1985) Oxygen in closed environmental systems. In: Gilbert DL (ed) Oxygen and living processes. Springer Verlag, New York, pp 343–357.
15. Kafer ER (1971) Pulmonary oxygen toxicity. A review of the evidence for acute and chronic oxygen toxicity in man. Br J Anaesth 43:687–95.
16. Holm BA, Matalon S, Finkelstein JN, Notter RH (1988) Type II pneumocyte changes during hyperoxic lung injury and recovery. J Appl Physiol 65:2672–2678.
17. Holm BA, Notter RH, Leary JF, Matalon S (1987) Alveolar epithelial changes in rabbits after a 21-day exposure to 60% O_2. J Appl Physiol 62:2230–36.
18. Hansen TN, Gest AL (1984) Oxygen toxicity and other ventilatory complications of treatment of infants with persistent pulmonary hypertension. Clin Perinatol 11:653–72.
19. Huber GL, Drath DB (1985) Pulmonary oxygen toxicity. In: Gilbert DL (ed) Oxygen and living processes. Springer Verlag, New York, pp 273–342.
20. Yam J, Frank L, Roberts RJ (1987) Oxygen toxicity: Comparison of lung biochemical responses in neonatal and adult rats. Pediatr Res 12:115–19.
21. Saari H, Suomalainen K, Lindy O, Konttinen YT, Sorsa T (1990) Activation of latents human neutrophil collagenase by reactive oxygen species and serine proteases. Biochem Biophys Res Commun 171:979–987.
22. Nogee LM, Wispe JR, Clark JC,Weaver TE, Whitsett JA (1991) Increased expression of pulmonary surfactant proteins in oxygen exposed rats. Am J Respir Cell Mol Biol 4:102–107.
23. Horowitz S, Dafni N, Shapiro DL, Holm BA, Notter RH, Quible DJ (1989) Hyperoxic exposure alters gene expression in the lung. Induction of tissue inhibitor and metalloproteinases mRNA and other mRNAs. J Biol Chem 264:7092–7095.
24. Northway WH, Rosan RC, Porter DY (1967) Pulmonary disease following respirator therapy of hyaline-membrane disease. Bronchopulmonary dysplasia. N Eng J Med 276:357–68.
25. Gerschman R, Gilbert DL, Nyl SW, Dwyer P, Fen WO (1954) Oxygen poisoning and x-ray irradiation: a mechanism in common. Science 119:624–26.
26. McCord JM, Fridovich I (1968) The reduction of cytochrome C by milk xanthine oxidase. J Biol Chem 243:5753–5760.
27. Babior BM, Kipnes RS, Curnutte JT (1973) Biological defense mechanisms. The production of superoxide – A potential bactericidal agent. J Clin Invest 52:741–744.

28. Grisham MB, Hernandez LA, Granger DN (1986) Xanthine oxidase and neutrophil infiltration in intestinal ischemia. Am J Physiol 251: G567-G574.
29. Kugo M, Sano K, Uetani Y, Nakamura H (1989) Superoxide dismutase in polymorphonuclear leukocytes of term newborn infants and very low birth weight infants. Pediatr Res 26:227.231.
30. Sherman MP, D'Ambola JB, Aeberhard EE, Barrett CT (1988) Surfactant therapy of newborn rabbits impairs lung macrophage bactericidal activity. J Appl Physiol 65:137–145.
31. Sherman MP, Condiotti R (1987) Hyperoxia damages phagocytic defenses of neonatal rabbit lung. J Appl Physiol 62:684–690.
32. Crowell JW, Jones CE, Smith EE (1969) Effect of allopurinol on hemorrhagic shock. Am J Physiol 216:744–748.
33. Granger DN, Rutili G, McCord, JM (1981) Superoxide radicals in feline intestinal ischemia. Gastroenterology 81:22–29.
34. Saugstad OD (1996) Role of xanthine oxidase (XO) and its inhibitor in hypoxia–reoxygenation injury. Pediatrics in press
35. Vettenranta K, Raivio KO (1990) Xanthine oxidase during human fetal development Pediatr Res 27:286–288.
36. Bratteby LE, Swanstrom S (1982) Hypoxanthine concentration in plasma during the first two hours after birth in normal and asphyxiated infants. Pediatr Res 16:152–155.
37. Aasen AO, Saugstad OD (1979) Washing out of hypoxanthine in terminal endotoxin shock in dogs. Circ Shock 185:6:277–283.
38. Rootwelt T, Almaas R, Øyasæter S, Moen A, Saugstad OD (1995) Release of xanthine oxidase to the systemic circulation during resuscitation from severe hypoxemia in newborn pigs. Acta Paediatr 84:507–511.
39. Supnet MC, David-Cu R, Walther FJ (1994) Plasma xanthine oxidase and lipid hydroperoxide levels in preterm infant. Pediatr Res 6:283–287.
40. McCord JM, Fridovich I (1969) Superoxide dismutase. An enzymatic function of erythrocuprein (hemocuprein). J Biol Chem 244:6049–55.
41. Wayner DDM, Burton GW, Ingold KU, Barclay LRC, Locke SJ (1987) The relative contributions of vitamin E, urate, ascorbate and proteins to the total peroxyl radical-trapping antioxidant activity of human blood plasma. Biochim Biophys Acta 924:408–19.
42. Cutler RC (1986) Aging and oxygen radicals. In: AE Taylor, S. Matalon, PA Ward (eds) Physiology of oxygen radicals: American Physiology Society, Bethesda, pp 251–285.
43. Sullivan JL (1988) Iron, plasma antioxidants and the „Oxygen radical disease of prematurity“. Am J Dis Child 142:1341–1344.
44. Stocks J, Gutteridge JMC, Sharp RJ, Dormandy TL (1974) Assay using brain homogenate for measuring the antioxidant activity of biological fluids. Clin Sci Mol Med 47:215–222.
45. Stocks J, Gutteridge JMC, Sharp RJ, Dormandy TL (1974) The inhibition of lipid autoxidation by human serum and its relation to serum proteins and alpha tocopherol. Clin Sci Mol Med 47:223–233.
46. Gutteridge JMC, Stocks J (1981) Caeruloplasmin: physiological and pathological perspectives. CRC Crit Rev Clin Lab Sci 14:257–329.
47. Hildebrand DC, Faluin Z, James E, Fahim M (1974) Ceruloplasmin and alkaline phosphatase levels in cord serum of term, preterm, and physiological jaundiced neonates. Am J Obstet Gynecol 118:950–954.
48. Scott PH, Berger HM, Kenward C, Scott T, Wharton RA (1975) Effect of gestational age and intrauterine nutrition of plasma transferrin and iron in the newborn. Arch Dis Child 50:796–798.
49. Stocker R, Yamamoto Y, McDonagh AF, Glazer AN, Ames BN (1987) Bilirubin is an antioxidant of possible physiological importance. Science 235:1043–1046
50. Stocker R, Glazer AN, Ames BN (1987) Antioxidant activity of albumin-bound bilirubin. Proc Natl Acad Sci 84:5918–5922.

51. Bracci R, Buonocore G, Talluri B, Berni S (1988) Neonatal hyperbilirubinemia. Evidence for a role of the erythrocyte enzyme activities involved in the detoxification of oxygen radicals. Acta Paediatr Scand 77:349–356.
52. Lindeman JHN, Van Zoeren-Grobben D, Schrijver J, Speek AJ, Poorthuis BJHM, Berger HM (1989) The total free radical ability of cord blood plasma in preterm and term babies. Pediatr Res 26:20–24.
53. Hågå P, Lunde G (1978) Selenium and vitamin E in cord blood from preterm and full term infants. Acta Paediatr Scand 67:735–739.
54. Owens WC, Owens EU (1949) Retrolental fibroplasia in premature infants. II. Studies on the prophylaxis of the disease: the use of alpha tocopherol acetate. Am J Opthalmol 32:1631–1637.
55. Phelps DL, Rosenbaum AL, Isenberg SJ, Leake RD, Dorey FJ (1987) Tocopherol efficacy and safety for preventing retinopathy of prematurity: a randomized, controlled, double-masked trial Pediatrics 79:489–500.
56. Chiswick ML, Johnson M, Woodhall C et al (1983) Protective effect of vitamin E (DL-alpha-tocopherol) against intraventricular haemorrhage in premature babies. British Med J 287:81–84.
57. Inan C, Kilic I, Kilinc K, Kalayci O, Kotiloglu E (1995) The effect of high fdose antenatal vitamin E on hypoxia-induced changes in newborn rats. Pediatr Res 38:685–689.
58. Tapppel AL (1968) Will antioxidant nutrients slow aging processes? Geriatrics 23:97–105.
59. Packer JE, Slater TF, Wilson RL (1979) Direct observation of a free radical interaction between vitamin E and C. Nature 278:737–738.
60. Frank L, Groseclose EE (1984) Preparation for birth into an O_2-rich environment: The antioxidant enzymes in the developing rabbit lung. Pediatr Res 18:240–44.
61. Hayashibe H, Asayama K, Dobashi K, Kato K (1990) Prenatal development of antioxidant enzymes in rat lung, kidney, and heart: marked increase in immunoreactive superoxide dismutase, glutathione peroxidase, and catalase in the kidney. Pediatr Res 27:472–475.
62. Vlessis A, Mela-Riker L (1989) Perinatal development of heart, kidney, and liver mitochondrial antioxidant defense. Pediatr Res 26:220–226.
63. Mishra OP, Delivoria-Papadopoulos (1988) Anti-oxidant enzymes in fetal guinea pig brain during development and the effect of maternal hypoxia. Develop Brain Res 42:173–179.
64. Ripalda MJ, Rudolph N, Wong SL (1989) Developmental patterns of antioxidant defense mechanisms in human erythrocytes. Pediatr Res 26:366–369.
65. Phylactos AC, Leaf AA, Costeloe K, Crawford MA (1995) Erythrocyte cupric/zink superoxide dismutase exhibits reduced activity in preterm and low–birthweight infants at birth. Acta Paediatr 84:1421–1425.
66. Frank L, Sosenko IRS (1991) Failure of premature rabbits to increase antioxidant enzymes during hyperoxic exposure: increased susceptibility to pulmonary oxygen toxicity compared with term rabbits. Pediatr Res 29:292–296.
67. Frank L (1985) Effects of oxygen on the newborn. Fed Proc 44:2328–2334
68. Frank L, Bucher JR, Roberts RJ (1978) Oxygen toxicity in neonatal and adult animals of various species. J Appl Physiol 45:699–704.
69. Sullivan JL, Newton RB (1988) Serum antioxidant activity in neonates. Arch Dis Childh 63:748–57.
70. Goetzman BW (1986) Understanding bronchopulmonary dysplasia. Am J Dis Child 140:332–34.
71. O'Brodovich HM, Mellins RB (1985) Bronchopulmonary dysplasia. Unresolved neonatal acute lung injury. Am Rev Respir Dis 132:694–709.
72. Philips AGS (1975) Oxygen plus pressure plus time: The etiology of bronchopulmonary dysplasia. Pediatrics 55:44–50.
73. Johnson KJ, Fantone JC, Kaplan J, Ward PA (1981) In vivo damage of rat lungs by oxygen metabolites. J Clin Invest 67:983–993.

74. Pitkanen OM, Hallman M, Andersson SM (1990). Correlation of free oxygen radical-influenced lipid peroxidation with outcome in very low birth weight infants. J Pediatr 116:760–764.
75. Varsila E, Pitkanen OM, Hallman M, Andersson S (1994) Immaturity-dependent free radical activity in premature infants. Pediatr Res 36:55–59.
76. Gladstone IM jr, Levine RL (1994) Oxidation of proteins in neonatal lungs. Pediatrics 93:764–768.
77. Varsila E, Pesonen E, Andersson S (1995) Early protein oxidation in the neonatal lung is related to development of chronic lung disease. Acta Paediatr 84:1296–1299.
78. Clement A, Chadelat K, Sardet A, Grimfeld A, Tournier G (1988) Alveolar macrophage status in bronchopulmonary dysplasia. Pediatr Res 23:470–473
79. Cross KW (1973) Cost of preventing retrolental fibroplasia? Lancet 2:954–956.
80. Lucey JF, Dangman B (1984) A reexamination of the role of oxygen in retrolental fibroplasia. Pediatrics 73:82–96.
81. Phelps DL (1982) Neonatal toxicity – Is it preventable? Pediatr Clin North Am 19:687–91.
82. Saugstad OD, Rognum TO (1988) High post mortem vitreous hypoxanthine levels in newborns with the respiratory distress syndrome (RDS). Pediatrics 31:395–398.
83. Parks DA, Granger DN (1986) Contributions of ischemia and reperfusion to mucosal lesion formation. Am J Physiol 250:G749-G753.
84. Grøgaard B, Parks DA, Granger DN, McCord JM, Forsberg O (1982) Effects of ischemia and oxygen radicals on mucosal albumin clearance in intestine. Am J Physiol 242:G448-G454.
85. Hernandez LA, Grisham MB, Granger DN (1987) A role for iron in oxidant-mediated ischemic injury to intestinal microvasculature Am J Physiol 253:G49–G53
86. Scheuch C, Berndt C, Gross J, Poulsen JP, Saugstad OD, Haberland A (1989) Influence of the hypoxanthine/xanthine oxidase system on striatal (3H) dopamine uptake. Biomed Biochim Acta 48:212–216.
87. Palmer C, Vannucci RC, Towfighi J (1990) Reduction of perinatal hypoxic–ischemic brain damage with allopurinol. Pediatr Res 27:332–336.
88. Tate RM, Morris HG, Schroeder WR, Repine JE (1984) Oxygen metabolites stimulate thromboxane production and vasoconstriction in isolated saline-perfused rabbit lungs. J Clin Invest 74:608–13.
89. Clyman RI, Saugstad OD, Mauray F (1989) Reactive oxygen metabolites relax the lamb ductus arteriosus by stimulating prostaglandin production. Circ Res 64:1–8
90. Sanderud J, Norstein J, Saugstad OD (1991) Reactive oxygen metabolites produce pulmonary vasoconstriction in young pigs. Pediatr Res 29:543–547.
91. Saugstad OD (1996) Mechanisms of tissue injury by oxygen radicals. Implications for neonatal disease. Acta Paediatr 85:1–4.
92. Ramji S, Ahuja S, Thirupuram S, Rootwelt T, Rooth G, Saugstad OD (1993) Resuscitation of asphyxic newborn infants with room air or 100% oxygen. Pediatr Res 34:809–812.
93. Poulsen JP, Øyasæter S, Saugstad OD (1993) Hypoxanthine, xanthine and uric acid in newborn pigs during hypoxemia followed by resuscitation with room air or 100% oxygen. Crit Care Med 21:1058–1065.
94. Rootwelt T, Løberg EM, Moen A, Øyasæter S, Saugstad OD (1992) Hypoxemia and reoxygenation with 21% or 100% oxygen in newborn pigs: changes in blood pressure, base deficit, and hypoxanthine and brain morphology. Pediatr Res 32:107–113.

Bronchopulmonary Dysplasia: Strategies for Therapeutic Intervention

A. K. Tanswell, M. Liu and M. Post

Introduction

Bronchopulmonary dysplasia (BPD), or chronic neonatal lung injury, is a chronic pneumopathy most commonly seen in preterm newborn infants requiring prolonged respiratory support. It was first described in the mid–1960's, following the introduction of effective and commercially available neonatal ventilators which allowed the extended survival of infants with severe pulmonary insufficiency. Bronchopulmonary dysplasia has become the commonest chronic lung disease seen in infancy, with there being some 7000 new cases per year in the USA in the early 1980s [1]. The increased survival of extremely low birth weight infants over the last decade is likely to have increased this number significantly. The increased representation of extremely low birth weight infants in the overall pool of infants developing BPD has also been associated with a change in the expected radiological and pathological features associated with evolving BPD. When first described, there appeared to be a fairly clear, and well correlated, sequence of changes on X-ray (XR) and in lung histology occurring in the relatively large infants surviving with BPD in that era. The XR changes were divided into four stages, with stage I having the characteristic features of neonatal respiratory distress syndrome (RDS), followed by an opacification of the lung fields in stage II, which was associated with thick airway exudates, necrosis of respiratory epithelium and evidence of early repair. Survival into stage III represented a transition stage into chronic lung injury with areas of emphysematous alveoli being adjacent to patches of alveolar atelectasis and fibrosis reflected in the XR by rounded areas of radiolucency superimposed on lung fields of increased radiodensity. Stage IV was the period of established chronic lung disease with hyper-expanded emphysematous lungs, right ventricular hypertrophy and pulmonary hypertension. The histological features were of emphysema and interstitial thickening, periarteriolar thickening, bronchial smooth muscle hyperplasia and airway epithelium showing ulceration and squamous metaplasia and an alveolar epithelium in which type I pneumocytes had been replaced by type II pneumocytes. In the current era, there appears to be two relatively distinct patterns of pulmonary lesions associated with the clinical evolution of BPD. One group has severe bronchiolar changes and emphysema with only modest interstitial fibrosis, while the other group has severe interstitial fibrosis with only mild airway and emphysematous changes. Chambers and van Velzen [2] have suggested that the group showing distinct bronchiolar lesions represent larger infants, comparable to those described in the original reports of the 1960s, while the group characterized by severe interstitial fibrosis is of lower birth weight and has changes related to their increased susceptibility to pulmonary interstitial emphysema. Van Lierde *et al.* [3], however, found an equal distribution of both profiles in their population of very low birth weight infants. The original groups of infants described with BPD had a alarming incidence of late pulmonary sequelae, but lung function tests of BPD survivors born in the late 1970s suggested that improvements in management had lessened the risk of long-term impairment of lung function in these relatively large preterm infants. Likely contributory factors include adoption of pressure limited ventilators, improved humidifiers to reduce particle deposition, heating of inspired gases and improved methods of parenteral nutrition.

This apparent improvement in outlook for infants with BPD is, however, unlikely to be sustained. It is widely recognized that there has been an overall increase in BPD due to the increased survival of infants of <1000 gm birth weight. The parenchymal injury seen in this population of patients in the 1990s is likely to be associated with a much greater long term impairment of alveolar and capillary growth than was seen in earlier decades [4]. At the present time there is no proven preventive or interventional therapy for BPD. Recent therapeutic advances, such as surfactant use to prevent RDS, may well increase survival with BPD even more as its use becomes more widespread. With occasional exceptions, multicenter clinical trials have not shown this therapy to have a major effect on the incidence of BPD. In contrast, trials from individual institutions have shown some preventive effect, particularly in larger infants. Postnatal steroid therapy has only had a clear short-term impact on IPPV and O_2 requirements. Despite apparently beneficial effects, such as reduced airway chemotaxis, inflammatory mediators and phagocytes, no long term benefits have yet been demonstrated. Indeed, the growth inhibitory properties of steroids raise particular concerns that the inhibition of lung growth seen in untreated BPD could be compounded by steroid treatment, particularly if repeated courses of steroids are used. In contrast, evidence is accumulating that steroid therapy to mothers in preterm labor does have some effect on the development of BPD after birth. Whether this is through enhanced surfactant synthesis reducing oxygen and ventilatory needs, induction of antioxidant enzyme synthesis to reduce susceptibility to oxidant injury, or structural changes in lung tissue which result in increased resistance to barotrauma or some as yet unrecognized effect is unknown.

BPD is widely recognized to be of multifactorial aetiology, but the specific contributions of individual factors remains unclear. An understanding of how individual aetiologic factors contribute to the disease process seems our best hope for developing management and therapeutic strategies which minimize the risks of extremely low birth weight infants developing severe BPD with a lifelong impairment of lung growth and function. Even after full term delivery, 80% of alveoli have yet to be formed during postnatal lung growth. That this process is drastically impaired in survivors of BPD has been confirmed in several reports of autopsy data from children subsequently dying from pulmonary and non-pulmonary causes. These data support experimental evidence that arrested septation during critical periods of alveolar formation may not be completely reversible. Our focus in this review will be the parenchymal changes which occur in BPD, and we will not address issues surrounding the development of pulmonary hypertension or its management. Figure 1 offers a scheme showing interactions between putative primary and secondary contributing factors.

Oxygen Toxicity

It is our belief, which we recognize is not universally shared, that oxidant injury is the initiator of the injury process which ultimately results in the parenchymal pathological features of BPD. This injury may be compounded or amplified by other factors perhaps, in some instances, through the same intracellular pathways. The hypothesis that oxygen plays a significant role in the parenchymal injury of BPD is supported by several lines of evidence: (i) A clear relationship between oxygen exposure and the development of BPD has been shown by retrospective analysis of putative contributory factors in preterm

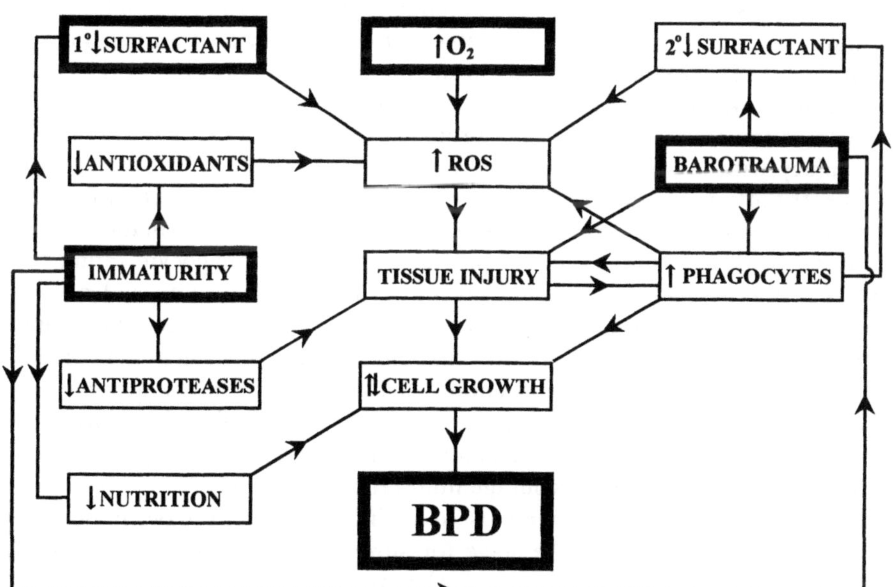

Fig. 1. The major etiological factors contributing to the development of BPD, hyperoxia, barotrauma, functional surfactant insufficiency and organ immaturity have a complex set of interaction which can contribute to an increase in reactive oxygen species (ROS), tissue injury and altered cell growth.

ventilated infants. (ii) Inhalation of high concentrations of oxygen results in lung injury and/or death in all mammalian species studied, including the adult human. (iii) BPD can occur in oxygen-treated but unventilated infants. (iv) The sequence and qualitative cellular changes in the lungs of infants with BPD are similar to those observed in oxygen-exposed animals.

It is generally recognized that the immediate cytotoxic effects of pulmonary oxygen toxicity are mediated through an increased formation of reactive oxygen species (ROS). Concentrations of ROS are, under normal circumstances, kept small by the antioxidant enzymes superoxide dismutases (SODs) and, for H_2O_2, catalase or glutathione peroxidase (GPx). This balance can be perturbed either by an increased oxygen formation leading to increased radical production or by reduced antioxidant defenses. We, and others, have shown in small animal models that the immature lung has reduced activities of antioxidant enzymes. This has led us to speculate that the very premature infant may be in a situation of double jeopardy with respect to increased ROS formation, because of both an elevated oxygen requirement and reduced antioxidant defenses. This limitation of antioxidant defenses in premature tissues extends beyond the primary enzymatic defenses to include a number of other molecules which serve a secondary line of antioxidant defense, such as α-tocopherol. Infants destined to develop BPD have lower glutathione concentrations in their bronchoalveolar lavage fluid, on the first day of life, than do infants not destined to develop BPD. Despite all of the available small animal data, an increased susceptibility of the preterm lung to oxygen toxicity relative to the adult lung has not been supported by studies in preterm baboons, and the issue in human infants is moot. Whether the preterm human is at any greater risk than the adult is, perhaps, of more academic interest than of practical importance. Whatever the maturity of the lung exposed to high concentrations of oxygen, if the balance of ROS and antioxidants is lost in favor of the former, cell injury with loss of epithelial and endothelial integrity will result. This allows entry of serum into the air spaces, which can result in surfactant inactivation, while oxidation of serum components can result in the formation of chemotaxins with a secondary influx of phagocytes. This phagocyte influx may play a critical role in subsequent tissue injury. There is also some evidence that when serum leak is nonhomogeneous, it is at sites of leakage where pulmonary fibrosis is most likely to occur. Another immediate consequence of oxidant injury, and loss of epithelial and endothelial integrity, is impaired lung compliance due to surfactant inactivation and both interstitial and peribronchial edema. Increased deposition of structural components, such as hyaluronan, in early lung injury may also encourage fluid retention. These changes lead to an increase in ventilation requirements to maintain adequate oxygenation and CO_2 clearance, thus setting the stage for superimposed barotrauma. Chronic diuretic therapy has long been a standard component of the routine therapy for infants with BPD, despite evidence that any short-term effects on lung mechanics are not sustained during chronic therapy. Chronic therapy does, however, appear to have some effect on survival which has to be attributed to other properties of loop diuretics such as furosemide. Furosemide is known to have several direct effects on lung cells, and careful study of these properties may allow any specific beneficial effect to be targeted.

If our hypothesis is correct, prevention of the initial radical-mediated injury should, if completely effective, abort the cascade described above and prevent lung injury. We, and others, have shown that the lethal effects of pulmonary oxygen toxicity *in vivo* can be prevented by pretreatment with antioxidant enzymes encapsulated in liposomes or conjugated to polyethylene glycol. Subsequent *in vitro* studies have shown that while combined liposomal SOD/catalase therapy does prevent cell death, it does not prevent disruption of cell function. The probable reason is that even though catalase is a more potent enzyme for converting H_2O_2 to H_2O than GPx in the test tube, GPx appears to be a more effective scavenger within the cell. GPx, but not catalase, is required to protect against hyperoxia and lipid peroxidation *in vitro*. A trial of SOD therapy in human infants, while affecting their XR findings had no effect on oxygen or positive pressure ventilation requirements [5]. As reviewed elsewhere, effective antioxidant therapies are likely to require either combination therapy or development of synthetic antioxidant compounds combining the properties of two or more natural antioxidants [6]. Recent animal studies with a group of synthetic antioxidants known as lazeroids have shown them to be potent antioxidants. The observation that lazeroids protect neonatal animals against hyperoxic inhibition of lung growth [7] is particularly encouraging.

While the acute cytotoxic effects of extreme oxygen exposures can lead to loss of cellular metabolic functions and cell death, lesser or brief exposures can mediate lung injury through less obvious pathways. Upregulation of gene expression for several growth factors, *e.g.* platelet-derived growth factor, and matrix components such as collagen and fibronectin are likely to contribute to the final pathological changes seen in the injured lung. Increased airway fibronectin concentrations and urinary elastin degradation products in infants receiving supplemental oxygen may reflect a direct degrading effect of oxygen, an oxygen-mediated induction of gene expression and protein synthesis, or a combination of both factors.

Barotrauma

Shortly after the original description of BPD, the probability that barotrauma contributed to the development of the disease was widely expounded. However, confirmation in experimental animals was slow to appear. Studies in adult animal conducted in the 1960's and 1970's, which compared lung injury from ventilation with oxygen *vs.* ventilation with air, did not show any convincing BPD-like lesions attributable to intermittent positive pressure ventilation. More recent studies using healthy young animals have confirmed parenchymal injury with the use of high peak airway pressures and large tidal volumes [8]. Nilsson *et al.* [9] used premature animals to show that bronchial epithelial lesions were produced by ventilation of the surfactant-deficient lung. More recently (10), it has been appreciated that airway injury in the surfactant-insufficient lung is phagocyte mediated and is attenuated by neutrophil depletion. The extremely low birth weight human infant is likely to receive exogenous surfactant in the present era, but that surfactant may be inactivated by serum components or by overstretching of the surfactant film, resulting in a secondary surfactant insufficiency. A contribution of barotrauma to the extensive airway lesions seen in some infants with barotrauma seems likely, and is consistent with the reported relationship between low arterial CO_2 concentrations and the subsequent development of BPD. Prevention relies on the continued search for improved methods of mechanical ventilation. Many infant ventilators now include an optional mode to allow infant-triggered assisted ventilation. This is an appealing approach, in that it should limit episodes of occluded expiration and lung over-distension. Documentation of any reduced risk of BPD with this approach awaits appropriate clinical trials. At least some human studies with high frequency oscillatory ventilation suggest that this mode of ventilation reduces the subsequent incidence of BPD, provided an adequate mean airway pressure is used, perhaps by limiting the shear forces experienced by the epithelium of the ventilated airways. These observations support data from a number of experimental models. In at least one surfactant-insufficient model high frequency oscillatory ventilation has been shown not to result in the phagocyte influx seen with conventional ventilation [11]. Liquid ventilation with perfluorocarbon solutions offers obvious theoretic advantages with respect to minimizing shear forces and may, in the future, prove to be a valuable tool in the prevention of the barotrauma component of developing BPD.

Over the last several years, we have conducted a series of studies with an *in vitro* model of the ventilated immature lung. Dispersed fetal lung cells applied to a gelatin sponge will reaggregate to form epithelial alveolar-like structures surrounded by mesenchymal cells. This sponge, and the alveolar-like structures therein, can be cyclically stretched to emulate various ventilation patterns. While our primary focus has been on how fetal breathing movements may play a critical role in normal lung development, it also became clear that exceeding a fairly narrow band of optimal settings can arrest cell growth, as shown in Figure 2.

These observations suggest that excessive ventilator settings may also play a role in alveolar changes seen in BPD. These may be a direct effect of barotrauma alone, or may be a consequence of additive effects between oxygen toxicity and barotrauma which may lessen the threshold for either. Stimulatory effects of intermittent stretch on lung cell growth appear to be mediated by a signal transduction pathway involving protein kinase C [12], which has also been shown to transduce a number of cellular responses mediated by ROS. In support of this hypothesis are a variety of *in vivo* studies in which animals made to chronically increase their minute ventilation, by exercise or hypobaric pressure, which show an increase in lung size as a consequence of such maneuvers.

Better known, perhaps, are studies with fetal animals in which upper airways have been ligated or occluded. These fetuses have consistently shown a very marked acceleration of parenchymal lung growth distal to the obstruction.

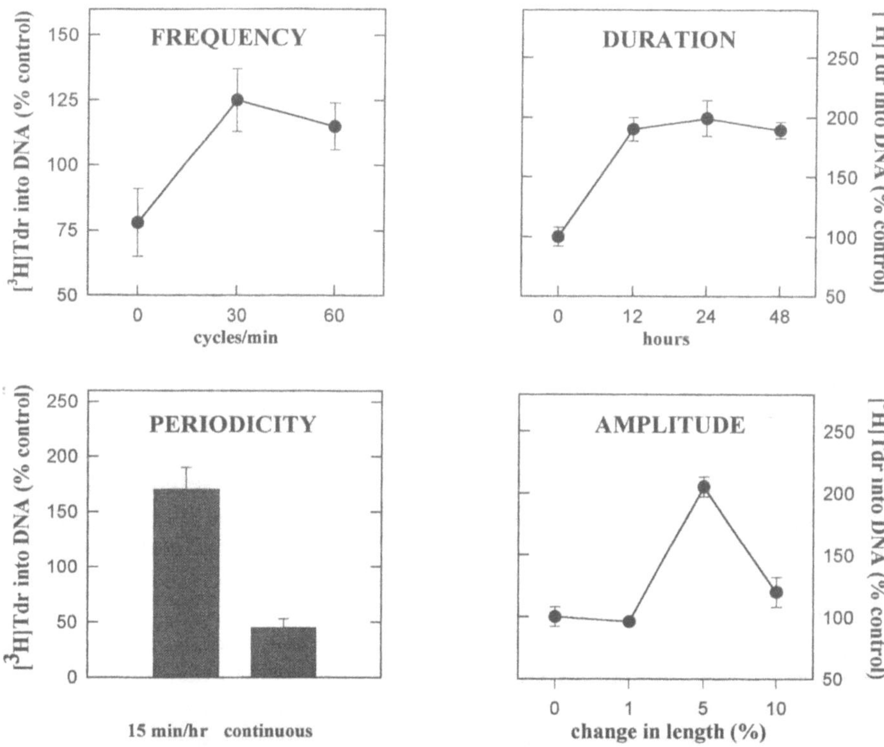

Fig. 2. Organotypic cultures of lung cells from preterm fetal rat lung were subjected to episodic stretch to emulate respiratory excursions, and the effect of various ventilatory patterns on [^{3}H]thymidine (Tdr) incorporation into DNA, as an index of cell division, was studied. Simulated respiratory movements had a significant impact on lung cell growth which was dependent upon the frequency, duration, periodicity and amplitude of the respiratory movements. Cell division was inhibited at high amplitudes which was associated with measurable cytotoxicity.

These observation strongly implicate alveolar distension as a regulator of distal lung cell growth which could be adversely affected during the process of mechanical ventilation.

The infant with established and —healing— BPD is required to generate a significantly increased driving pressure to establish airflow. As measured by the peak-to-peak esophageal pressure change in normal and affected infants this pressure may be double normal values in infants with established BPD. Such pressure changes may be outside the normal range for postnatal acini and may adversely affect normal alveolar growth and development if postnatal lung cell proliferation is as sensitive to pressure changes as is fetal lung. It is also possible, of course, that raised intra-alveolar pressures serve as a compensatory mechanism to encourage alveolar development in the injured postnatal lung. The relationship between transpulmonary pressure and postnatal lung growth rates is an area of investigation which has been regrettably neglected.

Immaturity

There is a clear inverse relationship between gestational age at the time of birth and the risk of developing BPD. It is likely that there are multiple contributors to this increased risk in the most immature infants. The smallest infants are the group likely to require the longest exposure to ventilatory support and supplemental oxygen. Adequate nutrition, sufficient to maintain a growth rate close to that which would have been seen *in utero*, is particularly difficult to achieve in this population and chronic malnutrition may have irreversible consequences on lung growth. The additive effects of undernutrition and pulmonary oxygen toxicity are well recognized. Tissue lipid peroxidation, as assessed by expired ethane and pentane, is directly correlated to the degree of immaturity at birth. The issue of the immaturity of the primary enzymatic antioxidant defense system has been discussed earlier. A number of secondary antioxidants, such as vitamins A, C and E, β-carotene and ceruloplasmin accumulate in fetal tissues in the latter part of the third trimester, as a result of maternal-fetal transfer. The immature lung is more friable than the mature lung and more prone to rupture and air leak. Diffuse pulmonary interstitial emphysema may result in a need for increased ventilator support and oxygen supplementation in addition to direct adverse effects.

Airway anti-protease activity is gestation dependent, and the α1-proteinase inhibitor is subject to oxidative inactivation as well as degradation and inactivation by macrophage elastase. The ratio of elastase to α1-proteinase inhibitor is increased in the airways of infants with BPD. A net increase in elastase has been shown to increase fibroblast migration into airway epithelium in experimental models. Significant protection against the pulmonary vascular and parenchymal effects of oxygen toxicity has recently been demonstrated in neonatal rats receiving parenteral α1-anti-protease [13].

The role of endogenous and exogenous surfactants in the immature lung developing BPD is far from clear, but there have been several recent observations which may help clarify a confusing, and sometimes apparently contradictory, series of experimental observations. Hyperoxia has been variously reported to increase, decrease or have no effect on lung surfactant content in various models with different exposure protocols. It has been recently appreciated that any effects on lung surfactant pools may be of less functional importance than changes in surfactant apoprotein expression [14] or the physical state of surfactant vesicles [15] which can affect surface activity. Protective effects of exogenous surfactant may act by minimizing these effects, but surfactant preparations have also been report to minimize phagocyte influx, suppress the respiratory burst of alveolar macrophages, have antioxidant activity and can extend antioxidant enzyme activity half-life as well as attenuate elastase-mediated lung injury.

Growth Factors

While the late consequence of severe BPD is pulmonary undergrowth with a reduction in alveolar number and gas exchange surface area, there are some cell types which proliferate during the initial injury process. Type II pneumocytes proliferate during the epithelial repair process, fibroblasts proliferate at sites of pulmonary fibrosis and smooth muscle cells proliferate around both airways and blood vessels. This is superimposed upon the situation of generally reduced acinar development.

There has been a considerable body of information generated for growth factor expression in various experimental adult lung injuries in recent years. Taking our own studies with the adult rat exposed to 85% O_2 as an example, we have observed increased expression of platelet derived growth factor-BB and its β-receptor in association with fibroblast hyperplasia, basic fibroblast growth factor and its (*flg*) receptor in association with pneumocyte hyperplasia and insulin-like growth factor I and its (type I) receptor in association with smooth muscle hyperplasia. These factors are likely to contribute to the various cellular hyperplasias seen in this, and other, models of adult lung injury. In the 85% O_2-exposed adult rat lung, as in other lung injuries, transforming growth factor βs (TGFβs) appear to play a key role in increased collagen deposition. Adult lung injury models have the distinct advantage that any observed proliferative responses are superimposed on an essentially non-proliferative basal state. This same property makes them of dubious value for predicting mediators of cell proliferation in the injured neonatal lung.

In the uninjured neonatal lung there is in a state of active proliferation. In BPD, and in animal models of BPD, the injury process is heterogeneous, with growth arrest and emphysema in some areas of the lung and patchy areas of interstitial thickening and proliferation elsewhere. Whether the pneumocyte, fibroblast and smooth muscle cell hyperplasias seen as part of the acute injury process represent a continued, but discoordinate response to the growth factors which mediate normal postnatal lung growth is unknown. Indeed, while there has been considerable information gathered over the last several years about growth factor and tissue interactions which control normal prenatal lung development there is, as yet, little available information about normal or abnormal postnatal lung growth controls. It is known that the epidermal growth factor receptor is found on bronchiolar epithelium of infants with BPD, and it may be assumed that one or both of its ligands, epidermal growth factor and transforming growth factor α, acts at that site and may play a role in the airway epithelial metaplasia seen in BPD. Gastrin-releasing peptide, a mitogen for airway epithelium, also increases in airway epithelium of infants with BPD. We have recently reviewed the available information on growth factors in prenatal lung development and lung injury in depth [16, 17] and will not discuss the issue at great length herein. There are three specific points relevant to potential therapeutic interventions worth mentioning. One is the apparently central role of successful re-epithelialization in the determination of whether lung injury will be successfully repaired or whether fibrosis will develop. One model that fits with the observation that interventions to slow re-epithelialization are associated with fibrosis in areas adjacent to areas of denuded epithelial basement membrane is a tonic release of a fibroblast growth inhibitor by epithelial cells. Loss of chronic inhibitory tone would allow fibroblast hyperplasia. This concept is important for several reasons. Firstly, sustained exposure to high concentrations of oxygen after an epithelial injury is known to slow re-epithelialization. Secondly, the epithelium is an easily accessible target for interventions. If interventions to protect against epithelial injury were unsuccessful or delayed it may still be possible to stimulate re-epithelialization by use of appropriate growth factors, or limit fibroblast hyperplasia by use of an appropriate inhibitor of fibroblast growth during epithelial recovery. It should be remembered that growth factors which primarily target mesenchymal cells of the adult lung may primarily target epithelial cells in the fetal lung. The situation in the postnatal lung is uncertain. Secondly, the role of TGFβs in the excessive matrix deposition of various tissue injuries, including lung, is becoming increasingly recognized. At least in some lung injuries, the primary source of TGFβs is the epithelium. Antibodies to TGFβs have been shown to limit collagen deposition in at least one lung injury model, and suggests a possible approach to intervention. Such an approach would need to be carefully evaluated and optimized in a good animal model, such as the preterm baboon, because TGFβs could play a role in matrix deposition in normal postnatal lung growth and sustained disruption of normal matrix deposition can by itself arrest alveolar development. TGFβs may also have a parallel beneficial effect by decreasing protease secretion and increasing protease inhibitor activity.

Phagocyte Influx

Neutrophils and alveolar macrophages increase significantly in the lungs of infants with evolving BPD [18]. While they serve an important and beneficial role in clearing debris derived from injured tissue they may, and probably do, contribute to tissue injury by releasing proteolytic enzymes and ROS. The neutrophil chemoattractants leukotriene B_4, interleukin-8 and C5a are all increased in tracheobronchial aspirates of infants with BPD. Other cytokines such as interleukin-6 and tumor necrosis factor α also increase in tracheobronchial aspirates of infants with BPD, but their roles in the inflammation cascade are not yet clear. The inflammatory cascade has recently been shown to be regulated by a group of molecules known as adhesion molecules [19]. There are three subfamilies of adhesion molecules: selectins, the immunoglobulin supergene family, and integrins. Antibodies raised against these adhesion molecules have been shown to provide significant levels of protection in a number of experimental phagocyte-mediated tissue injuries and they provide an exciting potential therapeutic approach. It is likely that such approaches will first be tried in adult human patients with acute respiratory distress syndrome, but if they are found to be effective in clinical trials they will undoubtedly come to trial for BPD shortly thereafter.

Neutrophils are not a recognized source of growth factors, but there is good evidence that macrophage-derived growth factors contribute to the pathological changes seen in a number of lung injuries. A series of studies in recent years have demonstrated the release of growth factors for fibroblasts by alveolar macrophages from injured lungs. At least in the neonatal and adult rat, we have found a minimal influx of phagocytes with exposed to elevated oxygen concentrations and these are limited to perivascular and peribronchial areas. The recruitment of macrophages into the interstitial and alveolar compartment of the human infant with BPD may reflect species differences or some other mechanism, such as barotrauma, which is responsible for initiating their influx.

Abnormal Matrix Deposition

The matrix changes which occur with pulmonary fibrosis have been subject to a recent comprehensive review (20). In fibrotic lungs fibronectin is increased beneath hyperplastic type II pneumocytes, perhaps reflecting an early stage of differentiation to type I pneumocytes. Collagen types I and III accumulate in the expanded interstitium with type III collagen initially predominant in alveolar septa and interstitium, while type I collagen becomes the principal collagen late in the process. At the onset of bleomycin-induced pulmonary fibrosis there is a marked accumulation of laminin at pericapillary sites of fibrosis, while there is also an association between fibronectin distribution and fibrosis in the same model. Fibroblasts from lungs with active fibrosis demonstrate an increased rate of cell division, compared with fibroblasts derived from normal, or densely fibrotic, lungs. Subcellular matrix composition has been shown to have both permissive and non-permissive actions on cell growth. *In vitro* studies have shown that the response of cells to growth factors is determined by their substratum, which is related in some way to their shape. Also, matrix can have direct effects on responsivity to growth factors, and indirect effects by binding growth factors to act as a reservoir. Conversely, growth factors may alter expression of matrix genes in responsive cells. Therapeutic interventions targeted at matrix molecule synthesis are feasible, but this approach is subject to the same concern as targeting TGFβs in that matrix deposition required for normal alveolar growth and development may also be inhibited.

Unresolved Issues

Preterm infants that develop BPD have low circulating levels of vitamin A, a differentiation factor for airway epithelium. Vitamin A deficiency is associated with the development of squamous metaplasia of the tracheobronchial epithelium. An initial trial of supplementation appeared to have a beneficial effect, but a subsequent trial at a different center did not reproduce the effect. The loss of effect may have been due to masking by other interventions such as steroid use and surfactant therapy. The role of vitamin A supplementation remains unresolved, but it is often provided in parenteral nutrition solutions and such benefits as there are may be unwittingly provided through normal nutritional practices.

A direct relationship between colonization with *Ureaplasma urealyticum* and the development of BPD has been postulated by a number of investigators. While there seem to be clear relationships between immaturity and colonization, and between immaturity and BPD, a cause-and-effect relationship between colonization and the development of BPD is unproven [21].

The role of a patent ductus arteriosus to subsequent development of BPD remains unclear, with various trials showing benefit of closure or no beneficial effect.

Conclusion

BPD has long been recognized to be of multifactorial origin. Immaturity increases susceptibility to oxygen toxicity, barotrauma and the consequences of inflammation. Our understanding of the cellular mechanisms by which these factors exert their toxic effects, and interact, has increased dramatically over the last several years. Maintaining an intact epithelium appears to be critical to the prevention of the cascade which ultimately leads to pulmonary fibrosis. For this to be achieved it is likely that a multifaceted approach to intervention will be required. Potent synthetic antioxidants have recently been developed which protect against oxygen toxicity. The recent appreciation of the critical role of functional surfactant in preventing phagocyte mediated barotrauma to the distal airways can be targeted through improved ventilation strategies, maintaining surfactant activity or by antibodies to adhesion molecules to prevent phagocyte influx. Now that a good animal model of human BPD has been developed, specifically the preterm baboon, estimating the relative individual and additive benefits of each approach, under tightly controlled laboratory conditions, has become a realistic goal which should benefit the human infant within the not too distant future.

References

1. Farell PM, Palta M (1986) Bronchopulmonary dysplasia. In: Farell PM, Tausig LM (eds) Bronchopulmonary dysplasia and isolated chronic respiratory disorders, Ross Laboratories, Columbus, Ohio, pp 1–7.
2. Chambers HM, van Velzen D (1989) Ventilator-related pathology in the extremely immature lung. Pathology 21:79–83.
3. Van Lierde S, Cornelis A, Devlieger H, Moerman P, Lauweryns J, Eggermont E (1991) Different patterns of pulmonary sequelae after hyaline membrane disease: heterogeneity of bronchopulmonary dysplasia? Biol Neonate 60:152–162.
4. Wohl MEB (1990) Bronchopulmonary dysplasia in adulthood. N Eng J Med 323:1834–1836.

5. Rosenfeld W, Evans H, Concepcion L, Jhaveri R, Schaeffer H, Friedman A (1984) Prevention of bronchopulmonary dysplasia by administration of bovine superoxide dismutase in preterm infants with respiratory distress syndrome. J Pediatr 105:781–785.
6. Tanswell AK, Freeman BA (1995) Antioxidant therapy in critical care medicine. New Horizons 3:330–341.
7. Frank L, McLaughlin GE (1993) Protection against acute and chronic hyperoxic inhibition of neonatal rat lung development with the 21-aminosteroid drug U74389F. Pediatr Res 33:632–638.
8. Tsuno K, Miura K, Takeya M, Kolobow T, Morioka M (1991) Histopathologic pulmonary changes from mechanical ventilation at high peak airway pressures. Am Rev Respir Dis 143:1115–1120.
9. Nilsson R, Grossmann G, Robertson B (1980) Pathogenesis of neonatal lung lesions induced by artificial ventilation: evidence against the role of barotrauma. Respiration 40:218–225.
10. Kawano T, Mori S, Cybulsky M, *et al.* (1987) Effect of granulocyte depletion in a ventilated surfactant-depleted lung. J Appl Physiol 62:27–33.
11. Matsuoka T, Kawano T, Gamsu HR (1994) Role of high-frequency ventilation in surfactant-depleted lung injury as measured by granulocytes. J Appl Physiol 76:539–544.
12. Liu M, Xu J, Liu J, Kraw ME, Tanswell AK, Post M (1995) Mechanical strain-enhanced fetal lung cell proliferation is mediated by phospholipases C and D and protein kinase C. Am J Physiol 268:L729-L738.
13. Koppel R, Han RNN, Cox D, Tanswell AK, Rabinovitch M (1994) α_1-antitrypsin protects neonatal rats from pulmonary vascular and parenchymal effects of oxygen toxicity. Pediatr Res 36:763–770.
14. King RJ, Coalson JJ, deLemos RA, Gerstmann DR, Seidner SR (1995) Surfactant protein-A deficiency in a primate model of bronchopulmonary dysplasia. Am J Respir Crit Care Med 151:1989–1997.
15. Clements JA, Goerke J, Wright JR, Beppu O (1984) Turnover of lung surfactant. Prog Respir Res 18:133–142.
16. Post M (1996) Tissue interactions. In: Crystal RG, West JB, Weibel E, Barnes PJ (eds) The lung: Scientific foundations, 2nd edn. Raven Press, New York, *In Press.*
17. Tanswell AK, Buch S, Liu M, Post M (1996) Factors mediating cell growth in lung injury. In: Bland RD, Coalson J (eds) Chronic lung disease in early infancy. Marcel Dekker, New York, *In Press.*
18. Bonikos DS, Bensch KG, Northway WH, Edwards DK (1976) Bronchopulmonary dysplasia: the pulmonary pathological sequel of necrotizing bronchiolitis and pulmonary fibrosis. Human Pathol 7:643–666.
19. Hamacher J, Schaberg T (1994) Adhesion molecules in lung disease. Lung 172:189–213.
20. Crouch E (1990) Pathobiology of pulmonary fibrosis. Am J Physiol 259:L159–L184.
21. Jonsson B, Karell A-C, Ringertz S, Rylander M, Faxelius G (1995) Neonatal *Ureaplasma urealyticum* colonization and chronic lung disease. Acta Paediatr 83:927–930.

Adverse Effects of Dexamethasone Treatment in Preterm Neonates

A. F. Bos and S. Bambang Oetomo

Introduction

Corticosteroids are frequently used in the perinatal period. In case of imminent preterm birth prenatal dexamethasone or betamethasone therapy has been shown to decrease the incidence of respiratory distress, periventricular hemorrhage and necrotizing enterocolitis [1]. Long-term adverse effects on neurodevelopmental outcome have not been demonstrated. On the contrary, a favorable effect on neurological abnormality at follow-up seems present [1].

Postnatally high dose dexamethasone therapy is used in preterm infants at risk for chronic lung disease. Several studies have demonstrated a positive effect on lung function, duration of artificial ventilation and oxygen requirements [2–8]. These effects, however, appear to be short-term, lasting several weeks at most. Although some recent studies suggest a reduced incidence of chronic lung disease at a postmenstrual age of 36 weeks [7, 8], long-term pulmonary sequelae are not different from controls in studies with a longer duration of follow-up [9–11].

The favorable findings of prenatal therapy are thus in contrast to those of postnatal therapy. It has to be taken into account that prenatally very short courses of corticosteroids are used. In general only one or two doses are given. Postnatally on the other hand, chronic administration of high dose dexamethasone for the prevention of chronic lung disease is common practice. Courses last at least one week, but frequently longer. It is possible that the discrepancy found is due to potential adverse effects of prolonged high dose corticosteroid therapy. In this review we will discuss the complications and side effects of dexamethasone therapy that have been reported in preterm infants.

Complications

Several complications in preterm infants are attributed to the steroid therapy they receive. Frequently these are rare complications, but some may be important enough to be cautious with steroids. One of these is the finding of new brain ultrasound abnormalities after the start of dexamethasone therapy [12]. After this single observation however, the occurrence of these abnormalities have not been confirmed by others.

In early studies concern has been raised about an increased incidence of sepsis [2]. In several later investigations however, this finding was not confirmed [5, 6, 8]. Although immunosuppressive effects are suggested in several reviews, this has in fact not well been studied in human preterm infants. Only one recent in-vitro study shows an immunosuppressive effect of dexamethasone on neonatal lymphocyte proliferation [13]. Other evidence is indirect and comes from in-vitro studies in animals or adults.

An association between dexamethasone treatment and an increased incidence of retinopathy of prematurity (ROP) has been found in two retrospective studies [14, 15]. The rapid improvement of oxygenation, and hence an increased arterial PO_2, is given as the explanation. In this respect we have to consider that the infants with the most severe chronic lung disease are treated with corticosteroids. Of course these infants are also more prone to development of ROP than less ill infants of similar gestational age. In none of the randomized studies an increased incidence of ROP in the dexamethasone treated groups has been confirmed.

An increased incidence of gastro-intestinal perforations is another frequent reported complication of steroid therapy [16, 17]. The increased susceptibility for gastric or duodenal ulcers due to treatment with high dose corticosteroids is held responsible for these life-threatening complications. Again, this might be a reflection of the severity of the clinical situation in which the infants with a severe bronchopulmonary dysplasia are, rather than a direct effect of the corticosteroids. In large randomized trials no difference of occurrence of gastrointestinal bleeding or necrotizing enterocolitis between groups has been found [5, 7].

Side Effects

In this section side effects are reviewed that occur in most infants on dexamethasone therapy. As indication, dosage regimes, timing of initiating and duration of corticosteroid therapy vary widely between studies, comparison between studies of the extent and impact of side effects are difficult. Furthermore, these effects may be transient and are not necessarily adverse effects. For systematical purposes a subdivision in cardiovascular, metabolic and central nervous system-effects has been made.

Cardiovascular Effects

In most studies on dexamethasone a transient and mostly insignificant hypertension is found [4–6, 8, 18]. Treatment is seldom required. A potential more serious effect is cardiac muscle hypertrophy, especially of the left ventricle and septum [19–21]. This occurs after several weeks of dexamethasone therapy, and resolves spontaneously after therapy is discontinued. Circulatory insufficiency is rare. The cause of the left ventricle hypertrophy is unknown.

Changes in heart rate and heart rate variability under the influence of steroid treatment have been established [22, 23]. Heart rate decreases and heart rate variability increases, already 12 to 24 hours after dexamethasone therapy was started. In human fetuses an increase of heart rate and decrease of heart rate variability is found 24 and 48 hours after the mothers had been given betamethasone for imminent preterm birth [24]. The significance of these findings remain unclear.

Metabolic Effects

Most studies report hyperglycemia, that sometimes is so severe that treatment with insulin is required [5, 7, 8, 18, 22, 25]. A significant and substantial rise of plasmalevels of aminoacids have been shown to occur as early as 24 hours after the start of therapy [26–28], indicative of breakdown of protein [29]. The enhanced catabolism is reflected in poor somatic growth [4, 12, 18], and concern has been raised on the potential adverse effects on lung growth, especially on alveolar development [30]. This might be one of the explanations why long-term pulmonary outcome in infants treated with corticosteroids is not different from controls. It is unclear whether the growth impairment is irreversible, as data on long-term development are scarce and contradictory.

The enhanced catabolism is further demonstrated by an increase in serum urea in several days [26, 31]. This might be one of the causes of the enhanced diuresis that has been observed following dexamethasone therapy [3, 22, 31], along with pressure diuresis induced by the increase in arterial blood pressure and glucosuria due to hyperglycemia.

Adrenal suppression has been demonstrated up to one month duration, even after 1 week of dexamethasone therapy [4, 6]. The clinical relevance of this finding is questioned, but may be of minor importance [6, 12]. In none of the studies clinical adrenal insufficiency is described.

Effects on the Central Nervous System

There exists a large discrepancy between the vast amount of literature on known negative effects of corticosteroids on the developing central nervous system in animals, especially rats, and the lack of studies on this topic in humans. In animals administration of glucocorticoids in the perinatal period has been shown to lead to serious and permanent negative effects on brain growth and behavior. Of course, the animal experiments need to be treated with great caution as a rat and human are only to a certain extent comparable; especially the degree of maturation is different. Still this is one of the important issues regarding perinatal steroid therapy, as adverse effects might be long-term and irreversible.

In Table 1 data of several animal studies are summarized that have investigated the effects of perinatal corticosteroid administration on the central ner-

Table 1. Effects of perinatal corticosteroid administration on the central nervous system in animals

Reference [number]	Animal	Cortico-steroid[a]	Age, dose and duration[b]	Effects
Howard 1968 [32]	mice	cortisone	2d pp, in cholesterol pellets; 0.4–0.6 grams in 14 days	impaired growth of cerebrum and cerebellum
Howard 1968 [36]	mice	cortisone	2d pp; in cholesterol pellets, 0.4–0.6 grams in 14 days	impaired gross motor coordination as adults
Schapiro 1968 [37]	rats	cortisol	1d pp; 1 mg once	delayed dendritic spine formation in cortex diminished locomotor activity
Benesova 1989 [33]	rats	dxa	7d pp; 0.2, 1 or 3 mg/kg once	acceleration of some developmental landmarks deficits in motor coordination and performance as adults permanent decreased cerebellum weight
Tsuneishi 1991 [34]	rats	dxa	3d pp; 1 mg/kg for 7d	suppression of genes involved in myelination of cerebrum and cerebellum
Barks 1991 [39]	rats	dxa	7d pp; various doses (0.001–0.5 mg/kg) various schedules (1–3d)	neuro-protective effect of pretreatment (>0.01 mg/kg) after hypoxia-ischemia
Fujii 1993 [38]	fetal rats	cortisol	12d or 8d ap; 10 mg/kg for 3d	delayed development of ambulatory behavior
Zahalka 1993 [35]	fetal rats	dxa	4d ap; 0.05, 0.2 or 0.8 mg/kg for 3d	dose dependent retardation of brain growth enhanced development of central cholinergic differentiation

[a] dxa = dexamethasone
[b] d = days; pp = post partum; ap = ante partum

vous system. At the moment of corticosteroid administration growth impairment of brain regions with a high mitotic activity of neurons and glia cells is found, with doses similar as are used in preterm infants [32–35]. During late gestation in rats the fetal forebrain exhibits a high mitotic activity [35], whereas the cerebellum shows the same mitotic and differentiating activity during the first postnatal days [33]. Effects are therefore dependent on the age and developmental stage of the animals. Changes in behavior, with at first acceleration of some developmental landmarks, but later impaired development and coordination is a consistent finding in most of these studies [33, 36–38]. This might be explained by the simultaneous inhibition of cell replication and enhanced cell differentiation, a well-known effect of glucocorticoids on cells [35].

One study shows a favorable, neuroprotective effect [39]. Recent studies on the other hand indicate that glucocorticoids exacerbates the neurotoxicity of a number of different metabolic insults, such as hypoxia, ischemia or hypoglycemia [40].

As already mentioned, adverse effects on the central nervous system in human preterm infants have scarcely been investigated. Long-term neurodevelopmental outcome of infants with bronchopulmonary dysplasia is poor, irrespective of the use of corticosteroids [41].

In Table 2 human studies are summarized that have investigated the neurodevelopmental outcome of infants treated with dexamethasone [9–11, 25, 42–44]. No clear difference between treated and non-treated infants is found. Most studies however, are not randomized controlled, and those that are, have allowed dexamethasone treatment in the control group at a later stage [11]. Up to 40% of control infants eventually received a dexamethasone course, and this makes comparison of long-term effects difficult.

Table 2. Effects of postnatal dexamethasone treatment in infants with chronic lung disease on neurodevelopmental outcome

Reference [number]	n	Study type[a]	Age at follow-up	Outcome[b]	Comment[b]
Mammel 1978 [42]	16	C	1 year	No difference	Dxa- and non-dxa treated infants differed
Ferrara 1990 [25]	107	C	15 months	No difference	Retrospective
Satish 1991 [43]	22	C	18 months	Neuromuscular delay in dxa group	Dxa- and non-dxa treated infants differed
Cummings 1992 [44]	23	RC	4 years	Improved cognitive and neurological outcome in dxa group	3 groups, small number in each group
O'Shea 1993 [9]	94	S, C	1 year	No difference	Historic controls
Furman 1995 [10]	83	S, C	20 months	Cognitive and psychomotor impairment in dxa group	Dxa and non-dxa treated infants differed
Jones 1995 [11]	209	RC	3 years	No difference	40% of controls received dxa later

[a] C = controlled, RC = randomized controlled, S = sequential observations

[b] dxa = dexamethasone

Only few studies have reported on acute effects of dexamethasone on the central nervous system in human infants. In one study marked irritability occurred in a few infants [25]. In another case-report changes in spontaneous motility have been observed [45]. By means of assessment of spontaneous motor behavior the function of the central nervous system in preterm infants can be studied [46]. Using this method, acute profound effects of dexamethasone therapy on spontaneous movements have been demonstrated in a prospective study during the first week after the dexamethasone course was started. All movement patterns decreased in number, particularly the fast ones. Furthermore, at detailed analysis of the quality of general movements, a reduction of speed and amplitude was found [47]. A reduction of motility has also been found in fetuses, after the mother was treated with betamethasone [24]. The significance of these findings for later development are not clear.

How can we explain the discrepancy between the absence of clear-cut effects on development in humans and the obvious negative effects on neurodevelopment in animals? First of all, as mentioned already, the effects of dexamethasone treatment on neurodevelopmental outcome in human infants have not been studied well. Effects might be present, only to become apparent after several years. A second explanation lies in the natural course of bronchopulmonary dysplasia. Recurrent, sometimes severe and undetected episodes of hypoxia are common. It might well be that corticosteroid treatment improves the occurrence and severity of episodes of hypoxia in these infants. The eventual damaging effect of corticosteroid treatment then outweighs the maybe even more damaging effects of recurrent episodes of hypoxia. The net effect is a poor outcome in comparison to healthy infants, as all studies demonstrate, but no difference between dexamethasone and non-dexamethasone treated infants.

Conclusion

Systemic neonatal dexamethasone therapy is associated with several, sometimes severe side effects. Concern continues to exist regarding the long-term efficacy and neurological effects of this treatment. More research is necessary to elucidate the optimal time to start, duration of therapy, and dosage regimen. A recent promising study showed a good effect on chronic lung disease with minimal side effects, using recurrent pulse therapy of short duration [7]. Another promising development is the use of inhalation steroids, thus avoiding systemic side effects [30]. Again, research is needed to establish the optimal time to start, duration of treatment and optimal distribution in the lungs. Until more is known about long-term neurological sequelae, a cautious use of systemic dexamethasone therapy in preterm infants is recommended. To our opinion it is only indicated in ventilator-dependent infants at risk for rather severe chronic lung disease, and this therapy should be as short as possible.

References

1. Crowley PA. (1995) Antenatal corticosteroid therapy: A meta-analysis of the randomized trials, 1972 to 1994. Am J Obstet Gynecol 173:322–335.
2. Avery GB, Fletcher AB, Kaplan M, Brudno DS. (1985) Controlled trial of dexamethasone in respirator-dependent infants with bronchopulmonary dysplasia. Pediatrics 75:106–111.
3. Gladstone IM, Ehrenkranz RA, Jacobs HC. (1989) Pulmonary function tests and fluid balance in neonates with chronic lung disease during dexamethasone treatment. Pediatrics 84:1072–1076.
4. Cummings JJ, D'Eugenio DB, Gross SJ. (1989) A controlled trial of dexamethasone in preterm infants at high risk for bronchopulmonary dysplasia. N Engl J Med 320:1505–1510.
5. Collaborative Dexamethasone Trial Group (1991) Dexamethasone therapy in neonatal chronic lung disease: an international placebo-controlled trial. Pediatrics 88:421–427.
6. Kari MA, Heinonen K, Ikonen RS, Koivisto M, Raivio KO. (1993) Dexamethasone treatment in preterm infants at risk for bronchopulmonary dysplasia. Arch Dis Child 68:566–569.
7. Brozanski BS, Jones JG, Gilmour CH, et al (1995) Effect of pulse dexamethasone therapy on the incidence and severity of chronic lung disease in the very low birth weight infant. J Pediatr 126:769–776.
8. Durand M, Sardesai S, McEvoy C. (1995) Effects of early dexamethasone therapy on pulmonary mechanics and chronic lung disease in very low birth weight infants: A randomized, controlled trial. Pediatrics 95:584–590.
9. O'Shea TM, Kothadia JM, Klinepeter KL, Goldstein DJ, Jackson B, Dillard RG. (1993) Follow-up of preterm infants treated with dexamethasone for chronic lung disease. Am J Dis Child 147:658–661.
10. Furman L, Hack M, Watts C, et al (1995) Twenty-month outcome in ventilator-dependent, very low birth weight infants born during the early years of dexamethasone therapy. J Pediatr 126:434–440.
11. Jones R, Wincott E, Elbourne D, Grant A. (1995) Controlled trial of dexamethasone in neonatal chronic lung disease: A 3-year follow-up. Pediatrics 96:897–906.
12. Noble-Jamieson CM, Regev R, Silverman M. (1989) Dexamethasone in neonatal chronic lung disease: pulmonary effects and intracranial complications. Eur J Pediatr 148:365–367.
13. Schwarze J, Bartmann P. (1994) Influence of dexamethasone on lymphocyte proliferation in whole blood cultures of neonates. Biol Neonate 65:295–301.
14. Batton DG, Roberts C, Trese M, Maisels MJ. (1992) Severe retinopathy of prematurity and steroid exposure. Pediatrics 90:534–536.
15. Ramanathan R, Siassi B, deLemos RA. (1995) Severe retinopathy of prematurity in extremely low birth weight infants after short-term dexamethasone therapy. J Perinatol 15:178–182.
16. Ng PC, Brownlee KG, Dear PR. (1991) Gastroduodenal perforation in preterm babies treated with dexamethasone for bronchopulmonary dysplasia. Arch Dis Child 66:1164–1166.
17. Wolf YG, Reyna T, Schropp KP, Harmel RP, Jr. (1991) Steroid therapy and duodenal ulcer in infants. J Pediatr Gastroenterol Nutr 12:269–271.
18. Yeh TF, Torre JA, Rastogi A, Anyebuno MA, Pildes RS. (1990) Early postnatal dexamethasone therapy in premature infants with severe respiratory distress syndrome: a double-blind controlled study. J Pediatr 117:273–282.
19. Werner JC, Sicard RE, Hansen TW, Solomon E, Cowett RM, Oh W. (1992) Hypertrophic cardiomyopathy associated with dexamethasone therapy for bronchopulmonary dysplasia. J Pediatr 120:286–291.
20. Brand PLP, van Lingen RA, Brus F, Talsma MD, Elzenga NJ. (1993) Hypertrophic obstructive cardiomyopathy as a side effect of dexamethasone treatment for bronchopulmonary dysplasia. Acta Paediatr 82:614–617.

21. Evans N. (1994) Cardiovascular effects of dexamethasone in the preterm infant. Arch Dis Child 70:F25–30.
22. Ohlsson A, Calvert SA, Hosking MC, Shennan AT. (1992) Randomized controlled trial of dexamethasone treatment in very-low-birth-weight infants with ventilator-dependent chronic lung disease. Acta Paediatr 81:751–756.
23. Bos AF, van Asperen RM, Van Eykern LA, Zijlstra WG, Okken A. (1994) Heart rate, heart rate variability and metabolic rate in preterm infants with bronchopulmonary dysplasia in the first week of dexamethasone treatment. J Physiol 479:23P–24P (Abst)
24. Mulder EJH, Derks JB, Zonneveld MF, Bruinse HW, Visser GHA. (1994) Transient reduction in fetal activity and heart rate variation after maternal betamethasone administration. Early Hum Dev 36:49–60.
25. Ferrara TB, Couser RJ, Hoekstra RE. (1990) Side effects and long-term follow-up of corticosteroid therapy in very low birthweight infants with bronchopulmonary dysplasia. J Perinatol 10:137–142.
26. Williams AF, Jones M. (1992) Dexamethasone increases plasma amino acid concentrations in bronchopulmonary dysplasia. Arch Dis Child 67:5–9.
27. Brownlee KG, Ng PC, Henderson MJ, Smith M, Green JH, Dear PR. (1992) Catabolic effect of dexamethasone in the preterm baby. Arch Dis Child 67:1–4.
28. Bos AF, van Asperen RM, Reijngoud DJ, Okken A. (1994) Plasma amino acid levels in preterm infants with bronchopulmonary dysplasia on the first days of dexamethasone treatment. Pediatr Res 36:7A. (Abst).
29. Van Goudoever JB, Wattimena JLD, Carnielli VP, Sulkers EJ, Degenhart HJ, Sauer PJJ. (1994) Effect of dexamethasone on protein metabolism in infants with bronchopulmonary dysplasia. J Pediatr 124:112–118.
30. Silverman M. (1994) Chronic lung disease of prematurity: are we too cautious with steroids? Eur J Pediatr 153:S30–S35.
31. Bos AF, Reitsma-Bierens WWC, Okken A. (1994) Effects of dexamethasone treatment on diuresis, serum urea and arterial blood pressure in preterm infants with bronchopulmonary dysplasia. Pediatr Res 36:7A. (Abst).
32. Howard E. (1968) Reductions in size and total DNA of cerebrum and cerebellum in adult mice after corticosterone treatment in infancy. Exp Neurol 22:191–208.
33. Benesova O, Pavlik A. (1989) Perinatal treatment with glucocorticoids and the risk of maldevelopment of the brain. Neuropharmacology 28:89–97.
34. Tsuneishi S, Takada S, Motoike T, Ohashi T, Sano K, Nakamura H. (1991) Effects of dexamethasone on the expression of myelin basic protein, proteolipid protein, and glial fibrillary acidic protein genes in developing rat brain. Brain Res Dev Brain Res 61:117–123.
35. Zahalka EA, Seidler FJ, Slotkin TA. (1993) Dexamethasone treatment in uteroen hances neonatal cholinergic nerve terminal development in rat brain. Res Commun Chem Pathol Pharmacol 81:191–198.
36. Howard E, Granoff DM. (1968) Increased voluntary running and decreased motor coordination in mice after neonatal corticosterone implantation. Exp Neurol 22:661–673.
37. Schapiro S. (1968) Some physiological, biochemical and behavioral consequences of neonatal hormone administration: cortisol and thyroxin. Gen Comp Endocrinol 10:214–218.
38. Fujii T, Horinaka M, Hata M. (1993) Functional effects of glucocorticoid exposure during fetal life. Prog Neuro-psychopharmacol & Biol Psychiat 17:279–293.
39. Barks JD, Post M, Tuor UI. (1991) Dexamethasone prevents hypoxic-ischemic brain damage in the neonatal rat. Pediatr Res 29:558–563.
40. Raley-Susman KM, Sapolsky RM. (1994) Glucocorticoid effects on neuronal development and vitality. In: Lou HC, Greisen G, Falck Larsen J, eds. Brain lesions in the newborn. Munksgaard, Copenhagen, pp 257–271.
41. Bregman J, Farrell EE. (1992) Neurodevelopmental outcome in infants with bronchopulmonary dysplasia. Clin Perinatol 19:673–694.
42. Mammel MC, Fiterman C, Coleman M, Boros SJ. (1987) Short-term dexamethasone therapy for bronchopulmonary dysplasia: acute effects and 1-year follow-up. Dev Pharmacol Ther 10:1–11.

43. Satish M, Schwartz P, Urrutia J, Krishnan V, Basting C. (1991) Developmental outcome of dexamethasone treated infants. Pediatr Res 29:1564A. (Abst).
44. Gross SJ and Cummings JJ. (1992) Four year follow-up of a controlled trial of dexamethasone (DEX) in ventilator dependent preterm infants. Pediatr Res 31:204A. (Abst).
45. Bos AF. (1993) Differential effects of brain lesions and systemic disease on the quality of general movements: a preliminary report. Early Hum Dev 34:39–45.
46. Prechtl HFR. (1990) Editorial: Qualitative changes of spontaneous movements in fetus and preterm infant are a marker of neurological dysfunction. Early Hum Dev 23:151–158.
47. Bos AF, van Asperen RM, Prechtl HFR, Okken A. (1994) Effects of dexamethasone treatment on spontaneous motor behaviour in preterm infants with bronchopulmonary dysplasia. Pediatr Res 36:7A. (Abst).

Neonatal Metabolism of surfactant Phosphatidylcholine: Therapeutic Implications

L. J. I. Zimmermann

Introduction

Neonatal respiratory distress syndrome (RDS), also known as hyaline membrane disease, is an important cause of neonatal and infant mortality. Together with congenital malformations, it is the leading cause of death in preterm infants and responsible for serious morbidity in survivors, associated with high costs to society.

Since 1959 it has been known that RDS is caused by lung immaturity with concomitant surfactant deficiency [1]. Numerous small studies and large multicenter trials have demonstrated decreased death rates and complications from RDS as a result of treatment with exogenous surfactant [2]. Despite its success however, surfactant therapy is not a panacea. Recent meta-analyses do not show a consistent decrease in long term pulmonary complications such as bronchopulmonary dysplasia, nor in the major non-pulmonary complications such as intraventricular hemorrhage [2]. Several issues are still unresolved such as the optimal timing, dosing and repetition of the treatment with exogenous surfactant. During the last few years these issues have been addressed in two types of studies: on the one hand animal and human studies have been designed to increase our understanding of surfactant metabolism and pharmacokinetics and on the other hand large clinical trials directly compared different treatment protocols. The results of these two complimentary approaches will be discussed.

As surfactant substitution therapy did not, and most likely will not, solve all pulmonary (and non-pulmonary) problems related to RDS, it will also be necessary to concentrate on attempts to increase fetal lung maturation. Antepartum corticosteroid therapy is more effective than postnatal surfactant therapy in reducing mortality and complications from RDS [3]. In recent surfactant trials, only 15–20% of the babies at risk of developing RDS could be given antenatal steroids [4]. Maternal administration of steroids is not without complications [5], it can impair lung growth [6], and can cause long term adverse effects, potentially into adulthood, which are only recently being recognized [7]. Thus, major problems remain.

At the moment, the benefits of prenatal corticosteroids outweigh the disadvantages, and are strongly recommended but insufficient reduction in bronchopulmonary dysplasia is achieved in the entire group of very preterm infants, presently seen in neonatal intensive care units. Enhancing lung maturation seems more effective than surfactant therapy in reducing RDS and its complications, but faster, safer, more efficient, and more specific ways to increase lung maturation and surfactant production are clearly needed.

Therefore, it is necessary to understand more about the mechanisms of morphological and biochemical lung maturation and their regulation. More specific, a better understanding of the regulation of surfactant synthesis during lung development is needed. New insights into the regulation of surfactant lipid synthesis will be discussed.

The Composition and Function of Surfactant

The main function of surfactant is to decrease the surface tension at the air-liquid interface in the alveoli in a manner that depends on alveolar surface area. The reduction of surface tension at this very extensive alveolar surface promotes lung expansion on inspiration and prevents lung collapse on expiration. Thus, surfactant plays a major role in the pressure–volume characteristics of the lung and in gas exchange. The importance of surfactant is best illustrated by RDS where an inadequate amount and dysfunction of surfactant leads to an almost general alveolar collapse while the intratracheal administration of exogenous surfactant leads to a dramatic improvement in lung expansion and gas exchange.

It is generally assumed that two surfactant pools exist in the lung. One is the intracellular pool, which consists of the lamellar bodies, the characteristic organelles of type II cells. Lamellar bodies are secreted by type II cells into the second pool, the alveolar pool. In the alveolus, surfactant exists in many different morphological forms which are converted into each other [review 8]. Lamellar bodies unravel to form tubular myelin which most likely is a direct precursor of the surfactant monolayer, the functional form of surfactant. "Used surfactant" then leaves the monolayer as small vesicular structures which are taken up again by the type II cells. A large part of this material can be re-used by the type II cell for secretion. Thus, surfactant recycling is at least as important as de novo synthesis of surfactant in the adult lung. In the newborn lung, recycling is quantitatively even much more important (about 15 times) than de novo synthesis [8].

The composition of surfactant is somewhat variable depending on the animal species. In general, it consists of about 90% lipid, 5–10% protein and small amounts of carbohydrate. Four specific surfactant-associated proteins have been described. Surfactant protein A (SP–A) is the most abundant surfactant-associated protein and accounts for 3–4% of the surfactant mass. It is a large collagen-like glycoprotein which is synthesized in type II cells but also in Clara cells of the respiratory bronchioles. The synthesis of SP-A is developmentally and hormonally regulated. SP-A plays a role in tubular myelin formation, in the regulation of re-uptake and secretion of surfactant by type II cells, in the adsorption of surfactant phospholipids at the air-liquid interface (together with

SP-B and SP-C). Especially intriguing is its role in non-immunological pulmonary defence. Surfactant protein B (SP-B) and surfactant protein C (SP-C) are smaller and very hydrophobic proteins. Together they account for 1–2% of the surfactant mass. SP-B plays a role in the formation of the tubular myelin structure but the most important function of both SP-B and SP-C is to promote the phospholipid adsorption at the air-liquid interface in the alveoli. Surfactant protein D (SP-D) is a more recently characterized surfactant protein which has several characteristics and functions in common with SP-A. The surfactant lipids mainly consist of phospholipids (80–90%). Cholesterol is the major neutral lipid. Phosphatidylcholine (PC) represents about 80% of surfactant phospholipids and is thus by far the most abundant phospholipid and surfactant component [9]. Approximately 60% of the PCs contain saturated fatty acids in both positions. This desaturated phosphatidylcholine (DSPC) is almost entirely dipalmitoylphosphatidylcholine (DPPC), which is the main surface tension lowering component of surfactant. Therefore adequate amounts of this surfactant component are essential for proper lung function immediately after birth. Phosphatidylglycerol is the second most abundant phospholipid in surfactant, accounting for 10% of total lipids in mature surfactant. However, in immature infants with RDS phosphatidylglycerol is almost absent. Phosphatidylglycerol and the other phospholipids promote the spreading of DSPC at the alveolar lining, but their precise function is not completely resolved.

Biosynthesis of Surfactant Phosphatidylcholine

It is now firmly established that the alveolar type II cells are the producers of surfactant [review 9]. Several experimental models have been used to study surfactant synthesis such as whole animal studies in vivo, isolated perfused lung and lung slices in vitro, lung explants in culture and finally isolated type II cells in primary culture. Each model has certain advantages and disadvantages. For physiologic studies the intact animal is usually best suited. In vitro models however, overcome the problem of the possible indirect effect mediated via other organs on the lung. The lung consists of more than 40 cell types and only a small percentage of these are type II cells. Thus, isolated type II cell studies are the only model to overcome this problem of cell heterogeneity, and offer many advantages over other models in the study of surfactant metabolism [6, 9]. The use of primary cultures of fetal type II cells or pre-type II cells is especially suited to study the biosynthetic pathways of surfactant lipids and to investigate the regulation of the important regulatory enzymes in these pathways. However, we have to realize that isolated type II cells in primary culture cannot be considered a physiologic model and that the data from such studies cannot be extrapolated directly to the whole animal and especially not to the human situation without further validation.

As PC is the major surfactant lipid, we will focus on the synthesis of this component and its intracellular regulation in type II cells. Abundant evidence indicates that the synthesis of surfactant PC increases during late gestation [9,

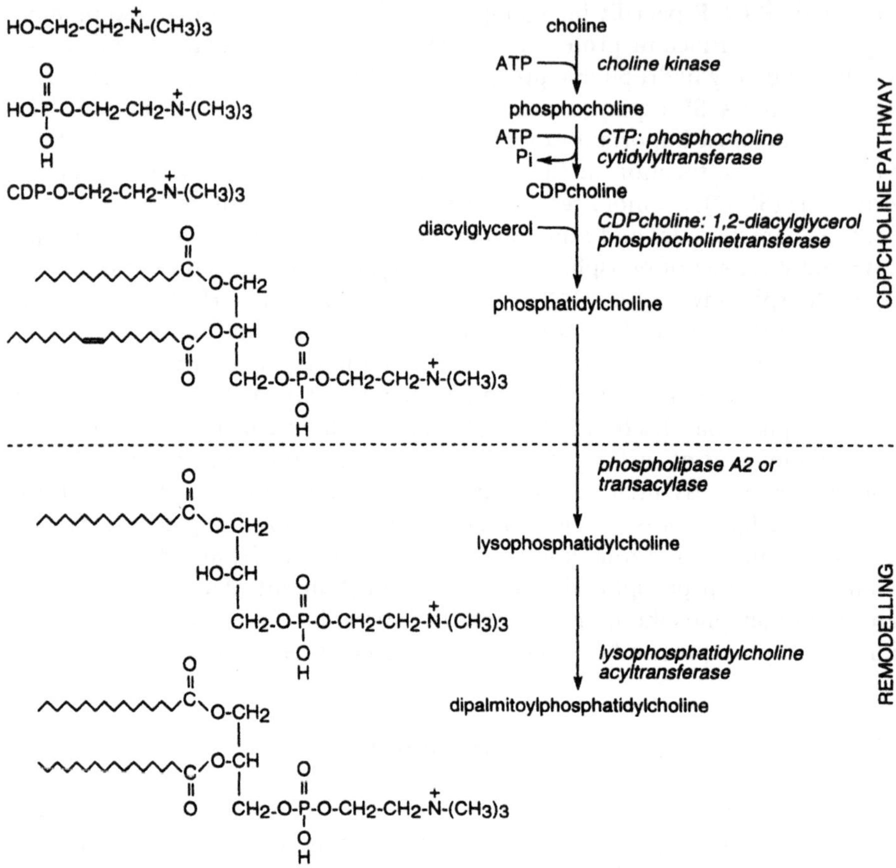

Fig. 1. *CDPcholine pathway and remodelling of phosphatidylcholine.* The CDPcholine pathway for de novo PC synthesis is shown in the upper part of the figure. About half of the newly synthesized PC is disaturated, the other half contains an unsaturated fatty acid in the 2-position. Further remodelling of unsaturated PC to dipalmitoyl-PC is shown in the lower part of the figure.

10]. The CDPcholine pathway is the primary pathway for de novo PC synthesis in the developing lung [reviewed in 9] (Fig. 1).

Choline is taken up by the cell through a facilitated transport system, and is phosphorylated by choline kinase. The synthesis of the activated intermediate, CDPcholine, is catalyzed by the CTP:phosphocholine cytidylyltransferase (CT) (EC 2.7.7.15). Finally, the phosphocholine moiety is transferred to diacylglycerol by the CDPcholine:1,2-diacylglycerol phosphocholinetransferase (Fig. 1). Studies with whole lung have shown an increased activity of the CDPcholine pathway during late gestation [9]. Pool size studies have demonstrated that the reaction catalyzed by the CT is a rate-limiting step in the CDPcholine pathway in fetal lung and isolated fetal type II cells. In addition, many studies indicate that CT is an important target for developmental [9, 10] and hormonal regulation in alveolar type II cells of the developing lung [6]. Although under most circumstances CT has indeed been shown to be the rate-regulating step, we have to realize that an entire pathway is never regulated by the activity of one single enzyme under all circumstances.

It has been suggested that in type II cells only approx. 50% of the DSPC is being synthesized directly by the de novo pathway by using saturated diacylglycerols as precursors [9, 10]. A considerable part of the desaturated species of PC is formed by remodelling of de novo synthesized unsaturated (in the 2-position) PC (Fig. 1). The most important mechanism for this remodelling is a deacylation of PC at the 2-position by a phospholipase A_2 or by a transacylation with another phospholipid, followed by a reacylation step of the resulting lysophosphatidylcholine by the lysophosphatidylcholine acyltransferase [reviewed in 9] (Fig. 1). The activity of the latter enzyme has been shown to be higher in type II cells than in whole lung, to increase during development and to exhibit specificity towards palmityl-CoA as a substrate in fetal type II cells [9]. The remodelling of the de novo synthesized PC to a high proportion of DSPC is also under hormonal control. It is known to be stimulated by glucocorticosteroids [6].

Recently, important progress has been made in the understanding of the regulation of CT activity. This was mainly made possible by the purification of the enzyme [11], followed by the availability of antibodies against the enzyme and the cloning of the cDNA for CT from rat liver [12] and lung [13]. These recent advancements have important implications for the understanding of the regulation of CT in developing fetal lung [reviewed in 14].

CT is essentially inactive without lipids. The amphipathic α-helical domain of the CT protein is involved in the binding of the enzyme to lipid membranes. In the type II cell, the most important binding sites involved in the activation of CT are the microsomal membranes and the lipids of the cytosolic H-form. The currently available data are indeed most compatible with an activation of both cytosolic and microsomal CT activity during fetal lung development and after corticosteroid administration. Cytosolic CT activity is regulated by phospholipids. The activation of cytosolic CT is accompanied by a conversion of a low molecular weight L-form to a high molecular weight H-form, which is a lipoprotein complex consisting of aggregated CT complexed with (phospho-)lipids. The H-form is the predominant form in the adult lung. Fatty acids, either in free form or possibly after incorporation into (phospho-)lipids, induce the conversion from L-form to H-form and are shown to be a very important regulator of CT activity after corticosteroid administration and, most likely, also during normal lung development. Translocation of CT from cytosol to the membranes of the endoplasmic reticulum activates the enzyme. This mechanism is also regulated by fatty acids and plays an important role during lung development. Recent evidence demonstrates that the cytosolic interconversion from L-form to H-form and the translocation of CT from cytosol to endoplasmic reticulum are closely related.

CT contains several potential sites for phosphorylation by protein kinases. There is now convincing evidence that CT is phosphorylated and dephosphorylated in intact cells and that the phosphorylation state of the enzyme regulates its activity. The phosphorylation state of the enzyme is correlated with its location: when the enzyme translocates from membranes to cytosol it becomes subsequently phosphorylated, when it translocates from cytosol to membranes it becomes dephosphorylated and active but the order of events and the precise significance is not yet clear. Protein phosphatases 1 and/or 2A have been shown to dephosphorylate the enzyme, but which protein kinase is involved in the phosphorylation is still unclear. Protein kinase C and cAMP-dependent protein kinase are very unlikely candidates as is demonstrated by recent studies, also involving fetal type II cells. The number of studies about the phosphorylation and dephosphorylation mechanism in developing lung are still very limited, and clearly further studies are required to elucidate the precise role of this mechanism in the regulation of CT activity.

In several cell types the regulation of CT activity by diacylglycerols was demonstrated but no convincing evidence exists for the fetal lung. The feedback inhibition of CT activity by increased PC in membranes or in general, the regulation of CT activity by altered membrane composition, may be a very important mechanism. Some evidence for this exists in type II cells.

From recent experiments, it has become very clear that all mechanisms in the regulation of CT activity are very closely interrelated. The precise role of these mechanisms and its interdependence has to be further investigated in the developing lung and isolated type II cells. Recent studies show that not only the activity of CT is regulated, but also that CT protein expression is regulated at a pre-translational level in the II cells of the developing lung. It is expected that the gene sequence for CT will be known soon, which will make it much easier to study the regulation of gene expression. Structure-function relationships will be further investigated with the help of site-directed mutagenesis and transgenic animals.

Apart from the molecular mechanisms of regulation of CT in fetal type II cells, it is important to understand how hormonal factors, growth factors, extracellular matrix and other extracellular influences effect CT activity through these intracellular pathways of CT regulation. Fetal type II cell-fibroblast interactions have been shown to be very important in modulating the effect of hormones and growth factors on CT activity and thus PC synthesis. There is good evidence for the following sequence of exogenous corticosteroid stimulation in fetal lung (Fig. 2) [reviewed in 15]: corticosteroids induce the production of fibroblast-pneumocyte factor (FPF) in lung fibroblasts adjacent to the alveolar epithelial cells at a pre-translational level; this FPF induces fatty acid synthase and other enzymes involved in fatty acid synthesis in fetal type II cells at a pre-translational level; this leads to an increase in fatty acid biosynthesis, and fatty acids, their metabolites, or lipids into which they become incorporated ultimately activate CT by increasing cytosolic H-form and possibly translocation of CT from cytosol to microsomes. Our study using a rat model for CDH [14], demonstrates that this sequence can be disturbed by an abnormal lung development and reinforces the idea that it is at least as important to study mesenchyme and epithelial–mesenchymal interactions as it is to study epithe-

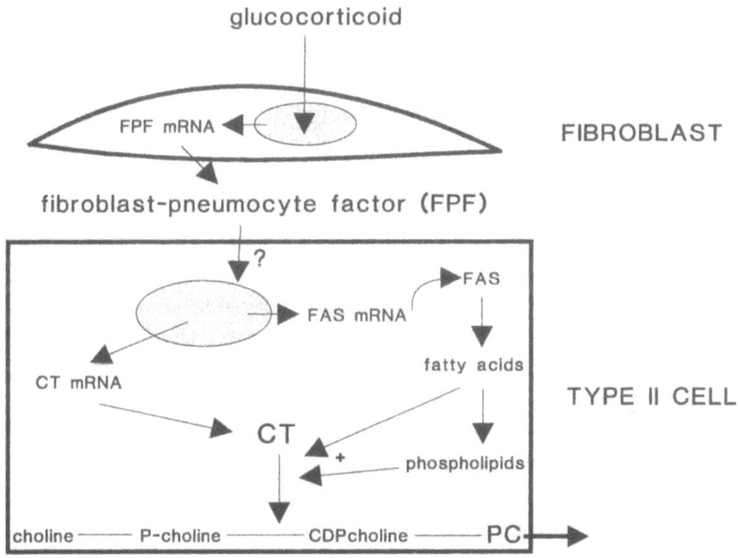

Fig. 2. *A model for the regulation of CTP:phosphocholine cytidylyltransferase (CT) in fetal lung after glucocorticosteroid administration.* Fetal type II cell–fibroblast interactions have been shown to play a very important role in this regulation. FPF: fibroblast-pneumocyte factor; P-choline: phosphocholine; PC: phosphatidylcholine; FAS: fatty acid synthase.

lial cell functions. Several other hormones such as thyroid hormones, insulin and sex hormones, and also several growth factors such as epidermal growth factor (EGF) and transforming growth factor beta (TGF-β) have been shown to influence this sequence of events either by influencing the production of FPF in lung fibroblasts or by modulating the effect of FPF on fetal type II cells [for review see 6]. That such regulatory mechanisms are not only important in cell culture or organ culture systems but also in clinical practice is illustrated by the success of the prenatal use of corticosteroids to prevent respiratory distress syndrome in premature infants [editorials 16, 17]. The antenatal administration of thyrotropin-releasing hormone (TRH) in combination with corticosteroids to accelerate lung maturity [18-20] originates from the insight gained from culture work and subsequent animal studies [review 6]. The recent suggestion to use antenatal TRH and corticosteroids for lung maturation in CDH [21] also originates from laboratory data showing lung immaturity in different models of CDH. The same is true for the possible use of EGF [review 6] as is currently being tested in baboons. The increased incidence of RDS in infants born to women with diabetes can also be explained, at least in part, by the insulin inhibition of the glucocorticoid-induced production of FPF by fetal lung fibroblasts [6].

It is clear that a better understanding of the mechanisms of regulation of surfactant PC synthesis can lead to more specific therapies. For now, it is wise to use antenatal corticosteroid therapy for women at risk of premature delivery. As this cannot be stressed enough I repeat the recent recommendations as given by the NIH Consensus Conference [22]:

- The benefits of antenatal administration of corticosteroids to fetuses at risk of preterm delivery vastly outweigh the potential risks. These benefits include not only a reduction in the risk of RDS but also a substantial reduction in mortality and intraventricular hemorrhage (IVH).
- All fetuses between 24 and 34 weeks gestation at risk of preterm delivery should be considered candidates for antenatal treatment with corticosteroids.
- The decision to use antenatal corticosteroids should not be altered by fetal race or gender or the availability of surfactant replacement therapy.
- patients eligible for therapy with tocolytics should also be eligible for treatment with antenatal corticosteroids.
- Treatment consists of two doses of 12 mg betamethasone given intramuscularly 24 hours apart or four doses of 6 mg of dexamethasone given intramuscularly 12 hours apart. Optimal benefit begins 24 hours after initiation of therapy and lasts 7 days.
- Because treatment with corticosteroids for less than 24 hours is still associated with significant reductions in neonatal mortality, RDS, and IVH, antenatal corticosteroids should be given unless immediate delivery is anticipated.
- In "preterm premature rupture of membranes" (PPROM) at less than 30 to 32 weeks gestation in the absence of clinical chorioamnionitis, antenatal corticosteroid use is recommended because of the high risk of IVH at these early gestational ages.
- In complicated pregnancies where delivery prior to 34 weeks gestation is likely, antenatal corticosteroid use is recommended unless there is evidence that corticosteroids will have an adverse effect on the mother or delivery is imminent.

These guidelines clearly take into account that corticosteroids do not only stimulate surfactant synthesis but have a much wider spectrum of beneficial effects such as the structural maturation of the lungs, brain and other organs.

Currently, other ways to increase lung maturation are being studied clinically. Thyroid hormones are known to accelerate fetal lung maturation in animal studies. However, the thyroid hormones T3 and T4 do not cross the placenta. This problem has been circumvented by maternal administration of thyrotropin-releasing hormone (TRH).

TRH, via an increase in thyroid hormones, seems to have some theoretical disadvantages [6] in that it inhibits maturation of anti-oxidant enzymes at least in the rat, does not stimulate (or even inhibits) surfactant protein production, and inhibits fatty acid synthesis. Clinical studies with maternal administration of a combination of thyrotropin-releasing hormone (TRH) and corticosteroids suggested a slight advantage over corticosteroids alone in the prevention of bronchopulmonary dysplasia [18, 19], but a recent multicenter trial found a worse outcome after prenatal corticosteroids and TRH compared to corticosteroids alone [20]. Further studies are clearly required before this therapy can be generally recommended.

The Pool Size of Surfactant Phosphatidylcholine at Birth and Postnatal Changes

As discussed above, surfactant synthesis increases with advancing gestation. From approximately 20 weeks gestation in the human, surfactant is accumulating within the primitive type II cells. Significant secretion from the type II cells into the alveolar space does not occur until approximately 34–35 weeks. The surfactant can be detected in the amniotic fluid and this can be used as a measure of fetal pulmonary maturity. The alveolar pool size of surfactant is difficult to measure in the human. From animal studies involving monkeys [reviewed in 23], it is known that at term the alveolar surfactant pool is about 100 mg/kg. Adult animals however, have an alveolar pool size of about 5–15 mg/kg. In several preterm animal models with RDS (rabbit, sheep, monkeys) the amount of surfactant in alveolar washes was about 5 mg/kg. In preterm monkeys an increase in pool size was found from day 1 to day 3–4 when levels of more than 60 mg/kg were reached. Thus, although secretory pathways are intact in the premature animal, the de novo synthesis is initially insufficient but accelerates in the first few days after birth. This increase correlates with the well known clinical improvement of RDS after 48–72 hours of live. In human infants with RDS similar but less reliable pool sizes of alveolar surfactant have been found. Adams et al [24] found around 5 mg/kg of surfactant in alveolar washes of infants with RDS who had died. Hallman et al [25] used phosphatidylglycerol as a marker to measure the surfactant phospholipid pool. As had been demonstrated earlier, the amount of phosphatidylglycerol is below the detection limit in tracheal aspirates of infants with RDS. When such infants are treated with a known amount of exogenous surfactant containing phosphatidylglycerol, the phospholipid pool size can be calculated from the dilution of phosphatidylglycerol, as measured in tracheal aspirates. A pool size of <10 mg/kg was found. As phospholipids are taken up by type II cells and re-secreted (recycling), the pool size measured consists of the alveolar and cellular compartment together.

No reliable data exist on the change of the surfactant pool size after birth in humans. However, several recent studies reported on PC concentrations in tracheal aspirates during the first few days of live in infants with RDS. These PC concentrations can be expressed in different ways, depending on the denominator used. Commonly used are PC concentration per ml aspirate (dependent on the amount suctioned and the dilution with normal saline), or per mg albumin or total protein (influenced by leakage of proteins into the alveoli in damaged immature lungs), or corrected for the sphingomyelin concentration (lecithin/sphingomyelin or L/S ratio) or for total phospholipid concentration (reflects composition more than amount of surfactant). The two most promising ways of expressing PC concentrations seem to be the correction for dilution with the urea-method and the use of the secretory component of IgA (SC-IgA) as a reference protein. There is little experience so far with the use of SC-IgA as a correction for PC concentration in tracheal aspirates [26]. In the urea-method advantage is taken from the fact that the urea concentration in plasma and alveolar fluid is equal. Thus PC concentration in tracheal aspirates is multiplied by $[\text{urea}]_{\text{serum}}/[\text{urea}]_{\text{aspirate}}$ to calculate the concentration of PC in "epithelial lining fluid" (ELF). Although this method also has some flaws, it is simple and correlates quite well with data obtained from alveolar washes [27]. Hallman et al [27] demonstrated a low $[\text{PC}]_{\text{ELF}}$ in tracheal aspirates of infants with RDS on day 1 (mean <1 mM compared to 6.1 mM in infants without RDS) and an increase of $[\text{PC}]_{\text{ELF}}$ from day 1 to day 4 to values comparable to those of infants without RDS. These data are consistent with clinical improvement of RDS after 2–3 days and with animal data.

Surfactant Replacement Therapy: The Initial Dose

Premature infants with RDS have a relative surfactant deficiency (5 mg/kg) compared to term infants (100 mg/kg) and this deficiency is temporary (about 4 days). Therefore, it seems logical to treat infants with RDS once with exogenous surfactant at a dose of approximately 100 mg/kg to overcome the critical period when there is not enough surfactant synthesis yet. Indeed, in clinical trials [28] with natural surfactants an initial surfactant dose of around 100 mg/kg body weight was optimal. In a study with Alveofact®, 100 mg/kg turned out to give better results than 50 mg/kg, and similarly Surfactant TA at a dose of 120 mg/kg did better than 60 mg/kg [29]. Clinical trials with Curosurf®, a porcine lung surfactant, suggest that 200 mg/kg could even be better than 100 mg/kg.

Prophylaxis or Rescue Treatment

From a theoretical point of view, prophylactic treatment before the first breath of infants at risk for developing RDS is best. Surfactant deficiency exists immediately after birth and lung damage is initiated fast once alveolar collapse is allowed to occur. The distribution of surfactant in the lungs will be better if surfactant is administered soon after birth. However, surfactant treatment may interfere with initial delivery room resuscitation of the infant. This may be a disadvantage, especially if the infant was not surfactant deficient. Therefore, an argument can be made for the administration of surfactant after stabilization in the more controlled environment of the NICU and once early signs of RDS are present (rescue treatment). A few studies have directly compared prophylaxis versus rescue treatment in a randomized way [reviewed in 2]. The results are somewhat contradictory, but overall no advantage of prophylaxis was found compared to rescue therapy. Using, subgroup analysis however, two studies suggested that the smallest infants (<26 weeks) who are at the highest risk of developing RDS, may benefit from prophylactic surfactant treatment. Another interesting finding was revealed in the large OSIRIS trial [4] which compared (random assignment) 1344 infants judged to be at high risk for RDS and treated before two hours of age with 1346 infants who received surfactant treatment only when symptoms of RDS developed at a mean age of about 3 hours. A significant difference in death or oxygen dependency at "term date" was found favoring the early treatment. From these data together with animal data that show lung damage from RDS within a few hours, we have to conclude that prophylactic therapy is not necessary, except maybe for the smallest infants, but when rescue therapy is used it should be used early, as soon as clinical signs of RDS appear (preferably before 2 hours of age).

Recycling of Surfactant Phosphatidylcholine and Metabolism after Surfactant Therapy

Surfactant is secreted as lamellar bodies by the type II cells. Lamellar bodies unravel to tubular myelin which forms the precursor to the surfactant monolayer at the air-liquid interface. The surface film is dynamic with cyclic area expansion and compression with ventilation. During cycling, small vesicular forms of surfactant are generated from the monolayer. These vesicles have poor surface properties and are thought to be destined for clearance. Most of this surfactant is taken up by the type II cells. Part is degraded by macrophages or lost from the airways. The surfactant which is taken up in the type II cell can be degraded or recycled back into the lamellar bodies. In animal studies [review 8, 23], it is estimated that in the adult about 50% of the surfactant is degraded and about half recycled. In the (term) newborn animal however, recycling efficiency is much higher (about 90–95%). De novo synthesis and catabolism of PC are very low compared to recycling. Surfactant PC will thus remain in the lung for a long time. The metabolism of saturated PC was very similar in the lungs of preterm animals. There is a long time from synthesis to secretion of surfactant PC as studied with the use of intravenously injected radiolabeled precursors. When a tracer dose of radiolabeled surfactant PC was injected into the airways of preterm lambs, 40% became rapidly "lung associated" (could not be recovered by alveolar wash). By 24 hours, about 80% was lung associated, probably because of uptake/recycling. However, almost 100% of the label could be recovered from the lung (alveolar wash and lung tissue together). A turnover time of approximately 13 hours was calculated for alveolar PC in these preterm lambs. The turnover time for the total surfactant pool (including lamellar bodies) was however several times longer.

When radiolabeled treatment doses of surfactant (100 mg/kg) were used instead of tracer doses, the results were not so different in these preterm lambs, despite a large increase in the surfactant pool [review 8, 23]. Sixty percent of the label became quickly lung associated, and after 24 hours about 20% could be recovered by alveolar wash. However, little of the label disappeared from the lung. That recycling takes place was also demonstrated by the intratracheal injection of labelled lysoPC, which was converted to PC and could be recovered from the alveolar wash. Again, adult animals may behave differently. In adult rabbits the clearance of surfactant was increased up to 5-fold proportionally to the surfactant dose administered.

In the human infant, little information regarding surfactant PC metabolism is available. The few data that are available seem to be consistent to the animal data. The half life of surfactant DPPC was studied by Hallman et al [28] with the use of deuterium labelled DPPC which was mixed with the surfactant administered endotracheally. The half live of DPPC was 39 to 59 hours. We studied fatty acid composition of PC from tracheal aspirates of infants with RDS who received surfactant. Fatty acids in PC consisted for 60–65% of palmitic acid before surfactant therapy. After treatment with Survanta®, palmitic acid was 85%. The return to baseline composition occurred exponential and allowed us to calculate a half live of 76 hours (mean of 4 patients). Hallman et al [25] were able to calculate the half live of phosphatidylglycerol after the administration of surfactant to infants with RDS and the analysis of phospholipids in tracheal aspirates at various time points thereafter. They found an half life of 31 hours.

These data suggest low synthesis and clearance rates for surfactant PC in human infants with RDS, and are compatible with animal data.

Individual Response to Surfactant Therapy and the Transient Effect

If the exogenous surfactant remains in the lung for a long time and disappears with a half life of more than 50 hours, then one dose of 100 mg/kg surfactant should be enough to cover the entire period from birth till the endogenous synthesis is high enough. However, primary surfactant deficiency is not the only factor which plays a role in RDS. In premature infants with RDS, the lungs are structurally immature and will can be damaged by asphyxia, infection, ventilation and high oxygen concentrations etc.; especially because the anti-oxidant systems are also immature. Because of this, surfactant function can be inhibited by several proteins that leak into the alveolar space and surfactant can be inactivated by oxygen radicals and enzymes or by transformation into small vesicular surfactant forms.

Thus, there is individual variability in the way infants respond to surfactant treatment. Charon et al [30] found that gross maldistribution of surfactant did not explain the variability in clinical response to surfactant therapy, but pathophysiologic conditions associated with the RDS, such as early air leaks and patent ductus arteriosus, did. We found a good to mild initial response in 24 of 28 infants, but 9 had a relapse with a worsening clinical condition. The 4 patients with a poor initial response to surfactant had either an associated asphyxia or infection. Before, but also after surfactant therapy, there was a negative correlation between the concentration of PC in tracheal aspirates and the oxygen need. Infants with a relapse had high PC levels in their tracheal aspirates after surfactant therapy but these decreased again at the moment of the clinical relapse. Hallman et al [27] showed similar findings earlier. Infants requiring 2 doses of surfactant instead of 1 showed a smaller increase in PC concentration in their tracheal aspirates after the first dose. Dunn et al [31] demonstrated that the effect of one single dose of surfactant on the decrease in oxygen need was transient while the effect of multiple doses of surfactant (100 mg/kg/dose) was more sustained. It seems that the amount of surfactant which remains in the alveolar compartment after one dose of 100 mg/kg surfactant is not always enough to cope with other factors such as surfactant inhibition and inactivation.

Speer et al [32] were able to show increased survival of infants with RDS after 3 doses of Curosurf® (up to 400 mg/kg total) compared to one dose (200 mg/kg). A study with Exosurf®, a synthetic surfactant, found that one prophylactic dose was less effective in reducing mortality than 3 doses. Thus it is clear that more doses of surfactant are better than one. But it is not clear yet that more than two doses are beneficial. In the OSIRIS trial [4] with Exosurf^R no difference in outcome was demonstrated between two and up to four doses.

Conclusion

Surfactant deficiency is the main cause of neonatal respiratory distress syndrome (RDS), an important cause of neonatal and infant mortality. Phosphatidylcholine (PC) is a major component of surfactant. In order to optimize the treatment for infants with RDS it is important to understand the metabolism of surfactant PC. CTP:phosphocholine cytidylyltransferase (CT) is a rate regulatory enzyme in the de novo synthesis of PC. New insights into the regulation of this enzyme can lead to more specific and safer ways to stimulate surfactant synthesis. For now, the antenatal use of corticosteroids is strongly recommended for women at risk of premature delivery. Once early signs of RDS are present, rescue treatment with an initial dose of (at least) 100 mg/kg surfactant is recommended. Prophylactic treatment may useful for very premature infants. Exogenous surfactant PC disappears very slowly from the lung in premature infants. Theoretically, one dose of 100 mg/kg should therefore be enough to cover the critical period till the endogenous PC production is sufficient, which is around day 3–4. However, as complex factors such as lung immaturity and surfactant inhibition/inactivation plays an important additional role, the response of the individual infant to surfactant therapy can vary, and frequently additional doses of surfactant are required.

References

1. Avery ME, Mead J (1959) Surface properties in relation to atelectasis and hyaline membrane disease. Am J Dis Child 97:517–523.
2. Jobe AH (1993) Pulmonary surfactant therapy. N Engl J Med 328:861–868.

3. Crowley P, Chalmers I, Keirse MJ (1990) The effect of corticosteroid administration before preterm delivery: an overview of the evidence from controlled trials. Br J Obstet Gynaecol 97:11–25.
4. The OSIRIS collaborative group (1992) Early versus delayed neonatal administration of synthetic surfactant – the judgment of OSIRIS. Lancet 340:1363–1369.
5. Ballard RA, Ballard PL (1992) Prevention of neonatal respiratory distress syndrome by pharmacological methods. In: Robertson B, Van Golde LGM, Batenburg JJ, eds. Pulmonary surfactant: from molecular biology to clinical practice. Amsterdam: Elsevier, pp 539–560.
6. Post M, Smith BT (1992) Hormonal control of surfactant metabolism. In: Robertson B, van Golde LMG, Batenburg JJ, eds. Pulmonary surfactant: from molecular biology to clinical practice. Amsterdam: Elsevier, pp 379–424.
7. Benediktsson R, Lindsay RS, Noble J, Seckl JR, Edwards CRW (1993) Glucocorticoid exposure in utero: new model for adult hypertension. Lancet 341:339–341.
8. Jobe AH, Rider ED (1992) Catabolism and recycling of surfactant. In: Robertson B, van Golde LMG, Batenburg JJ, eds. Pulmonary surfactant: from molecular biology to clinical practice. Amsterdam: Elsevier, pp 313–337.
9. Post M, Van Golde LMG (1988) Metabolic and developmental aspects of pulmonary surfactant systems. Biochim Biophys Acta 947:249–286.
10. Zimmermann LJ, Hogan M, Carlson KS, Smith BT, Post M (1993) Regulation of phosphatidylcholine synthesis in fetal type II cells by CTP:phosphocholine cytidylyltransferase. Am J Physiol 264:L575–L580.
11. Feldman DA, Weinhold PA (1987) CTP:phosphorylcholine cytidylyltransferase from rat liver. Isolation and characterization of the catalytic subunit. J Biol Chem 262:9075–9081.
12. Kalmar GB, Kay RJ, Lachance A, Aebersold R, Cornell RB (1990) Cloning and expression of rat liver CTP: phosphocholine cytidylyltransferase: an amphipathic protein that controls phosphatidylcholine synthesis. Proc Natl Acad Sci USA 87:6029–6033.
13. Hogan M, Zimmermann LJ, Wang J, Kuliszewski M, Liu J, Post M (1994) Increased expression of CTP:phosphocholine cytidylyltransferase in maturing type II cells. Am J Physiol 267:L25–L32.
14. Zimmermann LJI (1995) The regulation of CTP:phosphocholine cytidylyltransferase in fetal type II cells [PhD thesis]. Erasmus University Rotterdam, The Netherlands, 277 p.
15. Rooney SA (1989) Fatty acid biosynthesis in developing fetal lung. Am J Physiol 257:L195–L201.
16. Avery ME (1995) Historical overview of antenatal steroid use. Pediatr 95:133–135.
17. Ryan CA, Finer NN (1995) Antenatal corticosteroid therapy to prevent respiratory distress syndrome. J Pediatr 126:317–319.
18. Morales WJ, O'Brien WF, Angel JL, Knuppel RA, Sawai S (1989) Fetal lung maturation: the combined use of corticosteroids and thyrotropin-releasing hormone. Obstet Gynecol 73:111–116.
19. Ballard RA, Ballard PL, Creasy RK, et al. (1992) Respiratory disease in very-low-birthweight infants after prenatal thyrotropin-releasing hormone and glucocorticoid. TRH Study Group. Lancet 339:510–515.
20. ACTOBAT Study Group (1995) Australian collaborative trial of antenatal thyrotropin-releasing hormone (ACTOBAT) for prevention of neonatal respiratory disease. Lancet 345:877–882.
21. Suen HC, Bloch KD, Donahoe PK (1994) Antenatal glucocorticoid corrects pulmonary immaturity in experimentally induced congenital diaphragmatic hernia in rats. Pediatr Res 35:523–529.
22. NIH Consensus Conference (1995) Effect of corticosteroids for fetal maturation on perinatal outcomes. JAMA 273:413–418.
23. Jobe AH, Ikegami M (1993) Surfactant metabolism. Clin Perinatol 20:683–696.
24. Adams FH, Fujiwara T, Emmanouilides GC, et al. (1970) Lung phospholipid of the human fetus and infants with and without hyaline membrane disease. J Pediatr 77:833.

25. Hallman M, Merritt TA, Pohjavuori M, Gluck L (1986) Effect of surfactant substitution on lung effluent phospholipids in respiratory distress syndrome: Evaluation of surfactant phospholipid turnover, pool size, and the relationship to severity of respiratory failure. Pediatr Res 20:1228–1235.
26. Dargaville PA, McDougall PN, South M (1995) Comparison of tracheal aspirate and bronchoalveolar lavage for collection of surfactant specimens in ventilated infants. Appl Cardiopulm Pathophysiol 5:18–19 (abstr)
27. Hallman M, Merritt TA, Akino T, Bry K (1991) Surfactant protein A, phosphatidylcholine, and surfactant inhibitors in epithelial lining fluid. Am Rev Respir Dis 144:1376–1384.
28. Hallman M, Merritt TA, Bry K (1994) The fate of exogenous surfactant in neonates with respiratory distress syndrome. [Review]. Clin Pharmacokinet 26:215–232.
29. Konishi M, Fujiwara T, Nalto T, et al. (1988) Surfactant replacement therapy in neonatal respiratory distress syndrome. A multi-centre, randomized clinical trial: comparison of high- versus low-dose of Surfactant TA. Eur J Pediatr 147:20–25.
30. Charon A, Taeusch HW, Fitzgibbon C, Smith GB, Treves ST, Phelps DS (1989) Factors associated with surfactant treatment response in infants with severe respiratory distress syndrome. Pediatr 83:348–354.
31. Dunn MS, Shennan AT, Possmayer F (1990) Single- versus multiple-dose surfactant replacement therapy in neonates of 30 to 36 weeks gestation with respiratory distress syndrome. Pediatr 86:564–571.
32. Speer CP, Robertson B, Curstedt T, et al. (1992) Randomized European Multicenter Trial of surfactant replacement therapy for severe neonatal respiratory distress syndrome: single versus multiple doses of Curosurf. Pediatr 89:13–20.

The Lung in Congenital Diaphragmatic Hernia (CDH)

D. Tibboel, T. Okazaki and T. Miyano

Introduction

Growth and development are fundamental processes and understanding of the mechanisms resulting in abnormal growth and development form the core of pediatrics and pediatric surgery.

Many acute problems in the perinatal period arise from prematurity and congenital anomalies. Although mortality is steadily decreasing due to progress in treatment modalities and prenatal diagnosis, remaining life-long morbidity is increasingly important. In many of these children such as premature newborns with respiratory distress syndrome (RDS), abnormal pulmonary development in case of congenital diaphragmatic hernia or oligohydramnios associated with prolonged rupture of membranes and renal anomalies the lungs are the target organ for treatment.

Pathology

It is generally accepted that the lung in CDH is hypoplastic, although large variability exists in the amount of hypoplasia. The same holds through for the contralateral lung. Structural changes have been demonstrated in the pulmonary parenchyma of CDH patients such as delayed maturation of alveolar structures and a decreased number of bronchial branches [1, 2]. At routine pathology a significant lower lung bodyweight ratio (< 0.012) and a decreased radial alveolar count (RAC) are common denominators of pulmonary hypoplasia.

An ongoing discussion is related to the functional maturation of the lung in CDH and contradictory results have been published. These are either based on measurement of surfactant components derived from bronchoalveolar lavage fluid or consecutive lecithin/sphingomyelin (L/S) ratio in prenatally diagnosed congenital diaphragmatic hernia patients with or without polyhydramnios [3, 4]. Prenatal ultrasound to predict the amount of pulmonary hypoplasia has not revealed simple measurements. A recently published manuscript on 44 fetuses with CDH, using a combination of sonographic parameters (lung/head ratio two dimensional area of right lung at the level of the right atrium / head circumference), looks promising [5].

The structural changes in the lungs of CDH patients, are not restricted to the respiratory unit. Well determined pulmonary vascular abnormalities are present as well. These consist of a decrease in total size of the pulmonary vascular bed, increased thickness of the pulmonary arterial smooth muscle coat and a decreased number of vessels per unit of lung [6, 7].

Clinical Consequences

One of the major problems following birth of a child with CDH is to predict outcome. The changed attitude towards timing of the operative repair of the diaphragmatic defect has revealed decreased compliance following repair of the diaphragm [8,9, 10]. But an absolute value of compliance predicting 100% mortality is not available. The same holds through for the reaction of the lung on artificial ventilation for which a variety of treatment modalities has been proposed to influence outcome ranging from gentle ventilation, high frequency oscillation with or without nitric oxide and extracorporeal membrane oxygenation [11–16].

Partial liquid ventilation is the last therapeutic modality; however no prospective randomized trials are available on any of these treatment modalities proving one to be superior compared with other treatments. We do know that following conventional artificial ventilation a high incidence of chronic lung disease is documented [17].

Animal Models for CDH Mimicking the Human Situation

Various animals are used for surgical induction of CDH; the lamb is the most widespread used, but also monkeys and rabbits have been tested [18–22].

The timing of CDH induction in lambs is, as in rats, important; the earlier in fetal life the lesion is produced the more severe the hypoplasia. Because this model is based on penetration of a balloon or bowels through an already closed diaphragm there is a limit in the advancing of the operation time; Adzick et al. created CDH in lambs at gestational day 60–63. In the lamb it is possible to evaluate hemodynamics and the influence of ventilation on blood gas values and morphology. Moreover the CDH lamb is surfactant deficient [23]. Recently Wilcox et al. reported on the effect of exogenous surfactant replacement therapy on gas exchange; both lung mechanics and gas exchange were markedly improved [24].

Harrison's group used the lamb model to study pulmonary hypoplasia that accompanies CDH and the possibility of reversing these changes by correcting the diaphragmatic defect in utero. In this view fetal therapy is the logical culmination of progress in fetal diagnosis. This influenced the ideas of Harrison's group on the embryological aspects of CDH: pulmonary hypoplasia was caused by migrated bowels during fetal development and could be corrected by retracting these loops out of the thoracic cavity in an as early as possible stage of development. The lungs will show a compensatory growth which will beneficially influence survival. The results of the animal experiments conducted by Harrison et al. proved, at least partially, their ideas.

Pulmonary hypoplasia in humans can also be associated with other anomalies such as renal dysplasia and oligohydramnios. Animal experiments in sheep revealed a relation between pulmonary fluid dynamics and pulmonary growth [25–27]. Tracheal ligation in the fetus accelerates lung growth beyond normal limits, even in the absence of kidneys [28–30]. Ligation of the trachea (PLUG technique) of CDH lambs during fetal development, resulted in an improved survival of the lamb with CDH after birth [31, 32]. This plugging is considered to provide a less invasive way of intra-uterine CDH treatment. Wallen et al. showed that fetal surgery sham operation had an adverse effect on lung growth: there was a significant decrease in DNA, protein and saturated phosphatidylcholine, but no significant change in lung volume was observed [33].

In the rat model of CDH the lungs are biochemically immature or hypoplastic with regard to DNA and phospholipid levels but not for antioxidant enzyme activity. Also morphologic measurements show hypoplasia: lowered lung weight, volumes and radial saccular count or immaturity evidenced by a retarded differentiation of cuboid type II cells into squamous type I cells [34–36].

Whether these animal models really contribute to the understanding of the morphological and functional abnormalities of the lung in CDH remains questionable.

The rat model of CDH enables investigators to study the natural history of the defect together with the biochemical maturation of the lung at different stages of development, with respect to type II cell differentiation, surfactant levels, anti-oxidant enzyme activity, neuroendocrine cell body (NEB) distribution, nitric oxide synthase activity as well eicasenoid levels. However it is very hard to perform interventions which mimic the clinical situation in the human, although short periods of artificial ventilation are possible [37–40].

In contrast to the rat model the sheep model offers great advantages in studying the pathophysiology of the lung and pulmonary vessels during different therapeutic interventions following birth [41]. Major differences exist between the lung developmental pattern in the sheep and the human while this animal model does not provide any insight into the pathogenesis of the defect or the natural history of the lung in CDH. Very few comparative studies are available in human cases of CDH describing surfactant levels, eicasenoid levels in BAL fluid, neuroendocrine body (NEB) distribution etc. For a better understanding of the specific aspects of the abnormal lung in CDH, a developmental biological approach may provide key answers in the future.

Developmental Biological Aspects of the Lung

Epithelial branching is one of the major events in lung morphogenesis. The branching process depends on the interaction of the epithelium with the mesenchyme; the amount of mesenchyme as well as its source (lung versus non-lung, terminal versus proximal) is shown in in vitro studies to be of importance [42–45].

The Significance of the Mesenchyme

It seems likely that mesenchyme supports the morphogenesis and differentiation of the respiratory epithelium in part through the type of matrix that it synthesizes and deposits [46]. Among the components of the extracellular matrix that have been indicated as being necessary for branching are collagens III and IV fibronectin and laminin [47–53]. In a recent study we evaluated in vivo expression of these extracellular matrix factors in normal and in Nitrofen-exposed fetal rat lungs. The expression patterns found correspond with those described by other authors for collagens, and fibronectin. For laminin a different staining pattern was found in addition to basal lamina staining, we also found staining of primordial epithelial cells and cuboid alveolar type II cells. Schuger et al. described that both lung epithelium and mesenchyme produce complete laminin molecules, shown by immunohistochemistry and in situ hybridization studies [54].

In another set of experiments fetal type II cells or lung fibroblasts were isolated on day 21 of gestation. Phosphatidylcholine (PC) and desaturated PC (DSPC) synthesis were lower in CDH than in control (no Nitrofen) type II cells. The activity of CTP: phosphocholine cytidylytransferase, a rate regulatory step in the novo PC synthesis, was lower in type II cells from severe CDH than in controls or than in a milder form of CDH. No difference was found in lysoPC acyltransferase activity or protein/DNA ratio. Conditioned medium from fetal lung fibroblasts stimulated with cortisol (FCM) is known to increase DSPC synthesis in fetal type II cells. FCM from control fibroblasts stimulated PC and DSPC synthesis in both control and CDH fetal type II cells, but FCM from CDH fibroblasts did not. These data suggest that decreased PC and DSPC synthesis in CDH can be explained by a lower cytidylytransferase activity in fetal type II cells due to a decreased production of fibroblast pneumocyte factor by lung fibroblasts. (submitted)

Hormonal Effects on Lung Development Relevant to CDH

It has long been known that thyroid hormone and glucocorticoids influence pulmonary development, especially type II cell differentiation.

Because thyroid hormone acts via its receptors, it is necessary to demonstrate the (nuclear) thyroid hormone receptor (THR) in early development. We have studied the spatio-temporal expression of the different isoforms of THR mRNAS both in the developing rat and mouse, using in situ hybridization techniques.

In rat THRalpha and THRbeta mRNAS were first detectable at embryonic day (ED) 13 and increased in cellular concentration up to ED 18, i.e. 4 days before birth, when organ maturation has come to proceed rapidly. THR-alpha is exclusively present in the mesenchyme. After ED 18, THRalpha and THRbeta mRNAS gradually decline so that by 1 week after birth, both receptors have reached their definitive (adult) levels.

In both mouse and rat, an expression comparable to that of the THRs was found for one of the partners of the THRs with which they from heterodimers, the 9-cis retinoic acid receptors (RXRs), RXR-alpha being concentrated in the developing epithelium and RXR–beta in the supporting mesenchyme of the lung.

The importance of thyroid hormone for pulmonary development and the structural resemblance of Nitrofen and thyroid hormone originated research into a possible inhibition of T3 receptor-binding by Nitrofen showing a non-competitive inhibition at receptor level.

Subsequently the spatio-temporal expression pattern was investigated of the THR, GCR (glucocorticoid) and RXR (retinoic acid) receptor during abnormal pulmonary development following induction of CDH by Nitrofen. No differences are observed suggesting that abnormal development is not mediated by a change in receptor expression in the developing lung. In other words, differences in expression pattern of thyroid hormone receptor can not be held responsible for the abnormal development of the lung in CDH. (unpublished observations)

In the developing rat lung, mRNA expression of all components of the IGF system (IGFs, IGFBPs and the type I IGF receptor) have been reported [55–58]. In addition, gene disruption strategies have demonstrated that both IGFs and the type I IGF receptor are indispensable for normal embryonic and postnatal growth. Type I IGF receptor mutants and some IGF-I mutants died at birth of respiratory failure [59]. This suggests that these proteins may participate in lung development in a paracrine or autocrine way.

Vascular Development in CDH

The morphological abnormalities in the pulmonary vasculature are well documented from a pathological point of view. The question remains whether these morphological features are directly correlated to the response of the pulmonary vasculature on hypoxia, metabolic acidosis and other stressful events. Moreover the reaction on the variety of vasoactive drugs including inspiratory NO-therapy used in a clinical practice is highly unpredictable.

Much attention has been paid to the increased muscular coat observed at birth and the peripheral extension of the muscularity in CDH [6, 7]. In contrast detailed descriptions on the development of the vasculature in CDH are almost non existing. This means that no direct correlation can be made between a well characterized stage in development in which this type of muscularization is a normal feature and the morphological features of the pulmonary vasculature in

CDH. Do the described abnormalities in the CDH lung represent a developmental delay only?

For the development of the blood vessels in the lung, angiogenesis and vasculogenesis are important morphogenetic processes. A close correlation is observed between the development of the airways and arteries. The synchronization of airway and vessel branches suggest that there is a response to common mediators or they exchange messenger molecules [for review, see 60].

Following the initial stage of vasculogenesis and angiogenesis, control of vascular proliferation is determined by the local production and action of growth factors.

TGB-beta1; platelet derived growth factor receptor ligand system and the insulin-like growth factors (IGFs) have been documented especially in in vitro culture systems as well as in tissue sections using in situ hybridization techniques and RT-PCR.

In the near future the effect of specific growth factors, able to induce angiogenesis in vivo like vascular endothelial growth factors (VEGF) will be elucidated especially because hypoxia has been shown to be a potent inducer of VEGF expression implicating his direct role in the hypoxia mediated angiogenesis [61, 62].

Besides the endothelial cell growth, normal vascular development acquires a muscular coat consisting of smooth muscle cells and extracellular matrix. The smooth muscle is essential for the development of vascular tone. Especially the group of Stenmark has contributed to the understanding of the interaction between the smooth muscle cells and the extracellular matrix using the high altitude calf as an animal model to study the cell biological features underlying pulmonary hypertension, review Stenmark [60].

Smooth muscle cells do contain different forms of myosin heavy chain molecules. In a number of species, including rabbit, rat and human, at least three types of MHC are isolated. Using cDNA probes and isoform specific isoforms Sm1 (204 kD), SM2 (200 kD) and SM embryo (200kD) are know to be developmentally regulated [63]. No studies are available during abnormal lung development but translation of the developmental biological knowledge of vasculogenesis and angiogenesis towards models of abnormal lung development is on its way.

In Conclusion

Many questions are unanswered at this moment. The significance of growth factors revealed by Northern blot analysis or differences in distribution pattern as shown by in situ hybridization or immunohistochemistry are hard to interpret either as cause or consequence of abnormal lung growth. The same holds true for the effects of hormones, especially the significance of thyroid hormone for (normal) lung growth, and differentiation of type II cells in particular. The use of transgenic mice models such as (conditional) knock out mutants for different genes relevant for lung development, such as THR alpha and the different surfactant proteins (surfactant protein B) are experimental approaches nowadays performed in different laboratories.

In the meantime experimental application of hormones like corticosteroids leads to an increase in SP A levels. Consequently prospective randomized trials are set-up evaluating the effect of prenatal administration of corticosteroids following prenatal diagnosis of CDH in humans. (Schnitzler, personal communication)

The release of vasoactive substances and the unpredictable reaction of the pulmonary vessels on inhaled nitric oxide is hardly understood. Whether the lungs are primarily abnormal in their vasoactive response, or these responses result from the insult of the lung during artificial ventilation is largely unknown.

Moreover, the significance of the described pathological features and the translation towards functional abnormalities is unclear. Especially the understanding of the reaction of the lung on the "insult" of pre or postnatal treatment modalities, such as different forms of artificial ventilation, the application of vasoactive drugs and the operative procedure, will take major efforts of a wide variety of investigators in the coming years.

The statement: the lung in CDH is just to small, is an oversimplification of an organ which has major endocrine and metabolic functions.

References

1. Nakamura Y, Yamamoto I, Fukuda S, Hashimoto T (1991) Pulmonary acinar development in diaphragmatic hernia. Arch Pathol Lab Med 115:372–376.
2. Kitagawa M, Hislop A, Boyden EA, Reid L (1971) Lung hypoplasia in congenital diaphragmatiuc hernia: a quantative study of airway, artery, and alveolar development. Br J Surg 58:342–346.
3. Moya FR, Thomas VL, Romaguera J, et al. (1995) Fetal lung maturation in congenital diaphragmatic hernia. Am J Obstet Gynecol 173:1401–1405.
4. Sullivan KM, Hawgood S, Flake AW, et al. (1994) Amniotic fluid phospholipid analysis in the fetus with congenital diaphragmatic hernia. J Pediatr Surg 29:1020–1024.
5. Harrison MR (1996) What's new in Pediatric Surgery. J Am Coll Surg 182:145–149.
6. Geggel RL, Murphy JD, Langleben D, et al. (1985) Congenital diaphragmatic hernia: arterial structural changes and persistent pulmonary hypertensions after surgical repair. J Pediatr 107:457–464.
7. Shochat SJ (1987) Pulmonary vascular pathology in congenital diaphragmatic hernia. Pediatr Surg Int 3: 331–335.
8. Sakai H, Tamura M, Hosokowa Y et al. (1987) Effect of surgical repair on respiratory mechanisms in congenital diaphragmatic hernia. J Pediatr 111:432–438.
9. Nakayama DK, Motoyama EK, Tagge EM (1991) Effect of preoperative stabilization on respiratory system compliance and outcome in newborn infants with congenital diaphragmatic hernia. J Pediatr 118:793–799.
10. Antunes MJ, Greensoan JS, Cullen JA, et al. (1995) Prognosis with Preoperative Pulmonary Function and Lung Volume Assessment in Infants With Congenital Diaphragmatic Hernia. J Pediatr 96:1117–1122.
11. Breux CW, Rouse TM, Cain WS et al. (1991) Improvement in survival of patients with congenital diaphragmatic hernia using a strategy of delayed repair after medical and/or extracorporeal membrane oxygenation stabilization. J Pediatr Surg 26:333–338.

12. Wilson JM, Lund DP, Lillhei CW et al. (1992) Delayed repair and preoperative ECMO does not improve survival in high risk congenital diaphragmatic hernia. J Pediatr Surg 27:268–375.
13. Wung JT, Sahni R, Moffitt ST, et al. (1995) Congenital diaphragmatic hernia: survival treated with very delayed surgery, spontaneous respiration, and no chest tube. J Pediatr Surg 30:406–409.
14. Stolar CJH, Dillon PW, Reyes C et al. (1988) Selective use of extracorporeal membrane oxygenation in the management of congenital diaphragmatic hernia, J Pediatr Surg 23:207–211.
15. Heiss KF, Clark RH (1995) Prediction of mortality in neonates with congenital diaphragmatic hernia treated with extracorporeal membrane oxygenation. Crit Care Med 23:1915–1919.
16. Müller W, Kachel W, Lasch P et al. (1996) Inhaled nitric oxide for avoidance of extracorporeal membranc oxygenation in the treatment of severe persistent pulmonary hypertension of the newborn. Int Care Med 22:71–76.
17. Bos AP, Hussain SM, Hazebroek FWJ et al. (1993) The incidence of bronchopulmonary dysplasia in high-risk congenital diaphragmatic hernia survivors. Pediatric Pulmonology 19:231–234.
18. Harrison MR, Bressack MA, Churg AM et al. (1980) Correction of congenital diaphragmatic hernia in utero. II. Simulated correction permits fetal lung growth with survival at birth. Surgery 88:260–268.
19. DeLorimier AA, Tierney DF, Parker HR (1967) Hypoplastic lungs in fetal lambs with surgically produced congenital diaphragmatic hernia. Surgery 62:12–17.
20. Kent GMK, Olley PM, Vreighton RE, et al. (1972) Hemodynamic and pulmonary changes following surgical creation of a diaphragmatic hernia in fetal lambs. Surgery 72:427–433.
21. Harrison MR, Anderson J, Rosen M et al. (1982) Fetal Surgery in the primate. I Anesthetic, surgical and tocolytic management to maximize fetal-neonatal survival. J Pediatr Surg 17:115–120.
22. Ohi R, Suzuki H, Kato T, Kasai M (1976) Development of the lung in fetal rabbits with experimental diaphragmatic hernia. J Pediatr Surg 11:955–959.
23. Glick PL, Stannard VA, Leach CL, et al. Pathophysiology of congenital diaphragmatic hernia II: the fetal lamb CDH model is surfactant deficient. J Pediatri Surg 27:383–388.
24. Wilcox DT, Glick PL, Karamanoukian H et al. (1994) Pathophysiology of congenital diaphragmatic hernia. V. Effect of exogenous surfactant therapy on gas exchange and lung mechanics in the lamb congenital diaphragmatic hernia model. J Pediatrics 124:289–293.
25. Docimo SG, Luetic T, Crone RK et al. (1989) Pulmonary development in the fetal lamb with severe bladder outlet obstruction and oligohydramnios: a morphometric study. J Urology 142:657–660.
26. Moessinger AC, Harding R, Adamson TM et al. (1990) Role of lung fluid volume in growth and maturation of the fetal sheep lung. J Clin Invest 86:1270–1277.
27. Peters CA, Reid LM, Docimo S et al. (1991) The role of the kidney in lung growth and maturation in the setting of obstructive uropathy and oligohydramnios. J Urology 146:597–600.
28. Adzick NS, Harrison MR, Glick PL et al. (1984) Experimental pulmonary hypoplasia and oligohydramnios: relative contributions of lung fluid and fetal breathing movements. J Pediatr Surg 19:658–663.
29. Wilson JM, DiFiore JW, Peters CA (1993) Experimental fetal tracheal ligation prevents the pulmonary hypoplasia assocated with fetal nephrectomy: possible application for congenital diaphragmatic hernia. J Pediatr Surg 28:1433–1440.
30. DiFiore JW, Fauza DO, Slavin R et al. (1994) Experimental fetal tracheal ligation reserves the structural and physiological effects of pulmonary hypoplasia in congenital diaphragmatic hernia (1994) J Pediatr Surg 29:248–257.

31. Hedrick MH, Estes JM, Sullivan KM et al. (1994) Plug the lung until it grows (PLUG): a new method to treat congenital diaphragmatic hernia in utero. J Pediatr Surg 29:612–617.
32. DiFiore JW, Wilson JM (1995) Lung liquid, fetal lung growth, and congenital diaphragmatic hernia. Pediatr Surg Int 10:2–9.
33. Wallen L, Perry SF, Alston J, Maloney JE (1994) Fetal lung growth. Influence of pulmonary arterial flow and surgery in sheep. Am J Respir Crit Care 149:1005–1011.
34. Kluth D, Kangah, R, Reich P et al. (1990) Nitrofen-Induced diaphragmatic hernia in rats: an animal model. J Pediatr Surg 25:850–854.
35. Kluth D, Tenbrinck R, Von Ekesparre M et al. (1993) The natural history of congenital diaphramatic hernia and pulmonary hypoplasia in the embryo
36. Sluiter W, Bos AP, Silvis F et al. (1992) Nitrofen-induced diaphragmatic hernias in rats: pulmonary antioxidant enzyme activities. Pediatr Res 32:394–398.
37. Scheffers EC, IJsstelstijn H, Tenbrinck R et al. (1994) Evaluation of lung function changes before and after surfactant application ventilation in newborn rats with congenital diaphragmatic hernia. J Pediatr Surg 29:820–824.
38. IJsselstijn H, Perrin DG, de Jongste JC et al. (1995) Pulmonary Neuroendocrine cells in neonatal rats with congenital diaphragmatic hernia. J Pediatr Surg 30:413–415.
39. Tenbrinck R, Scheffers EC, IJsselstijn H et al. (1995) Nitrofen induced diaphragmatic hernia: pressure-volume registration and artificial ventilation in newborn rats. Cardiopulmonary Pathophysiology 5:257–264.
40. North AJ, Moya FR, Mysore MR et al. (1995) Pulmonary endothelial nitric oxide synthase gene expression is decreased in a rat model of congenital diaphragmatic hernia. Am J Respir Cell Mol Biol 13:676–682.
41. Wilcox DT, Glick PL, Karamanoukian HL et al. (1995) Perfluorocarbon-associated gas exchange improves pulmonary mechanics, oxygenation, ventilation, and allows nitric oxide delivery in the hypoplastic lung congenital diaphragmatic hernia lamb model. Crit Care Med 23:1858–1863.
42. Gross I (1990) Regulation of fetal lung maturation. Am J Physiol 259:L337–L344.
43. Hilfer SR, Rayner RM, Brown JW (1985) Mesenchymal control of branching pattern in the fetal mouse lung. Tissue Cell 17:523–538.
44. Masters JR (1976) Epithelial-mesenchymal interaction during lung development: the effect of mesenchymal mass. Dev Biol 51:98–108.
45. Taderera JV (1976) Control of lung differentiation in vitro. Dev Biol 16:489–512.
46. Brody JS (1985) Cell-to-cell interactions in lung development. Pediatr Pulmonol 1:S42–S48.
47. Arden MG, Spearman MA, Adamson IYR (1993) Degradation of type-IV collagen during the development of fetal rat lung. Am J Respir Cell Mol Biol 9:99–105.
48. Chen JM, Little CD (1987) Cellular events associated with lung branching morphogenesis including the deposition of collagen type IV. Dev Biol 120:311–321.
49. Heine UI, Munoz EF, Flanders KC (1990) Colocalization of TGF-beta 1 and collagen I and III, fibronectin and glycosaminoglycans during lung branching morphogenesis. Development 109:29–36.
50. Chen WT, Chen JM, Mueller SC (1986) Coupled expression and colocalization of 140K cell adhesion molecules, fibronectin, and laminin during morphogenesis and cytodifferentiation of chick lung cells. J Cell Biol 103:1073–1090.
51. Roman J, Mcdonald JA (1992) Expression of Fibronectin, the Integrin alpha5, and alpha-Smooth Muscle actin in Heart and Lung Development. Am J Resp Cell Mol Biol 6:472–480.
52. Rosenkrans WA Jr, Albright JT, Hausman RE et al. (1983) Light-microscopic immunocytochemical localization of fibronectin in the developing rat lung. Cell Tissue Res 233:113–123.
53. Schuger L, O'Shea S, Rheinheimer J et al. (1990) Laminin in lung development: effects of anti-laminin antibody in murine lung morphogenesis. Dev Biol 137:26–32.

54. Schuger L, Varani J, Killen PD et al. (1992) Laminin Expression in the Mouse Lung Increases with Development and Stimulates Spontaneous Organotypic Rearrangement of Mixed Lung Cells. Dev Dynam 195:43–54, 1992.
55. Stylianopulou F, Efstratiadis A, Herbert J et al. (1988) Pattern of the insulin-like growth factor II gene expression during rat embryogenesis. Development 103:497–506.
56. Werner H, Woloschak M, Adamo M et al. (1989) Developmental regulation of the rat insuling-like growth factor I receptor gene. Proceedings of the National Academy of the Sciences of the USA 86:7451–7455.
57. Pietrzowski Z, Sell C, Lammers R et al. (1992) Roles of insulin-like growth factor I (IGF-I) and the IGF-I receptor in epidermal growth factor-stimulated growth of 3T3 cells. Molecular and Cellular Biology 12:3883–3889.
58. Price WA, Moats-Staats BM, D'Ercole AJ et al. (1993) Insulin-like growth factor binding protein production and regulation in fetal rat lung cells. Am J Resp Cell Mol Biol 8:425–432.
59. Liu JP, Baker J, Perkins et al. (1993) Mice carrying nul mutations of the genes encoding insulin-like growth factor I (gf–1) and type 1 IGF receptor (Igflr). Cell 75:59–72.
60. Morin FC, Stenmark KR (1995) Persistent Pulmonary Hypertension of the Newborn. Am J Resp Crit Care Med 151:2010–2032.
61. Leung DW, Cachianes G, Kuang WJ et al. (1989) Vascular endothelial growth factor is a secreted angiogenic mitogen. Science 246:1306–1312.
62. Sharma HS, Tan ZH, Gho BCG et al. (1995) Nucleotide sequence and expression of the porcine vascular endothelial growth factor. Biochim Biophys Acta 1260:235–238.
63. Aikawa M, Sivam PN, Kuro-o M et al. (1993) Human smooth muscle myosin heavy chain isoforms as molecular markers for vascular development and atherosclerosis. Circ Res 73:1000–1012.

Congenital Diaphragmatic Hernia, a Defect beyond Surgical Repair

J. C. Molenaar

Introduction

Over the years, congenital diaphragmatic hernia (CDH) has slowly, but in our days definitely, escaped the scope of surgical repair. Its high mortality, as appears now, is not caused by the anatomic defect of the diaphragm, but by a complex disorder involving hypoplasia of the lungs complicated by high resistance of the pulmonary vascular system, which leads to pulmonary hypertension, right-left shunting and ultimately to death on account of persistent serious hypoxia.

There seem to be two types of newborns with congenital diaphragmatic hernia: the one asphyctic immediately at birth, the other born with no or mild and late presenting respiratory distress. This difference in presentation is not related to the gross anatomic nature of the defect, but to other, so far unknown causes.

Puri and Gorman [1] reported that in a consecutive series of 15 stillborn infants with CDH all had associated anomalies. The commonest were neural tube defects, but major anomalies of other systems (cardiac) were observed as well. In another consecutive series, of 116 liveborn cases of CDH, it was found that 40 of 64 patients who died during resuscitation and stabilization before surgery showed 79 associated anomalies, whereas only 4 of the 52 patients who were stable enough to undergo operation, had associated anomalies. Here again cardiac and neural tube defects were the predominant anomalies [2]. These data suggest that, while multifactorial inheritance of CDH seems most likely, [3] CDH associated with specific patterns of other anomalies might be linked with serious lung hypoplasia and high pulmonary vascular resistance, resulting in a high mortality rate.

Stillbirth and immediate postnatal death seem to be the major forces that keep the rate of CDH with associated malformations among surviving infants as low as possible. Doctors who attempt to salvage CDH patients prenatally by fetal surgery or immediately postnatally by vigorous resuscitation ought to be constantly aware of this.

Prenatal Management

The value of prenatal ultrasound diagnosis lies mainly in allowing the parents to be prepared for the possible outcome and having the opportunity to transfer the mother to a center where optimal facilities for postnatal care are available. Vaginal delivery is preferred unless obstetric criteria indicate a cesarean section.

Postnatal Management

Each newborn baby showing respiratory distress and dextrocardia should be suspected of having CDH. Postnatal management depends largely on the available facilities. One thing is certain: immediate postnatal surgical repair is out of the question. Prospective studies [4, 5] have shown that the operative procedure itself has a negative impact on pulmonary circulation and lung compliance. Although CDH has been considered a surgical emergency for decades, delayed surgery for CDH has definitely found its place in modern-day treatment [6, 7]. Whether delayed surgery indeed contributes to better survival, remains controversial.

When artificial ventilation is not available, avoid the temptation of mask ventilation. This fills the stomach and bowels with air, resulting in more compression of the lungs. Continuous suction of the stomach by nasogastric tube, nursing in a incubator supplied with oxygen-rich air, and emptying the bowels by means of a mild enema might improve the child's condition. If it should not improve, there is no need for hurried surgical correction as this will not contribute to a better outcome.

If intubation of the trachea is possible and convential artificial are feasible, they should be given a chance. High inspiratory pressures (peaks $>$ 30mm Hg) must be avoided, because neonatal lungs, and the hypoplastic lungs in CDH the more so, are very susceptible to barotrauma and high oxygen [8]. There is also the danger of pneumothorax. If, after some improvement has been achieved, the condition of the child deteriorates again, think of pneumothorax and insert a chest tube starting with the right side, which is most likely to have a pneumothorax in left-sided CDH.

If survival seems to be likely, all efforts should be aimed at avoiding pulmonary hypertension, the first and foremost cause of death in CDH. Ventilatory conditions that produce alkalosis are favorable in this respect, but persistent hypercapnia often prevents reaching that goal.

A variety of drugs have been tried to treat increased pulmonary vascular resistance. Most of them do lower the pulmonary pressure, but also effect the systemic resistance likewise. None of them has proven to have selective dilating effects on the pulmonary vascular bed or to improve survival. If a drug lowers the systemic pressure as much as it lowers the pulmonary pressure, then the effective gradient across the ductus remains the same, and the right-to-left shunt will remain unaffected, leaving the child equally hypoxic and additionally hypotensive [8]. Inhaled nitric oxide has been shown to influence the regulation of pulmonary vascular resistance in the animal model [9]. However, in the treatment of increased pulmonary vascular resistance the effect of its endotracheal application in newborns is unpredictable and so far its use has not contributed to a better survival.

When, despite conventional ventilation, refractory hypoxemia and hypercapnia persist, other options are available to combat these symptoms. Both high-frequency oscillation ventilation and extracorporeal membrane oxygenation (ECMO) have shown to be equal in producing an approximately 15% improvement of salvage [10, 11]. This could but lead to the conclusion that ECMO might no longer have a place in the treatment of CDH, as ECMO produces a 15–20% additional morbidity [12].

Other new treatment modalities are surfactant replacement therapy [13] and liquid ventilation [14]. They are both – like all the others mentioned above – symptom-combating treatments.

Conclusion

The continued high mortality rate will not improve as long as the real cause of the mortal symptoms is not known. Research aiming at the prenatal prevention of lung hypoplasia and concomitant increased pulmonary vascular resistance is the only way to solve this problem and to salvage newborns born asphyctic owing to congenital diaphragmatic hernia [15].

References

1. Puri P, Gorman WA (1987) Natural history of congenital diaphragmatic hernia: implication for management. Pediatr Surg Int 2: 327–330.
2. Sweed Y, Puri P (1994) Congenital diaphragmatic hernia: the influence of associated malformations on survival. Arch Dis Child 69:68–70.
3. Norio R, Kaamaimen H, Rapola J. Herva R, Kekomaki M (1984) Familial congenital diaphragmatic defects: aspects of etiology, prenatal diagnosis and treatment. Am J Med Genet 17:471–483.
4. Bos AP, Tibboel D, Hazebroek FWJ, Stijnen T, Molenaar JC (1990) Congenital diaphragmatic hernia: impact of prostanoids in the perioperative period. Arch Dis Child 65:994–995.
5. Tibboel D, Bos AP, Pattenier JW, Hazebroek FWJ, Madern GC, Molenaar JC (1989) Preoperative stabilization with delayed repair in congenital diaphragmatic hernia. Z Kinderchir 44:139–143.
6. Langer JC, Filler RM, Bohn DJ et al (1988) Timing of surgery for congenital diaphragmatic hernia: is emergency operation necessary? J Pediatr Surg 23:731–734.
7. Hazebroek FWJ, Tibboel D, Bos AP et al (1988) Congenital diaphragmatic hernia: impact of preoperative stabilization. A prospective pilot study in 13 patients. J Pediatr Surg 23:1139–1146.
8. Weinstein S, Stolar CJH (1993) Congenital diaphragmatic hernia and extracorporeal membrane oxygenation. Pediatr Clin N Am 40:1315–1333.
9. Lipsitz EC, Weinstein S, Smerling AJ, Stolar CJH (1996) Endogenous nitric oxide and pulmonary vascular tone in the neonate. J Pediatr Surg 31:137–140.

10. Azarow K, Pearl R, Messineo A, Filler R, Bohn D (1996) The Toronto experience. 12th Annual CNMC symposium on ECMO & Advanced Therapies for Respiratory Failure:43 (Abst)
11. Wilson JM, Lund DP, Lillehei CW, Fauz DO, Vacanti JP (1996) The Boston experience. 12th Annual CNMC symposium on ECMO & Advanced Therapies for Respiratory Failure:44 (Abst)
12. Lund DP, Mitchell J, Kharason V, Quigley S, Kuehn M, Wilson JM (1994) Congenital diaphragmatic hernia: the hidden morbidity. J Pediatr Surg 29:258–264.
13. Bos AP, Tibboel D, Hazebroek FWJ, Molenaar JC, Lachmann B, Gommers D. Surfactant replacement therapy in high-risk congenital diaphragmatic hernia (1991) Lancet 338:1279.
14. Fauza DO, DiFiore JW, Hines MH et al (1995) Continuous intrapulmonary distension with perfluorocarbon accelerates postnatal lung growth: possible applications for congenital diaphragmatic hernia. Surg Forum 46:666–669.
15. Tibboel D, Keijzer R, Okazaki T, Miyano T (1996) The lung in congenital diaphragmatic hernia. This issue.

Neonatal Intensive Care and Neurodevelopmental Outcome

N. Weisglas-Kuperus

Introduction

The introduction of modern neonatal intensive care units (NICUs) and the technological advances, used in these NICUs, have markedly improved the survival rates for all neonates. Improved survival has been most dramatic for very low-birth-weight (VLBW, <1500g) infants. During the last 20 years, the survival rate in our own neonatal intensive care unit increased from 60 to 90% for infants with birthweights of 1000 to 1500 grams and from 25 to 70% for infants with birthweights <1000 grams (ELBW). New treatment techniques, like for example extracorporal membrane oxygenation (ECMO), have also been developed for the fullterm infant with intractable respiratory failure secondary to a variety of disorders that have common a high mortality rate (>80%) and a potential for reversibility. Mortality has traditionally been the tool used to evaluate the success of NICU treatment. With the increasing survival rate the interest in the quality of survival was growing and consequently follow-up studies were undertaken. Adverse outcome in survivors was first mostly described in terms of major handicap and defined as "the presence of impairments that will prevent the child from leading a normal daily life". Most major handicaps can be detected in the first year of life. Less severe impairments may go undetected until later in childhood, but may also be more amenable to intervention. Therefore, today both shortterm and longterm neurodevelopmental outcome must be evaluated in the NICU graduate.

Infants who need neonatal intensive care are not only at risk for neonatal cerebral damage but are also at psychosocial risk. Being treated by neonatal intensive care, their early environment is different. Neonatal intensive care also includes many caretakers and separation from the parents. Parents have to relate to their newborn infant in the high tech environment of a NICU. Moreover, the parents may be uncertain for a very long time whether their child will survive or die, whether it will survive healthy or handicapped. This may affect the parent-child relationship.

Prevention of morbidity in the neonatal period as well as later in life has now become an important goal of neonatal intensive care and pediatricians are faced with questions related to the quality of life of NICU graduates. In this paper I will therefore review the short- and longterm neurodevelopmental outcome of the preterm as well as the fullterm NICU graduate.

The Preterm Infant

The preterm infant is not ready for extrauterine life. Preterm infants are therefore at risk for a wide range of hazards such as chronic lung disease (CLD), retinopathy of prematurity (ROP) and hemorrhagic and ischemic cerebral lesions:

- Periventricular-intraventricular hemorrhage (PIVH) is almost exclusively a lesions of the preterm infant. Hemorrhages are initially subependymal. Intraventricular hemorrhage results when the ependyma ruptures. The presence of parenchymal blood corresponds not to the extension of the bleeding but to hemorrhagic infarction associated with PIVH and can result in a porencephalic cyst. Progressive posthemorrhagic hydrocephalus is a not uncommon sequel to PIVH [1].
- Periventricular leucomalacia (PVL) is of ischemic origin and refers to bilateral ischemic white matter injury. The lesions may be extensive enough to evolve into multiple small cystic lesions. Transient densities not evolving into cystic lesions, when persisting for at least a week, may represent a mild degree of leucomalacia [2].
- Ventriculomegaly may be either secondary to periventricular cerebral atrophy, that develops slowly over several weeks or secondary to progressive posthemorrhagic hydrocephalus with the development of increased intracranial pressure or rapid head growth [1].

Hemodynamic factors are essential in the development of PIVH. Critically ill preterm infants lack autoregulation of brain vessels. Systematic changes in arterial blood pressure, which have been shown to occur in preterm infants even during crying, or ordinary caretaking procedures such as feeding or suctioning, are passively transmitted to the cerebral vessels and may precipitate the bleeding. In addition hypercarbia, decreased haemoglobin, decreased glucose and alternations in the venous side of the cerebral circulation may also play a role in the pathogenesis of PIVH [1]. Abrupt decreases in blood pressure, secondary to such events as perinatal asphyxia, circulatory disturbances, severe pulmonary disease, myocardial failure, sepsis, patent ductus arteriosus and apneic spells, are essential in the pathogenesis of PVL [3]. The two major pathological conditions in the preterm infant, hemorrhagic and ischemic cerebral lesions, are therefore not totally separate entities. They share some common causes and they often coexist.

Handicaps such as cerebral palsy, mental retardation, severe visual and hearing impairments are found in up to 15% (minor handicaps 8%, major handicaps 6,5%) of the surviving VLBW infant [4]. Serial neonatal cerebral ultrasound scanning is very useful in the detection of PIVH and PVL and in the prediction of neurodevelopmental outcome. Infants with normal neonatal cerebral ultrasound scans or with uncomplicated PIVH will almost invariably have a normal neurological outcome. Of the infants with ventriculomegaly, without parenchymal damage, on neonatal cerebral ultrasound scans 43% have a normal neurological outcome, 47% have minor neurological dysfunction and 10%

have cerebral palsy at 3 1/2 years of age. Neonatal neurological examinations have additional value in predicting neurological outcome especially in this group of infants with ventriculomegaly. Intraparenchymal damage, either due to periventricular hemorrhagic infarction or cystic periventricular leucomalacia, is associated with a high incidence of cerebral palsy as well as other (mental and sensory) handicaps (86%) [5]. Infants with localized intraparenchymal echodensities have a more favorable outcome than infants with extensive intraparenchymal lesions. A distinction should also be made between cysts in the periventricular white matter and cysts in the deep white matter, as the later carries higher risk for cerebral visual impairment [2]. In posthemorrhagic hydrocephalus outcome appears to relate to the occurrence of parenchymal injury consequent to preceding hemorrhagic and/or ischemic insults [1]. Serial cranial ultrasound scanning is mandatory, since the maximum extent of hemorrhagic lesions may not develop until after the first week of life and ischemic lesions may only become visible after the first two weeks of life.

The predictive value of the neurodevelopmental assessments in the first year of life for later outcome is low. The neurological classification can change in time and mild cerebral palsy can only reliably be diagnosed after 18 months of age. Only 1/3 of the children with a mental delay at 2 years of age will have a mental handicap at 3 1/2 years of age and 1/3 of the children with a mental delay at 2 years of age will have normal cognitive outcome. This is not surprising since development is a process of continuous change. Pediatricians therefore should be cautious in the interpretation of developmental test results in infancy in order to prevent unnecessary parental concern [6].

From the second year onwards most follow-up studies on VLBW children show a decline in mean cognitive indices. Growing older, the environment becomes increasingly important in the cognitive development of the VLBW child. Except in extreme cases of neonatal cerebral damage, children at high biological risk are able to catch up on their cognitive delay in a highly stimulating home environment. Children at low as well as high biological risk in a less stimulating home environment show a decline in cognitive development [7]. In addition VLBW children at preschool age have more problem behavior than healthy fullterm preschool children. Emotional and conduct problems might be associated with parental reactions to the birth of a VLBW child [8].

To stimulate the development of the child and to prevent behavioral problems, early intervention programs, that involve the child as well as its parents, are important. Extensive educational and family support in the first 3 years of life, as for example in "The Infant Health and Developmental Program" can enhance the development of premature infants from 2 years onwards [9]. More specific and less extensive early intervention programs focussed on the mother-infant interaction in the first 3 months of life, such as the Mother Infant Transaction Program [10], are also very effective. At 9 years of age the LBW children in the Mother Infant Transaction Program scored significantly higher on intelligence tests and had also advanced more rapidly in school than the LBW children in the control group [11].

As the school curriculum places increasingly heavier demands on cognitive processing further evidence of learning difficulties may emerge. Attention problems might be linked indirectly to brain damage via cognitive impairments [8] and may contribute significantly to the risk of these academic difficulties [12]. In VLBW children the prevalence of learning problems and of cognitive and motor impairments is very high. In the Scottish very low birthweight population at 8 years of age 15% of ELBW and 6% of VLBW children attended special schools. In addition 52% of the ELBW and 37% of VLBW children required learning support on mainstream schools. Families may then, for the first time, find themselves in need of professional support and advice long after it has been assumed that their children had survived low birthweight unimpaired [13].

Preterm infants have to adapt earlier to extra-uterine life. Given the rapid development and differentiation of the brain from 26 to 40 weeks of gestational age, especially of the cortical areas, concerns has been raised that this unsuspected activation of the premature infant's immature brain, may inhibit developing neuronal pathways and interfere with full differentiation. Changing the NICU environment may positively influence neurodevelopmental functioning and may help to improve neurodevelopmental outcome. The Newborn Individualized Developmental Care and Assessment Program [14, 15] gives an individualized approach to NICU care. This early intervention program modifies the extrauterine environment and supports the individual infant's own efforts towards self-regulation and competent functioning. In healthy preterm infants the use of individualized developmental care appears to prevent frontal lobe and attentional difficulties in the newborn period, the possible causes of behavioral and learning problems often seen in low-risk preterm infants at later ages [16]. Newborn individualized care in high risk ventilated VLBW infants resulted in a significantly shorter duration of mechanical ventilation and supplemental oxygen use, a reduced incidence of pneumothorax and severe bronchopulmonary dysplasia. These infants also had better daily weight gain, a shorter hospital stay and a better neurodevelopmental outcome compared with infants in a control group [17].

The Fullterm Infant

Hypoxic-ischemic brain injury is the major recognized perinatal cause of neurological morbidity in both the premature as well as the fullterm infant. Hypoxic-ischemic insults resulting in damage may also occur antepartum and in the postnatal period. In the pathogenesis of neonatal hypoxic-ischemic encephalopathy insults primarily related to antepartum events (e.g. maternal hypotension) account for approximately 20% of the cases. Insults primarily related to intrapartum events (e.g. traumatic delivery) account for approximately 35% of cases. In an additional 35% of infants, evidence for intrapartum disturbances (e.g. fetal heart alterations, meconium stained amniotic fluid) is present; however in a substantial number of these patients, evidence for antepartum difficulty (e.g. maternal diabetes, pre-eclampsia, intrauterine growth retardation) is also present. Finally, approximately 10% (or less) of fullterm infants experience primarily postnatal insults (e.g. severe recurrent apneic spells, cardiac failure or pulmonary disease) [3].

There are five neuropathological varieties of hypoxic ischemic brain injury [3]:
1. Selective neuronal necrosis is characterized by neuronal injury at specific sites in the cerebral cortex, diencephalon, brainstem, cerebellum and spinal cord.
2. Status marmoratus is distinctive because of the prominence of neuronal loss, astrocyte response and hypermyelinsation of the basal ganglia and thalamus.
3. Parasagittal cerebral injury is the major ischemic lesion in fullterm infants. The area of necrosis are the border zones between the end fields of the anterior, middle and posterior cerebral arteries.
4. Periventricular leucomalacia (PVL), the major ischemic lesion in the preterm infant, may also occur in the fullterm infant. Necrosis occurs in areas that represent arterial border zones and end zones.
5. Focal and multifocal ischemic brain necrosis occur usually within the distribution of single or multiple major vessels.

Hypoxic-ischemic encephalopathy (HIE) is the neonatal neurological syndrome that accompanies serious perinatal asphyxia. The main grades can be described as mild (Stage 1), moderate (Stage 2) or severe (Stage 3) HIE. Infants with severe HIE are stuporous, flaccid with absent primitive reflexes. Moderate HIE is marked by lethargy, hypotonia and suppressed primitive reflexes. Mild HIE is characterized by hyperalertness, hyperexcitability and various tone abnormalities [18]. Most infants who experience perinatal hypoxic-ischemic insults do not exhibit abnormal neurological features or subsequent evidence of brain injury. Individual factors commonly used as markers of perinatal asphyxia do not predict outcome well. It is the occurrence of a sequence of indicators of exposure, response and impact on the brain and other organ function that carries predictive weight. For this reason a definition consistent with the American Academy of Pediatrics-American College of Obstetrics and Gynecology Guidelines for Perinatal Care requires multiple biochemical and clinical indices for perinatal asphyxia [19]:
1. Profound umbilical artery metabolic or mixed acidemia (Ph < 7.00).
2. Persistence of an Apgar score of 0 to 3 for longer than 5 minutes.
3. Clinical neurological sequelae in the immediate neonatal period to include seizures, hypotonia, coma or HIE.
4. Evidence of multiorgan system dysfunction in the immediate neonatal period.

It is generally agreed that the prognosis of HIE in fullterm infants depends mainly on the severity and the duration of the clinical neurological syndrome. Unfortunately the severity of HIE can only be diagnosed retrospectively after symptoms have developed and can therefore not be used as an early predictor of outcome. Repetitive seizures and severe abnormalities on the electroencephalogram or cerebral function monitor (including burst suppression, sustained low voltage, and isoelectric activity) in the first 24 hours appears to predict accurately bad outcome [20]. In the first week of life, somatosensory evoked potentials (SEPs) and visual evoked potentials (VEPs) are both of value in the early assessment of the full-term infant with HIE. Abnormal VEPs guarantee abnormal outcome while normal SEPs virtually guarantee normal outcome [21]. Supplementary evaluations, including neonatal cerebral ultrasound, computed tomography (CT) and magnetic resonance imaging (MRI) are important in the detection of a treatable complications of asphyxia (such as subdural hemorrhage) and in the determination of the site and extent of the injury for prognosis:

- Neonatal cerebral ultrasound scanning is especially of value in the identification of periventricular white matter injury. Abnormal cerebral blood flow velocity by Doppler ultrasound in the first 24 hours of life has a positive predictive value for adverse outcome [20].
- A CT scan is useful in the evaluation of both the premature and fullterm infant with hypoxic-ischemic injury as well as in the detection of associated hemorrhagic complications. MRI, however, provides superior imaging resolution for delineation of hypoxic-ischemic lesions on follow-up. A now growing experience of MRI in neonates may make this the investigation of choice in the future [22].

Asphyxia sets up a cascade of intracellular events which causes primary and secondary neuronal injury. During the primary process there is degradation of intracellular ATP with lactic acid production. Secondary injury occurs as the result of a number of complicated processes culminating in cell death. New techniques such as magnetic resonance spectroscopy suggests that there is progressive and permanent degradation of high energy ATP molecules within the brain and may be useful for the prognosis of HIE in fullterm infants in the future [20].

In infancy the emphasis of most follow-up studies of HIE has been on major handicaps, including cerebral palsy, with in some cases mental retardation, seizures and sensory loss. The prognosis of severe HIE is poor (75% death and 100% handicap in survivors). The prognosis of moderate HIE is unpredictable (5% death and 21% handicap in survivors). The prognosis for mild HIE is favorable and no sequelae are to be expected in such cases [3]. At 4 years of age major developmental dysfunction, in fullterm infants with documented HIE at birth, still depends more on the prospectively established clinical categories of HIE than on other perinatal or social factors. All surviving infants with severe HIE have major handicaps, of the children with moderate HIE 1/5 is handicapped and children with mild HIE are free of major deficits at toddler age [23]. At 8 years of age again, children with severe HIE have a poor outcome and of the children with a moderate HIE 1/5 is handicapped. Children with mild HIE continue to be free from neurological impairment and have schoolperformance quite similar to those in a comparison group. For children with moderate HIE, without a major handicap, schoolperformance is reduced. Of the non-handicapped children with moderate HIE, 42% are delayed on school readiness tests particularly for tests involving the auditory pathway, attention and short term recall [24]. These findings suggests that after an asphyxial insult, there is a group of children who will not have a major handicap but may have minor disturbances. It seems unlikely however that learning difficulties or behavioral problems can be sequela to perinatal asphyxia not clearly manifested in the neonatal period.

Extracorporal membrane oxygenation (ECMO) is a technique of cardiopulmonary bypass utilized for term and near-term infants who have pulmonary failure that is potentially reversible but has not responded to conventional or high-frequency ventilation. ECMO therapy is used in meconium aspiration syndrome, persistent pulmonary hypertension, respiratory distress syndrome, sepsis and congenital diaphragmatic hernia. The short-term benefits of ECMO are apparent, showing an overall survival rate of more than 80% in infants with predicted mortality of more than 80%. In most intensive care units, ECMO is carried out by venoarterial technique. The venoarterial bypass technique requires cannulation of both the right carotid artery and the internal jugular vein and after decannulation these vessels are permanently ligated. Anticoagulation therapy with heparin is administered systematically for the duration of the bypass procedure to prevent clotting in the ECMO circuit. Alterations in cerebrovascular hemodynamics accompanying carotid ligation and reperfusion are implicated in the pathogenesis of the cerebral damage. In most studies 25% to 50% of infants treated with ECMO exhibit intracranial abnormalities. Approximately 40% of these abnormalities are purely hemorrhagic lesions, approximately 20% hemorrhagic complicating apparent ischemic lesions and approximately 40% nonhemorrhagic ischemic lesions. Ischemic lesions consists primarily of periventricular leucomalacia, cerebral infarction and selective neuronal necrosis. Hemorrhagic lesions in infants treated with ECMO are often observed in unusual locations i.e. beyond the confines of the anterior circulation and in the temporal and occipital lobes. The laterality of hemorrhagic lesions in infants treated with ECMO has been the subject of controversy. Some reports suggests a preponderance of hemorrhagic cerebral lesions on the left side others did not describe a left side preponderance. Focal cerebral infarctions in infants treated with ECMO, however, preferentially affect the right hemisphere [25].

Rough comparison for all the cohorts of neonates that received ECMO or conventional neonatal intensive care treatment from january 1980 to july 1992 suggests equivalent amounts of morbidity within the first years of life [26]. Adverse neurological and cognitive outcome is approximately twice as common in ECMO treated infants who exhibit parenchymal injury or seizures in the neonatal period than in ECMO treated infants who do not exhibit such evidence of major abnormalities. The absence of intracranial hemorrhage, cerebral infarct or cerebral atrophy usually correlates with normal outcome in the latter group of infants [27]. Outcome must also be evaluated as a function of birthweight. ECMO treated infants with birthweights of 2000 to 2500 grams do less well than heavier and more mature ECMO treated infants. The mortality rate is significantly greater in ECMO treated infants with lower (2000 to 2500 grams, 34%) than in ECMO treated infants with higher (>2500 grams, 11%) birthweights. The overall incidence of any neuro-imaging abnormality is also significantly greater in ECMO treated infants with lower birthweights, primarily because of the higher incidence of major intracranial hemorrhage. Developmental delay was found in 38% of the ECMO treated infants with lower and in 8% of the ECMO treated infants with higher birthweight [28]. The number of infants followed to school age has been relatively small. At 5 years of age 11% of ECMO treated children are mentally retarded and mild cerebral palsy is diagnosed in 5%. In addition a higher rate of academical difficulties (49%) and behavioral problems (42%) are also reported in ECMO treated children [29].

ECMO treated infants with congenital diaphragmatic hernia have a lower survival rate and encounter a greater number of neurodevelopmental, respiratory and feeding abnormalities, during the first year of life than infants into the other primary diagnostic categories. These differences may be related to the variables associated with prolonged ECMO therapy or with the severity of the primary illness itself [30]. There are some indications that, in newborns with other serious congenital malformations that require neonatal surgical intervention, there is also a tendency for verbal IQ deficiency at school age especially in children with anorectal anomalies [31].

Conclusion

In contrast with the sparse literature on the neurodevelopmental outcome of newborns with serious congenital malformations, the dramatic increase in survival rate of VLBW and ECMO treated infants resulted in a flood of papers. In these patients the detection of parenchymal damage, with neuroimaging techniques, is most useful for the early identification of children at risk for neurodevelopmental disabilities and neonatal neurological examinations are of additional value. In fullterm infants with perinatal asphyxia the clinical neurological syndrome of moderate and severe HIE is most useful for the early identification of children at risk for neurodevelopmental disabilities and neuroimaging techniques and electroencephalography are of additional value. Environmental factors can modulate the effect of neonatal cerebral damage, particularly in the preterm child. An individualized perspective on neonatal intensive care, modifying the extrauterine environment and putting medical procedures in a developmentally appropriate framework of care, shows clear benefits. Early intervention programs that promote the parent child interaction are important in the prevention of developmental and behavioral problems in later life of all NICU graduates. The increased risk for subsequent school failure among non-handicapped NICU graduates is worrying and supports the need for long-term follow-up to increase our knowledge on the effects of improved survival in NICU graduates and to organize timely intervention.

References

1. Volpe JJ (1995) Intracranial Haemorrhage: Geminal matrix-intraventricular hemorrhage of the premature infant. In: Volpe JJ Neurology of the newborn, 3rd edition. Saunders Company, pp403–453.
2. de Vries LS, Eken P, Dubowitz LM (1992) The spectrum of leucomalacia using cranial ultrasound. Behav Brain Res 49(1):1–6.
3. Volpe JJ (1995) Hypoxic-ischemic encephalopathy: Clinical aspects. In: Volpe JJ Neurology of the newborn, 3rd edition. Saunders Company, pp 315–367.
4. Veen S, Ens-Dokkum MH, Schreuder AM, Verloove-Vanhorick SP, Brand R, Ruys JH (1991) Impairments, disabilities, and handicaps of very preterm and very-low-birthweight infants at five years of age. The Lancet 338;33–36.
5. Weisglas-Kuperus N, Baerts W, Fetter WP, Sauer PJ (1992) Neonatal cerebral ultrasound, neonatal neurology and perinatal conditions as predictors of neurodevelopmental outcome in very low birthweight infants. Early-Hum-De 31(2);131–48.
6. Weisglas-Kuperus N, Baerts W, Sauer PJ (1993) Early assessment and neurodevelopmental outcome in very low-birth-weight infants: implications for pediatric practice. Acta-Paediatr. 82(5):449–53.
7. Weisglas-Kuperus N, Baerts W, Smrkovsky M, Sauer PJ (1993) Effects of biological and social factors on the cognitive development of very low birth weight children. Pediatrics 92(5):658–65.
8. Weisglas-Kuperus N, Koot HM, Baerts W, Fetter WP, Sauer PJ (1993) Behaviour problems of very low-birthweight children. De. Med. Child Neurol. 35(5):406–16.
9. Brooks-Gunn J, Kato P, Liauw F, Spiker D (1993) Enhancing the outcome of low birthweight premature infants; results from the Infant Health and Development Program. Child De. 64:736–53.
10. Rauh VA, Nurcombe B, Achenbach T, Howell C (1990) The Mother-Infant Transaction Program: The Content and implications for the Mothers of Low-Birthweight Infants. Clinics in Perinatology 17: 31–47.
11. Achenbach TM, Howell CT, Aoki MF (1993) Nine-Year Outcome of the Vermont Intervention Program for Low-Birthweight Infants. Pediatrics 91: 45–55.
12. McCormick M, Gortmaker SL, Sobol AM (1990) Very low birthweight children: Behavior problems and school difficulty in a national sample. J Pediatr. 117:687–93.
13. Hall A, McLeod A, Counsell C, Thomson L, Mutch L (1996) School attainment, cognitive ability and motor function in a total scottish very-low -birthweight population at eight years: a controlled study.
14. Als H (1986) A synactive model of neonatal behavioral organization: Framework for the assessment and support of the neurobehavioral development of the premature infant and his parents in the environment of the neonatal intensive care unit. In J.K. Sweeney (Ed.), The high-risk neonate: Developmental therapy perspectives. Physical and Occupational Therapy in Pediatrics 6/(3/4):3–55.
15. Als H (1991) Manual for the Naturalistic Observation of Newborn Behavior. The Children's Hospital Boston, MA 02115.
16. Buehler DM, Als H, Duffy FH, McAnulty GB, Liederman J (1995) Effectiveness of Individualized developmental care for low risk preterm infants: behavioral and eletrophysiologic evidence. Pediatrics 96:923–938.
17. Als H, Lawhon G, Duffy FH, McAnuity GB, Gibes-Grossman R, Blickman JG (1994) Individualized developmental care for the Very Low- Birth-Weight Preterm Infant. JAMA 272:853–858.
18. Sarnat HB, Sarnat MS (1976) Neonatal Encephalopathy Fetal Distress. A clinical and electroencephalographic study. Arch. Neurol. 33:696–705.
19. Carter BS, Haverkamp AD, Merenstein GB (1993) The definition of acute perinatal asphyxia. Clinics in perinatology 20:287–304.
20. Levene MI (1993) Management of the asphyxiated full term infant. Archives of disease in childhood 68:612–616.

21. Taylor MJ, Murphy WJ, Whyte HE (1992) Prognostic relaibility of somatosensory and visual evoked potentials of asphyxiated term infants. De. Med. Child Neurol. 34:507–15.
22. Rutherford MA, Pennock JM, Scwieso JE, Cowan FM, Dubowitz LMS (1995) Hypoxic ischaemic encephalopathy: Early magnetic resonance imaging findings and their evolution. Neuropediatrics 26:183–191.
23. Low JA (1993) The relationship of asphyxia in the mature fetus to long-term neurological function. Clinical obstetrics and gynecology 36(1):82–90.
24. Robertson CMT, Finer NN (1993) Long-term follow-up of term neonates with perinatal asphyxia. Clinics in perinatology 20:287–304.
25. Volpe JJ (1995) Intracranial hemorrhage: Subdural, primary subarachnoid, intracerebellar, intraventricular (term infant), miscellaneous. In: Volpe JJ Neurology of the newborn, 3rd edition. Saunders Company, pp396–399.
26. Page J, Frisk V, Whyte H (1994) Developmental outcome of infants treated with extracorporal membrane oxygenation (ECMO) in the neonatal period: is the evidence all in? Pediatr Perinat Epidemiol 8(2):123–139.
27. Griffin MP, Minifee PK, Landry SH, Allison PL, Swischuk LE, Zwischenberger JP (1992) Neurodevelopmental outcome in neonates after extracorporal membrane oxygenation: cranial magnetic resonance imaging and ultrasonography correlation. J Pediatr Surgery 27 (1):33–35.
28. Revenis ME, Glass P, Short BL (1992) Mortality and morbidity rates among lower birth weight infants (2000 to 2500 grams) treated with extracorporal membrane oxygenation. J Pediatrics 121:452–458.
29. Glass P, Wagner AE, Papero PH, Rajasingham SR, Civitello LA, Kjaer MS, Coffman CE, Getson PR (1995) Neurodevelopmental status at age five years of neonates treated with extracorporal membrane oxygenation. J Pediatr 127 (3):447–4457.
30. Bernbaum J, Schwartz IP, Gerdes M , D'Agostino JA, Coburn CE, Polin RA (1995) Survivors of extracorporal membrane oxygenation at 1 year of age: The relationship of primary diagnosis with health and neurodevelopmental sequelae. Pediatrics 96 (5):907–913.
31. Kato T, Kanto K, Yoshino H, Hebiguchi T, Koyama K, Arakawa Y, Hishikawa Y (1993) Mental and intellectual development of neonatal surgical children in long-term follow-up. Journal of Pediatric Surgery 28 (2):123–129.

Organization

Outcome Assessment and Quality Assurance in Pediatric Intensive Care

R. J. B. J. Gemke, G. J. Bonsel and A. J. van Vught

Introduction

In the last decades, technological developments facilitating advanced medical care, have contributed much to the success of the management of complex diseases. More recently, however, the heterogeneity in applications and results of numerous new technologies, in combination with financial constraints have made systematic evaluation of outcome and quality of medical care imperative [1]. In response to this demand for evidence based medicine, methods to assess the effectiveness of new and existing medical technologies including long-term functional outcome have emerged rapidly. This new area of research is expected to provide knowledge to facilitate evidence based future choices in health care and has been called "the third revolution in medical care" [2]. Related to outcome assessment are quality assessment and quality assurance. The most concise and appropriate definition of quality of care is 'doing the right thing and doing the thing right'. Particularly in intensive care medicine, where costs are invariably high and effectiveness of care is sometimes challenged, systematic assessment of outcome has become mandatory.

The primary goal of intensive care medicine is to diagnose and treat patients with acute life threatening illness in order to prevent avoidable death and to restore their previous health and quality of life [3]. If a previously healthy patient with an acute life-threatening illness survives restlessly due to treatment in an intensive care unit (ICU), this goal is met completely. However, if a similar patient survives but continues to live with a severely impaired health, this goal is only partially met, if at all. Comparison of outcome in different (pediatric) ICUs is hampered by differences in severity of illness and case-mix patterns. To circumvent these problems various clinical scoring systems have been developed, facilitating objective and uniform assessment of severity of illness adjusted mortality in order to address questions of effectiveness, efficiency, and quality of intensive care. As mortality is not the only endpoint for effectiveness of care, instruments to assess (changes in) health status or health related quality of life have been introduced. In addition to mortality, simultaneous inclusion of effects on health status allows a more comprehensive assessment of the merits of advanced medical care. Furthermore, for survivors it is the overall final outcome that counts, although it will not always be possible to detach the contribution of different aspects of a complex therapy, in which treatment in the ICU might only have had an ancillary role. Hence quality of life after advanced medical care constitutes an important overall measure of quality of care, while change thereof may not be solely attributed to treatment in the ICU.

In the following sections of this chapter we will address the principles of effectiveness and efficiency of pediatric intensive care, assess the merits of severity of illness measures, discuss how outcome of pediatric intensive care should (not) be compared between units and finally address the role of long-term survival and health status after advanced medical care in children.

Effectiveness and Efficiency

Effectiveness and efficiency constitute the core attributes of outcome and quality assessment. Their most important characteristics are schematically shown in Table 1.

Efficacy can be defined as the result of a health care program under optimal circumstances; i.e. a controlled clinical trial with homogenous patient groups, experienced physicians, and excellent facilities. The core question to be answered is: "Can it work?"

Effectiveness can be defined as the result (benefit) of a medical technology in comparison to a competing alternative or a golden standard technology. The core question to be answered is: "Does it work"? In this respect it should be realized that, when efficacious technologies diffuse to average conditions of employment, benefits realized under strictly controlled conditions may no longer apply. Particularly in case of potentially life-saving treatment modalities, as is often the case in intensive care medicine, comparison with alternative options is frequently hampered, if not precluded, on ethical grounds.

Table 1. Attributes of outcome and quality assessment

Attribute	Aim of measurement	Outcome measure
1. Efficacy	Result of a technology under optimal conditions	improved health
2. Effectiveness	Result of a technology under average conditions	improved health
3. Efficiency	The relation between costs and consequences	ratio of marginal costs to marginal benefits:
– Cost-benefit	Comparison of costs with monetary revenue attributed to health outcome	monetary units
– Cost-utility	Comparison of costs with length and quality of survival	quality adjusted life years (QALYs)
– Cost-effectiveness	Comparison of costs with improved health	health events

In absence of large randomized studies, comparing intensive care with normal ward care, effectiveness of intensive care may be challenged. Certain patient categories may be to ill to benefit from intensive care, while others may be not ill enough to justify admission to the ICU. Lacking an absolute standard, effectiveness of intensive care is usually expressed as the ratio of observed mortality and expected mortality, adjusted for severity of illness. This ratio is called the standardized mortality rate (SMR). If the observed mortality is lower than expected mortality, adjusted for severity of illness (SMR < 1), this suggests a superior performance with respect to ICU mortality. As such, the SMR constitutes a measure of relative effectiveness of care as compared to a large reference population in which the instrument to assess severity of illness has been developed and validated.

Although intensive care probably has reduced acute short term mortality, survival to hospital discharge is not the only endpoint of effectiveness of advanced medical care. Particularly because there are indications that decreased mortality is accompanied by an increasing proportion of patients with chronic residual morbidity [4–7]. Therefore, functional outcome and longitudinal assessment of length and quality of survival have become crucial supplementary parameters of outcome after intensive care, in addition to plain ICU and hospital mortality. In adult intensive care, assessment of health related quality of life, using established health status measures, has gradually become a well acknowledged concept. In several recent evaluation studies a rather poor long-term outcome was found, with cumulative 1 year mortality rates ranging from 23–63%, while health status after 1 year was conserved or improved in 10–74% of survivors (Table 2).

There are a number of factors that hamper straightforward assessment of efficacy and effectiveness of (pediatric) intensive care:

1. The heterogeneity of treated patient groups. To solve this problem, robust clinical scoring systems for objective and uniform assessment of severity of illness in (pediatric) ICU patients have enabled comparison among heterogenous patient groups.
2. The basic difference of patients who are primarily admitted to the (pediatric) ICU following an acute insult, and those in whom admission to the (pediatric) ICU is ancillary to another therapeutic strategy, e.g. after major elective surgery. Particularly in the group of patients who are not primarily admitted to the (pediatric) ICU, it may be difficult to distinguish the contri-

Table 2. Long-term outcome of adults discharged from ICUs

Author	Outcome after 1 year Mortality	Equal or improved health status
Goldstein, 1986 [4]	23%	61%
Yinnon, 1989 [5]	63%	68%
Mata, 1992 [6]	30%	10%
Konopad, 1995 [7]	25%	74%

butions of therapies inside and outside the ICU to the eventual outcome of the patient. Pseudo-experimental studies, comparing intensive care with standard ward care, using historical control groups have lost their validity because of the rapid development of intensive care medicine. Consequently studies which systematically assess the technology and quality of (pediatric) intensive care are scarce and their results are divergent.

3. The heterogeneity of (pediatric) ICUs. In specialized tertiary care ICUs, usually all advanced treatment options will be available. This will not always be the case in non-tertiary hospitals in which ICUs might function partly as post-operative recovery, predominantly admitting patients for monitoring purposes.
4. The fact that in numerous countries children are (still) admitted to multidisciplinary „adult" ICUs where often the numbers of children are too low and expertise is primarily focussed on the majority of adult patients.

Beside effective, being a high cost health care facility, intensive care should also be employed in an efficient manner. Efficiency of a health care program can be defined as the relation between the costs and the consequences (benefits or drawbacks) of that program. The core question to be answered is: "Do the marginal (incremental) benefits outweigh the marginal costs?" In the absence of conclusive data for absolute effectiveness of intensive care, and without a reliable estimate of incremental costs of intensive care, straightforward determination of the cost-effectiveness of intensive care is not feasible. Nevertheless, a unit can be considered cost-*in*effective if it utilizes more resources, while producing the same results as others with respect to severity of illness corrected mortality under analogous conditions. Stated conversely, for patients who may derive similar benefits from a non-ICU setting, the preference of this alternative strategy (treatment in the regular ward) with respect to cost-effectiveness is obvious. Consequently, in order to assess what results in an ICU are obtained with available resources, expressed as ICU bed-days, objective criteria to assess the justification of admission or stay in the ICU may be adopted [8]. These criteria comprise a lower limit of mortality risk and a number of active, ICU dependent therapies to determine whether admission or stay on each consecutive day was warranted.

1. Admission to the ICU can be regarded as efficient if the mortality risk of a patient exceeds an arbitrary value *or* the patient undergoes at least one ICU dependent therapy on the day of admission.
2. Stay in the ICU can be regarded efficient if the patient underwent at least one ICU dependent therapy.

Important prerequisites for the implementation of these criteria are validated and robust severity of illness measures and appropriate application of ICU dependent therapies. The latter comprise 21 therapeutic options (as opposed to monitoring facilities) that reasonably cannot be given in a normal ward. All of these can be derived from the Therapeutic Intervention Scoring System (TISS) [8].

Schematically, inefficient ICU days can be incurred by:

1. patients whose mortality risk was too low *and* who never used an ICU dependent therapy; so called „low risk monitoring patients".
2. patients whose mortality risk was above the arbitrary value *or* who used one or more ICU dependent therapies, however not during all consecutive ICU days (usually not during the last day(s) preceding discharge); so called „potential early discharge patients".

As it might not always be clear whether a patient will sustain substantial risk of dying and/or require an ICU dependent therapy, particularly in the Western world a considerable number of patients are admitted for safety reasons [9, 10]. In retrospect, these patients only use monitoring facilities and/or standard care, while never requiring ICU dependent interventions. Although this uncertainty can never be eliminated completely, unnecessary (pediatric) ICU admissions occur and may contribute significantly to health care cost.

Studies in adult ICU populations have determined that a large proportion of resources is spent on a relatively small subgroup of patients with a high probability of an unfavorable outcome. The opposite conclusion may be drawn from neonatal intensive care, because particularly the respiratory distress syndrome is a reversible disorder with a good chance of acceptable functional recovery with an overall favorable long-term prognosis and because infant non-survivors tend to have a shorter hospital course than adult non-survivors [11].

There is a paucity of information with respect to cost-effectiveness and resource utilization in pediatric intensive care and the results are divergent. Some authors have suggested a relation between severity of illness (mortality risk) and resource utilization. Glass *et al.* demonstrated that resource utilization among pediatric ICU patients was highest in 3 categories: (1) children undergoing palliative or temporizing therapy, (2) children with acute disease from congenital origin and (3) infants of less than 1 month of age. Significant chronic disease was not associated with increased resource utilization [12]. Pon *et al.* showed that diagnosis-related group (DRG) based reimbursement resulted in a negative financial balance, suggesting that the DRG classification inadequately reflects expected costs of pediatric ICU services [13]. Gemke *et al.* demonstrated that a high proportion of average daily and total ICU resource utilization per admission was determined by a concise set of basic clinical characteristics (severity of illness, surgical status, the presence of substantial chronic comorbidity, emergency admission and transfer from another hospital). High resource utilization in high risk patients was probably warranted, as effectiveness of prolonged intensive therapy was demonstrated by a relatively low standardized mortality in this category [14].

Severity of Illness Measures; Potentials and Limitations

One of the first objective measures for aggregated severity of illness was the system developed in the early 1950s by Virginia Apgar to evaluate newborns.

This quantitative scoring instrument gained nearly universal acceptance and is still in common use today. Since then an exponential proliferation of clinical scoring systems that quantify severity of illness in an objective and unequivocal manner, based on parameters of acute physiologic dysfunction, has evolved. Identification of relevant variables for mortality risk assessment, which therefore may be included in a mortality probability model, can be determined by advanced statistical techniques (multivariate analysis; logistic regression). Fundamental in the methodology to devise a mortality probability model is the utilization of two independent multicenter patient data sets for the development and validation of the model, respectively.

Objective description of acute severity of illness with these measures is accomplished by the weighted contributions of a selection of significant parameters to overall physiologic instability. For each parameter that diverts from a defined normal range, its weighted contribution is included in the total score. In a number of well established severity of illness measures, the total score can subsequently be converted into a mortality risk by means of a logistic regression technique.

For each age category mortality probability models have been introduced:

1. *Adults.* The Acute Physiology and Chronic Health Evaluation (APACHE) stands out as the most extensively studied and applied model in adult ICU patients, [15] although several other general systems are used. These include the Mortality Probability Model (MPM) [16] and the Simplified Acute Physiology Score (SAPS) [17]. Most authors agree that advancement in prognostication should be achieved by further refinement of these readily accepted and diffused models, although new models have been suggested recently.
2. *Infants and children.* For pediatric patients similar generic severity of illness and mortality prediction models have been developed and are widely used. The first was the Physiologic Stability Index (PSI), followed by a refined version called the Pediatric Risk of Mortality (PRISM) score [18]. A further update, called PRISM III, also devised by the group of Pollack *et al.* will become available in the near future. In addition to 16 variables for acute physiology, this model will also include a number of variables for chronic health status before admission to the pediatric ICU.
3. *Newborns.* For (premature) newborns several scoring systems have been developed in order not to rely only on birthweigth or gestational age for assessment of mortality probability. The most important systems are the Clinical Risk Index for Babies (CRIB) [19], the Score for Neonatal Acute Physiology (SNAP) [20].

Apart from the above mentioned generic mortality probability models, several disease specific scoring systems have been introduced such as the combined Trauma Score and Injury Severity Score (TRISS) and several predictive scores for meningococcal infection in children.

Severity of illness measures are used in ICUs to facilitate comparison in heterogenous patient groups for different purposes. Applications include:

Table 3. Performance of clinical scoring systems in predicting hospital mortality in independent cohorts of intensive care patients

Patient group	Score	Sampling period	Number of variables	Area under ROC curve
Adults	APACHE III	24 h	19	0.90
Adults	MPM II	0, 24, 48, 72 h	15	0.79–0.84
Children	PRISM score	24 h	14 (+2)	0.92
Children	PRISM III	12 or 24 h	16 (+8)	0.95
Newborns	CRIB	12 h	6	0.90
Newborns	SNAP	24 h	29	0.93

1. Stratification of patients for research in clinical trials. One of the most important controls is the ability to define severity of illness of each included patient in an objective and unequivocal manner.
2. Quality assessment and medical audit. Another important application of mortality prediction models is quality assessment, either between ICUs or within a single ICU over an extended period of time. A probability of mortality based on a model is estimated for each patient, which represents the likelihood of mortality of a similar patient in the ICUs where the original model was developed. Significant differences in standardized mortality rates require further explanation of probable discrepancies in quality of care.
3. Hospital reimbursement. In some countries, hospital reimbursement is based on Diagnostic Related Group (DRG), although this approach has been demonstrated to be inadequate [13]. Severity of illness based reimbursement is expected to be more appropriate.
4. Discussion of prognosis. Mortality probability is an objective measure that can contribute to discussions about prognosis with the patient's relatives and among physicians in clinical decisions as a supplement to clinical judgement.
5. Management purposes, such as assignment of personnel and resource allocation.

When adopting a mortality probability model that was developed elsewhere, its validity in a particular unit should be assessed by the discrimination and calibration of the model. If discrepancies are found it may be possible to customize the model for a particular unit to enhance model performance. The discrimination of a model can be determined by the concordance between overall observed and expected outcomes (death and survival, respectively) by means of a 2×2 classification table. Subsequently a Receiver Operating Characteristic (ROC) curve can be constructed, which reflects the relation of sensitivity (correct prediction of death) and specificity (correct prediction of survival) of the model. The shape and area under the ROC curve (A_z) is an important measure of overall discriminatory performance of the mortality prediction model. An A_z of 0.5 corresponds to chance performance whereas an A_z of 1.0

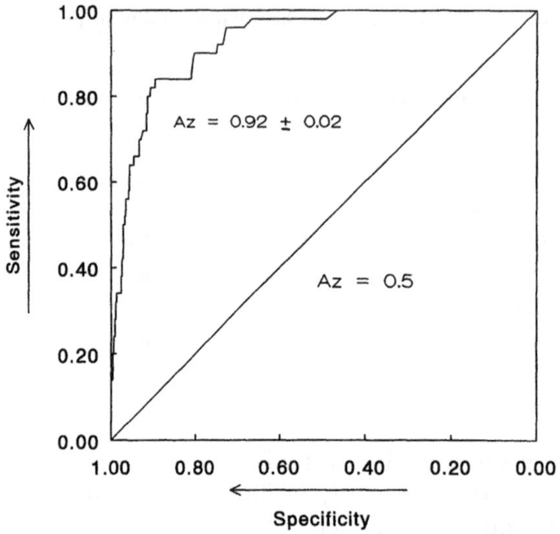

Fig. 1. Receiver Operating Charateristic (ROC) curve, relating the true positive rate (sensitivity; correct prediction of death) to the false positive rate (specificity; correct prediction of survival). The area under the curve (A_z) is an overall measure for the discriminatory performance of a mortality probability model. (Reproduced from Gemke *et al.* [21] with permission from the publisher.)

Table 4. Classification table based on an arbitrary mortality risk cutoff point. (Reproduced from Gemke et al. [21] with permission from the publisher)

Predicted outcome	Pediatric ICU discharge status Observed died	Observed survivor	Total
Non-survivors	18	13	31
Survivors	32	530	562
Total	50	543	593

Specificity (correct prediction of survival) 530/593 = 0.976
Sensitivity (correct prediction of death) 18/50 = 0.36
Predictive value of death 18/31 = 0.581
Predictive value of survival 530/562 = 0.943
Correct classification rate (18 + 530)/593 = 0.924

corresponds to perfect prediction. Good mortality risk prediction models have an $A_z > 0.85$. An example of a ROC curve is shown in Figure 1.

Appropriate model performance may not only be based on a high sensitivity and specificity in classification tables as these are highly dependent on the chosen cut-off points, selected to predict survival and death from the probabilities derived from the model. Assessment of the accuracy (or calibration) of the model compares the number of expected deaths as determined by the model to the number of patients who actually die within 5–10 subgroups of patients. Typically, a 2 × (5–10) table is made by using deciles of mortality risk as cut-off points between the 10 groups. Subsequently, using formal goodness-of-fit tests, the expected mortality in each interval is compared with the observed mortality in that interval.

Potential weaknesses in the day-to-day application of clinical scoring systems are the compliance with the original model including its rules of application, artefact rejection (especially in automated data acquisition from Patient Data Management Systems) and inter-observer reliability.

Although severity of illness adjusted hospital mortality, expressed as standardized mortality rate constitutes an important indicator of outcome, it is not the only measure of quality of intensive care. Reduction of mortality among complex diseases due to advanced medical care is accompanied by an increasing morbidity, hence probably a decreased health related quality of life in survivors. This indicates that although severity of illness corrected mortality is *indispensable* to assess quality of intensive care, it does not *suffice*.

The most established objective severity of illness measure for pediatric ICU patients is the PRISM score which quantifies severity of illness, based on 14 routinely measured clinical and laboratory parameters of physiological instability. For each parameter, an abnormal range represented by a number of scoring points is assigned, reflecting its weighted contribution to overall severity of illness. The number of points corresponding to the most abnormal recorded value from each of the 14 parameters on the admission day are summed to obtain the total PRISM-score. The overall mortality probability in the pediatric ICU can be subsequently predicted by a logistic regression equation with the PRISM score as main covariate, while age and operative status are included as additional covariates.

$P = \exp(R)/(1 + \exp[R])$ P = probability of PICU death $0 < P < 1$

$R = a \cdot \text{PRISM} + b \cdot \text{age (in months)} + c \cdot \text{operative status (0 or 1)} + d$

In the validation series: $a = 0.207$, $b = -0.005$, $c = -0.433$, $d = -4.782$

In a multicenter study of tertiary pediatric ICUs in the USA the predictive power of the PRISM score was established as an institutional independent measure of severity of illness with a high predictive accuracy for ICU mortality [18].

In the near future PRISM III will made available by the group of Pollack *et al.* This enhanced update was developed and validated in 32 pediatric ICUs in the USA. The 16 included variables of acute physiology are heart rate, systolic blood pressure, temperature, mental status, pupillary reflexes, blood gas analysis (pH, PCO_2, P_aO_2, total CO_2), glucose, potassium, creatinine, BUN, white blood cell count, platelet count and prothrombin time or partial thromboplastin time. Moreover, eight indicators of chronic health status are included (chromosomal anomaly, cancer, acute diabetes, previous pediatric ICU admission, pre-ICU CPR, post-operative, nonoperative cardiovascular disease, and admission from an inpatient unit). Whether its broader application will be hampered by the fact that regression equations will not become part of the public domain and the author's decision to charge a license fee for PRISM III software and algorithms remains to be established.

For (premature) newborns the Clinical Risk Index for Babies (CRIB) score has been developed in 4 UK tertiary hospitals. Scores are given for birthweight, gestational age, minimum and maximum FiO_2, and maximum base excess during the first 12 h, and the presence of congenital malformations. The area under the ROC curve was substantially greater for CRIB than for birthweight alone (0.90 and 0.78, respectively). The Score for Neonatal Acute Physiology (SNAP), developed in 3 USA tertiary neonatal ICUs, proved to be of similar prognostic value as the CRIB score, although the rather high number of variables (26 or 29, depending on the SNAP version) has hampered its broader application.

In a study by the International Neonatal Network, with birthweight alone, risk-adjusted hospital mortality was lower in tertiary hospitals than in non-tertiary hospitals [19]. This does not prove that the non-tertiary hospitals' performance was worse, because of the potentially confounding effects of disease severity. With CRIB however, the difference in risk-adjusted mortality between the types of hospitals was even greater, and it persisted when the comparison was confined to inborn infants. The difference was thus not explained by increased severity of illness in infants treated in non-tertiary hospitals, which suggests that they performed less successfully.

Despite considerable differences in the provision of care for critically ill children among countries, few authors have attempted to validate the model outside the group of hospitals in the United States where the model was developed. In a Dutch multidisciplinary pediatric ICU for medical, cardiovascular surgical and other surgical patients the performance of the model (discrimination and calibration) was good. No significant difference between observed and expected mortality was found in the total population, nor in a number of mortality risk strata; the area under the ROC curve was 0.92. Mortality was most reliably predicted in medical patients; in surgical patients somewhat less optimal, yet very satisfactory performance was found [21].

Probabilities of hospital mortality provide meaningful information in many contexts. However, use of probabilities as dichotomous predictors can be misleading for making treatment decisions for individual patients, even when the performance of the model is overall good. In adults alternative models for estimating severity of illness in ICU patients, while demonstrating good agreement for describing patients in aggregate, have been shown to differ considerably for individual patients. This suggests that identifying patients unlikely to benefit from intensive care by using mortality probability models must be approached with considerable caution.

Despite the advantages of the PRISM score for assessment of ICU mortality in children, so far it does not include aspects of chronic health status and, alike adult mortality probability models, it does not address functional outcome. Recently an important advancement has been made by the incorporation of functional outcome several months after ICU discharge in a prognostic model assessing the merits of advanced medical care in adults. This Study to Understand Prognosis and Preferences for Outcome and Risks of Treatments (SUPPORT) concluded that functional outcome varied substantially in patients after hospitalization for serious illness and that a small amount of readily available clinical information can estimate the probability of severe functional limitations [22].

Comparison of (Pediatric) Intensive Care

As controlled trials, in which patients are randomly assigned to an ICU or a normal ward are precluded for ethical reasons, quality of (pediatric) intensive care can only be assessed by comparing the performance of different units. In these studies, differences in effectiveness of care, confined to standardized ICU mortality rate, and efficiency of utilization of ICU capacity can be analyzed. Multicenter studies among tertiary pediatric ICUs have demonstrated that differences in crude mortality rates were largely explained by differences in severity of illness. In a US multicenter study, acutely ill children were demonstrated to have a better chance of survival when they were admitted to a tertiary pediatric ICU instead of to a district hospital's ICU. Despite the usually less stabile transport conditions and longer time before arrival, severity of illness corrected mortality was lower in tertiary pediatric ICUs, this advantage being more prominent in children with higher mortality risks [23].

Transport of acutely ill children may constitute an important pitfall in quality assurance of pediatric intensive care. Although in most countries the medical team of the referring hospital is responsible for safe and expedite transport, in practice this responsibility can only be met by dedicated and specially trained transport teams, recruited from tertiary centers. Only then adverse events occurring during interhospital transfer of critically ill children can be prevented, enabling maximal profit from tertiary care facilities.

In a recent Dutch multicenter study, in which outcome of 10 pediatric intensive care units was compared, observed and expected mortality in the total population were similar. Among the participating centers, despite wide fluctuations in crude mortality (mean 7.1%, range 1–10%), standardized mortality rates were similar (mean SMR 0.99, range 0.8–1.5). Subsequent analysis showed that in tertiary pediatric ICUs, severity of illness adjusted mortality in high-risk patients was superior to the reference population used for model development, while paradoxically, in low-risk tertiary care patients observed mortality was higher than expected [24]. The former finding warrants the existence of independent tertiary pediatric ICUs and supports the concentration of severely ill patients there. The latter, paradoxical finding was probably due to the relatively great proportion of low-risk tertiary care patients suffering from severe, incurable chronic disease. This emphasizes that other factors than acute derangements should be taken in account when assessing outcome of intensive care in children.

Studies assessing the circumstances of dying in hospitalized children have indicated that in 30–40% of non-survivors, death was associated with limitations of life supporting therapies [25]. In neonatal intensive care even higher figures are found. Consequently, future studies should also address chronic (co)morbidity and decisions regarding limitation of life supporting treatment in addition to acute severity of illness when assessing outcome of intensive care.

Apart from differences in effectiveness with respect to severity of illness corrected mortality, efficiency of the utilization of intensive care capacity may show wide fluctuations. Previous studies in adult ICUs have suggested that low risk monitoring patients could be readily identified and nursed outside the ICU; some indicated a relation between limited bed capacity and better selection of patients [9]. For instance, in countries with a relative scarcity of (pediatric) ICU beds, intensivists appear to be more capable to select those patients that, in retrospect, actually needed acute life supporting therapies [9, 10]. In the USA, being the country with the highest health care expenditure, Pollack *et al.* assessed daily efficiency in 8 tertiary care pediatric ICUs. Using the criteria mentioned before, on average 77.8% of ICU bed-days were justified, however figures varied widely between units (55–89%) [8]. In another multicenter study comparing outcome of pediatric intensive care, overall efficiency of bed usage was 72.2%, also with a wide fluctuation (22–95%) [24]. On balance the figures of pediatric ICU efficiency compare favorably with those published on adult ICUs in the USA and several other western countries, where average daily efficiency rates were 53.9% and 49.5%, respectively, using the same criteria [26]. This confirms that substantial inter-institutional differences in thresholds for ICU admission and discharge exist. These may be influenced by ICU bed capacity, hospital bed capacity, availability of a "step down unit", monitoring facilities, medical and/or nursing expertise on the ward. In general an average daily efficiency between 0.70 and 0.90 would be regarded acceptable. Indeed, a mean efficiency rate of 0.80 suggests an overall appropriate admission and discharge policy as well as sufficient total bed capacity to support (national) needs, although temporarily (regional) over- and undercapacity might still exist. The high efficiency rates in combination with adequate effectiveness found in some centers indicate that temporary capacity constraints might be solved by well structured referral patterns and improved admission and discharge policies, particularly in the less efficient centers.

Quality of Life as Indicator of Overall Quality of Care

As stated in the introduction, the aim of intensive care medicine is not only to prevent avoidable death but also to restore a patient's previous health and quality of life. Hence, preservation of health related quality of life, also denoted as health status, constitutes an important overall indicator of effectiveness of advanced medical care. A major handicap in assessing the effectiveness of intensive care is to detach the contribution of intensive care to the patient's final outcome from other contributions within a broader medical or surgical therapy. In previously healthy patients with an acute devastating illness (e.g. meningococcal septicemia), length and quality of survival may be primarily ascribed to the merits of intensive care. However, particularly in patients where intensive treatment is ancillary to a much broader therapy (e.g. in a complex surgical case) the contribution of intensive care to length and quality of survival cannot be assessed independently. Nevertheless, especially in patients with complex diseases, assessment of length and quality of survival is mandatory. Although it may not be possible to detach specific contributions within a broader therapeutic regimen, ultimately (parents of) patients regard survival and quality of life the final measures by which the merits of medical care should be judged.

Assessment of health related quality of life or health status tries to establish in quantitative terms the concept, denoted health. Usually 3–7 health domains are distinguished, which together are regarded to encompass the essential core of health. Although a considerable variety of health status measures has emerged in recent years, there is broad consensus about the core of various established instruments.

Well recognized health status measures mostly include the following domains [27]:
- physical function (mobility, self care)
- psychosocial function (social support, anxiety, communication)
- role performance (work, household, school)
- cognitive function

Factors that influence the selection of instruments are methodological requirements (feasibility, reliability and validity), the type of instrument (generic *versus* disease specific), the method of administration (self or proxy questionnaire, interview) and whether descriptive or valued aggregation of the health status is desired. For populations with heterogenic diseases, such as ICU patients, only generic health status measures are appropriate. Generic health status measures are intended to be applicable to a broad population, while capturing a wide range of health problems. Some well established generic health status classification systems for adults are the Nottingham Health Profile, Quality of life index, the Sickness Impact Profile, the Quality of Well-being, the Short Form 36 (SF-36) [28].

In pediatrics, despite the ubiquitous employment of the terms health status and quality of life, its contents are barely substantiated. Particularly the paucity and complexity of health status measuring in children has contributed to this detainment. Nevertheless assessment of health status gradually becomes more important as an increasing number of children are now surviving formerly incurable diseases, while continuing to live with substantial chronic disorders. For outcome assessment of heterogenous groups of children undergoing advanced medical care, also generic rather than disease specific health status measures are the most appropriate. These include the Functional Status II,[29] the Pediatric Overall Performance Category (POPC) and Pediatric Cerebral Performance Category (PCPC),[30] although their coarseness has hampered broader application. A pediatric adaptation of the SF-36, called the Child General Health Survey, is currently developed at the New England Medical Center, Boston, USA.

Multi-attribute health status measures, intended for clinical application in heterogenous categories of children, have been introduced and recently reviewed by the group of Torrance *et al.*[31] From a total of 15 health domains, six that were found to be the most important by parents of schoolage children were selected for inclusion in health status classification. Each domain comprised 4–5 levels of functioning; sensory functions (4 levels), mobility (5 levels), emotional and social function (5 levels), cognition (4 levels), self-care (4 levels), pain and discomfort (5 levels). Any specific combination of 6 domain levels constitutes a health status. Subsequently this so-called Health Utility Index (HUI) was applied in analysis of health status of survivors of neonatal intensive care and childhood cancer [32]. The reliability and validity of this classification to assess health status in pediatric intensive care patients has been established [33]. A special feature of the HUI is the possibility to convert the system to a health status index score by weighing and aggregating the scores of all domains. This enables to derive the number of quality adjusted life years (QALYs) gained by a particular intervention for cost-utility analysis. For that purpose, a selection of health states was used to estimate health status preferences from a random sample of parents of school aged children. Despite the attractiveness of a single summary score for health status, involvement of disparate dimensions makes its interpretation hazardous, particularly in non-epidemiologic use.

In a study assessing survival and health status one year after discharge of 468 children admitted to a Dutch intensive care unit, ICU mortality was 7.5%, cumulative hospital mortality 8.3% and 1 year mortality 10.5%. Hospital mortality primarily was found in previously healthy children, suffering from an acute devastating illness. With the HUI, health status before admission and after 1 year were assessed. After 1 year, of the 254 patients eligible for analysis, 80 (31.5%) had no overall health impairment preceding admission; of these 11 had died in ICU and 69 were long-term survivors of whom 45 recovered to perfect health. A high proportion of patients experienced some form of health deficits before ICU admission. Expressed as overall health impairment, 174 of 254 patients (68.5%) had 1 affected health domains before admission. However, after one year overall health status was improved or equal to pre-admission health in 164 of 226 survivors (72.6%). With respect to domain specific health, the proportion who improved or was identical varied from 77.9% (emotional functions) to 89.4% (mobility and pain). Consequently, despite the large number with health impairment before admission, cumulative 1 year survival was favorable and health status in three quarters of the population was preserved [34].

In a retrospective Australian study, assessing long-term outcome of admission to pediatric ICU, Butt et al. found a cumulative mortality of 14.3% and overall health impairment on follow up in 58% [35]. Health status remained unchanged in 68.7%, deteriorated in 8.3% and improved in 8.7% as compared to pre-admission. The higher morbidity, both on admission and after 1 year, and the more frequent changes in health status that were found in the Dutch study are probably related to the more refined health status measure and the prospective design.

Conclusion

We have reviewed methods for assessment of quality of advanced medical care in children, using uniform, well designed and validated measures for acute severity of illness and chronic health status. In general, children with severe acute illnesses have a higher chance of survival in tertiary centers which justifies the independent existence of pediatric ICUs and the concentration of severely ill children there. Although severity of illness adjusted hospital mortality, expressed as standardized mortality rate, constitutes an important indicator of performance, mortality is not the only endpoint of quality of intensive care. ICU mortality is probably also affected by decisions regarding the limitation of life supporting treatment, implementation of which may not only be based on imminent death due to acute illness but also on poor long-term prognosis associated with chronic (co)morbidity. This indicates that, although severity of illness adjusted mortality is *indispensable* to assess quality of intensive care, it does not *suffice*. Long-term survival and health status as well as decisions regarding the limitation of life supporting treatment should also be incorporated in future studies that aim at comprehensive assessment of the merits of advanced medical care in children.

References

1. Roper WL, Winkenwerder W, Hackbarth GM, Knakaven H (1988) Effectiveness in health care; an initiative to evaluate and improve medical practice. N Engl J Med 319:1197–1202.
2. Relman AR(1988)Assessment and accountability. The third revolution in medical care. N Engl Med 319:1220–1222.
3. Suter P, Armaganidis A, Beaufils F, *et al* (1994) Predicting outcome in ICU patients consensusconference. Intensive Care Med 20:390–397.
4. Goldstein RL, Campion EW, Thibault GE, Mulley AG, Skinner E (1986) Functional outcomes following medical intensive care. Crit Care Med 14:783–787.
5. Yinnon A, Zimran A, Hershko C (1989) Quality of life and survival following intensive medical care. Q Med J 264:347–357.
6. Mata GV, Fernandez RR, Carmora AG *et al* (1992) Factors related to quality of life 12 months after discharge from the intensive care unit. Crit Care Med 20:1257–1262.
7. Konopad E, Noseworthy TW, Johnston R, Shustack A, Grace M (1995) Quality of life measures before and one year after admission to an intensive care unit. Crit Care Med 23:1653–1659.
8. Pollack MM, Getson PG, Ruttimann UE *et al* (1987) Efficiency of intensive care; a comparative analysis of eight pediatric intensive care units. JAMA 258:1481–1486.
9. Sirio CA, Tajimi K, Tase C *et al* (1992) An initial comparison of intensive care in Japan and the United States. Crit Care Med 20:1207–1215.
10. Pollack MM, Ruttiman UE, Glass NL, Yeh TS (1985) Monitoring patients in pediatric intensive care. Pediatrics 76:719–724.
11. Prano JR, Teres D, Lemeshow S, Brown RB (1992) Hospital charges and long-term survival of ICU versus non-ICU patients. Crit Care Med 10:569–574.
12. Glass NL, Pollack MM, Ruttimann UE (1986) Pediatric intensive care: Who, why and how much. Crit Care Med 14:222–226.
13. Pon S, Notterman DA, Martin K (1993) Pediatric critical care and hospital costs under reimbursement by diagnosis-related group: Effect of clinical and demographic characteristics.J Pediatr 123:355–64.
14. Gemke RJBJ, Bonsel GJ, McDonnell J, van Vught AJ (1994) Patient characteristics and resource utilisation in paediatric intensive care. Arch Dis Child 71:291–296.
15. Knaus WA, Wagner DP, Draper EA *et al* (1991) The APACHE III prognostic system. Risk prediction of hospital mortality for critically ill hospitalized patients. Chest 100:1619–1636.

16. Lemeshow S, Teres D, Klar J, Spitz-Avrunin J, Gehlbach SH, Rapoport J (1993) Mortality Probability Models (MPM II) based on an international cohort of intensive care unit patients. JAMA 270:2478–2486.
17. LeGall, Loirat P, Alperovich A (1984) A simplified acute physiology score for ICU patients. Crit Care Med 12:975–982.
18. Pollack MM, Ruttiman UE, Getson PR (1988) Pediatric risk of mortality (PRISM) score. Crit Care Med 16:1110–1116.
19. International neonatal network (1993) The CRIB (Clinical Risk Index for Babies) score: a tool for assessing initial neonatal risk and comparing performance of neonatal intensive care units. Lancet 342:193–198.
20. Richardson DK, Gray JE, McCormick MC, Workman K, Goldmann DA (1993) Score for neonatal acute physiology: a physiologic severity of illness index for neonatal intensive care. Pediatrics 91:617–623.
21. Gemke RJBJ, Bonsel GJ, van Vught AJ (1992) Effectiveness and efficiency of a dutch pediatric intensive care unit: validity and application of the pediatric risk of mortality (PRISM) score. Crit Care Med 22:1477–1484.
22. Wu AW, Damiano AM, Lynn J *et al* (1995) Predicting future functional status for seriously ill hospitalized patients. The SUPPORT prognostic model. Ann Int Med 122:342–350.
23. Pollack MM, Alexander SR, Clarke N, Ruttimann UE, Tesselaar HM, Bachulis AC (1991) Improved outcomes from tertiary center pediatric intensive care: A statewide comparison of tertiary and non-tertiary care facilities. Crit Care Med 19:150–159.
24. Gemke RJBJ, Bonsel GJ, the Pediatric Intensive Care Assessment of Outcome (PICASSO) study group (1995) Comparative assessment of pediatric intensive care: A national multicenter study. Crit Care Med 23:238–245.
25. Levetown M, Pollack MM, Cuerdon TC *et al* (1994) Limitation and withdrawal of medical intervention in pediatric critical care. JAMA 272:1271–1275.
26. Apache Medical Systems, Inc (1992) Report to the Foundation for Research on Intensive Care in Europe. In: Reis Miranda D, Spangenberg JFA (ed) Quality, efficiency and organisation of intensive care units in the Netherlands. Foundation for Research Intensive Care in Europe (FRICE); Groningen, The Netherlands, pp 112–129.
27. Fitzpatrick R, Flechter A, Gore S, Jones D, Spiegelhalter D, Cox D (1992) Quality of life measures in health care. BMJ 305:1074–1077:1145–1148:1205–1209.
28. McDowell I, Newell C (1987) Measuring health: a guide to rating scales and questionnaires. Oxford University Press, Oxford, UK.
29. Stein REK, Jessop JD. Functional status II(R) (1990) A measure of child health status. Med Care 28:1041–1055.
30. Fiser DH (1992) Assessing the outcome of pediatric intensive care. J Pediatr 121:68–74.
31. Feeny D, Furlong W, Torrance GW (1993) Multi-attribute health status classification systems. In: Patrick DL, Erickson P. Health status and health policy: Quality of life in health care evaluation and resource allocation. Oxford University Press, Oxford, pp 381–389.
32. Saigal S, Rosenbaum P, Stoskopf B *et al* (1994) Comprehensive assessment of the health status of extremely low birth weight children at eight years of age: Comparison with a reference group. J Pediatr 125:411–417.
33. Gemke RJBJ, Bonsel GJ (1996) Reliability and validity of a comprehensive health status measure in a heterogenous population of children admitted to intensive care. J Clin Epidem (in press)
34. Gemke RJBJ, Bonsel GJ, van Vught AJ (1995) Long term survival and health status after paediatric intensive care. Arch Dis Child 73: 196–201.
35. Butt W, Shann F, Tibballs J *et al* (1990) Long-term outcome of children after intensive care. Crit Care Med 18:961–965.

Effectiveness and Efficiency in Pediatric Intensive Care

F. Shann

Introduction

Pediatric intensive care makes a substantial contribution to the health of children in developed countries. For example, in Victoria, a state of Australia with a population of 4.5 million, one child in 70 (1.5% or 15 per 1000) is admitted to the pediatric intensive care unit at the Royal Children's Hospital. A conservative estimate is that half the children admitted would die without intensive care ($15 \times 0.5 = 7.5$ per 1000), so Victoria's under 15 years mortality rate would double from 7.1 to 14.6 deaths per 1000 live births without pediatric intensive care.

It is only recently that systematic attempts have been made to assess how well intensive care is being given to children and how efficiently it is being given – it is most important that these assessments be as accurate as possible. To demonstrate the effectiveness of pediatric intensive care, patients would have to be randomized to receive either intensive care or standard ward care – but this would be unethical. In lieu of such a trial, quality of care is assessed by comparing mortality rates adjusted for severity of illness between ICUs. Efficiency cannot be quantified unless the effectiveness is known, so assumptions have to be made about effectiveness – for example that intubated patients would not survive without intensive care, and that unintubated patients would survive.

Do Children Benefit from Intensive Care?

There is only limited empirical evidence for the effectiveness of pediatric intensive care, but there is a considerable amount of evidence relating to neonatal intensive care and some relating to adult intensive care.

Neonatal Intensive Care

Most neonatal deaths are caused by just a few diseases, and the risk of death can be defined fairly easily – so the impact of intensive care can be assessed more easily in newborn babies. There has been one randomized controlled trial of intensive care in neonates – it was performed in Melbourne before the introduction of neonatal ventilation [1]. In the last two years of the study, mortality was only 18.3% in the intensive care group compared to 35% in the control group ($p < 0.05$); there was no difference in mortality in the first two years of the four-year study, which suggests that the experience of those delivering intensive care is important.

When assessing the impact of neonatal intensive care, it is important to compare the outcome of entire populations rather than just subgroups that did or did not get intensive care [2]. Studies that have done this [3–14] have consistently shown a substantial improvement in outcome with intensive care for newborn babies – see Table 1. The exception is a study of all births in New Zealand in 1978–81 [10] that found that small rural maternal hospitals had lower perinatal mortality rates than larger hospitals for babies weighing more than 1500g, but higher mortality rates for babies less than 1500g. The authors suggest that the difference in mortality in larger babies was probably due to the fact that perinatal care in New Zealand is highly regionalized, and high-risk mothers and babies were referred to larger hospitals before delivery; in these circumstances, they were unable to detect a volume threshold below which obstetric care was unsafe.

Budetti [15] has reviewed the effectiveness of neonatal intensive care and its cost- effectiveness [16]. He concluded that the evidence supports the conclusion that intensive neonatal care has played a significant role in bringing about the impressive reduction in infant mortality that has taken place in the United States since 1965.

Table 1. Hospital of birth (tertiary or non-tertiary) and perinatal mortality in defined populations

References	Place	Years	No. births	Type of birth
Bokketeig [3]	Norway	1967–73	454358	All singleton
Bowes [4]	Colorado	1977–78	319040	Live births
Cooke [5]	Liverpool	1980–83	201	<1001 g
Forbes [6]	Norway	1979–81	4692	<2500 g
Horwood [7]	Ontario	1964–77	638	500–1499 g
Kitchen [8]	Victoria	1979–87	911	500–999 g
Paneth [9]	New York	1976–78	13560	501–2250 g
Rosenblatt [10]	New Zealand	1978–81	206054	All births
Saigal [11]	Ontario	1977–84	521	501–1000 g
Verloove-Vanhorick [12]	The Netherlands	1983	1338	<32 wk or <1500 g
Williams [13]	California	1960–73	3441448	All births
Yankaner [14]	New York	1945–54	1489175	All births

Adult Intensive Care

In 1984, Bereson [17] reviewed the clinical outcome and costs of intensive care for the United States Congress. He concluded that the effectiveness of ICU varies according to the underlying disease (p34–35), and that "conditions which respond well to ICU are reversible illnesses without significant underlying chronic illness (eg respiratory arrests as a result of drug overdoses, major trauma, reversible neuromuscular diseases such as Guillain-Barre syndrome, and diabetic ketoacidosis). Conditions which generally do not respond well are exacerbations of chronic conditions for which there has been no definitive treatment (eg cirrhosis with gastrointestinal hemorrhaging, and advanced cancer)". The advantages and disadvantages of intensive care are summarized on page 12 of Berenson's review.

Pediatric Intensive Care

I do not know of any controlled trials of paediatric intensive care. However, extrapolation of the evidence from neonatal and adult experience, and empirical observation, strongly suggests benefit for many children admitted to intensive care. For example, there can be little doubt that properly performed endotracheal intubation benefits children with severe airway obstruction caused by epiglottis or croup, or that intensive care benefits many children after severe trauma or major surgery for congenital heart disease.

Indeed, children admitted to intensive care have much higher survival rates than low-birthweight babies or adults in intensive care – children stay a shorter time in intensive care than neonates or adults, and the survivors have a much greater life- expectancy than adults. Tables 2 and 4 show a comparison of the costs and benefits of neonatal, pediatric and adult intensive care at three large teaching hospitals affiliated to the University of Melbourne. Table 2

Table 2. Victoria: outcome 2 years after intensive care in 1983

	Neonates birthweight <1000 g[a]	Children >28 days of age[b]	Adults[c]
Dead	60%	15%	55%
Severe handicap	10%	10%	10%
Mild handicap[d]	10%	10%	20%
Functionally normal	20%	65%	15%

[a] Data from references [18, 19], and Kitchen WH personal communication
[b] Data from reference [20] and unpublished data
[c] Proc 9th Aust and NZ Int Care Soc Meeting, Perth 1984, and Cade JF personal communication
[d] Handicapped, but likely to lead an independent life

Table 3. Cost per independent survivor and per year of life saved for neonatal, pediatric and adult intensive care

	ICU cost per intubated patient*	Years of independent life saved/100 patients (see Table 5)	ICU cost per independent survivor	ICU cost per year of independent life saved	Comment
Neonates (<1000 g birthweight)	$28650	Dead 60 × 0 yr Severe 10 × 0 yr Mild 10 × 50 yr Normal 20 × 70 yr 1900 yr	$95500	$1500	Survivors live many years, *but* high mortality and prolonged ICU stay (therefore a fairly high ICU cost per year of independent life saved)
Children (over 28 days old)	($18 m × 72)/(596 × 1138) = $8600	Dead 15 × 0 yr Severe 10 × 0 yr Mild 10 × 50 yr Normal 65 × 70 yr 5050 yr	$11500	$170	Survivors live many years, *and* need only a short period in ICU (therefore a low ICU cost for each year of independent life saved)
Adults (mean age 55 years)	($151 m × 60)/(1300 × 715) = $9750	Dead 55 × 0 yr Severe 10 × 0 yr Mild 20 × 10 yr Normal 15 × 20 yr 500 yr	$27850	$1950	Need only a short period of ICU, *but* survivors have limited life expectancy (therefore a high ICU cost for each year of independent life saved)

* Neonates: From reference [20]. Children and adults: (Hosp budget × ICU nurse EFT)/(Hosp nurse EFT × intubated admissions)
These calculations assume that intubated patients would not survive without intensive care, and that unintubated patients would survive without intensive care

shows the outcome two years after neonatal, pediatric and adult intensive care: neonatal and adult intensive care had high mortality rates and only 15–20% functionally normal survivors, while pediatric intensive care had a low mortality rate and 65% functionally normal survivors.

Table 3 calculates the ICU cost per year of independent life saved for adult ($ 1950 per year of independent life saved), neonatal ($ 1500) and pediatric ($ 170) intensive care. The cost is very low for pediatric intensive care because children have short stays in intensive care, a low mortality rate and a low handicap rate after intensive care.

Table 4 is a cost-benefit analysis for neonatal, pediatric and adult intensive care. The analysis shows substantial savings from pediatric intensive care, and small losses from neonatal and adult intensive care.

These analyses (Tables 2 to 4) are hospital-based rather than community-based, and the cost–benefit analysis (Table 4) uses some very broad assumptions. Nevertheless, the analyses suggest that pediatric intensive care is highly cost effective because children have a shorter stay in ICU and most of them survive – with most of the survivors likely to lead an independent existence for many years.

Assessing Severity of Illness

Objective measures of severity of illness are needed for several purposes, including the assessment of effectiveness and efficiency. Severity of illness scores have usually been derived by using logistic regression analysis to determine which variables predict mortality in a group of patients, and then assuming that risk of mortality is equivalent to severity of illness. This is a reasonable assumption for most types of patients in intensive care, but it is not true for groups of patients that need intensive care but have a very low risk of dying (for example, severe croup). The available severity of illness scores are accurate enough to be used to describe groups of patients, but they should not be used to determine the management of individual patients – although it has been suggested that a low score might be used to suggest that a patient is ready for discharge from ICU [25].

The only validated score for prediction of outcome in pediatric intensive care is the Pediatric Risk of Mortality (PRISM) score [26], which is calculated from the most abnormal values of 14 physiological variables in the first 24 hours after admission, as well as the child's age and postoperative status. This score has excellent predictive power, but the method of calculating the latest version of the score (PRISM 3) is not in the public domain and the license fee is US 750 per annum. PRISM does not perform optimally in all groups of patients - it has been suggested that it underestimates the risk of death in postcardiovascular surgery patients [27, 28], and overestimates risk in other postoperative surgical patients [28] and infants [29].

PRISM (or its predecessor, the PSI) has been used to estimate the efficiency of ICU [30], the relationship between severity of illness and cost [31], rationing

Table 4. Cost-benefit analysis (discounted at 5% per annum) for neonatal, pediatric and adult intensive care in Victoria, 1989

		Neonate <1000 g	Child >28 days old	Adult (mean 55 years)
COSTS				
Died	Hospital	0.6 × \$39 954 = \$23 972	0.23 × \$8 612 = \$1 981	0.55 × \$12 185 × 3 = \$20 105
Severe	Hospital	0.1 × \$39 954 = \$3 995	0.1 × \$8 612 × 3 = \$2 584	0.1 × \$12 185 × 3 = \$3 651
	Institution	0.05 × \$50 000 × 20yr = \$32 713	0.05 × \$50 000 × 17yr = \$29 594	0.05 × \$50 000 × 5yr = \$11 365
	Medical/Educ	0.05 × \$15 000 × 20yr = \$9 814	0.05 × \$15 000 × 17yr = \$8 878	0.05 × \$15 000 × 5yr = \$3 409
Mild	Hospital	0.1 × \$39 954 = \$3 995	0.1 × \$8 612 × 3 = \$2 584	0.2 × \$12 185 × 3 = \$7 310
	Medical	0.1 × \$20 000 = \$2 000	0.1 × \$20 000 = \$2 000	0.2 × \$20 000 = \$4 000
Normal	Hospital	0.2 × \$39 954 = \$7 990	0.65 × \$8 612 × 3 = \$16 793	0.15 × \$12 185 × 3 = \$5 480
		\$84 479	\$64 414	\$55 320
EARNINGS				
Mild		0.1 × \$29 335 × 30yr = \$20 659	0.1 × \$29 335 × 30yr = \$23 915	0.2 × \$29 335 × 3yr = \$16 776
Normal		0.2 × \$29 335 × 42yr = \$46 829	0.65 × \$29 335 × 42yr = \$176 184	0.15 × \$29 335 × 5yr = \$20 003
		\$67 488	\$200 099	\$36 779
BALANCE		−\$16 991	+\$135 685	−\$18 541

Calculations based on reference [21]
If En is the amount earned in year n, the discounted present value is $En/(1.05)^{n-1}$
Proportion died/severe/mild/normal: Table 2
Cost of intensive care for children and adults: Table 3
Cost of neonatal hospital care: reference [18] (+16% for inflation)
Life expectancy of severely handicapped child (e.g. Down's syndrome): reference [22]
Cost of institutional and medical care with severe handicap: Dr D Reddihough, personal communication
Proportion of severely handicapped in institutional care: RCH ICU followup data (unpublished)
Total medical cost for 6 months from time of admission to ICU = 3 × ICU cost: reference [23]
Average annual earnings: and age employment began and ended: reference [24]

of intensive care [32], quality of care in tertiary versus non-tertiary ICUs [28, 33] and the quality of specialist versus nonspecialist interhospital transport [34].

Like all outcome scores that use information collected over the first 24 hours after admission, PRISM suffers from practical and methodological disadvantages. The practical disadvantage is that a considerable amount of effort is needed to collect the most abnormal values of 14 different variables so, in practice, many PICUs do not collect PRISM routinely. The methodological problems with worst-in-24-hour scores are considerable. First, such scores appear to be more accurate than they really are: about 40% of deaths in pediatric intensive care units occur in the first 24 hours after admission, so the score is really diagnosing death rather than predicting it. Second, one of the main purposes of outcome scores is to enable comparisons between units, but worst-in-24-hour scores are treatment dependent, so they blur the differences between units: a child admitted to a good ICU who rapidly recovers will have a score that suggests mild illness, but the same child who is mismanaged in a bad ICU will have a score that suggests severe illness – the bad unit's high mortality rate will be incorrectly attributed to it having sicker patients than the good unit.

The Mortality Prediction Model (MPM) is an outcome prediction model for adult intensive care that uses only data available at the time of admission; MPM has been found to have good predictive power [35]. The Paediatric Index of Mortality (PIM) score using only admission data has been developed at the Royal Children's Hospital, Melbourne, and is being tested in six Australian PICUs and one PICU in the United Kingdom.

Quality of Care

Whether a particular ICU is delivering effective care can be assessed by comparing the actual mortality rate for its patients to the expected mortality rate calculated using an outcome prediction model. For example, in 1000 admissions to a hypothetical ICU, suppose that 50 patients died (observed deaths) and that the risk of death (ranging from 0 to 1) calculated for each of the 1000 patients using PRISM sums to 46.2 (expected deaths); the standardized mortality rate (SMR) is then 46.2/50, or 92.4% of the PRISM standard. The significance of the observed difference (50 versus 46.2) can be tested using Flora's Z test [36].

Most of the published literature assesses only mortality in intensive care or in hospital. However, it is also important to assess mortality over several years, and to examine quality of life: this has been done for children in Melbourne [20] and Utrecht [37]. The Melbourne study showed that 30 to 36 months after admission, 80% of the 976 children were alive, and 91% of the survivors were likely to lead an independent life; most of the survivors who were not likely to lead an independent life were children with Down's Syndrome who had had surgical repair of congenital heart lesions [20].

A major study in 16 randomly selected PICUs in the USA [38] used PRISM to adjust for the severity of illness, and found that mortality was reduced by having a paediatric intensivist, and increased in teaching hospitals (this effect was probably due to the presence of residents caring for ICU patients). The study detected no reduction in mortality with larger ICUs, full time consultants or location in a children's hospital – but had sufficient power (alpha 0.05, beta 0.1) to detect only a change of more than 40% in mortality due to any given factor. Note that, to determine the effect of these risk factors (such as size of ICU) on mortality, the relevant sample size is the number of units in the study (which was only 16), *not* the number of patients (which was 5415).

Efficiency

Pollack [30] has suggested that the efficiency of paediatric intensive care can be measured by assuming that intensive care is justified if the risk of mortality is greater than 1% or an ICU-dependent treatment was given. This rule has the merit of allowing each admission (or every day of each admission) to be classified as efficient or inefficient. However, the choice of a 1% risk of mortality is entirely arbitrary (1.01% is not really different from 0.99%), and an ICU that uses excessive therapy for mildly ill patients will be inappropriately classified as efficient because of the reliance on ICU-dependent therapy.

An ICU is making efficient use of its resources if it has only sick patients who need intensive care, high bed occupancy rates (an ICU that is usually empty is inefficient), and short lengths of stay (an ICU that keeps patients longer than necessary is inefficient). These three factors can be combined into an Efficiency Index (EI):

$$\text{EI} = \text{mortality risk x\% occupancy / length of stay.}$$

However, occupancy is equal to (length of stay) × (admissions per year) / (number of ICU beds), so we have:

$$\begin{aligned}\text{EI} &= \text{mortality risk} \times (\text{LOS} \times \text{admissions / beds}) / \text{LOS} \\ &= \text{mortality risk} \times \text{admissions / beds}\end{aligned}$$

where mortality risk is the average risk of death for the patients calculated from an outcome prediction score such as PRISM, LOS is the average length of stay in ICU, admissions is the number of admissions to ICU and beds is defined in terms of the total full time equivalent (FTE) nurses available to the unit:

$$\begin{aligned}\text{Funded beds} &= \frac{(\text{nurse hours per wk}) \times (\text{weeks worked per yr}) \times (\text{nurse FTE})}{(\text{days in a year}) \times (\text{hours/day} + 2)} \\ &= \frac{38 \times 46 \times 61}{365 \times 26} = 11.2\end{aligned}$$

for our PICU in Melbourne – where a full time nurse works 38 hours a week for 46 weeks a year (4 weeks recreation leave and 2 weeks sick leave), and we have 61 FTE nurses; two hours is added to the number of hours in a day in the denominator to allow for handover time and administration. The Efficiency Index should be interpreted in conjunction with its individual components: average risk of mortality, bed occupancy rate and the mean length of stay.

In 1994, our PICU in Melbourne had an average risk of mortality of 0.070 (7.0%), a bed occupancy rate of 79%, and an average length of stay of 2.65 days. There were 1219 admissions in 1994, so we had an Efficiency Index of 0.070 × 1219/11.2, or 7.62.

Many ICUs do not collect the information needed to calculate PRISM, so I suggest that the Intubation Index (II) be used as a measure of efficiency in such units:

$$\text{II} = \text{intubated admissions} \,/\, \text{funded beds} = 841/11.2 = 75.1$$

for our PICU in Melbourne in 1994.

Quite appropriately, small ICUs often have a high proportion of nonintubated high dependency patients. To allow more accurate comparison between ICUs with different proportions of high dependency patients, I suggest that paediatric intensivists always give the number of admissions, the mortality risk and the mean length of stay in their ICUs for both intubated and nonintubated patients. The failure to allow for the difference in the proportions of high dependency patients has caused considerable confusion in the literature about the number of PICU beds required.

Regionalization of Pediatric Intensive Care

There is increasing evidence that children who need intensive care should be looked after in large specialist paediatric intensive care units, rather than in small pediatric units or in general ICUs with adult patients.

Direct evidence that mortality is lower in specialist pediatric ICUs comes from three separate studies. A study in Oregon and Washington [33] found that the standardized mortality rate was 102% of expected in three pediatric units, and 139% of expected in 71 general ICUs ($p < 0.05$). Teres [39] has criticized this study because Flora's Z test was used (but this is a valid test for this data), because there was not a significant difference in the standardized mortality rate between tertiary and non tertiary hospitals in children with a 5–30% risk of dying (but the difference was significant in the >30% group), and because the confidence intervals of the differences were very wide (which merely reflects the small number of deaths in some groups).

A study in Holland [40] found that mortality in high risk patients was 85% of expected in six tertiary pediatric units, and 143% of expected in four nontertiary units ($p < 0.05$). In low risk patients, the standardized mortality rate was actually higher in the tertiary units, but 60% of the 25 low risk children who died in a tertiary unit suffered from a severe and incurable disease with no prospect of long-term survival.

A third study, as yet unpublished, included all children who received intensive care in Victoria, a state of Australia, and in the Trent Region of the United Kingdom - both areas have a population of about 4 million. In Victoria, where almost all children receive intensive care in a large tertiary pediatric ICU, the standardized mortality rate was very much lower than in Trent, where children receive intensive care in small paediatric units or in general ICUs.

All these studies compared large specialist tertiary pediatric intensive care units with small non-specialist units, and it is not possible to be sure which of the differences between these two types of units (size of ICU, specialist or non-specialist pediatric unit, tertiary or nontertiary hospital) contributed to the difference in standardized mortality rates. However, taken together, these three studies provide strong evidence in favour of the regionalization of pediatric intensive care.

There is indirect evidence that ICUs that look after many children are likely, on average, to perform better than ICUs that look after few children: numerous studies in many specialties have found that units looking after many cases of a particular disease have better results than units with few cases [41, 42].

The American College of Critical Care Medicine and the Society of Critical Care Medicine [43], the British Paediatric Association [44], and the Australian National Health and Medical Research Council [45] have all said that children should receive intensive care in specialist pediatric units. The weight of authoritative opinion and direct and indirect evidence is strongly in favour of looking after children in regionalized dedicated pediatric ICUs.

Conclusion

Paediatric intensive care is highly cost-effective. Children have a short stay in intensive care, there is a low mortality rate, and most of the survivors are likely to lead an independent life. In Victoria, one child in 70 is admitted to paediatric intensive care, and the under 15 year mortality rate would approximately double from 7.1 to 14.6 deaths per 1000 live births without paediatric intensive care.

There are no randomized controlled trials of the overall effectiveness of paediatric intensive care, but there is strong epidemiological evidence of the effectiveness of neonatal intensive care - and paediatric intensive care is likely to be at least as effective as neonatal intensive care.

Objective methods for predicting the risk of mortality are needed to monitor the effectiveness and efficiency of paediatric intensive care. The only widely used paediatric scoring system, PRISM, is based on the most abnormal values of 14 physiological variables over a 24 hour period. There are strong practical and methodological reasons for preferring scores calculated from data available on admission rather than worst-in–24-hour scores.

The standardized mortality rate is used to assess the quality of care delivered by an individual ICU: the number of observed deaths is divided by the sum of the probabilities of death for each patient calculated from a mortality prediction model.

Efficiency can be assessed by assuming that intensive care is justified if the risk of mortality is greater than 1% or if an ICU-dependent treatment is given. However, this definition is arbitrary, and I suggest that an Efficiency Index be calculated from the average mortality risk, multiplied by the number of admissions, and divided by the number of funded beds. To adjust for differences between ICUs in the proportion of intermediate care patients, it is important to report results separately for intubated and nonintubated patients.

Numerous studies in many specialties have found that units that look after many cases of a particular disease have better results than units with few cases. Three separate studies have found lower standardized mortality rates when children are looked after in large specialist pediatric ICUs.

We are just beginning to develop suitable ways to measure effectiveness and efficiency in paediatric intensive care. Such tools are urgently needed to help decide the best ways to organize and deliver intensive care to children.

References

1. Kitchen WH, Ryan MM, Rickards A, et al (1978) A Longitudinal study of very low-birthweight infants: study design and mortality rates. Develop Med Child Neurol 20:605–618.
2. Mugford M (1991) Commentary. Arch Dis Child 66:410–411.
3. Bakketeig LS, Hoffman HJ, Sternthal PM (1978) Obstetric service and perinatal mortality in Norway. Acta Obstet Gyn Scand Suppl 77:1–19.
4. Watson AB (1981) A review of perinatal mortality in Colorado, 1971 to 1978, and its relationship to the regionalization of perinatal services. Am J Obstet Gynecol 141:1045.
5. Cooke RWI (1987) Referral to a regional centre improves outcome in extremely low birthweight infants. Arch Dis Child 62:619–21.
6. Forbes JF, Larssen KE, Bakketeig LS (1987) Access to intensive neonatal care and neonatal survival in low birthweight infants: a population study in Norway. Paed Perinatol Epidemiol 1:33–42.
7. Hopwood SP, Boyle MH, Torrance GW, Sinclair JC (1982) Mortality and morbidity of 500- to 1,499-gram birth weight infants live-born to residents of a defined geographic region before and after neonatal intensive care. Pediatrics 69:613–620.
8. Kitchen WH (1991) Improvement of outcome for infants of birth weight under 1000 g. Arch Dis Child 66:765–769.
9. Paneth N, Kiely JL, Wallenstein S, Marcus M, Pakter J, Sussre M (1982) Newborn intensive care and neonatal mortality in low-birth-weight infants. N Engl J Med 307:149–155.
10. Rosenblatt RA, Reinken J, Shoemack P (1985) Is obstetrics safe in small hospitals? Lancet 2:429–32.
11. Saigai S, Rosenbaum P, Hattersley B (1989) Decreased disability rate among 3-year-old survivors weighing 501 to 1000 grams at birth and born to residents of a geographically defined region from 1981 to 1984 compared with 1977 to 1980. J Pediatr 114:839–46.
12. Verloove-Vanhorick SP, Verwey RA, Ebeling MCA, Brand R, Ruys JH (1988) Mortality in very preterm and very low birth weight infants according to place of birth and level of care: results of a national collaborative survey of preterm and very low birth weight infants in the Netherlands. Pediatrics 81:405–411.

13. Williams RL (1979) Measuring the effectiveness of perinatal medical care. Med Care 17:95–110.
14. Yankauer A, Allaway NC (1958) An analysis of hospital neonatal mortality rates in New York State. AMA J Dis Child 95:240–44.
15. Budetti PP, McManus P (1982) Assessing the effectiveness of neonatal intensive care. Med Care 20:1027–39.
16. Budetti P, Barrand N, McManus P, Heinen LA (1981) The implications of cost-effectiveness analysis of medical technology: background paper 2; case study 10: the costs and effectiveness of neonatal intensive care. Office of Technology Assessment, Congress of the United States, Washington.
17. Bereson RA (1984) Intensive care units (ICUs): clinical outcomes, costs and decisionmaking. Health Technology Case Study 28. Office of Technology Assessment, Congress of the United States, Washington.
18. Doyle LW, Murton LJ, Kitchen WH (1989) Increasing the survival of extremely-immature (24- to 28-weeks' gestation) infants - at what cost? Med J Aust 150:558–568.
19. Kitchen WH, Doyle LW, Ford GW, et al (1991) Changing two-year outcome of infants weighing 500 to 999 grams at birth: a hospital study. J Pediatr 118:938–43.
20. Butt W, Shann F, Tibballs J, et al (1990) Long-term outcome of children after intensive care. Crit Care Med 18:961–965.
21. Boyle MH, Torrance GW, Sinclair JC, Horwood SP (1983) Economic evaluation of neonatal intensive care of very-low-birth-weight infants. N Engl J Med 308:1330–1337.
22. Bull C, Rigby ML, Shinebourne EA (1985) Should management of complete atrioventricular canal defect be influenced by co-existent Down syndrome? Lancet 1:1147–1149.
23. Chassin MR (1982) Costs and outcomes of medical intensive care. Med Care 20:165–179.
24. Castles I (1988) Year Book Australia. Australian Bureau of Statistics, Canberra.
25. Ruttimann UE, Albert A, Pollack MM, Glass NL (1986) Dynamic assessment of severity of illness in pediatric intensive care. Crit Care Med 14:215–221.
26. Pollack MM, Buttimann UE,Getson PR (1988) Pediatric risk of mortality (PRISM) score. Crit Care Med 16:1110–1116.
27. Balakrishnan G, Aitchison T, Hallworth D, Morton NS (1992) Prospective evaluation of the paediatric risk of mortality (PRISM) score. Arch Dis Child 67:196–200.
28. Gemke RJBJ, Bonsel GJ, van Vught JA (1994) Effectiveness and efficiency of a Dutch pediatric intensive care unit: validity and application of the pediatric risk of mortality score. Crit Care Med 22:1477–1484.
29. Goddard JM (1992) Pediatric risk of mortality socring overestimates severity of illness in infants. Crit Care Med 20:1662–1665.
30. Pollack MM, Getson PR, Ruttimann UE, et al (1987) Efficiency of intensive care. JAMA 258:1481–1486.
31. Klem SA, Pollack MM, Getson PR (1990) Cost, resource utilization, and severity of illness in intensive care. J Pediatr 116:231–237.
32. Stambouly JJ, Pollack MM, Ruttimann UE (1991) An objective method to evaluate rationing of pediatric intensive care beds. Intensive Care Med 17:154–158.
33. Pollack MM Alexander SR, Clarke N, Ruttimann UE, Tesselaar HM, Bachulis AC (1991) Improved outcomes from tertiary center pediatric intensive care: a statewide comparison of tertiary and nontertiary care facilities. Crit Care Med 19:150–159.
34. Edge WE, Kanter RK, Weigle CGM, Walsh RF (1994) Reduction of morbidity in interhospital transport by specialized pediatric staff. Crit Care Med 22:1186–1191.
35. Castella X, Artigas A, Bion J, Kari A (1995) A comparison of severity of illness scoring systems for intensive care unit patients: results of a multicenter, multinational study. Crit Care Med 23:1327–1335.
36. Flora JD (1978) A method for comparing survival of burn patients to a standard survival curve. J Trauma 18:701–705.
37. Gemke RJ (1994) Outcome assessment of pediatric intensive care: principles and applications. Gemke, Maarssen, 115–128.

38. Pollack MM, Guerdon TT, Patel KM, Ruttimann UE, Getson PR, Levetown M (1994) Impact of quality-of-care factors on pediatric intensive care unit mortality. JAMA 272:941–946.
39. Teres D (1991) Are we ready to regionalize pediatric intensive care? Crit Care Med 19:139–140.
40. Gemke RJBJ, Bonsel GJ (1995) Comparative assessment of pediatric intensive care: a national multicenter study. Crit Care Med 23:238–245.
41. Luft HS, Garnick DW, Mark DH, McPhee SJ (1990) Hospital volume, physician volume, and patient outcomes. Health Administration Press Perspectives, Ann Arbor.
42. Farley DE, Ozminkowski RJ (1992) Volume-outcome relationships and inhospital mortality: the effect of changes in volume over time. Med Care 30:77–94.
43. Thompson DR, Clemmer TP, Applefeld JJ, et al (1994) Regionalization of critical care medicine: task force report of the American College of Critical Care Medicine. Crit Care Med 22:1306–1313.
44. British Paediatric Association (1993) The care of critically ill children. British Paediatric Association, London.
45. National Health and Medical Research Council (1983) Management of seriously ill children in adult intensive care units. NH&MRC, Canberra.

Specialized Pediatric Interhospital Transfer

J. Britto, C. DeMunter, and P. Habibi

Introduction

Increasing medical technology and the need for specialized services has resulted in the delivery of pediatric intensive care in designated, centralized, regional units. Critically ill children managed in tertiary centre pediatric intensive care units (PICU) have improved outcomes when compared to children managed in non-tertiary care facilities [1]. The majority of children with life threatening conditions requiring intensive care are initially admitted to hospitals without pediatric intensive care facilities. If these children are to receive the benefits of pediatric intensive care they need to be transferred to a regional PICU.

Between October 1993 and January 1996 our specialized pediatric transfer team (SPTT) transferred 350 critically ill children to our PICU from referring hospitals in the south east of England. In this article, in addition to reviewing certain important aspects of pediatric transport medicine we have incorporated data based on 203 interhospital transfers by our SPTT.

Specialized and Nonspecialized Transport Teams

The transfer of an unstable, ill child is potentially hazardous. Besides the risk of deterioration from the primary illness there are the added risks of complications of therapy and secondary insults of the transfer process itself.

The interhospital transfer of critically ill children by personnel not trained in pediatric transport medicine (nonspecialized transfer teams) has been shown to be associated with unacceptable and largely preventable transfer related morbidity. In a study from Birmingham UK, 75% of 56 critically ill children transferred to a PICU by non-specialized referring hospital personnel, suffered serious clinical complications, 23% of which were considered life threatening [2, 3]. A study from the USA, by Kanter and Tompkins of 117 children transferred to a PICU by non-specialized referring hospital personnel, showed that 24 patients (21%) suffered physiological deterioration or equipment related adverse events during transfer [4].

There is strong evidence that teams trained in pediatric transport medicine (specialized pediatric transfer teams) can transfer critically ill children more safely than nonspecialized teams. In a study from Vancouver, Canada, Mcnab noted that 64 errors in management occurred in 34 transfers by untrained personnel compared to 25 errors in 96 transfers by personnel trained in pediatric transport [5]. Using the criteria of Kanter and Tompkins, a study in the USA by Edge et al comparing specialized (n = 47) and non-specialized (n = 92) pediatric transfers demonstrated that the SPTT significantly reduced the occurrence of equipment related adverse events (from 20% to 2%) but not the occurrence of physiological deterioration (12% to 11%) during transport [6]. Our own study evaluated the morbidity and severity of illness during the transfer of 51 critically ill children to our PICU by our SPTT. Using the same criteria we showed that physiological deterioration during transport occurred in 4% of patients and there were no instances of equipment related adverse events. Further, there was a significant decrease in the severity of illness measured by the PRISM score, in the majority of patients during stabilization and transport [7, 8].

On the basis of these studies the need for SPTTs to transfer critically ill children seems incontrovertible. The use of SPTTs has been recommended in several countries including the USA [9], Australia [10] and the UK [11].

Composition of the Transport Team

The composition of a SPTT is dictated by an accurate assessment of the nature and severity of illness of the child at the time of referral to the PICU and the anticipated need for major therapeutic interventions during stabilization prior to transport. The accuracy of information given on the telephone is usually dependent on the pediatric critical care experience of the observer and therefore is variable. In our experience, the use of a questionnaire in the form of a transfer log (Table 1) ensures that the right questions are asked and this can improve the accuracy of assessments over the telephone.

Although the pretransport PRISM score has been validated as an accurate predictor of hospital mortality it does not perform adequately as a triage tool in trying to decide transport team composition and the need for major therapeutic interventions during stabilization [12, 13, 14]. In the transport situation children with low PRISM scores remain at risk of morbidity and mortality and often need major therapeutic interventions prior to transport [13].

The problem of assessing severity of illness and the need for major therapeutic interventions on the telephone is compounded by the fact that the condition of the child could rapidly change at any stage of the transfer. Several studies have addressed the question of the need for a physician on transport teams and despite a lack of consensus the majority of SPTTs in the USA include a physician [15]. We believe that all interhospital transfers of critically ill children should be performed by a SPTT trained in pediatric transport medicine. Such a team should include a pediatric intensivist (attending physician or fellow) and an experienced pediatric intensive care nurse.

Table 1. The transfer log

Referring hospital and physician data	
Patient data	
Provisional diagnosis and reasons for transfer	
Brief history	
Patients initial clinical status at referring hospital	
Patients current clinical status at referring hospital	
Most recent investigations at referring hospital	
Recommendations:	Intubation & ventilation
	Colloid & crystalloid therapy
	Vasoactive drugs
	Sedatives & muscle relaxants
	Management of raised ICP & seizures
	Acid base, glucose & electrolytes
	Anti-infective agents
	Further investigations
Composition of SPTT:	Name of nurse
	Name of physician
Mode of transport	
Patient's clinical status at referring hospital assessed by SPTT	
Action taken by SPTT:	Endotracheal intubation/tube change
	Ventilatory support
	Central venous access
	Arterial access
	Bladder catheter
	Peritoneal dialysis/intercostal drain/others
	Colloid/crystalloid used
	Vasoactive drugs
	Metabolic corrections
	Anti-infective agents
Investigations/blood gases/ventilator settings during transfer	
Cardiorespiratory status and metabolic condition on arrival at PICU	
Problems/remarks during transfer	
OPERATIONAL DETAILS	
Time of initial referring phone call to the PICU	
Time transport nurse contacted	
Time transport physician contacted	
Time of departure of SPTT from the PICU	
Time of arrival of SPTT at the referring hospital	
Time of departure with patient from the referring hospital	
Time of arrival of patient at the PICU	
Distance travelled	

The Ethos of Mobile Intensive Care

The belief that a transport team should 'swoop and scoop' to get the patient back to the PICU as quickly as possible where intensive care is then initiated is no longer appropriate [16, 17]. The ethos of mobile intensive care implies that intensive care is established by the SPTT at the referring hospital. The level of therapy and monitoring that the child receives at the referring hospital during the period of stabilization and transport should be comparable to that received by the child had it been admitted directly to the PICU [18]. The need to anticipate and preempt clinical problems is more imperative during interhospital transfer than on a PICU. Major therapeutic interventions such as endotracheal intubation and vascular access, besides being hazardous are extremely difficult to accomplish within the confines of a moving ambulance or a helicopter.

In our series, the median stabilization time (interval from arrival of the SPTT at the referring hospital to departure from the referring hospital) was 165 minutes (Table 2). The mean stabilization time in other studies of SPTTs vary from 75 to 156 minutes [5, 18]. The major benefit of instituting intensive care at the referring hospital is that appropriate therapeutic interventions and monitoring by the SPTT, could lead not only to a decrease in the morbidity but also reduce the severity of illness during stabilization and transport [7].

Transfer of Trauma Patients

In a study by Sharples et al, 121 potentially avoidable factors that possibly or probably contributed to death were identified in 255 fatal head injuries in children [19]. 11 (9%) of these factors occurred during 68 interhospital transfers to a regional neurosurgical centre. 15 of these 68 children (22%) were described as being in a critical condition at the end of the transfer. The concept of the "golden hour" in trauma does not preclude appropriate stabilization of patients by a SPTT prior to transport. Studies on pretransport stabilization of trauma patients have shown improved outcomes in patients with a higher rate of therapeutic interventions such as endotracheal intubations, fluid resuscita-

Table 2. Operational time intervals

	Mobilization (a)	Journey out (b)	Response (c)	Stabilisation (d)	Journey in (e)	Extrication (f)
Median (min)	70	33	105	165	37	310
Range (min)	20–330	10–140	40–380	36–525	15–140	130–615

(a = Time from referral to departure of SPTT from PICU. b = Time from departure of SPTT from PICU to arrival at patient's bedside. c = Time from referral to arrival of SPTT at patient's bedside. d = Time from arrival of SPTT at the patient's bedside to departure of patient from the referring hospital. e = Time from departure of patient from referring hospital to arrival at tertiary centre. f = Time from referral to arrival of the patient at PICU)

tion, blood transfusions and thoracic decompressions [15, 16]. A child with a life threatening subdural/epidural hematoma or a penetrating injury of the chest or abdomen needs rapid transfer by a SPTT to a centre offering definitive surgery. A favorable outcome in such patients will ensue only if the ABC of pediatric resuscitation has been attended to. Depending on the clinical situation, appropriate pretransport stabilization in such children could include endotracheal intubation, controlled hyperventilation, the use of sedatives and muscle relaxants, osmotic diuretics, fluid and inotrope therapy.

Utilizing the Response Time

The time taken to deliver intensive care to the child awaiting transfer is crucial to patient outcome [20]. The median response time (interval from the initial referring phone call requesting transfer to the PICU until arrival of the SPTT at the referring hospital) for our urban based SPTT was 105 minutes (Table 2).

As a consequence of the inevitable length of the response time, the immediate institution of therapeutic measures by personnel at the referring hospital, while awaiting arrival of the SPTT, becomes crucial to patient outcome. It is therefore essential that the SPTT be involved in the patient's management from the time of the initial request for transfer. Depending on the clinical situation, this would include advice over the telephone regarding the airway, ventilatory support, fluid resuscitation, vasoactive therapy, correction of metabolic derangements, hematological support, anti-infective therapy, anti-convulsants, measures to control raised intracranial pressure (ICP), the need for further investigations and if appropriate, moving the child to a high dependency area/ adult ICU while awaiting the SPTT.

In order to facilitate initiation of intensive care at the referring hospital while the SPTT is being mobilized, requests from hospitals referring children for intensive care should be directed immediately to the pediatric intensivist at the tertiary centre designated to lead the SPTT. At the time of the initial phone call, clinical and laboratory data are recorded on the transfer log (Table 1). The transfer log accompanies the SPTT to enable documentation of morbidity, severity of illness and therapeutic interventions before, during and after stabilization and transport. Besides serving as a medico-legal document, the transfer log facilitates audit and research.

Equipment and Monitoring

The ethos of mobile intensive care implies that all the equipment essential for the resuscitation, stabilization and monitoring of a critically ill child needs to be carried by the SPTT. The referring hospital should not be relied upon to make up for deficiencies in equipment. Equipment should not only be dedicated for use on transfer but must meet the specific requirements of the transport environment.

We use a portable monitoring system that allows the following parameters to be monitored continuously and stored for subsequent printing and analysis: heart and respiratory rate, invasive and cuff blood pressure, central venous pressure, percutaneous oxygen saturation, end tidal CO2 and core and peripheral temperatures. In addition, urine output using a bladder catheter, neurological status including pupillary size and degree of muscle relaxation and blood sugars are also assessed periodically.

We believe tracheally intubated patients should be ventilated mechanically rather than manually. Portable mechanical ventilators (which function solely on pipe/cylinder oxygen) allows one to accurately set, deliver and measure peak inspiratory pressures and PEEP. In addition, minute volume, fractional inspired oxygen concentration, respiratory rate and disconnect / low pressure alarms can also be altered. New models of portable ventilators also offer variable inspiratory and expiratory times and synchronized intermittent mandatory ventilation or continuous positive airway pressure modes of ventilation. An oxygen cylinder (e.g., E size) to drive the portable ventilator with an attached flow meter capable of delivering upto 15 liters/min is a vital part of the SPTT's equipment. In the event of the transfer of an infant less than 5 Kg. we use a portable incubator (isolette) with a built-in time-cycled, pressure-limited ventilator. Battery powered syringe pumps capable of handling up to 50 ml syringes and of performing accurately at both slow rates (less than 1 ml/min) and fast rates (up to 99 ml/min) are indispensable on transfer. Useful warming devices on transfer include space blankets and chemical heat packs.

Communication in transit between the SPTT, the PICU and the referring hospital are vital. Cellular telephones are convenient but could interfere with electronics on board aircraft and in medical equipment.

Ground Versus Air Transport

The choice of the most appropriate mode of transport depends on the nature and severity of illness of the child (e.g., trauma needing definitive surgical management), the distance to and geographical location of the referring hospital (e.g., urban or rural based), the proximity of the referring and receiving hospitals to an helipad or an airport, weather and flying conditions and the number of personnel in the SPTT.

Ground ambulances are effective in transporting critical or unstable patients up to 50 km and stable patients upto 150 km [21]. The majority of tertiary centre PICUs are urban based and the obvious disadvantage of ground based transport is length of time spent on the road negotiating traffic congestion.

Helicopters are effective for transporting patients up to a 150 km radius and for distances greater than that fixed wing aircraft are preferred [21]. The absence of an helipad in close proximity to the hospital results in multiple transfers of the child between the referring hospital, ambulance, aircraft and PICU. Whichever mode of transport is used the most important consideration is the ability of the team travelling in the vehicle or aircraft to care for the child [17].

Familiarization with helicopter and fixed wing aircraft, training in aviation physiology and safety and the use of aircraft compatible monitoring equipment are essential for the safe and effective transfer of critically ill children by air.

Air Medical Physiology

Depending on the type of aircraft used changes in altitude, acceleration and deceleration forces, temperature, humidity, noise and vibration could have significant physiologic effects [22].

In fixed wing aircraft with increasing altitudes there is a decrease in the partial pressure of oxygen at the alveolus which could result in a fall in arterial oxygenation. The partial pressure of oxygen decreases by approximately 30% at an altitude of 7000 - 8000 feet. Patients with pulmonary problems and an increased alveolar-arterial gradient are at increased risk of developing hypoxia and will require increasing FiO2 with increasing altitude [22]. Children breathing spontaneously and requiring an FiO2 of 1 on the ground will require a change in ventilatory support prior to air transport [21]. The problems of hypoxia during air transport could be further compounded by a decrease in the hemoglobin and the oxygen carrying capacity of blood [22].

According to Boyle's law if temperature is constant, the volume of a gas varies inversely with the pressure. In fixed wing aircraft with increasing altitude, as the pressure of gas in a closed space decreases the volume increases (dysbarism). There are several important clinical implications of this phenomenon that need to be born in mind. The cuff on endotracheal tubes needs to be minimally inflated to allow for expansion. Small asymptomatic pneumothoraces or pneumatoceles at sea level could expand by approximately 30% at an altitude of 7000 - 8000 feet and therefore should be drained (and connected to Heimlich valves) prior to transport. Gastric distension and bowel gas should be treated prophylactically with gastric and rectal tubes. Air trapped in other closed spaces like the intracranial sinuses and ventricles (head injury) or bowel wall air (necrotizing enterocolitis) is likely to expand and cause morbidity at high altitudes.

Acceleration and deceleration forces could alter blood flow and cerebral perfusion during take off and landing in fixed wing aircraft. These factors need to be considered when transferring hemodynamically unstable patients and patients with raised ICP [21].

Airway and Ventilatory Intervention

Airway and ventilatory intervention is often the earliest and most important task the SPTT is called upon to perform. It is therefore mandatory for transport personnel to be skilled in airway management, ventilatory techniques, and the use sedatives and muscle relaxants.

Endotracheal Intubation

In keeping with the principles of pediatric resuscitation, the first priority of a SPTT on arrival at the referring hospital is assessment and management of the airway and breathing. Studies indicate that up to 43% of critically ill children require some form of airway management or respiratory support by the SPTT on arrival at the referring hospital [23]. In our series of 203 patients airway intervention by the SPTT was required in 129 (64%) patients.

173 (85%) patients transferred by our SPTT were endotracheally intubated and mechanically ventilated (Figure 1). In 65 (38%) of these patients rapid sequence tracheal intubation was performed by our SPTT immediately on arrival at the referring hospital. The indications for endotracheal intubation included shock [24], a Glasgow Coma Scale score of < 9 [25], and respiratory failure/ upper airway obstruction. Depending on the clinical situation, the drugs we use for rapid sequence tracheal intubations are a combination of anti-cholinergics (atropine), sedatives (thiopentone or ketamine) and muscle relaxants (suxamethonium or vecuronium). For tracheal intubation in the presence of upper airway obstruction we use the inhalational agent halothane.

Reintubation of the trachea by a SPTT is frequently necessary. In our series 64 (59%) of the patients that underwent endotracheal intubation by referring hospital physicians, were reintubated by the SPTT. The reasons for reintubation of the trachea include the need to replace an oral endotracheal tube for a

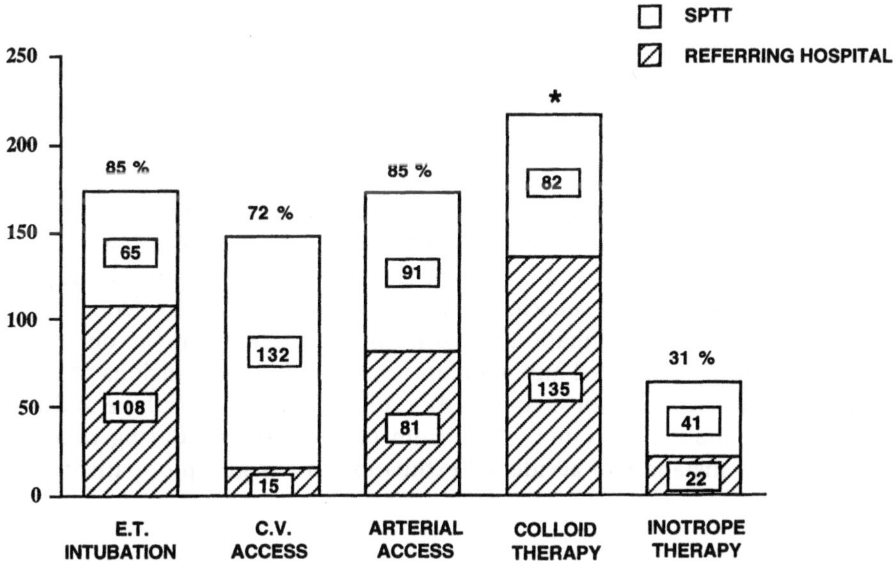

Fig. 1. Major therapeutic interventions by the referring hospital and the specialised pediatric transfer team (SPTT) in our series of 203 patients.
* Colloid therapy ≥ 20 ml/kg; 74 patients received this volume of colloid from both the referring hospital and the SPTT.
[ET = endotracheal, CV = central venous access].

nasal one (unless contraindicated) or to change to an endotracheal tube of a more appropriate diameter and/or length.

Route of Endotracheal Intubation

124 (72%) of the intubated patients in our series were transferred with nasotracheal tubes which were secured using a Tunstall connector. Although there are no published studies comparing the incidence of accidental extubation in children with orotracheal as opposed to nasotracheal tubes during pediatric transfer, it is generally considered that nasotracheal tubes are secured more easily and safely in children and are preferable for long term use [26]. It is our policy to change an oral endotracheal tube for a nasal one unless the patient is suspected to have a fracture of the cribriform plate with cerebrospinal fluid leak, has a nasal deformity or clinical evidence of a bleeding diathesis [27].

Endotracheal Tube Blockage

The incidence of endotracheal tube blockage has been reported at 8% for intubated patients during transfer by non-specialized pediatric teams [4]. To counter the effects of the cold dry gas that is used to ventilate patients during transfer, we perform frequent suction with saline and use an in-line thermal condenser with a humidifier filter. There was just one instance of endotracheal tube blockage in our series.

Accidental Extubation

The incidence of accidental extubation for all intubated pediatric patients has been reported to vary between 3% and 13% [26]. Inadequate sedation or muscle relaxants were implicated as common risk factors in these and the appropriate use of sedatives or muscle relaxants has been shown to decrease the incidence of accidental extubation [26, 28]. All intubated patients in our series were mechanically ventilated and maintained on continuous infusions of sedatives and analgesics (one, or a combination of: fentanyl or morphine and midazolam) and muscle relaxants (atracurium or vecuronium) during transfer. There were no instances of accidental extubation in our group of patients.

Ventilatory Intervention

In our series, the SPTT initiated mechanical ventilation in 42 (39%) of the patients already intubated by the referring hospital. In addition, controlled hyperventilation was used to treat raised ICP in 14%, we applied positive end expiratory pressure (PEEP) in 23% of patients and withdrew PEEP in 6% of patients with raised ICP and normal lungs.

Central Venous Access

Studies have shown that the incidence of loss or lack of intravenous access during transfer by nonspecialized teams to be as high as 10% [29]. We believe that central venous access should be obtained in any patient with established or potential hemodynamic instability especially in the context of transfer. Large bore (5 to 7 Fr) multi-lumen central venous catheters facilitate measurement of central venous pressure, rapid administration of colloid that is often not possible through peripheral venous lines [30], administration of vasoactive drugs and hypertonic or irritant solutions (bicarbonate / potassium /calcium) into the central circulation, and safe, sutured and secure venous access for the administration of multiple infusions i.e., dextrose, sedation and muscle relaxants.

There were no instances of loss of intravenous access in our study. Central venous catheters were inserted in 147 (72%) patients in our series (Figure 1). In the majority of instances we catheterize either the subclavian or internal jugular veins. Catheterization of the subclavian vein should be avoided in the presence of a bleeding diathesis.

Direct Blood Pressure Monitoring

In all critically ill, ventilated and/or hemodynamically unstable patients, mean, systolic and diastolic blood pressures should be monitored directly by pressure transduction of an indwelling intraarterial catheter as well as indirectly by oscillometry. Besides facilitating repeated steady state blood sampling, direct blood pressure monitoring also provides a continuous pulse-pressure wave form and an alternative source for measurement of the heart rate. Direct monitoring of heart rate and blood pressure during transfer is more accurate, reliable and practical than palpatory and auscultatory methods [31]. 172 (85%) patients underwent intra-arterial catheterization and direct blood pressure monitoring and none had any complication (Figure 1).

Colloid Therapy, Inotropic Support and Metabolic Correction

The aim of treatment of shock states in children is to optimize the perfusion of critical vascular beds and to prevent or correct metabolic abnormalities arising from cellular hypoperfusion [32]. To this end, besides airway and ventilatory intervention and achieving vascular access, among other major therapeutic measures that a SPTT will undertake are fluid resuscitation, institution or modification of vasoactive drug therapy and correction of metabolic derangements.

In our series, half of the patients suffered from meningococcal or other forms of septic shock and therefore colloid and inotrope therapy and correction of metabolic derangements were required in many of them. 82 (40%) received ≥20 ml/kg of colloid from the SPTT and in 41 (20%) patients a vasoactive drug was started by the SPTT (Figure 1). During stabilization and transport low plasma levels of potassium, bicarbonate and calcium were corrected in 71 (35%), 46 (23%) and 44 (22%) patients respectively by the SPTT.

Intrahospital Transfers

Critically ill children frequently need to be moved from one location in the hospital to another. This could include transfers from a general ward or the emergency room to the PICU or two way transfers from the PICU to a nonportable diagnostic facility or the operating theatre.

Intrahospital transfers can be associated with a surprisingly high incidence of serious transport related adverse events. In a recent study on intrahospital transfer of critically ill children, Wallen et al showed significant physiological deterioration in up to 72% of children and equipment related mishaps in up to 19% of children. Fourteen percent of children needed at least one major therapeutic intervention during transfer [33]. Studies such as this suggest that prior to every intrahospital transfer the benefits of the planned diagnostic test or surgery need to be weighed against the potential risks of the transfer.

If the morbidity during intrahospital transfers is to be minimized then the ethos of mobile intensive care needs to be extended to transfers within the hospital, however short the distance. The principles, philosophy, personnel and equipment that make up the interhospital SPTT, place the latter in an ideal situation to perform transfers within the hospital.

Conclusions

Critically ill children can be transferred by a SPTT with minimal transport related morbidity, mortality and with a decrease in the severity of illness. Involvement by a SPTT in the management of a critically ill child should begin at the time of the initial request for transfer. Throughout the transfer process the aim is to achieve a level of therapy and monitoring comparable to that of a PICU. The ethos of mobile intensive care should lead to a decrease in the eventual PICU morbidity and mortality.

Acknowledgement: We are grateful to the George John Livanos charitable trust for supporting of our research in pediatric transport medicine.

References

1. Pollack MM, Alexander SR, Clark N, Ruttimann UE, Tesselaar HM, Bachulis AC (1991) Improved outcomes from tertiary centre pediatric intensive care: a statewide comparison of tertiary and nontertiary care facilities. Crit Care Med 19:150–159
2. Barry PW, Ralston C (1994) Adverse events occurring during interhospital transfer of the critically ill. Arch Dis Child 71:8–11.
3. Britto J, Nadel S, Habibi P, Levin M (1994) Adverse events occurring during interhospital transfer of the critically ill. Arch Dis Child 71:559.
4. Kanter RK, Tompkins JM (1989) Adverse events during interhospital transport: Physiological deterioration associated with pretransport severity of illness. Pediatrics 84:43–48.
5. Macnab A (1991) Optimal escort for interhospital transport of pediatric emergencies. J Trauma 31:205–209.
6. Edge WE, Kanter RK, Weigle CGM, Walsh RF (1994) Reduction of morbidity in interhospital transport by specialized pediatric staff. Crit Care Med 22: 1186–1191.
7. Britto J, Nadel S, Machonochie I, Levin M, Habibi P (1995) Morbidity and severity of illness during interhospital transport: Impact of a specialized paediatric retrieval team. BMJ 311:836–839.
8. Britto J, Nadel S, Machonochie I, Levin M, Habibi P (1996) Impact of specialized paediatric retrieval teams. BMJ 312:121.
9. McCloskey KA (1995) Transport team training. In: McCloskey KA, Orr RA (ed) Pediatric transport medicine. Mosby Year Book Company, St. Louis, pp 100–107.
10. Shann F (1995) Should there be specialist paediatric transport services? NHS Centre for Review and Dissemination. Which way forward for care of critically ill children ? (CRD report No.1) University of York, York pp 49–50.
11. Transfer of critically ill children (1993) British Paediatric Association. The Care of Critically Ill Children. Report of the multidisciplinary working party on intensive care. British Paediatric Association. London, pp 62–65.
12. Pollack MM (1994) Pediatric transport research: It is improving (finally). Crit Care Med 22:1073–1074.
13. Orr RA, Venkataraman ST, Cinoman MI, Hogue BL, Singleton CA, McCloskey KA (1994) Pretransport pediatric risk of mortality (PRISM) score underestimates the requirement for intensive care or major interventions during interhospital transport. Crit Care Med 22:101–107.
14. Britto J, Nadel S, Habibi P, Levin M (1994) Pediatric risk of mortality score underestimates the requirement for intensive care during interhospital transport. Crit Care Med 22:2029–2030.
15. Ramsey CB, Holbrook PR (1993) Pediatric critical care transport. In: Holbrook PR (ed) Textbook of Pediatric Critical Care. Saunders. Philadelphia, pp 1108–1116.
16. Krug SE (1995) Principles and philosophy of transport stabilization. In: McCloskey KA, Orr RA (ed) Pediatric transport medicine. Mosby Year Book Company, St. Louis, pp 132–142.
17. Orr RA, McCloskey KA, Britten AG (1992) Transportation of critically ill children. In: Rogers MC (ed) Textbook of Pediatric Intensive Care. Williams & Wilkins. Baltimore, pp 1571–1587.
18. Whitfield JM, Buser MK (1993) Transport stabilization times for neonatal and pediatric patients prior to interfacility transfer. Pediatr Emerg Care 9:69–71.
19. Sharples PM, Storey A, Aynsley-Green A, Eyre JA (1990) Avoidable factors contributing to the death in children with head injury. BMJ 300:87–91.
20. Black RA, Mayer T, Walker ML, et al (1982) Air transport of pediatric emergency cases. N Engl J Med 307:1465–1468.
21. Brink LW, Neuman B, Wynn J (1993) Air transport. Pediatr Clin North Am 40:439–456.
22. Ackerman N (1995) Aeromedical physiology. In: McCloskey KA, Orr RA (ed) Pediatric transport medicine. Mosby Year Book Company, St. Louis, pp 143–157.
23. Fuller J, Frewen T, Lee R (1991) Acute airway management in the critically ill child requiring transport. Can J Anaesth 38:252–254.

24. Hussain SNA, Roussos C (1985) Distribution of respiratory muscle and organ blood flow during endotoxic shock in dogs. J Appl Physiol 59: 1802–1808.
25. Vera FT, Dean MJ, Hanley DF (1992) Evaluation of the comatose child. In: Rogers MC (ed) Textbook of Pediatric Intensive Care. Williams & Wilkins. Baltimore, pp 733–750.
26. Rivera R, Tibbals J (1992): Complications of endotracheal intubation and mechanical ventilation in infants and children. Crit Care Med 20: 193–199.
27. Backofen JE, Rogers MC (1992) Emergency management of the airway. In: Rogers MC (ed) Textbook of Pediatric Intensive Care. Williams & Wilkins. Baltimore, pp 52–74.
28. Scott PH, Eigen H, Moye LA, Georgitis J, Laughin JJ (1985) Predictability and consequences of spontaneous extubation in a pediatric ICU. Crit Care Med 13: 228–232.
29. Henning R (1992) Emergency transport of critically ill children: stabilization before departure. Med J Australia 156: 117–124.
30. Rosen KR, Rosen DA (1986) Comparative flow rates for small bore peripheral intravenous catheters. Pediatr Emerg Care 2: 153–156.
31. Runcie CJ, Reeve W, Reidy J, Dougall JR (1990) A comparison of measurements of blood pressure, heart rate and oxygenation during interhospital transport of the critically ill. Intens Care Med 16: 317–322.
32. Wetzel RC, Tobin JR (1992) Shock. In: Rogers MC (ed) Textbook of Pediatric Intensive Care. Williams & Wilkins. Baltimore, pp 563–613.
33. Wallen E, Venkataraman ST, Grosso MJ, Kiene K, Orr RA (1995) Intrahospital transport of critically ill pediatric patients. Crit Care Med 23: 1588–1595.

The Nursing Mutual Participation Model of Care

M. A .Q. Curley

Introduction

Family-centered care is considered "best practice" in most pediatric health care settings. Family-centered care is a philosophy of care that recognizes, respects, and supports the essential role of the family in the lives of children [1]. It is a philosophy that acknowledges and supports diversity among families - diversity that encompasses varied family structures and sociocultural backgrounds, family goals and priorities, strategies and actions, as well as diversity in family support, service, and informational needs [2]. Family-centered care strives to support families in their natural caregiving roles by building upon their unique strengths as individuals and as families. It is a philosophy that views parents and professionals as equals in a partnership committed to excellence at all levels of health care [1].

While pediatric nurses have long recognized the fundamental importance of caring for children within a family context, operationalizing family-centered care in the pediatric intensive care unit (PICU) is less clear, and often based on intuition and untested assumptions with few empirical guidelines [3, 4]. Nurses tend to intervene in a similar manner with all families whose needs are perceived to be essentially the same [5]. This is problematic because there is significant variability in family perceptions and experiences, stress levels, and needs that require individualized intervention. What may be helpful to one parent may not be helpful, or even useful, to another parent even within the same family.

Researchers have noted the incongruence between nurses' understanding of parental needs and parents' own understanding [6]. Indeed, additional parental stress may result from this mismatch [7]. At times, particularly in PICU settings, parents are considered "visitors" to their own children forcing temporary and perhaps permanent disruption in the parent-child relationship. Parental needs, their role with their critically ill child, and the basis for establishing therapeutic nurse-parent relationships are aspects of family-centered care that continue to present challenges to pediatric critical care nurses.

The Nursing Mutual Participation Model of Care (NMPMC) articulates family-centered care within pediatric acute care settings and provides a framework for supportive, psychosocial interventions intended to help parents of critically ill children alleviate their own levels of stress and cope with their child's critical illness. This article will present the major tenets of the NMPMC, review applications of the model within the PICU setting, discuss the strengths and limitations of the model, present several propositions of the model for further study, critically analyze the model, and suggest several methods for studying the model.

Overview of the Nursing Mutual Participation Model of Care

Szasz and Hollender [8] first described a "mutual participation" model of interaction for use with chronically ill adults. The model, fundamentally different from others practiced at the time, was based on the premise that the health care provider could not know what might be best for an individual. The search for what might be considered individually helpful was the essence of the therapeutic interaction. The individual was assisted to help themself as their own experiences and beliefs provided reliable and important clues to therapy.

Table 1. Nursing mutual participation model of care

Clarifying the Parental Role – Admission
Extend our care to include parents
Acknowledge their importance

Strengthen Parental Involvement – Daily Bedside Contact
Enabling strategies that provide parents with system savvy
1. Provide Information – instruct & clarify
2. Anticipatory guidance – illness trajectory
3. Provide pragmatic resources

Facilitate transition to "parent-of-a-critically-ill-child"
1. Enhance unique connectedness
2. Role model interactions
3. Invite participation in nurturant activity
4. Provide options during procedures

Communication Pattern
1. Establish a caring relationship with the parent
   How are you doing today?
2. Assess parental perception of the child's illness
   How does s/he look to you today?
3. Determine parental goals, objectives, and expectations
   What troubles you most?
4. Seek informed suggestions and preferences, and invite participation in care
   How can I help you today?

Data from:

Curley MAQ (1988). Effects of the nursing mutual participation model of care and parental stress in the pediatric intensive care unit. Heart & Lung 17(6,1); 682–688

Curley MAQ & Wallace J (1992) Effects of the nursing mutual participation model of care on parental stress in the pediatric intensive care unit – A replication. Journal of Pediatric Nursing 7(6); 377–385

In 1980, Brody [9] operationalized Szasz and Hollender's [8] mutual participation model into a four-step process for use with adults in outpatient settings. The foundation of the intervention was conceptualized as agenda seeking – the patient was enlisted and invited into the health care decision-making process by asking: How can I help you today?

Curley [10] adapted the model for use with parents of critically ill children as it provided a philosophical foundation for family-centered care within the acute care environment and accommodated the numerous interventions intended to decrease parental stress recommended from descriptive nursing research.

The model is congruent with Hill's [11] ABCX and McCubbin and Patterson's [12] double ABCX model of crises in that the individualized nature of PICU-related stress is acknowledged and in turn drives individualized nursing interventions. The model is based on the premise that nurses have something of value to offer parents, but also acknowledges that parents have something of value to contribute to themselves, the caregiving process, and to their children. Nurses, through their expertise, know what might be helpful to a population of parents of critically ill children, but they cannot specifically know what is best for an individual parent. Parents, on the other hand, know what might be helpful to them and their child, but are usually unfamiliar with the experience of critical illness within an acute care setting.

The NMPMC provides a framework for individualized interactions that seek to clarify a parental role in the PICU setting and strengthen the parent's confidence in performing their role in the foreign setting. The process is individually determined and evolves to meet the expressed needs of each parent. The goal of the nurse-parent relationship is to achieve mutuality – defined as a synchronous, co-constituting relationship that stimulates the process of personal becoming.

Clarifying the Parental Role

Admission is a very stressful time for parents during which they experience significant loss of control [13, 14]. Acknowledging the parent's valuable and irreplaceable role during this critical period helps to set the expectations for the entire PICU hospitalization. For example, saying "We believe parents to be very important to their children, especially when they're sick. We would like to work with you to help you find ways that you can continue to be important to your child while in the PICU." These words broaden the perspective of care to include parents. Right from the start, parents are invited as partners into the caregiving process which establishes an atmosphere in which parents feel that their contributions are essential.

If parent-child separation is necessary, parents are asked as to their preference about the level and frequency of nursing updates. If prolonged periods of separation are unavoidable, opportunities to provide parents with brief visits between procedures are sought. After any period of separation or change in their child's appearance and/or behavior, parents are prepared for the new experience. Given the high levels of parental stress, it is anticipated that information may need to be repeated or reframed at frequent intervals.

Strengthen Parental Involvement

After acknowledging the importance of the parental role, the NMPMC provides a framework for interventions that are supportive to and guided by the perceived individual needs of each parent. The model incorporates enabling strategies to equip parents with health care system savvy, helps the parent's transition to "parent-of-a-critically-ill-child," and delineates a consistent nurse-parent communication pattern.

Enabling Strategies that Provide Parents with System Savvy

Socializing parents to the PICU and hospital system, especially providing information that they need to cognitively appraise the situation will serve to empower them.

Provide Information that Instructs and Clarifies

Besides information about the child's illness and milieu (monitors, catheters, endotracheal tubes, etc.) specific information about changes in their child's appearance, behavior, and emotional reactions is essential. After addressing these immediate needs, parents require an understanding of the PICU and hospital environment. The process of how parents gain access to their child is particularly important as well as information about the units' routine, for example, who is in charge of their child's medical and nursing care and when and where to expect information. Only after sharing information about their child, providing information about the hospital environment, and answering any questions the parents might have, should dialogue progress to alterations in parental role and responsibility.

Provide Anticipatory Guidance About the Illness Trajectory

Uncertainty, that is, ambiguity and unpredictability over various aspects of the illness or outcome can be extremely stress provoking for parents [15–17]. Information about what parents will see or experience can be shared in an anticipatory manner. Describing the illness trajectory, and what can be reasonably predicted, is extremely helpful as it allows parents to understand and distinguish what is "normal and expected" from what is "life-threatening."

Provide Pragmatic Resources

Provision of adequate resources is necessary so that parents can maintain both physical and emotional accessibility to their child 24 hours/day. Necessary resources include sleep facilities, showers, telephones, nutritious food, transportation, and parking [18]. Physical barriers to the welcoming process, including activities that make parents feel like visitors to their own child are eliminated.

Facilitate Transition to Parent-of-a-Critically-Ill-Child

Alterations in parental role, and the subsequent disruption in the parent-child relationship are consistently identified as the most stressful aspect of the PICU environment [19–22]. Helping parents to formulate a role that they find personally comfortable and supporting them in their decision-making capacity helps parents successfully transition into their new role of parent-of–a-critically-ill-child.

Enhance Parent-Child Unique Connectedness

Due to changes in their child's appearance and behavior, parents may need help reconnecting to their child who appears so different. Strategies include finding at least one of the child's characteristics that has not changed, that is, some enduring feature and noting it to parents. Examples might include hair or eye color, or evidence of the child's increased heart rate in response to the parent's voice. Creativity is sometimes needed to help reestablish the unique parent-child connection when significant disfigurement is present.

Parents are encouraged to bring in their child's favorite blanket, toy, doll, or family pictures to comfort the child and individualize their bedspaces. These reminders of life at home provide nonverbal cues of the valued nature of the family, and are as important as direct communication.

Role Model Interactions

Parents have reported that their initial fears are lessened by observing and modeling nursing care activities [10]. Parents notice and sort nursing activities into two categories: what is familiar activity and what is different activity [21]. Acknowledging that one's nursing care activity is being observed (not to assure correctness as there is usually no basis for that distinction) provides an opportunity for the nurse to role model care through nonverbal communication. Parents may need "permission" to, and demonstrations of how to touch and interact with their critically ill child. Rubin's [23] maternal touch progression, for example, can be demonstrated in the PICU regardless of the age of the child.

Invite Participation in Nurturing Activity

Following the initial period of disorganization, [24] parents are usually readily able to identify activities that they wish participate in [25]. When offered options and opportunity, parents do provide care in an effort to renew their self-esteem and feel instrumental in their child's recovery. Suggesting ways parents can help their child cope will help to reduce parental anxiety [26]. Ideally, there are special aspects of parental care and comfort that can be distinguished from things that others can do for the child (e.g., provide breastmilk, voice, touch). Options include diversional, nurturing, comforting, caregiving, and monitoring activities.

Provide Options During Procedures

Considering that parental presence during procedures can potentially support a child's coping efforts and provide the child with a familiar source of comfort, [27, 28] parents are offered a choice regarding their presence and/or participation in PICU procedures. To be supportive parents need to know why the procedure is important, what to expect during the procedure, what normal age-related reactions might occur, and how they can best help. Parents are not placed in a position of restraining their child. Traditionally, forced separations, sometimes lasting hours, and related conflicts in values about the approaches used to obtain a child's cooperation have been a significant source of stress for parents [29].

Communication Pattern

With the goal of achieving mutuality, the NMPMC delineates a communication process that is helpful and displays caring toward the parent, assesses parental perceptions, determines the parental agenda, and invites participation in care. This communication process is congruent with the ABCX model of crisis in that parent's perception of the stressful event serves as an important guide to therapy. This communication strategy is helpful in the PICU as interventions can be specifically focused when time is limited. Also, when help is rationally directed and purposefully focused at the right time, it will be perceived as more effective than more help given at a period of less emotional accessibility.

Establish a Caring Relationship with the Parent

Dialogue is established with parents to convey a sense of care, warmth, and empathy. For example, asking "How are you doing? How are you holding up? Were you able to sleep?" extends the focus of care to include parents and communicates the message that parents, too, are important.

Assess Parental Perception of the Child's Illness

Parental responses to the PICU admission of their child cannot be predicted by objective measures of the child's severity of illness [30]. To assess parental perception of illness severity the parent is asked directly: "How does your child look to you today? Does s/he look more comfortable to you today than yesterday?" The nurse builds trust by clarifying misconceptions and providing accurate, concise, and complete information. Also, nurses often make assessments and judgments about a child's pain, activity, and behavior based upon experience, but unfamiliarity with an individual child. Parents are often well aware of their child's subtle behavioral and communicative cues that can be helpful in individualizing care. Nurses and parents working together can better understand an address the child's needs.

Determine Parental Goals, Objectives, and Expectations

The third step helps parents to prioritize their concerns. It also sanctions the expression of feelings that parents might otherwise consider inappropriate to express. Here, the nurse may ask "What troubles you most? Do you have any questions? Is this what you expected?" Interventions are then focused on parent specific issues rather than nurse speculated problems. Failure to address a parent's agenda may lead to an increase in stress and parental dissatisfaction.

Seek Suggestions and Preferences and Invite Participation in Care

The last step invites parental participation in caregiving activities. Here, the nurse may ask: "How can I help you? How can we do this together? Do you have any suggestions or preferences concerning the care your child is receiving? Is there anything that you personally want to do for your child?"

Clinical Applications

The effects of the NMPMC in helping parents alleviate their stress have been supported in three separate nursing research studies. In the first study, [10] the principal investigator, functioning in the role of a clinical nurse specialist implemented the model. Parents reported significantly less overall stress in the areas of child's behavior and emotions, parental role revision, child's procedures, and nursing communication and behavior. The second study replicated and supported the results of the first study [31]. In the third study, [32] primary nurses implemented the model. Parents who had the intervention reported significantly less stress associated with the hospitalization, particularly in the area of parental role alteration.

Advantages and Limitations of the NMPMC

Providing a humanistic PICU environment that recognizes parents as unique autonomous individuals who, when supported, are capable of providing vital elements of care to their critically ill child will help to alleviate parental stress. The effectiveness of the NMPMC in helping to decrease parental stress is related to its instrumentality in helping parents to formulate a role that is individually comfortable and supportive of them in their decision-making capacity. Not all parents will have the desire or capacity to actively participate in the care of their child, however, the NMPMC provides a means to assess and to individualize psychosocial interventions. Limitations of the model include the potential inconsistency in practice that may result when the model is implemented in a unit/hospital that does not fully support family-centered care. Furthermore, parental confusion and potentially additional stress may result when parents are subjected to various individuals practicing the NMPMC in an inconsistent manner.

Propositions for Study

- A child's PICU admission is stressful for parents.
- The individualized nature of PICU-related parental stress requires individualized nursing assessment and intervention.
- Nurses, through their expertise, know what is generally helpful to a population of parents of critically ill children but cannot specifically know what is best for an individual parent.
- Parents, through their experience, can contribute to the caregiving process and help their children cope with the PICU experience.
- Parental competence as parent-to-a-critically-ill-child will result from providing a role for parents and strengthen the parent's confidence in performing their role in the PICU setting.
- Parental stress related to alterations in parental role is inversely related to parental competence as parent-to-a-critically-ill-child.
- The degree of mutuality achieved within the nurse-parent relationship will have a direct and positive impact on patients' outcome, parent satisfaction, and nurse satisfaction.

Critical Analysis of the NMPMC

The Nursing Mutual Participation Model of Care is a practice theory because its scope is narrow, its concepts specific and concrete, and it can be directly applied to the clinical setting. According to Walker and Avant, [33] "The essence of practice theory is a desired goal and prescriptions for action to achieve the goal" (p. 12).

All four metaparadigm concepts: person, environment, health, and nursing, [34] are discussed within the NMPMC. Parents are considered unique autonomous individuals who are valued as equal participants in their child's care. The PICU environment is considered potentially stressful to parents. Health is seen as an optimal level of stress that enhances parents' ability to function within the PICU setting. Nurse-parent relationships are characterized as mutually empowering and helpful. Addressing the metaparadign propositions identified by Donaldson and Crowley, [35] the NMPMC deals with the life process of parent-to-a-critically-ill-child, the pattern of human behavior which results from parent interaction within the PICU environment, and the mutuality that can exist within nurse-parent relationships to affect a positive outcome.

Curley [10] developed the NMPMC in an effort to delineate several measurable outcomes of family-centered care within the PICU setting. The philosophical origins of the NMPMC were deduced from the Association of Care of Children's Health family-centered care framework [1] and the mutual participation model as first described by Szasz and Hollender [8] and further articulated by Brody [9]. Hill's [11] ABCX and McCubbin and Patterson's [12] double ABCX models of crisis informed the assessment strategy and communication framework. The interventions intended to clarify the parental role and strengthen the parent's confidence in performing their role in the PICU setting were inductively generated from many similar recommendations from descriptive nursing research on parental stress in the PICU, most notably, Jay [21], Miles and Carter [36], Jay's [21] work is based upon Rubin's [23] attainment of maternal role theory whereas Miles and Carter's work is based on Selye's theory of stress [37] and Roy's adaptation model [38].

The NMPMC has been supported in three separate nursing research studies to help decrease parental stress related to the PICU environment. Curley's [10] first study delineated and tested the communication framework. Curley and Wallace's [32] second research study added specific interventions intended to strengthen the parental role within the PICU setting. Although the critical features of the model have always included "equal status parent–professional relationships, mutual interdependency, and mutual satisfaction between nurses and parents" [10] (p. 683), the concept of "mutuality" is new to the model.

The meaning or language used within the NMPMC is clinically based. Concepts are clearly defined, internally consistent, and interrelated. The concept of parent-of-a-critically-ill-child is not new and builds upon previous research [21]. Parental stress is defined as stress unique to the pediatric intensive care setting and potentially within nursing's role to manipulate. Miles and Carter [36] delineated seven dimensions of the PICU environment that parents find stressful. These dimensions, derived from observational data, parent and staff nurse interviews, and the literature, form the basis of the PSS:PICU or the Parental Stressor Scale: Pediatric Intensive Care Unit [39]. All three research studies that supported the NMPMC used the PSS:PICU to measure PICU related parental stress. The concept of mutuality has been recently explicated and is congruent with the care literature [40, 41].

The NMPMC propositional statements are clear. Several statements have been supported by nursing research. Hypothesis can be generated from each propositional statement. Considering this, the NMPMC can be empirically tested to support its validity.

There is logical adequacy within the model. Intuitively the NMPMC makes sense and has been effective in decreasing parental stress within the PICU setting. The NMPMC is very useful for both novice and advanced practitioners within the critical care setting as it contributes to our understanding of the parent's experience of their child's critical illness. Novice staff appreciate the structure contained within the communication pattern. Expert nurses appreciate the framework for nursing interventions focused to optimize the parental role. Nurse educators find the videotape on the NMPMC [42] helpful in teaching staff about family-centered care in acute care settings. The NMPMC is relevant to nurse administrators in planning parent facilities. Although the NMPMC was constructed with a narrow focus, the basic principles of the model have broad application to other pediatric care settings. Further dissemination is unadvisable until the NMPMC has been supported outside the PICU.

Currently the model seems too parsimonious. Further work is necessary to explicate the phenomena and the short and long-term effects of family-centered care within acute care settings.

Further Questions for Study

Continued nursing research is needed to describe the possible differences in the utility of the NMPMC according to the changing demographics of parents, nurses, and health care system. The effects of the NMPMC may be different for parents of acute and chronically ill children. The NMPMC has only been tested in predominately white middle class Americans. Further testing is required in culturally diverse populations. Studies investigating the relationship between nursing staff attitudes toward parental involvement and participation in care is also needed. Adding to the science of family-centered care are studies specifically describing clinical situations that illuminate how parental involvement in their child's care in the PICU setting impacts child's recovery [43–45]. Finally, the long-term effects of parental involvement in PICU hospitalization on parents and children have yet to be investigated.

Conclusions

It is simply impossible to care for a child without caring for them in the context of their family. Intensive care hospitalization has traditionally violated the parents' usual role in caring for and protecting their child that may be experienced by parents as displacement, enforced passivity, and profound helplessness. The crisis inherent in hospitalization can severely impair parental sense of confidence and control, thereby compromising parental coping and performance. Helping parents to reduce their own levels of stress into the moderate range will enable parents to better fulfill their natural parenting role that can be therapeutically used at the bedside.

Nursing care must be inherently supportive to parents. Parental involvement must be encouraged and welcomed as family-centered care implies a partnership, not merely that 24-hour visitation is allowed. We must continue to accept the challenge of developing strategies that assess parental needs, establish therapeutic nurse-parent relationships, provide care that is flexible and individualized, and support the parents' role in the care of their critically ill child. Nurses can make a significant difference for parents of critically ill children. By providing care that is inherently supportive to parents nurses help to make the experience of "parent-to-a-critically-ill-child" tolerable.

References

1. Shelton TL, Jeppson ES, Johnson BH (1987) Family centered care for children with special health care needs. 2nd ed. Washington, DC: Association for the Care of Children's Health.
2. Ahmann E (1994) Family-centered care: The time has come. Pediatric Nursing 20:52–53.
3. Meyer EC, Bailey DB (1993) Family-centered care in early intervention: Community and hospital settings. In: Simeonsson JL & RJ (eds) Children with special needs: Family, culture, and society. New York: Harcourt Brace Jovanovich College Publishers.
4. Rushton CH (1990) Family-centered care in the critical care setting: Myth or reality? Children's Health Care 19:68–78.
5. Jacono J, Hicks G, Antonioni C, O'Brien K, Rasi M. (1990) Comparison of perceived needs of family members between registered nurses and family members of critically ill patients in intensive care and neonatal intensive care unit. Heart & Lung 19:72–78.
6. Johnson PA, Nelson GL, Brunnquell DJ (1988) Parent and nurse perceptions of parental stress in the pediatric intensive care unit. Child's Health Care 17:98–105.
7. Hayes VE, Knox JE (1984) The experience of stress in parents of children hospitalized with long-term disabilities. Journal of Advanced Nursing 9:333–341.
8. Szasz TS, Hollender MH (1956) A contribution to the philosophy of medicine. Archives of Internal Medicine 97:585–592.
9. Brody DS (1980) The patient's role in clinical decision making. Annals of Internal Medicine 93:718–722.
10. Curley MAQ (1988) Effects of the nursing mutual participation model of care and parental stress in the pediatric intensive care unit. Heart & Lung 17:682–688.
11. Hill R (1949) Families under stress. New York: Harper and Row.
12. McCubbin HI, Patterson JM (1983) Family transitions: Adaptation to stress. In McCubbin HI and Figley CR (eds) Stress and the Family: I Coping with Normative Transitions. Volume 1 (pp. 5–25). New York: Brunner/Mazel.
13. Skipper JK, Leonard RC (1968) Children, stress, and hospitalization. Journal of Health and Social Behavior 9:275–287.
14. Wolfer JA, Visintainer MA (1975) Pediatric surgical patients' and parents' stress responses and adjustment. Nursing Research 24:244–255.
15. Comoroff J, Maguire P (1981) Ambiguity and the search for meaning: Childhood leukaemia in the modern clinical context. Social Science Medicine 15B:115–123.
16. Mishel MH (1983) Parent's perception of uncertainty concerning their hospitalized child. Nursing Research 32:324–330.

17. Turner MA, Tomlinson PS, Harbaugh BL (1990) Parental uncertainty in critical care hospitalization of children. Maternal-Child Nursing Journal 19:45–62.
18. Fisher DH, Stanford G, Dorman DJ (1984) Services for parental stress reduction in a pediatric ICU. Critical Care Medicine 12:504–507.
19. Carter MC, Miles MS, Buford TH, Hassanein RS (1985) Parental environmental stress in pediatric intensive care units. Dimensions of Critical Care Nursing 4:180–188.
20. Eberly TW, Miles MS, Carter MC, Hennessey J, Riddle I (1985) Parental stress after the unexpected admission of a child to the intensive care unit. CCQ: Critical Care Quarterly 8:57–65.
21. Jay SS (1977) Pediatric intensive care involving parents in the care of their child. Maternal Child Nursing Journal 6:195–204.
22. Miles MS, Carter MC, Spicher C, Hassanein RS (1984) Maternal and paternal stress reactions when a child is hospitalized in a pediatric intensive care unit. Issues in Comprehensive Pediatric Nursing 7:333–342.
23. Rubin Reva. (1967) Attainment of maternal role: Parts I and II. Nursing Research 16:83–91:342–346.
24. Rothstein P (1980) Psychological stress in families of children in the pediatric intensive care unit. Pediatric Clinics of North America 27:613–620.
25. Kirschbaum MS (1990) Needs of parents of critically ill children. Dimensions of Critical Care Nursing 9:344–352.
26. Vulcan BM, Nikulich-Barrett M (1988) The effect of selected information on mothers' anxiety levels during their children's hospitalization. Journal of Pediatric Nursing 3:97–102.
27. Shaw EG, Routh DK (1982) Effect of mother's presence on children's reactions to aversive procedures. Journal of Pediatric Psychology 7:33–42.
28. Sevedra M. Parental responses to a painful procedure performed on their child (1981) In Azarnoff P, Hardgrove C (eds) The Family in Child Health Care. New York: John Wiley & Sons.
29. LaMontagne LL, Pawlak R (1990) Stress and coping of parents of children in a pediatric intensive care unit. Heart & Lung 19:416–421.
30. Youngblut JM, Shiao SYP (1992) Characteristics of a child's critical illness and parents' reactions: Preliminary report of a pilot study. American Journal of Critical Care 1:80–4.
31. Ohns M (1991) Effects of the nursing mutual participation model of care on parental stress in the pediatric intensive care unit: A replication and refinement. Unpublished master's thesis, University of Ohio, Toledo, Ohio.
32. Curley MAQ, Wallace J (1992) Effects of the nursing mutual participation model of care on parental stress in the pediatric intensive care unit – A replication. Journal of Pediatric Nursing. 7:377–385.
33. Walker LO, Avant KC (1995) Strategies for theory construction. 3rd ed. Norwalk, CT: Appleton & Lange.
34. Fawcett J. (1995) Analysis and evaluation of nursing theories. Philadelphia, PA: F.A. Davis Company.
35. Donaldson SK, Crowley DM (1978) The discipline of nursing. Nursing Outlook 26:113–120.
36. Miles MS, Carter MC (1982) Sources of parental stress in pediatric intensive care units. Children's Health Care 11:65–69.
37. Selye H (1956) The stress of life. NY, NY: McGraw-Hill Book Co.
38. Riehl JP, Roy SC (1980) Conceptual models for nursing practice. 2nd. ed. NY, NY: Appleton-Century-Crofts.
39. Carter MC, Miles MS (1983) Parental Stressor Scale: Pediatric Intensive Care Unit. Kansas City, KS: School of Nursing, University of Kansas.
40. Watson MJ. (1988) New dimensions if human caring theory. Nursing Science Quarterly 1:175–181.
41. Newman M (1994) Health as expanding consciousness. 2nd ed. NY, NY: National League for Nursing Press.

42. Curley MAQ (1989) Caring for parents of critically ill children [Videotape]. NY, NY: American Journal of Nursing.
43. Mitchell PH, Johnson FB, Habermann Little B (1985) Promoting physiologic stability: Touch and ICP. Communicating Nursing Research 18:93.
44. Anderson GC (1991) Current knowledge about skin-to-skin (kangaroo) care for preterm infants. Journal of Perinatology 11:216–226.
45. Zeskind PS, Iacino R (1984) Effects of maternal visitation to preterm infants in the neonatal intensive care unit. Child Development 55:1887–1893.

Neuroscience

The Role of Leukocytes in Global and Focal Brain Ischemia

C. L. Schleien and J. W. Kuluz

Introduction

The role of leukocytes in the pathogenesis of ischemia-reperfusion injury in the brain remains unclear. The weight of experimental data suggests that leukocytes are integrally involved in the development of ischemia-reperfusion injury at both the endothelial and neuronal level, and are not simply inflammatory respondents to the primary brain injury. In the text to follow we will review the evidence for leukocytes in cerebral vessels and brain tissue itself, and the pathophysiologic mechanisms of injury by leukocytes with its therapeutic implications.

Evidence for Leukocytes in Brain

Normally, leukocytes are not present within brain parenchyma and they are not normally adherent to cerebral vessels. Following ischemia-reperfusion injury, there is growing evidence that white blood cells interact with cerebral endothelial cells, adhere to their luminal membrane and occasionally transmigrate through the blood-brain barrier into the brain parenchyma. The transvascular infiltration of leukocytes into infarcted brain tissue has been generally regarded as a relatively late phenomenon following reperfusion, usually occurring after 24 hours or more [1]. More recently, however, the presence of leukocytes in cerebral vessels has been seen earlier following both focal [2, 3] and global brain ischemia [4]. Using a canine model in which focal ischemia was induced by air embolism, Hallenbeck et al found polymorphonuclear (PMN) leukocytes in the injured hemisphere after 4 hours of reperfusion [5]. Del Zoppo et al observed PMN leukocytes in baboon brain 60 minutes after a 3 hour period of reversible middle cerebral artery occlusion [6]. Dietrich et al demonstrated PMN leukocyte accumulation at 1 hour of resuscitation following 20 minutes of normothermic global ischemia [7]. We recently demonstrated widespread leukocyte adherence to vascular endothelium only 4 hours following cardiac arrest and reperfusion in piglets [8] (see Figure 1).

We observed PMN and mononuclear leukocytes in 33 of 36 brain regions within venules and capillaries. In some cases, physical interaction between leu-

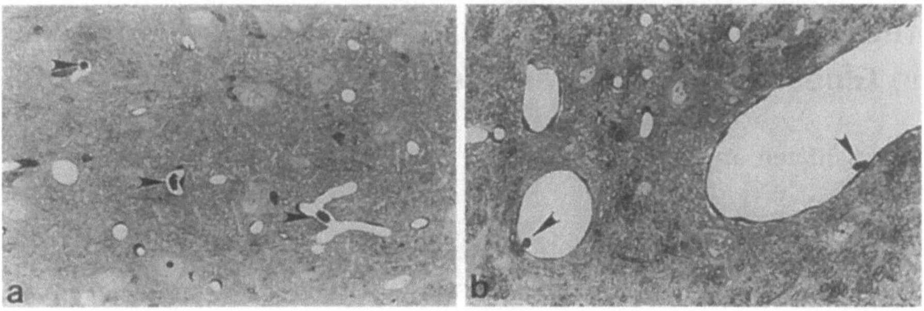

Fig. 1. Plastic sections of piglet brain (stained toluidine blue) 4 hours after cardiac arrest. (a) Luminal leukocytes *(arrowheads)* are present within brainstem microvessels. Note that the surrounding brain parenchyma appears normal. (b) Within the thalamus, adhering leukocytes are present within venules *(arrowheads)*. × 800. (From: Caceres MJ, et al: Acta Neuropathol 1995;90:582–591)

kocytes and endothelial cells occurred in the form of finger-like membrane projections from these cells towards each other (see Figure 2).

Pathophysiologic Mechanism of Injury By Leukocytes

The rapid appearance of leukocytes in post-ischemic cerebral microvessels implicates them in causing early microvascular injury and postischemic blood flow alterations. Micro-infarcts in areas of endothelial disruption and endothelial membrane blebs in the presence of leukocytes may reflect a no-reflow phenomenon in these areas [9]. Leukocytes can reduce local blood flow either by plugging vessels or by causing intense vasoconstriction. Leukocytes may indirectly cause vasoconstriction by releasing superoxide which binds to nitric oxide to form peroxynitrite. The absence of nitric oxide causes vasoconstriction [10] (Figure 3).

The no-reflow phenomenon, refers to the inability to reestablish microcirculatory blood flow in small regions throughout the brain after ischemia despite achieving adequate cerebral perfusion pressure [11]. No-reflow has been observed following both global and focal brain ischemia. Originally, obstruction of capillary blood flow was thought to be due to endothelial projections which impeded red blood cell movement. Other mechanism for the no-reflow phenomenon include extrinsic compression of vessels by interstitial edema, hemorrhage, glial swelling or dysfunction, and intravascular aggregates of leukocytes and platelets [6]. The mechanisms by which ischemia causes endothelial membrane abnormalities have not been elucidated, however, a likely mechanism includes lipid peroxidation due to the release of oxygen radicals formed by endothelial cells [14, 15] or leukocytes [12, 13] during ischemia or early reperfusion. In addition to the release of superoxide radicals, leukocytes also release cytokines, nitric oxide, and proteases, which can damage the cell membrane of endothelial cells as well as neurons and glia if they cross the blood-

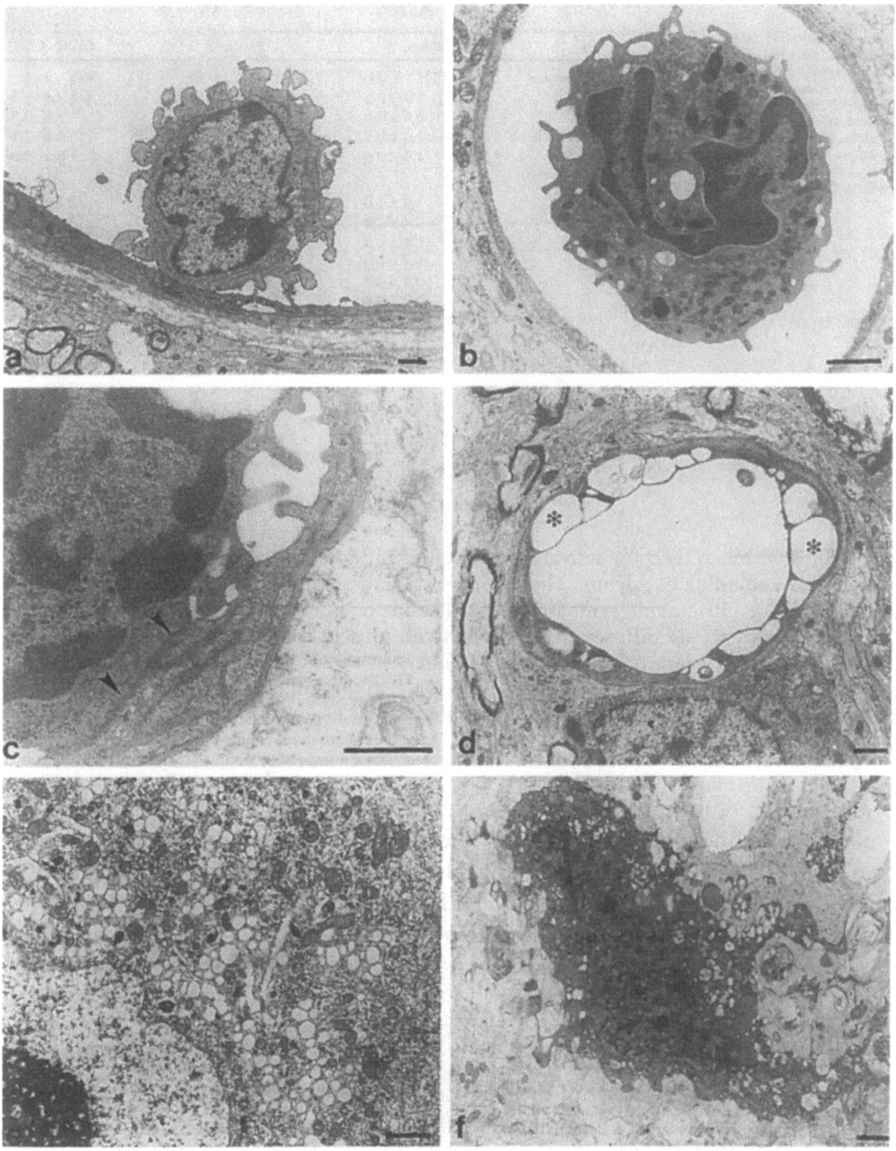

Fig. 2. Transmission electron micrographs of post-arrest piglet brains. (**a**) Adherent leukocyte which appears to be a monocyte is present within a cortical venule. The cell surface is irregular in contour. Note the site of membrane discontinuity on the intravascular endothelial surface. (**b**) Luminal polymorphonuclear leukocyte within caudate nucleus. (**c**) Leukocyte is shown adhering to vascular endothelium *(arrowheads)*. Endothelial cell and leukocyte demonstrate pseudopodia and microvilli. (**d**) Numerous endothelial vacuoles *(asterisk)* are present within this cortical microvessel. (**e**) Cortical neuron showing abnormally large numbers of perinuclear cytoplasmic vacuoles. (**f**) Dark shrunken neuron with pyknotic nucleus appears irreversibly injured. Bars a,b,d–f = 1 mM, c = 0.5 mM. a × 5,000; b × 9,700; c × 31,500; d × 6,300; e × 7,900; f × 6,300. (From Caceres MJ, et al: Acta Neuropathol 1995;90:582–591)

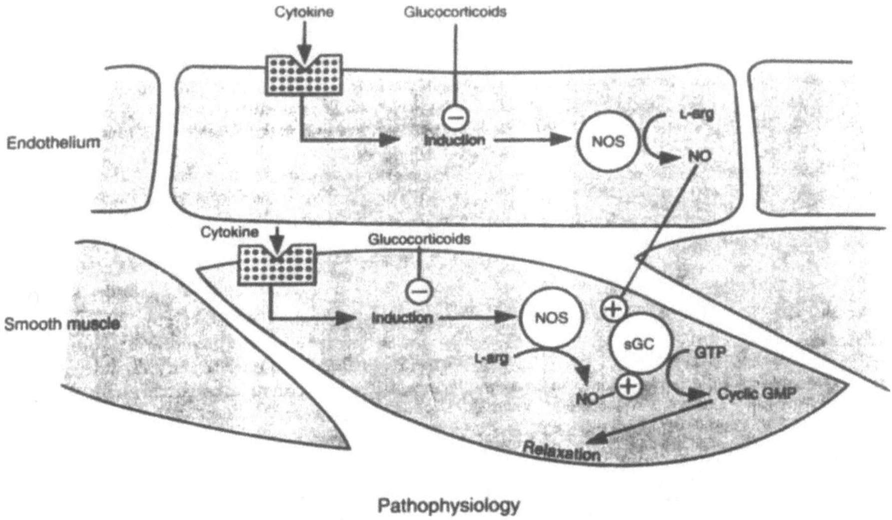

Fig. 3. Shear stress or receptor activation of vascular endothelium by bradykinin or acetylcholine results in an influx of calcium. The consequent increase in intracellular calcium stimulates the constitutive nitric oxide synthase (NOS). The nitric oxide (NO) formed from L-arginine (L-arg) by this enzyme diffuses to nearby smooth-muscle cells, in which it stimulates the soluble guanylate cyclase (sGC), resulting in enhanced synthesis of cyclic GMP from guanosine triphosphate (GTP). This increase in cyclic GMP in the smooth-muscle cells leads to their relaxation. (From Moncada S, et al: N Engl J Med 1993;329:2002–2012)

brain barrier. Another mediator, platelet activating factor is release from PMN leukocytes, monocytes, and platelets. Platelet activating factor promotes activation of granulocytes, monocytes, and platelets, and increases vascular permeability, thus merging the processes of inflammation and coagulation [16, 17].

Microvillus formation, representing more severe endothelial damage, can act as a nidus of attachment of blood elements including leukocytes and platelets. These cellular elements can then cause further release of toxic products which can injure endothelial cells and neurons, or release vasoactive compounds which can alter microcirculatory flow [7]. Four hours after cardiac arrest and CPR in infant piglets, we found that intraluminal leukocytes adherent to brain endothelium were often associated with morphologic changes in endothelial membranes which included blebs, membrane projections and infoldings and sites of membrane disruption that took on a "puff of smoke" appearance (Figure 4).

We also noted a high incidence of perivascular clearing with surrounding vacuolated parenchyma in areas of endothelial disruption [8]. This most likely represents vasogenic edema which occurs following global ischemia in a variety of animal species [18, 19]. The physical disruption of endothelial membranes may serve as a portal of entry into brain parenchyma for leukocytes, large endogenous molecules, as well as drugs that may be used for resuscitation [20, 21].

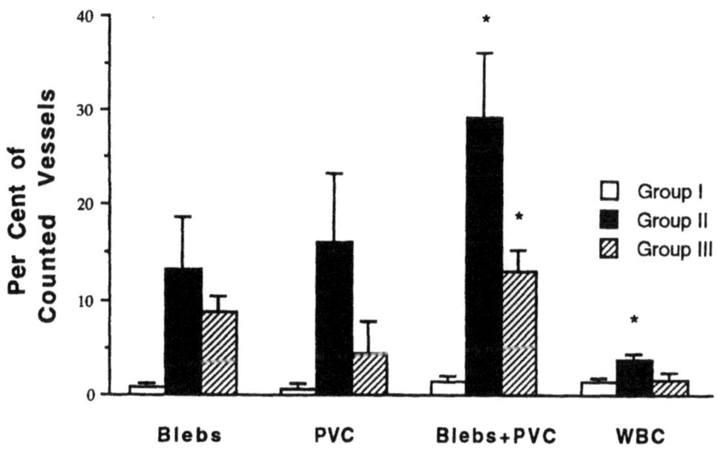

Fig. 4. Percentage of vessels counted for the three groups (see key) containing endothelial blebs. PVC, blebs plus PVC, or WBC. Data are shown as mean ± SEM, *$p<0.05$ compared with group 1 (PVC perivascular swelling, WBC leukocytes with either blebs or perivascular swelling). (From Caceres MJ, et al: Acta Neuropathol 1995;90:582–591)

The role of adhesion receptors in the interaction between endothelial cells and white blood cells has been well described. These receptors include (1) *selectins*, cell adhesion molecules found primarily on endothelial cells, platelets and leukocytes, (2) *integrins*, glycoprotein receptors expressed on the granulocyte surface and (3) *immunoglobulin-like adhesion receptors*, located on the endothelial surface (ICAM-intercellular adhesion molecule). (see Table 3) The family of selectins appears to induce rolling of leukocytes, a low-affinity adhesive interaction between leukocytes and endothelium where the force of blood flow acts on the leukocyte to induce a rotational motion. The selectins include P-selectin which provides the earliest adhesive mechanism, within 1 to 2 minutes of cellular stimulation [22–24]. The E-selectin and L-selectin support rolling, providing this function 1 to 2 hours after endothelial stimulation. E-selectin or endothelial leukocyte adhesion molecule-1 (ELAM-1) appears on endothelial cells stimulated by cytokines, promoting the adhesion of granulocytes and mononuclear cells. L-selectin or lymphocyte adhesion molecule-1 (LAM-1) promotes the binding of leukocytes to endothelium and the transmigration of white cells through endothelium [16].

The β_2 integrins CD11a-c/CD18, found on leukocytes, bind to immunoglobulin-like receptors on endothelium. This group of adhesion molecules promotes efficient stationary adhesion of leukocytes to endothelium. For example, the CD11b/CD18 complex (Mac-1) binds PMN leukocytes to endothelial cell ICAM-1 [25]. ICAM-1 serves as an adhesion ligand on the endothelial cell surface for leukocyte integrins (see Figure 5).

A large number of compounds, both endogenous and exogenous, are known to affect leukocyte-endothelial interactions. Most of these compounds alter these interactions by changing either the density or function of the above-

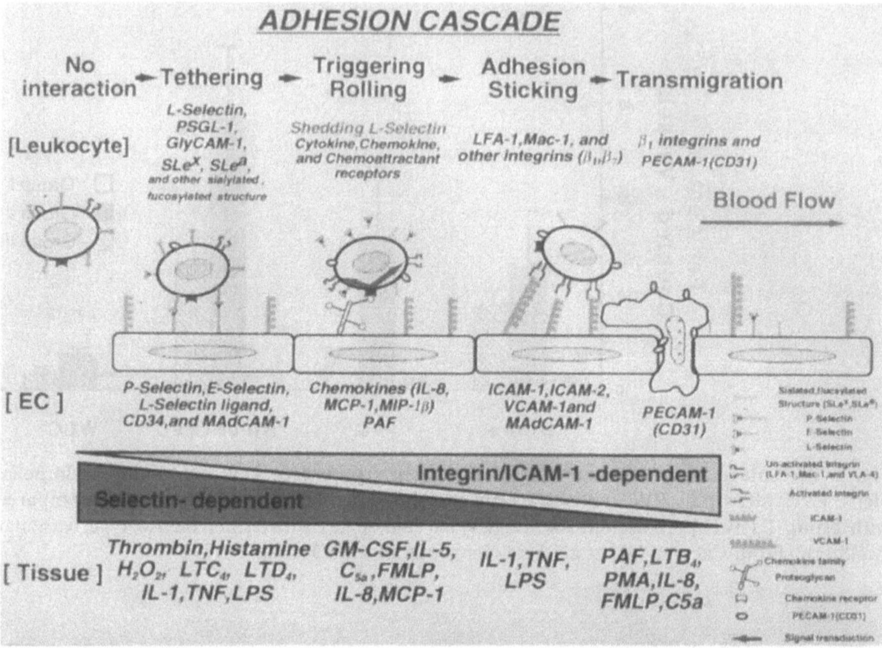

Fig. 5. The adhesion cascade beginning with tethering of the leukocyte to the endothelial cell (EC), triggering/rolling, adhesion/sticking and transmigration of leukocytes through the EC. The adhesion molecules located on leukocytes and EC are noted. Tissue activators are listed in the bottom row. (Y. Yasuma, personal communication)

mentioned adhesion molecules. Stimulants for leukocyte rolling include superoxide radical, interleukin-1 and histamine among others (see Table 1).

This early rolling effect is mediated primarily by the selectin family of cell adhesion molecules. In contrast, firm leukocyte adherence to endothelial cells can occur via adhesion receptor, or non-adhesion receptor mediated mechanisms. For example, leukotriene B4, an arachidonic acid metabolite produced after inflammation, platelet activating factor, and bacterial products such as formulated peptide (fMLP) increase adhesion via upregulation of β_2 integrin [26]. Leukocyte adhesion independent of integrin upregulation is seen with a number of substances such as administration of calcitonin gene-related peptide and substance P [27].

Therapeutic Modulation of Leukocyte-Endothelial Interactions

A number of methods have been used in animal models to reduce leukocyte-endothelial interactions in an effort to ameliorate ischemia-reperfusion injury in the brain. A marked reduction of the number in circulating neutrophils, to less than five percent of normal, can be achieved by pharmacologic suppression of bone marrow. This strategy has been shown to reduce cerebral infarct

Table 1. Agents or conditions that promote leukocyte rolling and/or adherence in postcapillary venules. (Adapted from: Granger DN, Kubes P. J Leuk Biol 1994; 55:662–675)

Rolling
- Superoxide
- Lactoferrin
- Histamine
- A23187 (calcium ionophore)
- Interleukin-1
- Hydrogen peroxide
- Compound 48/80
- Indomethacin
- Ischemia-reperfusion
- Low shear rates

Adherence
- C5a
- Platelet-activating factor
- Leukotriene B_4
- N-Formylmethionyl-leucyl-phenylalanine (fMLP)
- Hydrogen peroxide
- Oxidized low-density lipoprotein
- Cigarette smoke
- Aspirin
- Indomethacin
- Nitric oxide synthase inhibitors
- Compound 48/80
- Ischemia-reperfusion
- Endotoxin
- Monochloramine
- Acute systemic hypoxia

volume after transient middle cerebral artery occlusion in rats [28], and improve electrical conductive function after global forebrain ischemia in rats [29] and after air embolism in dogs [30]. This approach is not recommended for use in humans because of the risk of severe, prolonged and even permanent suppression of bone marrow function.

More recently, antibodies directed against specific adhesion molecules have been used to reduce leukocyte-endothelium interactions in a more controlled fashion. For instance, treatment with anti-CD18 antibody produced a significant reduction of neurologic deficits in a reversible model of spinal cord ischemia in rabbits [31]. In another model, anti-Mac-1 (anti-CD11b/CD18) antibody given to rats subjected to two hours of middle cerebral artery occlusion significantly reduced ischemic cell damage when given either immediately [32] or one hour after reperfusion [33]. These are just two examples of attempts at using specific antibodies to the various classes of selectins and integrins. (see Table 2).

Interestingly, classical anti-inflammatory drugs such as indomethacin and aspirin actually promote leukocyte adhesion in venules [34, 35]. A number of endogenous molecules, particularly those synthesized by endothelial cells may

Table 2. Agents that reduce leukocyte adherence in postcapillary venules. (Adapted from: Granger DN, Kubes P. J Leuk Biol 1994; 55:662–675)

Compound	Biological Action
Adenosine	Endogenous anti-inflammatory agent
Prostacyclin (PGI_2)	Endogenous anti-inflammatory agent
Iloprost	PGI_2 analogue
NO donors	Release nitric oxide
8-Bromo-cGMP	Cyclic GMP analogue
Superoxide dismutase	Scavenges superoxide
Catalase	Detoxifies H_2O_2
Quinacrine	Phospholipase A_2 inhibitor
WEB2086	PAF antagonist
Misoprostol	PGE_2 analogue
SC41930	LTB_4 antagonist
L663, 536, MK886	Lipoxygenase inhibitors
Dietary fish oil	?
Colchicine	Antirheumatic
Methotrexate	Antirheumatic
Ketotifen, cromolyn	Mast cell stabilizers
Cyclosporine, L683, 590	Immunosuppressive agents
Salicylate	Anti-inflammatory agent
Leumedins	Anti-inflammatory agent
L658, 758, Eglin C	Neutrophilic protease inhibitors
Dimethyl sulfoxide	Hydroxyl radical scavenger
Verapamil, diltiazem	Calcium antagonists
Hypothermia	

have important effects on leukocyte adhesion. Nitric oxide (NO) is thought to inhibit adherence of leukocytes to endothelial cells. This is supported by the finding that inhibition of NO synthase increases the postischemic accumulation of leukocytes in brain [36, 37] and that NO donors such as nitroprusside prevent leukocyte adherence. Superoxide radical produced by leukocytes and other cells after ischemia, promotes leukocyte adherence by inactivating NO [38]. As a result, the administration scavengers results in a decrease in leukocyte adherence by inactivating NO. We previously showed decreased permeability of the blood-brain barrier after 4 hours of reperfusion following cardiac arrest using polyethylene glycol conjugated superoxide dismutase and catalase. This effect may be due partially to the indirect beneficial effect of oxygen radical scavenging on leukocyte adherence [39] (Figure 6).

Another endogenous compound which has important effects on ischemia-reperfusion injury and leukocyte-endothelium interactions is adenosine. Adenosine inhibits several functions of PMN leukocytes including adherence via activation of A_2 receptors on leukocytes [40]. Since adenosine levels rise significantly in ischemic tissue due to limited washout by decreased blood flow, ad-

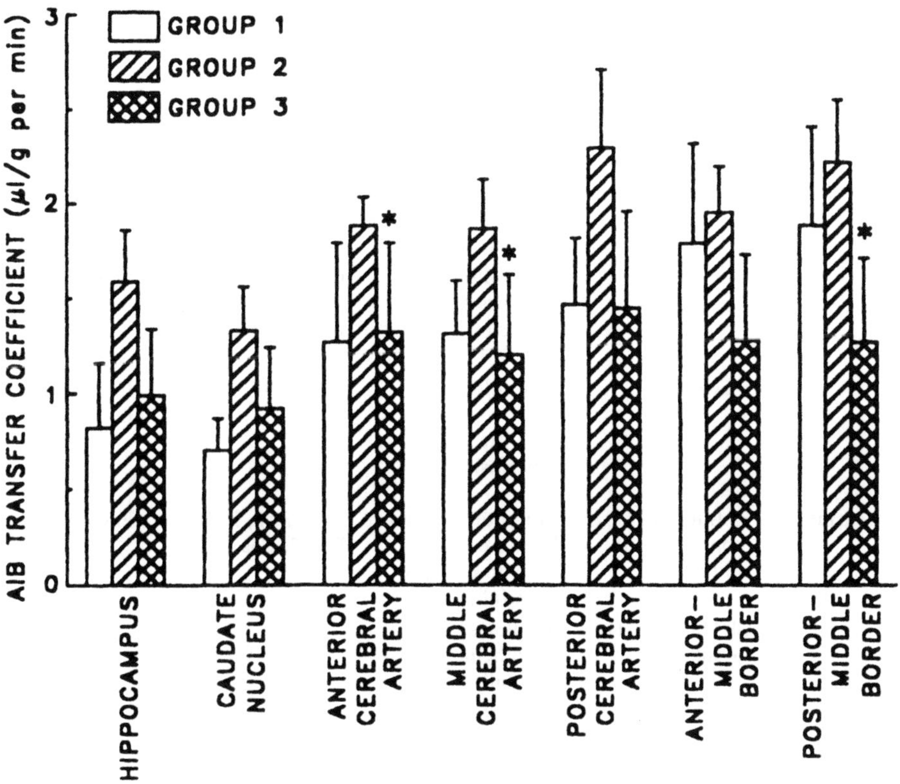

Fig. 6. Bar graph showing transfer coefficient of α-aminoisobutyric acid (AIB) from plasma to brain in hippocampus, caudate nucleus, and primary supply and border regions of cerebral arteries in nonischemic time controls (group 1; n=5), ischemia group treated with polyethylene glycol (PEG) (group 2; n=8), and ischemia group treated with PEG-superoxide dismutase and PEG-catalase (group 3; n=8). Error bars represent SEM. *$p<0.05$ between groups 2 and 3 by Mann-Whitney U test. (From Schleien CL, et al.: 1994;25:1830–1835)

enosine may have additional protective effects during reperfusion by reducing leukocyte-endothelial interaction [41]. Methotrexate, by increasing adenosine production [42], also has potent anti-adhesive leukocyte properties. The third endogenous compounds of leukocyte adherence is prostacyclin (PGI_2), a cyclooxygenase product of arachidonic acid metabolism [35].

Conclusion

There is currently a vast amount of experimental data which suggests that leukocytes accumulate in the brain soon after an ischemic insult, first in intraluminal sites adjacent to endothelial cell injury, and later in brain tissue. Whether the role of leukocytes is solely as an inflammatory responder to ischemia-reperfusion or they play a major role in causing the early damage seen in vas-

Table 3. Cell-adhesion molecules

Family	Specific Cellular Location	Action Subclass	Stimulated	Down-Regulated By:
Selectin:	P-Selectin	Early rolling	Histamine	PAF Endothelium
		(1–2 mins after reperfusion)	Thrombin, Bradykinin, LTC_4, H_2O_2	Platelets
	L-Selectin	Late rolling (1–2 hrs after reperfusion)	Cytokine, Chemokine, and Chemoattractant activation	Leukocytes
	E-Selectin	Late rolling	IL-1, TNF, LPS	IL-8 Endothelium
		(1–2 hrs after reperfusion)		
Integrin:	B_2 Integrins (contains α, β subunits)	Promotes firm adhesion of leukocytes to endothelium (all)	IL-8, PAF, LTB_4, FMLP, C5a	Endothelium
	CD11a (LFA-1) (α subunit)	Promotes transendothelial migration (all)		
	CD11b (Mac-1) (α subunit)	Supports adhesion of neutrophil to other neutrophils (CD11b)		
	CD18 (β subunit)	Promotes phagocytosis (CD11b) Promotes cell locomotion (CD11b)		
Intercellular Adhesion Molecules:	ICAM-1 ICAM-2 ICAM-3	Ligand for CD11a–b/CD18 Firm adhesion of leukocytes to endothelium (appears in 4 hrs; peaks 12–24 hrs) Transmigration of leukocytes through endothelium	IL-1, TNF	Endothelium Lymphocytes Monocytes

cular endothelium remains unknown at this time. Therapies aimed at either decreasing the number of leukocytes, decreasing the adhesion of leukocytes to cerebral vascular endothelium by specific adhesion molecule antagonists, enhancing the release of or administering mediators that decrease leukocyte adhesion, or decreasing the effects of the toxic products of leukocytes such as proteases and oxygen radicals require further experimental investigation and will warrant future clinical trials.

References

1. Petito CK (1979) Early and late mechanisms of increased vascular permeability following experimental cerebral infarction. J Neuropathol Exp Neurol 38:222–234.
2. Petito CK, Schaefer JA, Plum F (1977) Ultrastructural characteristics of the brain and blood-brain barrier in experimental seizures. Brain Res 127:251–267.
3. Pulsinelli WA, Brierley JB, Plum F (1982) Temporal profile of neuronal damage in a model of transient forebrain ischemia. Ann Neurol 11:491–498.
4. Chiang J, Kowada M, Ames A III, Wright RL, Majno G (1968) Cerebral ischemia. III. Vascular changes. J Neurosurg 52:455–465.
5. Hallenbeck JM, Dutka AJ, Tanishima T, et al. (1986) Polymorphonuclear leukocyte accumulation in brain regions with low blood flow during the early post-ischemic period. Stroke 17:246–253.
6. Del Zoppo GJ, Schmid-Schonbein GW, Mori E, Copeland BR, Chang CM (1991) Polymorphonuclear leukocytes occlude capillaries following middle cerebral artery occlusion and reperfusion in baboons. Stroke 22:1276–1283.
7. Dietrich WD, Busto R, Ginsberg MD (1984) Cerebral endothelial microvilli: formation following global forebrain ischemia. J Neuropathol Exp Neurol 43:72–83.
8. Caceres MJ, Schleien CL, Kuluz JW, Gelman B, Dietrich WD (1995) Early endothelial damage and leukocyte accumulation in piglet brains following cardiac arrest. Acta Neuropathol 90:582–591.
9. Siesjo BK (1981) Cell damage in the brain: a speculative synthesis. J Cereb Blood Flow Metab 1:155–185.
10. Lipton SA, Choi YB, Pan ZH, et al. (1993) A redox-based mechanism for the neuroprotective and neurodestructive effects of nitric oxide and related nitroso-compounds. Nature 364:626–632.
11. Ames A III, Wright RL, Kowada M, Thurston JM, Majno G (1968) Cerebral ischemia. II. The no-reflow phenomenon. Am J Pathol 52:437–453.
12. Babior BM, Curnutte JT, McMurrich BJ (1976) The particulate superoxide-forming system from human neutrophils: properties of the system and further evidence supporting its participation in the respiratory burst. J Clin Invest 58:989–96.
13. Jarasch E-D, Bruder G, Heid HM (1986) Significance of xanthine oxidase in capillary endothelial cells. Acta Physiol Scand [Suppl] 548:39–46.
14. Kontos HA, Wei EP (1986) Superoxide production in experimental brain injury. J Neurosurg 64:803–7.
15. Braughler JM, Hall ED (1989) Central nervous system trauma and stroke: I. Biochemical considerations for oxygen radical formation and lipid peroxidation. Free Rad Biol Med 6:289–301.
16. Del Zoppo GJ (1994) Microvascular changes during cerebral ischemia and reperfusion. Cerebrovasc Brain Metab Rev 6:47–96.
17. O'Flaherty JT, Surles JR, Redman J, Jacobsen D, Pianotadosi C, Wykle RL (1986) Binding and metabolism of platelet-activating factor by human neutrophils. J Clin Invest 78:381–8.
18. Dobbin J, Crockard HA, Ross-Russell R (1989) Transient blood-brain barrier permeability following profound temporary global ischemia: an experimental study using ^{14}C-AIB. J Cereb Blood Flow Metab 9:71–6.
19. Kuroiwa T, Ting P, Martinez H, Klatzo I (1985) The biphasic opening of the blood-brain barrier to proteins following temporary middle cerebral artery occlusion. Acta Neuropathol (Berl) 68:122–129.
20. Carre J-B, Morand O, Homayoun P, Roux F, Boure J-M, Baumann N (1989) Purified rat brain microvessels exhibit both acid and neutral sphingomyelinase activities. J Neurochem 52:1294–9.

21. Crowell RM, Olsson Y, Klatzo I, Ommaya A (1970) Temporary occlusion of the middle cerebral artery in monkey. Clinical and pathological observations. Stroke 1:439–48.
22. Geng J-G, Bevilaqua MP, Moore KL, et al. (1990) Rapid neutrophil adhesion to activated endothelium mediated by GMP140. Nature 343:757–60.
23. Larson E, Celi A, Gilbert GE (1989) PADGEM protein: a receptor that mediates the interaction of activated platelets with neutrophils and monocytes. Cell 59:305–12.
24. Palabrica T, Lobb R, Furie BC, et al. (1992) Leukocyte accumulation promoting fibrin deposition is mediated in vivo by P-selectin on adherent platelets. Nature 359:848–51.
25. Wright SD, Detmers PA (1988) Adherence promoting receptors on phagocytes. J Cell Sci [Suppl] 9:99–120.
26. Bienvenu K, Russell J, Granger DN (1992) Leukotriene B4 mediates shear rate-dependent leukocyte adhesion in mesenteric venules. Circ Res 71:906–11.
27. Zimmerman BJ, Anderson DC, Granger DN (1992) Neuropeptides promote neutrophil adherence to endothelial cell. Am J Physiol 263:G678–82.
28. Chen H, Chopp M. Bodzin G (1992) Neutropenia reduces the volume of cerebral infarct after transient middle cerebral artery occlusion in the rat. Neurosci Res Comm 11:93–99.
29. Vasthare VS, Heinel LA, Rosenwasser RH, Tuma RF (1990) Leukocyte involvement in cerebral ischemia and reperfusion injury. Surg Neurol 33:261–265.
30. Dutka AJ, Kochanek PM, Hallenbeck JM (1989) Influence of granulocytopenia on canine cerebral ischemia induced by air embolism. Stroke 20:390–395.
31. Clark WM, Madden KP, Rothlein R, Zivin JA (1991) Reduction of central nervous system ischemic injury in rabbits using leukocyte adhesion antibody treatment. Stroke 22:877–883.
32. Chen H, Chopp M, Zhang RL, et al. (1994) Anti-CD11b monoclonal antibody reduces ischemic cell damage after transient focal cerebral ischemia in rat. Ann Neurol 35:447–452.
33. Chopp M, Zhang RL, Chen H, Li Y, Jiang N, Rusche JR (1994) Postischemic administration of an Anti-Mac-1 antibody reduces ischemic cell damage after transient middle cerebral artery occlusion in rats. Stroke 25:869–876.
34. Asako H, Kukes P, Wallace JL, Wolf RE, Granger DN (1992) Modulation of leukocyte adhesion in rat mesenteric venules by aspirin and salicylate. Gastroenterology 103:146–152.
35. Asako H, Kubes P, Wallace JL, Gaginella T, Wolfe RE, Granger DN (1992) Idomethacin-induced leukocyte adhesion in mesenteric venules: role of lipoxygenase products. Am J Physiol 262:G903–908.
36. Kubes P, Kanwar S, Niu X-F, Gaboury J (1993) Nitric oxide synthesis inhibition induces leukocyte adhesion via superoxide and mast cells. FASEB J 7:1293–1299.
37. Kurose I, Kubes P, Wolfe RE (1993) Inhibition of nitric oxide production: mechanisms of vascular albumin leakage. Circ Res 73:164–171.
38. Del Maestro RF, Planker M, Arfors KE (1982) Evidence for the participation of superoxide anion radical in altering the adhesive interaction between granulocytes and endothelium in vivo. Int J Microcirc Clin Exp 1:105–120.
39. Schleien CL, Eberle B, Shaffner H, Koehler RC, Traystman RJ (1994) Reduced blood-brain barrier permeability after cardiac arrest by conjugated superoxide dismutase and catalase in piglets. Stroke 25:1830–1835.
40. Cronstein BN, Levin RI, Belanoff J, Weissman G, Hirschhorn R (1986) Adenosine: an endogenous inhibitor of neutrophil-mediated injury to endothelial cells. J Clin Invest 78:760–770.
41. Grisham MB, Hernandez LA, Granger DN (1989) Adenosine inhibits ischemia/reperfusion-induced leukocyte adherence and extravasation. Am J Physiol 257:H1334–1339.
42. Cronstein BN, Eberle MA, Gruber HE, Levin RI (1991) Methotrexate inhibits neutrophil function by simulating adenosine release from connective tissue cells. Proc Natl Acad Sci. USA 88:2441–2445.

Hypoxia and Acute Brain Insult

R. C. Tasker

Introduction

In practice, when an anoxia-associated brain insult has been extensive, patients do not recover consciousness despite adequate cardiopulmonary resuscitation. The persistence of acute neurological symptoms and signs reflect a significant period of impaired substrate delivery, which may or may not be associated with a depression in cerebral perfusion. In some of these patients diffuse cortical and basal ganglia changes may be seen on cranial CT or magnetic resonance imaging 24–72 hours after the cerebral insult. Interestingly the severity of such cerebral edema that occurs and its time course and association with cerebrovascular and cerebrometabolic dysfunction is influenced by the events around the time of the insult. For example, hypoxia-induced cardiac arrest, as may be seen in the child with a respiratory illness, is more commonly associated with the development of marked post-resuscitation cerebral edema when compared with the post-resuscitation features of patients suffering primary cardiac arrest. Specific basal ganglia changes which relate to later movement disorders in survivors may also be seen more commonly in patients suffering prolonged hypoxia without cardiac arrest, or cardiac arrest associated with low cerebral blood flow, protracted hypothermia and lactic acidosis.

Irrespective of the initiating cause of the acute life-threatening cerebral event, there are many pathophysiological similarities when considering what might be amenable to pharmacological intervention. Given that cerebral hypoxia and ischemia may result in a complex interaction between changes in cerebral energy metabolism, cerebral blood flow, blood-brain barrier function, neuronal depolarization, and glial-neuronal interaction, there now appears to be a variety of potential therapeutic approaches.

Rationale for Treatment: Present Practice and Potential Strategies

At present, so-called neurological intensive care is directed toward the prevention of secondary cerebral insult due to avoidable physiological or biochemical insults (e.g. hypoxia, hypotension, hyperglycemia), sometimes treatment of cerebral edema and raised intracranial pressure, and control of seizure activity.

Cerebral Edema and Raised Intracranial Pressure

Early on in its development many practitioners have observed a clinical response to fluid restriction, osmotic diuresis, and hyperventilation. Unfortunately, if the edema reflects a cytotoxic process as in hypoxic-ischemic injury outcome is unaffected by such measures.

Pharmacology and Protection Against Neuronal Injury

Many agents have been suggested as potential therapies to limit or prevent the development of brain damage attributable to an acute insult. Behind all such notions however, one should remember that there may be a variety of pathophysiological processes among the different types of injurious events. However, invariably poor cerebral perfusion of blood with substrates is a final common pathway. The particular emphasis of this review will be an outline of the phenomena of cerebral hypoperfusion – hypoxic-ischemic injury – and the potential mechanisms for protection in the developing brain.

From the neonatal period onwards significant developmental alterations occur in the brain. As well as increases in overall size and myelination there are changes in the brain's complexity: there are changes in the total number of neurons and synapses; established neural connections; and the distribution and number of excitatory amino acid receptors, e.g. the N-methyl-D-aspartate (NMDA) ionophore. Cerebrovascular control mechanisms are well developed, by the time of normal birth, and the healthy infant can regulate cerebral hemodynamics in the face of alterations in blood pressure and blood gas tension, although these mechanisms are easily disrupted by hypoxic-ischemic injury.

The metabolic cascades induced during and following ischemia, which may be interrupted by pharmacology, have been described in the experimental setting in detail by Siesjo and others [1]. The initiating event, a decrease in local cerebral blood flow below a critical threshold results in the following; energy failure, tissue acidosis, disturbed ion homeostasis (characterized by enhanced cellular K^+ efflux and a Na^+ and Ca^{2+} influx), membrane depolarization, and cytotoxic edema. A massive release of the excitatory amino acid (EAA) neurotransmitters, glutamate and aspartate, and the activation of glutamate receptors (including NMDA receptors) have been ascribed a major pathophysiological significance [2]. This triggers further membrane depolarization and additional accumulation of free cytosolic Ca^{2+} by cellular influx, release from intracellular compartments and disturbed extrusion mechanisms. The Ca^{2+} accumulation then seems to play a key role in propagation of the process eventually culminating in irreversible neuronal damage, in that it leads to an activation of a series of neurotoxic events, such as lipid peroxidation, free radical generation, activation of proteolytic enzymes and pathological gene activation [3]. In addition, microglial cells also seem to have a significant role, in that they are an important source of free radicals [4]. The relative importance of each of these factors depends highly upon the type and duration of the hypoxic-ischemic insult, and the age at which it occurs. Considering the relationship between EAA system activation and energy failure, the brain of immature animals is known to be generally more resistant to anoxia and ischemia than that of adults. This is attributed to low cerebral energy consumption in immature brains and to a more delayed energy failure [5, 6]. It has been suggested that when the severity of hypoxic-ischemic insult is comparable in the immature and adult brain, the former is less likely to develop energy failure severe enough to activate its EAA system; however, once the EAA system is activated in the immature brain, because of intrinsically exaggerated EAA postsynaptic activities, it could have more devastating effects than in the adult brain [7].

The potential role of glucose supplementation rescue-treatment should also be considered. Pretreating immature animals with glucose prolongs survival during hypoxia by maintaining brain ATP and phosphocreatine levels [8]. In marked contrast however, in juvenile and adult animals, elevated levels of blood glucose during ischemia aggravates the severity of the brain damage [9], which may lead to cerebral infarction when associated with an accumulation of lactic acid above a critical point (16–20 mmol/kg) [10]. Concerning the more clinically useful 'rescue-therapy', one neonatal animal model using posthypoxic glucose supplementation reduced hypoxic-ischemic brain damage [11] although the mechanism of protection was not fully understood and the 'window of opportunity' was not generally characterized.

The recognition of these complex cascades have provided a framework for the development of pharmacological and metabolic interventions before, during, and after cerebral hypoxia-ischemia, designed to prevent or ameliorate neuronal death or injury.

Inhibitors of Cerebral Metabolism

Hypothermia, which generally depresses metabolism, is currently by far the most effective and commonly used means of inhibiting cerebral metabolism. Hypothermia enhances the brain's tolerance of ischemia by slowing adenosine triphosphate depletion and lactic acid formation [12]. Hypothermia appears to depress general cerebral metabolism, whereas drugs, such as barbiturates, depress only that part related to active electrical function [13]. Midazolam, a short-acting water-soluble benzodiazepine, in sufficient dosage also profoundly depresses the cerebral metabolic rate for oxygen ($CMRO_2$). This has been demonstrated in dogs without severe hemodynamic depression or alteration of the cerebral energy state [14]. Accordingly, midazolam may be an alternative to barbiturates for cerebral protection. It has also been suggested that isoflurane, a volatile anaesthetic, may be used to protect the brain during incomplete ischemia [15]. Isoflurane produces an isoelectric EEG in humans at hemodynamically tolerable concentrations (2.4%).

The mechanism by which these agents protect the brain is believed to be by reducing $CMRO_2$. Isoflurane decreases $CMRO_2$, primarily by suppressing cortical electrical activity. Barbiturates, known to reduce $CMRO_2$ in a dose-dependent manner (but only down to the point of isoelectric EEG), have also been shown to protect the brain during incomplete ischemia [16, 17]: though other possible mechanisms of protection have been suggested [12].

Calcium Entry Blockers

There have been many studies of calcium's role in normal cellular function and during ischemia. In ischemia, extracellular calcium decreases - probably because it progressively enters the cells themselves. This knowledge has led to many investigations of calcium entry blocking drugs and their ability to protect or minimize neurological damage after ischemic events [18–20]. Nimodipine, one of the most extensively studied of the calcium entry blockers, consistently prevented the delayed hypoperfusion state that otherwise occurs in a canine model of ischemia [18]. It also improves neurological outcome when administered after complete cerebral ischemia in primates [19].

To date, the cerebral protective mechanism of calcium entry blockers, if it exists, has not been substantiated by any paediatric clinical series.

Other Specific Pharmacotherapies

A number of investigators are examining possible treatment of cerebral ischemia in animals by using pharmacological agents that are antagonists at EAA receptors. It has been postulated that pathological activation of these receptors contribute to the consequences of brain ischemia, though the role of the different receptors (i.e. NMDA *versus* non-NMDA) may be different in different models of ischemia [7, 21, 22]. The concept of such a so-called 'excitotoxic' mechanism for hypoxic-ischemic injury in the developing brain is supported by the neuroprotective efficacy of EAA receptor antagonists, particularly of selective noncompetitive NMDA receptor antagonists [23–25]. However, whilst trials of such receptor antagonists may be imminent for adult patients, in the developing brain exposure to NMDA receptor blockers may have lasting adverse effects on morphogenesis, and the potential for learning. Hence, such agents may, for the present, only be useful experimentally in elucidating underlying pathophysiological mechanisms [26], and will probably not be warranted for clinical use in children and neonates until more is known about there long-term functional effects.

Finally, other cerebroprotective agents, which are used clinically, include phenytoin and lignocaine. In animal models phenytoin has been shown to provide protection after global cerebral ischemia [27, 28]. Its mechanism of protection may be that it reduces the ion flux across membranes during hypoxia-anoxia and thereby decreases potassium accumulation. Pretreatment with lignocaine significantly reduced the neural decrement and enhanced neural functional recovery following acute cerebral ischemia induced by air embolism in cats [29]. In dogs in pentobarbital-induced EEG isoelectricity, lignocaine delayed the efflux of potassium and further reduced metabolism by 15–20% [30].

Conclusion

As our understanding of neuronal injury produced by acute cerebral insult has grown, experimenters have identified a variety of pharmacological strategies which may be of pathophysiological and therapeutic relevance. In the clinical realm, translation of these approaches are being applied firstly to adult patients. Irrespective of their potential benefit and application to children we should not forget the clinical context and perspective of intensive care, particularly with respect to appropriate patient selection and the identification of those individuals having a likelihood of recoverable post-resuscitation neurology.

References

1. Siesjo BK (1984) Cerebral circulation and metabolism. J Neurosurg 60:883.
2. Simon RP, Swan JH, Griffiths T, Meldrum BS (1984) Blockade of N-methyl-D-aspartate receptors may protect against ischemic damage in the brain. Science 226:850.
3. Siesjo BK, Bengtsson F (1989) Calcium fluxes, calcium antagonists, and calcium related pathology in brain ischemia, hypoglycemia, and spreading depression: A unifying hypothesis. J Cereb Blood Flow Metab 9:127.
4. Banati RB, Rothe G, Valet g, Kreutzberg GW (1991) Respiratory burst activity in brain macrophages: a flow cytometric study on cultured rat microglia. Neuropathol Appl Neurobiol 17:223.
5. Thurston JH, McDougal DB Jr (1969) Effect of ischemia on metabolism of the brain of the newborn mouse. Am J Physiol 216:348.
6. Duffy TE, Kohle SJ, Vannucci RC(1975) Carbohydrate and energy metabolism in perinatal rat brain: Relation to survival in anoxia. J Neurochem 24:271.
7. Hattori H, Wasterlain CG (1990) Excitatory amino acids in the developing brain: Ontogeny, plasticity, and excitotoxicity. Pediatr Neurol 6:219.
8. Holowach-Thurston J, Hauhart RE, Jones EM (1974) Anoxia in mice: reduced glucose in brain with normal or elevated glucose in plasma and increased survival after glucose treatment. Pediatr Res 8:238.
9. Pulsinelli WA, Waldman S, Rawlinson D, Plum F (1982) Moderate hyperglycemia augments ischemic brain damage: a neuropathologic study in the rat. Neurology 32:1239.
10. Plum F (1983) What causes infarction in ischemic brain?: the Robert Wartenberg lecture. Neurology 33:222.
11. Hattori H, Wasterlain CG (1990) Posthypoxic glucose supplement reduces hypoxic-ischemic brain damage in the neonatal rat. Ann Neurol 28:122.
12. Safar P, Bleyaert A, Nemoto EM, et al (1978) Resuscitation after global brain ischemia-anoxia. Crit Care Med 6:215.
13. Michenfelder JD (1974) The interdependency of cerebral functional and metabolic effects following massive doses of thiopental in the dog. Anesthesiology 41:231.
14. Nugent M, Artru AA, Michenfelder JD (1982) Cerebral metabolic, vascular and protective effects of midazolam maleate. Anesthesiology 56:172.
15. Newberg LA, Milde JH, Michenfelder JD (1983) The cerebral metabolic effects of isoflurane at and above concentrations that suppress cortical electrical activity. Anesthesiology 59:23.

16. Newberg LA, Michenfelder JD (1983) Cerebral protection by isoflurane during hypoxemia or ischemia. Anesthesiology 59:29.
17. Meyer FB, Sundt TM, Yanagihara T, Anderson RE (1987) Focal cerebral ischemia: Pathophysiologic mechanisms and rationale for future avenues of treatment. Mayo Clin Proc 62:35.
18. Steen PA, Newberg LA, Milde JH, Michenfelder JD (1983) Nimodipine improves cerebral blood flow and neurologic recovery after complete cerebral ischemiaa in the dog. J Cereb Blood Flow Metab 3:38.
19. Steen PA, Gisvold SE, Milde JH, et al (1985) Nimodipine improves outcome when given after complete cerebral ischemia in primates. Anesthesiology 64:406.
20. Deshpande JK, Wieloch T (1986) Flunarizine, a calcium entry blocker, ameliorates ischemic brain damage in the rat. Anesthesiology 64:215.
21. Simon RP, Swan JH, Griffiths T, Meldrum BS (1984) Blockade of N-methyl-D-aspartate receptors may protect against ischemic damage in the brain. Science 226:850.
22. Block GA, Pulsinelli WA (1987) Excitatory amino acid receptor antagonists: Failure to prevent ischemic neuronal damage. J Cereb Blood Flow Metab 7(suppl 1):S149.
23. McDonald JW, Silverstein FS, Johnston MV (1987) MK-801 protects the neonatal brain from hypoxic-ischemic damage. Eur J Pharmacol 140:359.
24. Hattori H, Morin AM, Schwartz PH, Fujikawa DG, Wasterlain CG (1989) Posthypoxic treatment with MK-801 reduces hypoxic-ischemic damage in the neonatal rat. Neurology 39:713.
25. Olney JW, Ikonomidou C, Mosinger JL, Frierdich G (1989) MK-801 prevents hypobaric-ischemic neuronal degeneration in infant rat brain. J Neurosci 9:1701.
26. Tasker RC (1992) Excitatory aminoacid neurotoxicity: a broader horizon for cerebral protection? Arch Dis Child 67:1327.
27. Artru AA, Michenfelder JD (1980) Cerebral protective, metabolic, and vascular effects of phenytoin. Stroke 11:377.
28. Artru AA, Michenfelder JD (1981) Anoxic cerebral potassium accumulation reduced by phenytoin: Mechanism of cerebral protection? Anesth Analg 60:41.
29. Evans DE, Kobrine AI, Le Grys DC, Bradley ME (1984) Protective effect of lidocaine in acute cerebral ischemia induced by air embolism. J Neurosurg 60:257.
30. Astrup J, Skovsted P, Gjerris F, Sorensen HR (1981) Increase in extracellular potassium in the brain during circulatory arrest: Effects of hypothermia, lidocaine, and thiopental. Anesthesiology 55:256.

Current Management of Seizures and Status Epilepticus in Children

R. Rivera Brenes and A. Baltodano Agüero

Introduction

The incidence of seizures in the general population is 50–100/100,000. 70–80% of all cases begin during the first 12 months of life. Between 0.5–5/1000 of all newborns will have at least one seizure during the first month of life [1]. In Europe and the United States of America (USA) between 2–4% of all children younger than 5 years old will have seizures associated with fever. The highest incidence is at 2 years of age [2]. The etiology of epilepsy is not clear and has been related to genetic factors as well as maturation of the cortex and subcortical regions of the brain. Etiology, clinical manifestations and prognosis of seizures in childhood are different of those presenting during the adult life [3].

Pathophysiology

The convulsion is the clinical manifestation of an electrical discharge that is abrupt, paroxysmic and self-limiting of a selected group of neurons. In order to have seizures a good number of cells must be recruited, therefore, the clinical manifestation will depend on the location of the discharging neurons on the cortex and the pattern of enrollment of adjacent cells through the Central Nervous System (CNS). There are many factors that may play a role in the beginning of a seizure: chemical excitatory and inhibitory stimuli, intersynaptic level of neurotransmitters and convulsive threshold. All this factors change with age and CNS development, therefore, they are different in the newborn, infant, adolescent and adult [4].

The cortex of the newborn is immature and not well organized for a seizure to be characteristic or similar to those of infants and children. Neurons are immature, apical dendrites are usually more developed than basilar, myelinization and connections within zones of the brain are also poor developed. Therefore, enrollment of fitting cells is slow at this age and the pathway is usually cortical-thalamic-cortical, following the reticular formation in the highest part of the bulb and the intralaminary system [4] where myelinization is good at this age. Inhibitory mechanisms are more mature than the excitatory ones, so it is difficult for the cortex to maintain activity. Subcortical structures are more mature and active at birth and so they are more sensitive to suffer damage due to hypoxia or abnormal stimuli [5].

In order to have seizures, it is necessary to reach the discharge threshold of a neuronal group. Why with some chemical, electrical or other stimuli, this group of cells reach this level is not known, nevertheless, it is clear that it depends on maturation, transmembrane ionic transport, size of membrane pores and the intrinsic process of repolarization and modulation [4, 5]. During infancy the development process reach a level where it is capable of maintaining activity with poor developed control zones or inhibitory mechanisms. This is the period of highest vulnerability for seizures and may be the reason for the high incidence of convulsions in this age group. It may also explain the frequency of febrile convulsions in the same group and why the incidence decreases once the cortex matures completely after 7–8 years of age [4].

Etiology

The etiology of seizures in children is multifactorial and they are precipitated by many external stimuli including fever, electrolyte and acid base disturbances, trauma etc. Genetic influence is also well documented [2]. The causes

Table 1. Etiology of seizures

Neonatal (<28 days)
- Asphyxia
- Intracranial hemorrhage
- Hypocalcemia
- Hypomagnesemia
- Hypoglycemia
- Hyponatremia/hypernatremia
- Infections (TORCHS)
- Congenital malformations of the CNS
- Congenital metabolic disorders
- Acute suppression of drugs

Infants (1 month–3 years)
- Chronic conditions of the newborn
- Infections (meningitis, encephalitis)
- Trauma
- CNS tumors
- Progressive encephalopathies
- Idiopathic

Children and adolescents
- Infections (meningitis, encephalitis)
- Trauma
- CNS tumors
- Progressive encephalopathies
- Idiopathic

also changes with age and development of the CNS. In about 30% of patients the etiology is never encountered and this group are called idiopathic [6]. Table 1 resumes the most frequent causes according to age.

Classification

The objectives to establish a classification are: to group the individual type, to follow the progression and to identify epileptic syndromes. Recent advances on etiology, pathophysiology, treatment and prognosis have made possible the establishment of such classification [6, 7]

Partial Crisis

In this group the first clinical and electroencephalographic (EEG) changes indicate that only a small number of neurons are active and they are located to one part of a hemisphere. They are also grouped in: partial simple, partial complex and partial and then tonic-clonic generalized.

Generalized Crisis

In this group the findings indicate that both hemispheres are active, there is usually depression of consciousness and the motor manifestation is bilateral. They include absences, myoclonic, clonic and tonic seizures, tonic-clonic and atonic.

Miscellaneous

Here we group all seizures not included in the above groups, such as those seen in the neonatal period. Some of these seizures are described as "subtle" like paddling, sucking, apnea and gaze abnormalities [8].

Febrile Convulsions

This type of seizures occur between 3 months and 5 years of age, and are associated to any febrile illness. It is the most frequent type of convulsions at this age. They are divided in two groups: with or without risk factors. Febrile seizures without risk factors are short duration and generalized seizures. They occur after an increase in body temperature in children with no evidence of CNS infection or poisoning [9]. EEG is normal one week after the episode and there is a familiar history of febrile convulsions in 10–30% of all cases. 50% of children have at least one first degree relative with history of febrile seizures.

4% of children have their first crisis before 6 months of age and 75% between 6 months and 3 years [10]. 95% of children who have febrile seizures will have their first episode before 5 years of age. The risk of recurrence is 30–50%, but if the first episode was before one year of age it is greater than 50%. The risk of presenting non febrile convulsions is 4%. If the episode is associated with risk factors such as prolonged crisis (more than 15 minutes), family history of non febrile seizures, low temperature and previous neurological abnormalities, the risk of non febrile seizures increases to 28% [9, 11].

Management of Febrile Seizures

Control of temperature either with medication or by physical means have failed to demonstrated any utility on prevention or treatment of febrile convulsions [12]. Only 10% of children who have seizures associated with a fever will have a bacterial infection that need to have specific treatment. There is controversy regarding lumbar puncture in these cases. Only 6% of all patients will have meningitis but 41% of all cases of meningitis will have seizures [12, 13]. In 503 cases of bacterial meningitis in children between 2 months and 15 years over a period of 20 years Green et al did not found a case in which seizures were the only manifestation of that illness [13]. The decision to do a lumbar puncture (LP) in children with seizures must be justified on clinical grounds, specially if there are signs of CNS infection. It must also be considered in presence of status epilepticus or if the recovery after the event takes longer than expected [14].

Long term prophylaxis with anticonvulsants is not indicated in children with febrile seizures without risk factors. In a randomized, controlled, double blind study Rosman and coworkers demonstrated that diazepam 0.33 mg/Kg given orally every 8 hours during a febrile illness decreased 44% the risk of recurrence [15]. It can also be administered rectally at 0.5 mg/Kg q8h during the first 48 hours of the febrile illness. Phenobarbital is the most popular drug used to prevent recurrence and seems to reduce the incidence of non febrile convulsions in patients with increased risk [16] when compared to placebo. Its use is controversial and not free of side effects such as delayed development, hyperactivity and sleep problems [17, 18]. Valproate (valproic acid) is equally effective, but because of its side effects (mostly hepatic) it is not the drug of choice specially in children under 2 years of age [19, 20].

Current indications for long term prophylaxis are basically for those patients with increased risk of recurrence (up to 28% when two or more are present) [21–23]:

- Developmental delay or previous neurological abnormalities.
- Prolonged crisis, focal or more than one in 24 hours.
- Familiar history of non febrile seizures in first degree relatives.
- In hospital stay longer than 28 days after birth.

The prognosis of febrile seizures is good when compared with non febrile convulsions. Verity and coworkers showed a rate of recurrence of 21% for children with febrile seizures compared to 82% for non febrile episodes. Long term development was also normal in 95% of children with febrile crisis [24].

Posttraumatic Seizures

Overall incidence of posttraumatic seizures is 10%. Lewis et al showed that in 194 patients with head injuries, 18 patients (9.3%) presented post-traumatic seizures. Risk factors included: loss of consciousness, Glasgow coma score (GCS) 3–8 (38% compared to 3.8% with GCS greater than 8), and abnormal CT scan (fractures, hematomas and contusions) [25]. The use of prophylactic phenytoin at 5 mg/Kg/day intravenously while the patient is paralyzed in the Intensive Care Unit decreases significantly its incidence [25]. It is not recommended to maintain long term prophylaxis once the patient is discharged.

Neonatal Seizures

Seizures during the neonatal period are usually an emergency because they reflect a severe neurological dysfunction or damage of an immature brain [26]. Incidence varies between term (0.5%) and preterm babies (20%) [27]. Establishing the diagnosis is difficult (clinical vs. EEG), as well as its etiology. Efficacy and side effects of anticonvulsants are not well studied in this particular group.

The management of seizures in the newborn period include: neutral thermal environment, general neurological assessment and ruling out metabolic problems like hypoglycemia or electrolyte disturbances (hyponatremia, hypocalcemia, hypomagnesemia). If hypoglycemia is documented then D10W (10% dextrose in water) should be administered at 2 mL/Kg intravenously over one minute (200 mg/Kg) followed by a continuous infusion of glucose. If there is evidence of sepsis, lumbar puncture is always indicated due to the high incidence of meningitis associated with sepsis of the newborn [26].

General Management of the Child with Seizures

To maintain good oxygenation and oxygen transport is the main goal of its management, therefore all measures to accomplish the ABC of resuscitation are the most important in this early phase of its treatment. Drug treatment is similar in children and adults but drugs should be carefully administered in small children and newborns in view of the increased side effects at this age, specially apneas [26].

Benzodiazepines are the usual initial drugs. They are very effective and have very little side effects. Diazepam at 0.3–0.5 mg/Kg intravenously (IV) and repeated every 5–10 minutes up to three times is the most commonly used [28]. Side effects include hypotension, respiratory depression, laryngeal spasm and cardiac arrest. This effects are more prominent if other drugs are given concomitantly. Lorazepam is 80–100% effective, has a larger duration of action and has less cardiorespiratory effect than diazepam. Its volume of distribution and half life are approximately half of diazepam. Body distribution of the drug is minimal so therapeutic levels remain within the CNS for several hours. Onset of action occurs within 3–5 minutes after a single dose and lasts for 2–8 hours. The usual dose is 0.05–0.2 mg/Kg/dose (maximum of 4 mg for children and 8 mg for adolescents and adults). It can be repeated every 15 minutes if necessary but its efficacy decreases with multiple doses. Lorazepam may be given rectally and is also very effective [29, 30].

Other drugs are clonazepam (0.5–1.0 mg/Kg IV) and midazolam (0.2–0.5 mg/Kg IV). They seem to be more effective and have less side effects [28]. When the drugs are given rectally it is recommended to use the highest dose as well as in newborns is good to begin with the lowest one. The effectiveness of midazolam has not been demonstrated in the newborn [31].

The next drug is Phenobarbital given at 20 mg/Kg (10 mg/Kg in newborns), then continue at 3–10 mg/Kg IV, PO once a day. There are reports of very high doses of phenobarbital (serum level of 70–340 mg/dL) to treat refractory seizures but is usually associated with severe side effects such as respiratory and cardiovascular depression and loss of consciousness [32].

Phenytoin is a second line drug due to its delayed onset of action. With a loading dose of 20 mg/Kg IV we have peak CNS levels at 10–30 minutes. It is very effective to control either generalized or partial seizures even in newborns [33]. Phenytoin does not decrease consciousness but must be given slowly (25 mg/Kg/min. in infants and 50 mg/Kg/min. in children). Side effects include hypotension and arrhythmia. Must not be given intramuscularly because of erratic absorption and may cause muscle necrosis [34].

Pyridoxine at 50–100 mg IV must be given in newborns or refractory seizures. In the case of metabolic derangement, once it is resolved anticonvulsants should be discontinued. If the etiology is not identified, it is recommended to continue with medication at least two years free of crisis [28, 32]

Status Epilepticus

Status epilepticus (SE) is a neurological emergency. Its incidence is 1/1000 in the USA being similar in other countries. It may occur at any age but is more frequent in children than adolescents and adults. If it is not treated promptly and aggressively may cause severe neurological damage and death [35].

The World Health Organization (WHO) defined status epilepticus as any seizure long enough or repeated so frequently that it produces a fix epileptic condition [36]. Now we know that any seizure longer than 30 minutes should be considered and treated like status epilepticus [37]. Other researchers define SE as any seizure that occurs so often that complete recovery between crisis is not achieved or the patient does not regain consciousness [38, 39]. Mortality of SE has been reported between 3–25% [40]. During the last 5 years the early recognition of the problem and aggressive treatment have decreased it to 3–10%, where most deads are related to the underlying disease [41]. Refractory seizures may be the first manifestation of epilepsy and it may appear at any time after the diagnosis. Its incidence among epileptic patients is 13–160/1000/year and is 10 times more frequent in children less than 1 year old [40].

Etiology varies according to age group. The most frequent cause is the sudden drop in plasmatic levels of anticonvulsants [41]. Precipitating factors include: CNS insult (ex. infection or trauma), metabolic disturbances, drug interaction by other drugs or illnesses (ex. theophylline, hepatic illness), anoxia, hormonal changes, electrolyte abnormalities, sleep problems, fever, ethanol intoxication, other toxics, tumors and cerebro-vascular problems [42].

Hypoxia if frequent during SE and it is responsible for most complications. It is secondary to the ventilation problems due to muscle spasms, salivation and increase tracheobronchial secretions. Oxygen consumption and extraction ratio are also increased because of increased metabolic demands of firing neurons and contracting muscles [43]. Prolonged convulsive activity produces cerebral damage and death. Several classic studies in the animal model have demonstrated the physiopathology of the SE [4, 43]. All chemical and clinical changes have been divided in two phases. Phase I occurs within 30 minutes of the beginning of the crisis and there is an increase in arterial blood pressure, heart rate and respiratory rate. Blood chemistry show increased lactate and glucose followed by a decrease in pH. Changes in PaO_2 and $PaCO_2$ depends on the type of seizure and the ventilatory status.

After the first few minutes, metabolic changes stabilize and there is a "plateau" during the beginning of phase II. In this phase there is a rapid drop in neuronal energy stores (ATP) due to an exaggerated increased in energy expenditure and metabolism. Blood glucose, lactate and pH return to normal or near normal levels due to compensation. It is also characteristic of this period the hyperthermia and hyperkalemia. Cardiac output decreases and perfusion pressure drops to levels that impair greatly the oxygen transport and consumption. This is the beginning of neuronal damage that increases along with the duration of the event. There is enough evidence indicating that cellular damage and death occurs in presence of electrical convulsive activity without clinical evidence of seizures (non convulsive status epilepticus) [44]. This process is related to the increased metabolism, poor oxygen and nutrients transport to very active firing cells. Finally there is an increment in the influx of calcium to the cytoplasm where many receptors are stimulated by means of nitric oxide. Membrane pores are opened and a massive influx of water and chloride produces cellular edema, mitochondrial dysfunction and neuronal death [45].

Management of Status Epilepticus

The initial assessment must be gradual but aggressive. The main objectives of the treatment are:

1. To prevent hypoxia: A(airway), B(breathing), C(circulation)
2. To control clinical seizures within the first 30 minutes and EEG activity within the first hour.
3. To prevent relapses.
4. To identify and control complications.
5. To optimize maintenance therapy.

To Prevent Hypoxia (Initial Assessment)

All patients must receive oxygen supplement. If the airway is not clear and the patient can not protect it or if it not breathing endotracheal intubation and assisted ventilation should be considered. All metabolic (electrolyte, glucose, acid base) disturbances must be corrected and prevented. Clinical history and physical examination must be quick to identify any precipitant or etiologic factor such as trauma or infection.

Vascular access must be accomplished and blood chemistry analyzed (glucose, sodium, calcium, magnesium, urea and blood gases) Further studies will be done according to the clinical picture and physical examination. If the patient was taken anticonvulsants, serum levels should be taken. If the initial vascular access is not possible or difficult, it is recommended to give the drugs (diazepam, midazolam, lorazepam or valproate) rectally [46, 47]. Benzodiazepines, barbiturates and phenytoin could also be given via an intraosseous catheter [48, 49].

Pharmacological Treatment

There are many drugs to treat SE, most of them have serious side effects and its use may aggravate the underlying problem. We should know this side effects and be prepared to prevent or treat them [50].

Pentobarbital was the most commonly used drug at this stage. It is a barbiturate, hypnotic and used during induction of general anesthesia. After a loading dose of 2–5 mg/Kg it is recommended to give a continuous infusion at 1–5 mg/Kg/hour [51, 52]. Despite the fact that it is very effective, pentobarbital has serious side effects. All patients will develop apnea, thus endotracheal intubation an assisted ventilation is mandatory. It also has a negative inotropic effect associated with a significant reduction in cardiac output, causing hypotension and drop in perfusion pressures. Its use has been associated with hypothermia and hypoglycemia that may increase morbidity and mortality of SE [53]. It is recommended to maintain the infusion for at least 24 hours then decrease it until its complete tapering. Pentobarbital remains in fat tissue for several days, small infants may need assistance for several days.

Thiopentone is another barbituric that shares the same properties as pentobarbital with less side effects. The loading dose is 5–15 mg/Kg IV followed by a continuous infusion at 1–3 mg/Kg/hour [52–54].

Lidocaine has been reported anecdotal to be useful in the treatment of refractory seizures but may be associated with arrhythmias or low cardiac output. It is rapid and effective but has a very short half life. Loading dose of 2–3 mg/Kg then infusion at 4–10 mg/Kg/hour [55].

Halothane and Isoflurane (1–4%) have also been reported anecdotal to treat severe status epilepticus [56]. Its administration requires costly equipment and experienced personnel.

Midazolam is a hydrosoluble benzodiazepine that has anxiolytic, muscle relaxant, anticonvulsant and hypnotic properties. It crosses the hemato-encephalic barrier (HEB) very quickly and has a short half life of 0.8 hours. Midazolam has hepatic metabolism and it is excreted via the urine [57]. Early in the animal model, then adults and children it has demonstrated that it is very safe and effective to treat seizures [58–61]. Current experience in children showed that it is very effective in terminating status epilepticus. An initial loading dose of 0.15–0.25 mg/Kg followed by a continuous infusion (1–18 μg/Kg/minute) was very effective in the treatment of status epilepticus in children [62–64]. It was also demonstrated that its use has very little side effects and most patients did not require endotracheal intubation nor ventilation. Cardiac output was not modified and other side effects such as delirium, muscle spasms and spasticity were not seen.

The pharmacological treatment of SE is summarized in the Table 2.

Table 2. Anticonvulsant drugs for status epilepticus

Type	Drug	Initial IV dose (velocity)	Max. dose (mg)	Repeated
First line	Diazepam	0.2–0.5 mg/Kg (2 minutes)	10	15 min
	Lorazepam	0.1–0.2 mg/Kg (1–2 min)	5–10	10–15 min
	Midazolam	0.15–0.50 mg/Kg (1–2 min)	5–10	CI (&) 1–18 μg/Kg/min
	Phenytoin	15–20 mg/Kg (max: 50 mg/min)	1250	
	Phenobarbital	10–20 mg/Kg (max: 30 mg/min)		20 min (once)
Second line	Thiopental	5 mg/Kg		CI (&)
	Pentobarbital	(1 min)		1–5 mg/Kg/h
	Phenobarbital	10 mg/Kg		q 30 min
	high doses			serum levels 120–370 mg/dl
Other drugs	Lidocaine	2–3 mg/Kg		CI (&) 4–10 mg/Kg/h
	Isofluorane	1–4%		

(&) CI: continuous infusion

Complications

Most complications of SE are related to either the underlying disease or the side effects of the treatment. Some of them such as neuronal damage, rhabdomyolysis or hyperthermia are closely related with the clinical or EEG convulsant activity. The most frequent encountered problems are: respiratory depression, loss consciousness, cardiac arrest, hypoxia, tachycardia, hypotension, pulmonary edema, rhabdomyolysis, acute renal failure, acidosis, and hyper/hypoglycemia.

Regarding prognosis, Aicardi and coworkers in 1970 found neurological sequelae in 50% of 239 children with status epilepticus longer than one hour. Hemiparesis was the most common but they also reported diplegia, microcephalia, cerebellar dysfunction and delayed development [35]. Recent studies show that when treatment is given aggressively, mortality and morbidity are low and usually related to the underlying disease [41]. In our own experience, this is true and mortality associated only to SE should be close to zero [61, 62].

Conclusions

Status epilepticus is a medical emergency that should be treated aggressively to avoid neurological sequelae and death. Initial assessment must be directed to the usual resuscitation techniques regarding airway, ventilation and hemodynamic status. Rapid intervention in the early phases of seizures avoid all complications derived of continuously firing neurons. Mortality must be low if treatment is instituted promptly and aggressively [65].

References

1. Evans OB (1987) Seizures and epilepsy. In: Manual of childhood Neurology. Churchill & Livingstone, New York, pp 435–441
2. Hauser WA (1994) The prevalence and incidence of convulsive disorders in children. Epilepsia 35 Suppl 2: S1–6
3. Bundey S (1987) The genetics basis of epilepsies. In: Hopkins A (ed) Epilepsy. Chapman & Xall, London, pp 137–149
4. Lothman E (1990) The biochemical basis and pathophysiology of status epilepticus. Neurology 40(s2):13–18.
5. Bundey S (1987) The genetics basis of epilepsies. In: Hopkins A (ed) Epilepsy. Chapman & Xall, London, pp 137–149
6. Dreifuss FE (1987) The different types of epileptic seizures and the International Classification of epileptic seizures and of epilepsies. In: Hopkins A (ed) Epilepsy. Chapman &Xall, London, pp 83–113
7. Dreifuss FE (1989) Clasificaci6n de las crisis epil6pticas y de las epilepsias. Clin Med North Am 2:289–303
8. Murphy JV, Dehkharghani F (1994) Diagnosis of childhood seizure disorders. Epilepsia 35: S7–17

9. Offringa M, Bossuyt PM, Lubsen J, Ellenberg JH, Nelson KB, Knudsen FU, et-al (1994) Risk factors for seizure recurrence in children with febrile seizures: a pooled analysis of individual patient data from five studies. J Pediatr 124:574–84
10. Leung A, Robson WL (1987) Febrile convulsions, how dangerous are they? Post Grad Med 89:63–71
11. Joint working group of the Research Unit of the Royal College of Physicians and the British Paediatric Association (1991) Guidelines for the management of convulsion with fever. British Med J 303:634–635
12. Schnaiderman D, Lahat E, Sheefer T, Aladjem M 1993 Antipyretic effectiveness of acetaminophen in febrile seizures: ongoing prophylaxis versus sporadic usage. Eur J Pediatr 152(9):747–749
13. Green SM, Rothrock SG, Clem KJ, Zurcher RF, Mellick L (1993) Can seizures be the sole manifestation of meningitis in febrile children? Pediatrics 92:527–534
14. Floret D (1993) Suppurative meningitis in infants and in children:adjuvant treatments and treatments of neurological forms. Pediatrie Bucur 48: 21–27
15. Rosman P, Colton T, Labazzo J, et al (1993) A controlled trial of diazepam administered during febrile illness to prevent recurrence of febrile seizures. N Engl J Med 329:79–84
16. Thilothammal N, Kannan V, Krishnamurthy PV, Kamala KG, Ahamed S, Banu K (1993) Role of phenobarbitone in preventing recurrence of febrile convulsions. Indian-Pediatr 30:637–642
17. Domizio S, Verrotti A, Ramenghi LA, Sabatino G, Morgese G (1993) Anti–epileptic therapy and behaviour disturbances in children. Childs Nerv Syst 9:272–274
18. Farwell J, Lee J, Hitz D, et al (1990) Phenobarbital for febrile seizures, effects on intelligence and on seizure recurrence. N Engl J Med; 322:364–368
19. Robinson R (1991) Febrile convulsion. Brit Med J 303:1345–1346
20. Pellock J (1989) Efficacy and adverse effects of antiepileptic drugs. Pediatr Clin North Am 36:435–448
21. Bethune P, Gordon K, Dooley J, Camfield C, Camfield P (1993) Which child will have a febrile seizure? Am J Dis Child 147:35–39
22. Van-Esch A, Steyerberg EW, Berger MY, Offringa M, Derksen-Lubsen G, Habbema JD (1994) Family history and recurrence of febrile seizures. Arch Dis Child 70:395–399
23. Kaplan RB (1987) Febrile seizures: When is treatment justified? Post Grad Med 82:63–71
24. Verity CM, Ross EM, Golding J (1993) Outcome of childhood status epilepticus in lengthy febrile convulsions: findings of national cohort study. B Med J 307:225–228
25. Lewis RJ, Yee L, Inkelis SH, Gilmore D (1993) Clinical predictors of post–traumatic seizures in children with head trauma. Ann Emerg Med 22:1114–1118
26. Painter MJ, Bergman I, Crumrine B (1986) Neonatal Seizures. Pediatr Clin North Am 33:91–109
27. Seay AR, Bray PF (1977) Significance of seizures in infants weighing less than 2500 grams. Arch Neurol 34:381–382
28. Tassinari CA, Daniele O, Michelucci R, Bureau M, Dravet C, et al (1983) Benzodiazepines: efficacy in status epilepticus. Adv Neurol 34:465–467
29. Leppik IE, Derivan AT, Homan RW, Walker JE, Ramsey RE, et al (1983) Double-blind study of lorazepam and diazepam is status epilepticus.JAMA 249:1452–1458
30. Kyriakopoulos AA, Greenblatt DJ, Shader RI (1978) Clinical pharmacokinetics of lorazepam: a review. J Clin Psychiatry 39:16–20
31. Volpe JJ (1987) In: Volpe JJ (ed) Neurology of the newborn. W.B. Saunders Company, Philadelphia, pp 716
32. Crawford TO, Mitchell WG, Fishman LS, Snodgrass SR (1988) Very high dose phenobarbital for refractory status epilepticus in children. Neurology 38:1035–1039
33. McWilliam PKA, Leeds MV (1958) IV phenytoin sodium in continous convulsions in children. Lancet 2:1147–1150
34. Wallis W, Kott M, McDowell F (1968) Intravenous difenildydantoin in treatment of acute repetitive seizures. Neurology 18:513–517

35. Aicardi J, Chevrie JJ (1970) Convulsive status epilepticus in infants and children: a study of 239 cases. Epilepsia 11:187–191
36. Roger J, Lob, Tassinari CA (1974) Status epilepticus. In: Vincent PJ, Bruyn GW, (eds) Handbook of clinical neurology. North-Holland, Amsterdam:145–154
37. Delgado-Escueta AV, Wasterlain CG, Treiman DM, Porter RJ (1983). Status epilepticus: summary. Adv Neurol 34:537–542
38. Delgado-Escueta AV, Wasterlain CG, Treiman DM, Porter RJ (1982) Management of status epilepticus. N Engl J Med 306:1337–1341
39. Frisby JR (1990): Status Epilepsy. In: Intensive Care Manual. Oh TE (ed) Butterworths, Sydney, pp 266
40. Hauser AW (1983) Status epilepticus: frequency, etiology and neurological sequelae. Adv Neurol 34:3–14
41. Maytal J, Shinnar S, Moshe SL, Alvarez LA (1989). Low morbidity and mortality of status epilepticus in children. Pediatrics 83:323–327.
42. Meldrum DS, Horton RW (1973) Physiology of status epilepticus in primates. Arch Neurol 28:8
43. Shields WD (1989) Status epilepticus. Pediatr Clin North Am 36:383–393
44. Delgado-Escueta AV, Bajorek JG (1982) Status epilepticus: mechanisms of brain damage and rational management. Epilepsia 23:29–34
45. Simon RP (1985) Physiologic consequences of status epilepticus. Epilepsia 26 (suppl 1):s58-s63
46. Albano A, Reisdorf EJ, Wiegenstein JG (1989) Rectal diazepam in pediatric status epilepticus. Am J Med;70:168–171
47. Nead O, Miles MV (1985) Treatment of status epilepticus in children with rectal valproate. J Pediatr 106:323–328
48. Orlowski JP, Eremberg G, Cruse RP, et al (1990) Comparison study of intraosseous, central intravenous and peripheral intravenous infusions of emergency drugs. Am J Dis Child 144:112–117
49. Walsh-Kelly CM, Berens RJ, Glaeser PW, Losek JD (1986) Intraosseous infusion of phenitoin. Am J Emerg Med 4:523–526
50. Browne TR (1990) The pharmacokinetics of agents used to treat status epilepticus. Neurology 40(suppl 2):s28-s42
51. Van Ness PC (1990) Pentobarbital and EEG burst supression in treatment of status epilepticus refractory to benzodiazepines and phenytoin. Epilepsia 31:61–67
52. Osorio J, Reed RC (1989) Treatment of refractory generalizewd tonic-clonioc status epilepticus with pentobarbital anesthesia after high dose phenytoin. Epilepsia 30:464–471
53. Tasker RC, Boyd SG, Harden A, Matthew DJ (1989) EEG monitoring of prolonged thipentone adminsitration for intractable seizures and status epilepticus in infants and young children. Neuropediatrics 20:147–150
54. Goldberg MA, McIntyre HB (1983) Barbiturates in the treatment of status epilepticus. In: Delgado-Escueta AV, Wasterlain CG, Treiman DM (eds): Advances in Neurology, Vol 34, Status Epilepticus. Raven Press, New York, pp 499–503.
55. Browne TR (1983) Paraldehyde, chlormethiozale and lidocaine for treatment of status epilepticus. Adv Neurol 34:509.
56. Kofke WA, Snider MT, Young RS, et al (1985) Prolonged low flow isofluorane anesthesia for status epilepticus. Anesthesiology 62:653–655
57. Amrein R, Hetzel W (1990) Pharamacology of Dormicum (midazolam) and Anexate (flumazenil). Acta Anaesthesiol Scand 34:6–25
58. Krutak-Krol H, Domino EF (1985) Comparative effects of diazepam and midazolam on paraoxom toxicity in rats. Toxicol Appl Pharmacol 81:545
59. Galvin GM, Jelinek GA. Midazolam: an effective agent for seizure epilepsycontrol. Arch Emerg Med 1987; 4:169–173
60. Galvin GM, Jelinek GA (1992) Successful treatment of 75 patients in status epilepticus with intravenous midazolam. Emergency Medicine 4:11–15
61. Mc Donagh TJ, Jelinek GA, Galvin GM (1992) Intramuscular midazolam rapidly terminates seizures in children and adults. Emergency Medicine 4:77–81

62. Rivera R, Segnini M, Baltodano A, Pérez V (1993) Midazolam in the treatment of status epilepticus in children. Crit Care Med 21:991–994
63. Rivera R, Baltodano A (1995) Acute management of seizures and status epilepticus. Acta Pediatrica Costarricense 9:7–13
64. Rivera R (1994) Status epilepticus. Actualizaciones en Pediatría 1:6–8
65. Gross-Tsur V, Shinnar S (1993) Convulsive status epilepticus in children. Epilepsia. 34:S12–20

Nursing Aspects of Head-Injured Children

P. A. Moloney-Harmon

Introduction

Every year in the United States, approximately 25,000 children die as the result of a traumatic brain injury [1]. The majority of these injuries are caused by motor vehicle accidents, either occupant or pedestrian. Overall, falls are second in frequency, most involving falls from heights. Sports and recreation activities are third in frequency, most commonly due to bicycle accidents not involving an accident with a motor vehicle [2]. Increasingly, firearms are a common cause of brain injury. One study showed that central nervous system injury was a leading cause of death in firearm incidents in children [3].

There is a strong correlation between age and brain injury in children. Approximately 80% of deaths from brain injury occur in children less than 2 years of age [4]. Children between the ages of 6 and 12 are victims of twice the number of motor vehicle accidents as younger children [5]. Males are affected twice as often as females [4].

Numerous studies from the last 20 years have demonstrated that mortality and morbidity associated with brain injury can be reduced with well-organized treatment. This article provides a comprehensive overview of the treatment of brain injury in children, emphasizing the important contribution of collaborative interventions.

Etiology

There are important anatomic considerations that predispose the child to brain injury. The cranial bones are thinner in children and offer less protection to the growing brain. In addition, the size of the infant head is large in proportion to body size. Children's response to head injury differs in that they have a lower incidence of mass lesions but a higher one of intracranial hypertension [6]. Children also more commonly suffer from "malignant brain edema," which is actually significant cerebral hyperemia. As many as 50 per cent of head-injured children may develop this [7]. Because children experience intracranial hypertension and cerebral hyperemia more frequently, they are more susceptible to a secondary head injury rather than a primary head injury.

Pathogenesis

Traumatic brain injury is characterized by primary and secondary injury. Primary injury is produced by the trauma itself. It occurs immediately in the CNS following impact and may cause damage and/or death of the neuronal cells. Axonal injuries, laceration of brain tissue, contusions, skull fractures, and scalp injuries are examples of a primary head injury. Hypoxic injury may also cause a primary head injury if any of the neurons or astrocytes are injured by hypoxia or ischemia. This can be seen following a cardiac arrest. Secondary injury is produced by the brain's response to trauma. Secondary injury is a dynamic process that evolves over a period of hours to days and generally peaks at 3 to 5 days after injury [6]. Secondary injury involves the loss of cerebral autoregulation, development of extracellular and intracellular edema, and a breakdown of the blood-brain barrier. Secondary injury is compounded by systemic hyper- and hypotension, hypoxia, and hypercarbia. Secondary injury can often be prevented.

Specific Head Injuries

There are a number of specific head injuries that may be seen in children. Even those these are discussed separately, each one may be an element of a more serious brain injury.

Scalp lacerations are common in infants and young children. Because of the vascularity of the scalp, a large amount of bleeding may result from a laceration. Once underlying pathology has been ruled out, treatment is minimal and consists of controlling bleeding, inspection, irrigation and suturing. An underlying skull fracture may be ruled out by palpation and possibly a skull film.

Many children with head trauma will have an accompanying skull fracture. Most of these will be linear fractures. The majority of linear fractures are uncomplicated and heal spontaneously in 2 to 3 months. However, there are some linear fractures that are considered serious, based on their location. A fracture that crosses a major vascular structure, such as the middle meningeal artery or the dural venous sinus, has the potential of bleeding into the subdural or epidural space. A complication of a linear fracture seen in children is where a portion of the arachnoid membrane becomes trapped between two edges of the fractures bone, producing a lepto–meningeal cyst. The child may present with a soft and pulsating skull defect, seizures, and other neurological defects [8]. This defect may resolve with age or surgical intervention may be necessary.

A depressed skull fracture is a fracture where the inner table of the skull is displaced by more than the thickness of the entire bone. This represents a severe injury since a major force is required to produce this situation. The treatment of a depressed skull fracture is debridement and elevation of the fragment within 4 hours [9].

A basilar skull fracture is a common type of skull fracture in children and represents a major blow to the head. A basilar skull fracture usually involves a break in the base of the frontal, ethmoid, sphenoid, temporal, or occipital bones. The diagnosis is generally made on clinical presentation. A history of impact at the back of the head raises the index of suspicion. There may also be a loss of consciousness, seizures, or other signs of neurological deficit. On physical examination, the child may show certain findings that are indicative of a basilar skull fracture. Rhinorrhea, raccoon eyes (periorbital ecchymosis), anosmia, and ocular motor palsies may occur with anterior fossa fractures. Hemotympanum, otorrhea, vertigo, Battle's sign (mastoid ecchymosis), or unilateral hearing loss may occur with middle fossa fractures. Hypotension, tachycardia, and changes in the respiratory pattern may be indicative of brainstem compression that can occur with posterior fossa fractures [7]. Cerebral spinal fluid (CSF) leakage from the ear indicates disruption of the leptomeninges and CSF leakage from the nose indicates leakage through the perinasal sinuses. Clear drainage from the ears or nose is tested for the presence of glucose, since glucose is present in CSF. However, since CSF is often mixed with blood and blood contains glucose, the presence of glucose does not always confirm that the fluid is CSF. If CSF is mixed with blood, as the blood dries, an xanthochromic or yellow halo will appear on a dressing as the blood dries. The presence of a halo confirms the presence of CSF. A serious potential complication of CSF leakage is the development of meningitis. This is unusual, however, and the use of prophylactic antibiotics is controversial. The trend has been to treat only documented cases of meningitis [9]. In general, most basilar skull fractures are uncomplicated.

Skull films identify basilar skull fractures in only 10% of cases. CT scans are indicated to identify the area of the fracture and any underlying brain injury. Because the cribriform plate is disrupted, insertion of nasotracheal and nasogastric tubes are avoided. Most children with basilar skull fracture require only 24–48 hours of observation with frequent neurological checks and can expect a full recovery.

Concussion is the mildest form of traumatic injury to the brain. With a concussion, the child momentarily loses consciousness at the time of injury. The loss of consciousness is the result of the stretching and shearing forces in the brainstem and may last from minutes to hours [9]. Diagnosis is usually made on a historical basis based on a temporary loss of consciousness.

The nature of concussion is varied based on the age group. Infants tend to have a less specific clinical presentation. They usually exhibit benign posttraumatic seizures, vomiting, diaphoresis, pallor and lethargy and do not usually experience a loss of consciousness [9]. In the older child, posttraumatic amnesia becomes an important finding. The child may also complain of headaches, dizziness, and fatigue and may show some behavioral changes. The child's neurological function usually normalizes in about 1 week though some symptoms may persist for months even to one year. This postconcussive syndrome is expected to resolve completely.

Cerebral contusion is defined as an actual bruising or microscopic bleeding of the brain, associated with temporary or permanent structural damage. A contusion is similar to a concussion in that a transient or actual loss of consciousness may occur, however, a contusion causes an actual disruption of cerebral tissue to varying degrees, often accompanied by parenchymal hemorrhage and focal edema. The contusion may occur at the site of impact (coup injury) or at a site opposite the impact (contrecoup injury). The degree of injury is reflected by alterations in the child's mental status. In a mild contusion, the return of consciousness is not as rapid as with a concussion and there is retrograde amnesia. With mild retrograde amnesia, the loss is only that of exact details of events occurring immediately before impact. More severe amnesia manifests itself by extending for a period of hours before the impact occurred. Children with more severe amnesia often have some disorientation, slowed reaction, headache, vomiting and other mild neurological abnormalities.

Diagnosis of contusion is made based on focal neurological signs and CT scan. The most common pattern seen on CT are multiple small hemorrhages surrounded by varying degrees of edema.

Return to consciousness following rapid neurological deterioration may be seen in children with a cerebral contusion. The cause in children is usually due to diffuse generalized cerebral swelling. The most common CT scan finding among all children with an acceleration/deceleration injury is diffuse cerebral swelling. This is produced by cerebral hyperemia rather than by an increase in cerebral water content.

The incidence of cerebral contusion in infants is rare compared to older children. This is attributed to several factors. The skull of the infant is more pliable and there are less convolutional markers on the inner table. Because the surface between bone and brain tissue is smoother, there is less resistance to movement and surface injury is minimized. Also, the infant's brain is less myelinized; and demyelinized brain tissue has a softer consistency, which may reduce injury [6].

Treatment of a cerebral contusion depends upon the severity of the contusion. Treatment may be supportive medical therapy, involving treatment of increased intracranial pressure (ICP) if it exists. Surgical treatment, removal of the contused tissue, may be necessary if medical management does not control increased ICP or if significant shifts are seen of CT scan.

An epidural hematoma refers to a collection of blood above the dura. Epidural hematomas are less common in children, especially infants, due to several reasons. The dura is tightly adherent to the inner table of the skull, especially at suture lines in infants and young children. Also, the fixation of the middle meningeal artery does not occur until approximately 2 years of age. Since the artery is not embedded into the temporal bone until fixation occurs, it can rotate and possible avoid injury.

An epidural hematoma is a readily correctable lesion if identified and removed before secondary injury to the brainstem occurs. The classic lucid interval between the initial loss of consciousness and subsequent rapid neurological deterioration is much less common in children [9]. More often the symptoms tend to be vague depending on the age of the child and the location of the bleeding. Infants may experience bulging fontanelles, separation of the sutures, decreased hematocrit, and shock with significant bleeding. In older children, an enlarging hematoma may cause herniation into other areas of the brain producing corresponding signs. The child may exhibit hemiparesis, hemiplegia, ipsilateral pupil dilatation, posturing, or contralateral limb weakness [8]. Symptoms may be delayed for hours or days, if the source of bleeding is venous rather than arterial. If the hematoma continues to enlarge and the compensatory mechanisms of the brain become exhausted, temporal lobe herniation and brainstem compression will occur. A progressive decrease in the level of consciousness is the most significant diagnostic sign for all age groups. If time permits, a CT scan can be done which will show a localized, high density lesion with mass effect. If the child demonstrates rapid clinical deterioration, immediate surgical intervention without the benefit of a CT scan is necessary.

Treatment of choice is surgical evacuation of the hematoma. This is done as quickly as possible to avoid increasing morbidity or mortality. Evacuation of the hematoma is by craniotomy with removal of the clot and control of bleeding. Burr holes are technically difficult but may be useful as a diagnostic procedure in the absence of CT scan evaluation [9]. With prompt surgical intervention, the prognosis for the child with an epidural hematoma is good.

A subdural hematoma is a collection of blood in the subdural space; often with associated cortical damage from lacerated vessels or direct contusion. Acute subdural hematomas are almost always caused by a traumatic incident. They are usually associated with a high mortality and morbidity due to the fact that the lesion is often caused by disruption of a cortical artery or a large bridging vein. The impact required to produce this type of injury is significant and is associated with severe contusion of the underlying vein. Common causes of a subdural hematoma are high speed motor vehicle accidents, falls, assaults and violent shaking.

The clinical presentation of a child with a subdural hematoma is routinely that of a child who has sustained a major head injury. The lucid interval seen with epidural hematoma is not seen here because the brain is so severely injured. The child will present with profound neurological deterioration and because of the force of impact, the mental status will almost always be affected. Confirmation of the diagnosis of subdural hematoma can be made with CT scan. The most effective treatment is evacuation of the clot with control of bleeding and possible resection of damaged brain tissue [10]. Even with aggressive treatment, the prognosis for the child with a subdural hematoma is less favorable than for the child with an epidural hematoma. This is due to the associated damage to the underlying brain tissue.

Collaborative Management

The final common pathway for the pediatric victim of brain injury is cerebral hypertension. Assessment is directed toward detection of clinical manifestations of increased intracranial pressure and include a history, physical examination and neurological examination.

A history is useful to be able to anticipate injuries associated with the traumatic incident. Since the majority of pediatric injuries are blunt, they may not be immediately obvious. Knowing that a child has been involved in a high speed motor vehicle accident or a long distance fall will raise the index of suspicion for a severe head injury.

Even with an obvious head injury, a general systems review takes place. Once airway, breathing, and circulation are adequate, the neurological assessment can take place. The most important component of neurological assessment is level of consciousness (LOC). The Glasgow Coma Scale (GCS) is a useful tool to evaluate LOC. The GCS is divided into three sections. These are eye opening which related to arousal and awareness, verbal ability which relates to content and mentation, and motor ability which reflects mentation as well as the functional integrity of the major CNS pathways. This score has been modified to take into account age-appropriate behaviors.

Ongoing assessment of the brain-injured child includes the systems review and the neurological examination. The GCS described above is useful for continuous evaluation of the child's LOC. Pupil size and responsiveness are evaluated at least every hour and documented carefully. Corneal, oculovestibular, and oculocephalic reflexes are also evaluated. Cognitive ability may be evaluated by assessing verbal and motor ability. If the child is capable of responding, there may be a claim not to remember the incident for fear of being punished. It is helpful to distinguish between "selective remembering" and posttraumatic amnesia, since the latter is an important finding that may indicate concussion.

Vital signs are taken routinely. Respiratory rate and pattern are carefully monitored since abnormal patterns may indicate the level of the lesion. In addition abnormal patterns may negatively affect the $PaCO_2/PaO_2$ ratio and alter cerebral blood flow and intracranial pressure. Auscultation of the lungs will help to detect the development of neurogenic pulmonary edema, often associated with intracranial hypertension. The exact mechanism of neurogenic pulmonary hypertension is not well understood, but a proposed etiology in a temporary, acute vasoconstriction mediated by central nervous system injury leading to hydrostatic edema and injury to the alveolar-capillary membrane causing pulmonary edema [11].

Posttraumatic seizures occur in a number of head-injured children. Hahn and colleagues found that factors associated with seizures were severe head injury (GCS 3–8), diffuse cerebral edema, and acute subdural hematoma. Seizure activity increases the metabolic demands of the cerebral tissue, which, if not met, can result in further injury. There is some controversy over the use of prophylactic anticonvulsants in these patients; however, if seizures develop, treatment is necessary with standard anticonvulsant agents. Posttraumatic seizures may occur for up to 1 to 2 years postinjury [12]. Seizure activity will not be evident in the chemically paralyzed child; therefore, close monitoring when the child is not paralyzed or an EEG evaluation will be necessary if seizures are suspected.

Neurodiagnostic evaluation is an important component of assessment of the head-injured child. Skull films are helpful in diagnosing depressed skull fractures and locating foreign bodies; and are always indicated for suspected child abuse. However, a computerized tomography (CT) scan is required for the child with significant intracranial lesions. A CT scan is a rapid, safe, non-invasive means of assessing brain injury which yields important information, including identification of intracranial hematomas, extent of subsequent mass effect, presence of cerebral edema or hyperemia, and the extent of depression of a skull fracture [6]. Teasdale and colleagues (1990) identified that the patients at highest risk for development of acute traumatic intracranial hematoma requiring surgical evacuation were those with a skull fracture documented by skull films or clinical evidence of a basilar skull fracture and who were in coma on arrival ($GCS \leq 8$). They suggested that all head-injured children with a $GCS < 15$ have a CT scan [10]. Humphreys et al (1990) recommend that patients with a GCS of 9–12 due to trauma, especially with a severe mechanism of injury, have an early CT regardless of signs of clinical improvement [13]. Kaufman and Dacey recommend A CT scan for any child with a head injury accompanied by a neurological deficit and a $GCS \leq 14$. They also recommend a CT scan regardless of GCS in children who have experienced a high force mechanism of injury, a history of a change in the level of consciousness, or who will be receiving an intervention where the ability to do a clinical examination will be lost for more than a brief period [14]. Patients with a GCS of 13 or higher and a history of loss of consciousness should be treated like patients with a GCS of 9–12 [15].

It is recommended that contrast enhanced CT scans be obtained, especially in children, despite ready visualization of larger hematomas without contrast [6]. Even some acute subdural and epidural hematomas will not be delineated and/or characterized without contrast. In addition, direct visualization of displaced vessels can improve the recognition of mass effects which may not be evident on non-contrast scan, which is often the case due to malignant brain syndrome [6].

Magnetic resonance imaging (MRI) is a newer technique for visualizing intracranial structures which relies on radio frequencies and magnetic fields. MRI is extremely useful in visualizing brain tumors, especially in the posterior fossa, spinal cord structures, and vascular lesions. Its use is limited by cost, long procedure time, and inability to directly visualize bone [8].

Most head-injured children will require intracranial pressure (ICP) monitoring. Two major purposes exist for monitoring ICP. One is the prevention of herniation since monitoring provide for early detection of the development of cerebral edema to prevent herniation from occurring. The other is preservation of cerebral perfusion. By monitoring ICP and preventing elevation, cerebral perfusion pressure (CPP) can be maintained and manipulated [16].

A difficulty with measuring CPP is that it is an estimated value and is an indirect index of the adequacy of cerebral oxygen delivery. This index comes into question when the autoregulation of the brain is disrupted as with severe head injury. A more direct method of monitoring the adequacy of cerebral oxygen delivery is jugular bulb oxygen monitoring. This provides a method for evaluation of cerebral oxygenation by measuring oxygenation of mixed cerebral venous blood [17].

The methods of treating intracranial hypertension include expert nursing care, ventilatory management, fluid restriction, diuretics, and barbiturates. Nursing care activities are important in the management of the head-injured child, however, some studies have demonstrated that these activities exacerbate intracranial hypertension. Mitchell and Mauss (1978) reported the first descriptive study on the effects of nursing care activities on intracranial pressure [18]. A number of other studies examining various positions and the effects of rest periods between nursing care activities have provided a basis for nursing care [19, 20, 21]. An important implication from all the studies is that nurses play an critical role in controlling the environment of the child experiencing intracranial hypertension.

Mitchell and colleagues (1985) conducted a study examining the effects of touch on children with intracranial hypertension. They found that touch alone never increased intracranial pressure to a life-threatening level. They emphasized that the fear of doing harm by gentle touch is not well-founded. They also suggested that nurses increase the amount of non-procedural touching and encourage parents to touch their children [22]. Another study found that emotionally-charged conversation increased intracranial pressure in critically ill patients [23].

The child with intracranial hypertension related to head injury is positioned with the head of the bed elevated and head midline to facilitate cerebral drainage. Activities that increase intrathoracic or intra-abdominal pressures are avoided or limited, along with extreme flexion of the hips and knees. Rest periods are provided between activities, and duration of procedures are limited as much as possible. Family members are encouraged to talk to and touch their child without fear of doing harm. Conversations about the child within hearing range are prevented.

Hyperventilation provides a rapid means for reducing intracranial pressure. An important nursing action is to monitor the $PaCO_2$ when using hyperventilation as an intervention since $PaCO_2$ levels of less than 20 mm Hg can have a negative effect on cerebral blood flow. Also, the respiratory alkalosis produced can interfere with tissue oxygenation. The CO_2 level can be continuously monitored by the use of an end-tidal CO_2 monitor to allow for optimal CO_2 control. Ventilatory management also includes prevention of hypoxia since this can also cause dramatic increases in cerebral blood flow and intracranial pressure.

Fluid restriction will depend on the severity of the child's condition. For minor head injuries, two-thirds normal maintenance fluid will be sufficient. For major head injuries, a fluid restriction of one-half to one-third normal maintenance may be appropriate as long as cardiac output and vital organ functions are maintained.

Diuretics are useful since cerebral hyperemia in children is such a common finding. Osmotic diuretics, such as mannitol, pull fluid from the normal brain and may worsen the edema if it extravasates into the edematous brain and pulls more fluid into the lesion with it. Mannitol is used with caution in the initial management of the head-injured child because it may worsen the cerebral hyperemia [7]. However, it is often used for pediatric patients to reduce brain bulk and intracranial pressure. A dose of 0.25 mg/kg of mannitol is recommended. Serum osmolality is assessed at least every 6 hours and should not exceed 320 mOsm/L since complications such as renal failure and systemic acidosis have been reported at those levels. Loop diuretics such as furosemide are useful for subacute and chronic prevention of edema. Furosemide may be administered with other modes of therapy, augmenting and prolonging the effect [24]. The recommended dose of furosemide is 0.5–1.0 mg per kg every 4 to 6 hours. Serum potassium levels are closely observed in the child receiving loop diuretics since they may cause potassium wasting.

The use of barbiturates in children to control intracranial hypertension remains controversial. Little evidence actually exists that barbiturates potentiate a good outcome in head injury, but they may be used to decrease intracranial hypertension refractory to other methods [25]. Multiple drugs such as thiopental, phenobarbital, and pentobarbital are available for use, though pentobarbital is most commonly used in children. A loading dose of 2.0 to 5.0 mg per kg is given with a continuous infusion of 1.0 to 3.0 mg per kg per hour to maintain a serum level of 20 to 40 mg per mL [26]. Thiopental is most commonly used to prevent acute increases in ICP associated with noxious interventions such as suctioning. A bolus of 1.5 to 5 mg/kg/dose is given immediately prior to the intervention. Children who are receiving barbiturate therapy will require ICP monitoring, hemodynamic support, and meticulous nursing care. An important nursing implication is that the ability to evaluate the child's neurological status by physical examination will be lost.

Suctioning has been demonstrated to cause increases in intracranial pressure in children [27]. The duration of this procedure is limited to no more than 10 seconds and some method of preoxygenation is provided. Certain drugs, such as lidocaine or thiopental, may be administered prior to suctioning to prevent an acute rise in intracranial pressure during this procedure.

The use of steroids remains controversial in treating or preventing cerebral edema. There is no clear-cut evidence that outcome is improved, and some studies have demonstrated higher morbidity in head-injured patients who received steroids [28]. Since there is no confirmed benefit from steroid use despite numerous trials, their use is not generally recommended [29].

The nutritional needs of the child with head injury cannot be overlooked. The child with head injury, as with any traumatic injury are at risk for the development of protein-calorie malnutrition. Following head injury, there is a metabolic response that includes an increased energy expenditure and a decreased serum albumin level [30]. Early nutritional assessment and support is critical.

Conclusion

Caring for the child with intracranial hypertension is a collaborative challenge. A critical aspect of care is to prevent or reduce the detrimental effects of secondary injury resulting from increased ICP, systemic arterial hypotension, hypoxia, impaired cerebral hemodynamics, and hypermetabolism. Children with brain injury have been shown to have a better potential for recovery than adults. The potential for a good outcome is maximized by the important contribution made by nursing care. Nursing care includes precise assessment and interventions guided by research-based practice.

References

1. Tepas J, Discala C, Ramenofsky, M (1990) Mortality and head injury: The pediatric perspective. J Pediatr Surg 25:29–32.
2. Kraus J, Rock A, Hemyari P (1990) Brain injuries among infants, children, adolescents, and young adults. AJDC 144:684–691.
3. Beaver BL, Moore VL, Peclet M, Haller JA, Smialek J, Hill JL (1990) Characteristics of pediatric firearm fatalities. J Pediatr Surg 25:97–100.
4. Allison M (1992) The effects of neurologic injury on the maturing brain. Headlines 3:2-7.
5. Dandrinos-Smith S. (1991) The epidemiology of pediatric trauma. Crit Care Nurs Clin North Am 3:387–389.
6. Walker ML, Storrs BB, Mayer TA (1985) Head injuries. In Mayer TA (ed) Emergency management of pediatric trauma. WB Saunders, Philadelphia, pp 272–286.
7. Bruce DA, Alavi A, Bilaniuk L, et al (1981) Diffuse cerebral swelling following head injuries in children:the syndrome of "malignant brain edema." J Neurosurg 54:170–178.
8. Vernon-Levett P (1991) Head injuries in children. Crit Care Nurs Clin North Am 3:411-421.
9. Davis RJ, Tait VF, Dean JM, Goldberg AL, Rogers MC (1992) Head and spinal cord injury. In:Rogers MC (ed) Textbook of pediatric intensive care, 2nd edn. Williams & Wilkins, Baltimore, pp 805–857.
10. Teasdale GM, Murray G, Anderson E, et al (1990) Risks of acute traumatic intracranial hematoma in children and adults:implications for managing head injuries. British Med J 300:363–367.
11. Royall JA, Matalon S (1992) Pulmonary edema and ARDS. In:Fuhrman BP, Zimmerman JJ (eds) Pediatric critical care. Mosby-Year Book, St. Louis, pp 445–458.
12. Hahn YS, Fuchs S, Flannery AM, Barthel MJ, McLone DG (1988) Factors influencing post-traumatic seizures in children. Neurosurgery 22:864–867.
13. Humphreys RP, Hendrick EB, Hoffman HJ (1990) The head-injured child who "talks and dies." Childs Nerv Syst 6:139–142.
14. Kaufman BA, Dacey RG (1994) Acute care management of closed head injury in childhood. Ped Ann 23:18–28.
15. Ackerman AD (1991) Current issues in the care of the head-injured child. Curr Opinions Ped 3:433–438.
16. Dean JM, Rogers MC, Traystman RJ (1992) Pathophysiology and clinical management of the intracranial vault. In:Rogers MC (ed) Textbook of pediatric intensive care, 2nd edn. Williams & Wilkins, Baltimore, pp 639–666.
17. Kerr ME, Lovasik J, Darby J (1995) Evaluating cerebral oxygenation using jugular venous oximetry in head injuries. AACN Clin Issues 6:11–20.
18. Mitchell P. and Mauss N. (1978) Relationships of patient/nurse activity to intracranial pressure variations:A pilot study. Nurs Res 27:4 – 10.
19. Mitchell P, Ozuna J, Lipe H (1980) Moving the patient in bed:Effects on intracranial pressure. Nurs Res 30:212–218.
20. Bruya M (1981) Planned periods of rest in the intensive care unit:Nursing care activities and intracranial pressure. J Neurosurg Nurs 13:184–186.

21. Snyder M (1983) Relation of nursing activities to increases in intracranial pressure. J Adv Nurs 8, 273–283.
22. Mitchell PH, Haberman-Little B, Johnson F, et al (1985) Critically ill children: The importance of touch in a high-technology environment. Nurs Admin Q 9:38–46.
23. McDonald-Jacobsen LS (1988) Intracranial pressure and the effects of conversation. Proceedings, Third International Intensive Care Nursing Conference, Montreal, Canada.
24. Wilkinson HA, Rosenfeld S (1983) Furosemide and mannitol in the treatment of acute experimental intracranial hypertension. Neurosurgery 12:403–405.
25. Pilmer SL, Duhaime A, Raphaely RC (1993) Intracranial pressure control. In Eichelberger MR (ed) Pediatric trauma: Prevention, acute care, rehabilitation. Mosby-Year Book, St. Louis, pp 200–216.
26. Fackler JC, Yaster M (1992) Multiple trauma in the pediatric patient. In Rogers MC (ed) Textbook of pediatric intensive care, 2nd edn, Williams & Wilkins, Baltimore, pp 1443-1475.
27. Fisher DM, Frewen T, and Swedlow DB (1982) Increase in intracranial pressure during suctioning: Stimulation vs. rise in $PaCO_2$. Anesthesiology 57:416–420.
28. Dearden NM, Gibson JS, McDowell DG, et al (1986) Effects of high-dose dexamethasone on outcome from severe head injury. J Neurosurg 64:81–88.
29. Ghajar J, Hariri RJ (1992) Management of pediatric head injury. Ped Clin North Am 39:1093–1125.
30. Phillips R, Ott L, Young B, et al (1987) Nutritional support and measured energy expenditure of the child and adolescent with head injury. J Neurosurg 67:846–850.

Sepsis

Neonatal Sepsis

H. Stopfkuchen

Introduction

Neonatal sepsis is a clinical syndrome characterized by systemic signs of infection and accompanied by bacteremia in the first days of life [1, 2].

Neonatal sepsis can be divided into early-onset and late-onset disease, each having distinct features.

Early-onset disease presents as a fulminant multisystemic illness during the first few days of life (4–7 days). These infants have a history of one or more significant obstetric complications such as prolonged rupture of maternal membranes, premature onset of labor, chorioamnionitis or peripartum maternal fever. Early-onset neonatal infections are typically transmitted from the mother to the infant, via infected amniotic fluid, or dy direct contact in passage through the birth canal.

Late-onset disease may occur as early as 5–7 days of age but is more commonly recognized beyond 7 days of life.

It may be caused by organisms from the maternal genital tract, but is more commonly acquired after birth from human contacts or from contaminated equipment or material.

Epidemiology

The incidence of neonatal sepsis is reported to be 1 to 8 cases per 1000 live births with 20–25% of those having associated meningitis.

A special problem is the apparent increase in the incidence of bacteremia in neonatal intensive care units. Overall rates are as high as 14%. In this context indwelling venous catheters are significant risk factors.

Etiology

The principal pathogens involved in neonatal sepsis vary in part from nursery to nursery. Most infections are caused by group B streptococci, Staphylococcus sp. or Escherichia coli but a number of other organisms may be involved, such as Enterococcus sp., Enterobacter sp., Klebsiella sp., Haemophilus sp. and Listeria monocytogenes. While B-Streptococci, Escherichia coli and Listeria monocytogenes may be responsible for early-onset and late-onset disease Staphylococcus sp. and Pseudomonas are mainly associated with late-onset sepsis.

Pathogenesis

The infant is usually colonized with organisms of the vaginal flora after rupture of maternal membranes, though organisms can also be acquired transplacentally via hematogenous routes.

But in most cases acquisition of pathogens is associated with the birth process by direct contact in passage through the birth canal. If delivery is delayed, vaginal bacteria may ascend to reach the amniotic fluid and fetus and may in some cases cause inflammation. Aspiration of infected amniotic fluid by the fetus or neonate may then result in fetal infection.

In contrast to infants delivered by cesarean section, skin and mucosa of newborns born per vagina are colonized with organisms from the birth canal, including Staphylococcus epidermidis and Escherichia coli. These bacteria can be inoculated through the skin or mucosa after abrasion of the skin or after traumatizing mucosal membranes resulting in local and/or systemic infection. Furthermore, bacteremia may follow multiplication of bacteria in the upper respiratory tract or other foci such as the umbilical stump.

It is not known why an individual newborn with predisposing factors is at high risk of sepsis. In principle a number of factors have an important role in the susceptibility of neonates to infection, including:
- inoculum size and virulence of the organisms
- immature function of phagocytes and immune response
- metabolic factors such as hypoxia and acidosis

Clinical Picture

Many newborns with early-onset sepsis already have clinical signs of infection before, at or soon after delivery. Signs of fetal distress, fetal tachycardia and/or a low Apgar Score may be indications of fetal infection that occurred some time before delivery.

The early signs and symptoms of septicemia in a term or preterm newborn may be minimal and nonspecific.

These signs include:
- lethargy
- mottled, pale skin
- change in feeding pattern
- vomiting

A few hours later more characteristic clinical signs and symptoms may evolve.

Hyperthermia (axillary temperature measured greater than 37.8°C) sustained for more than one hour and/or associated with other signs of infection must be considered as indicative of sepsis.

Respiratory distress or apnea occurs in 55% of septic infants, apnea being a rather late sign of sepsis. Gastrointestinal disturbances including unwillingness to feed, vomiting, regurgitation, diarrhea and abdominal distention are frequently early signs of sepsis.

Clinical signs of cardiovascular dysfunction including tachycardia, arrhythmia and poor peripheral perfusion are also very sensitive signs of sepsis.

With progression of the septic process the clinical signs become more obvious and characteristic.

Diagnosis

Since it is difficult to establish the diagnosis of systemic bacterial infection on the basis of clinical findings alone the diagnosis usually relies on:

- history including maternal history and relevant recent nursery history
- clinical signs (see above)
- and on the results of laboratory tests.

Besides the results of cultures, there is no single test to allow clear-cut differentiation between infected and noninfected newborns. Therefore, if there is suspected sepsis, material for cultures and for rapidly available laboratory tests should be obtained immediately.

Microbiologic Techniques

The most specific method to diagnose a systemic bacterial infection in a newborn infant is the recovery of the organism(s) from the blood or other significant sites such as spinal fluid, urine or other body fluids. In contrast, surface cultures from the nose, throat, skin or umbilicus only indicate colonization and do not establish the presence of active systemic infection.

Cultures of Blood

The most specific method of diagnosis of neonatal bacterial sepsis is the recovery of a pathogenic microorganism from the blood. Bacterial growth is evident in the vast majority of cultures of blood within 48 hours. Blood may be obtained from a peripheral vein or from the umbilical vessels immediately following sterile umbilical vessel catheterization.

Culture of Cerebrospinal Fluid

Because meningitis may accompany sepsis, a lumbar puncture should be considered for examination of the spinal fluid in any neonate with suspected sepsis, although clinical judgement must be used in determining the safety of lumbar puncture in infants at risk for respiratory or cardiac compromise or for intraventricular hemorrhage (in preterm infants). If the newborn seems to be endangered by the lumbar puncture, the procedure should be postponed until the infant is stabilized.

Cultures of gastric aspirate and from the middle ear may reflect the bacterial colonization of the birth canal.

Laboratory Tests

All diagnostic tests should have maximal (100%) sensitivity and maximal (100%) negative predictive accuracy.

Antigen Detection

A rather rapid (within minutes) and sensitive test for group B streptococcus is the latex particle agglutination test based on the agglutination of specific antibody coated latex particles by bacterial antigen. This test is also of value in the previously treated patient [3].

Leukocytes

- Total neutrophil count:(< 4000/mm)
- Total nonsegmented neutrophil count
- Neutrophil ratios:
  - Band to total neutrophil ratio: normal < 0.2
  - Immature (band and promyelocyte to total neutrophil ratio: normal < 0.16 for the first 24 hours; < 0.2 for all age groups [4, 5]).

Acute Phase Reactants

C-Reactive Protein (CRP): normal < 1 mg/dl

Increases of CRP-levels in neonates may be associated with either inflammation caused by infection or with noninfectious conditions causing tissue injury or inflammation such as fetal asphyxia, respiratory distress syndrome and meconium aspiration pneumonitis. This reduces the positive predictive value of CRP determinations and their usefulness in diagnosis.

Furthermore, there is a poor response of CRP elevation during the first 12–24 hours after infection. Therefore, CRP levels used alone as an initial test for neonatal sepsis are of limited value; approximately 10% of cases are missed. Nevertheless, determination of CRP levels may give practically relevant informations about the presence, the intensity and the response to therapy of a systemic bacterial infection in newborns.

Neither the determination of plasma fibrinogen, the sedimentation rate nor haptoglobin concentration has been shown to be diagnostically useful in neonates.

This has lead to a search for other perhaps better indicators for the early diagnosis of neonatal sepsis. These include alpha 1-antitrypsin, lactoferrin, the complex of elastase, transferrin and interleukin-6 [6].

Further clinical studies have to demonstrate the significance of these indicators.

The inability of any single laboratory test to provide rapid, reliable and early identification of neonates with bacterial sepsis has led to the strategy of combining data from several different adjunctive laboratory tests such as band to neutrophil ratio, immature to total neutrophil ratio, total neutrophil count, CRP, sedimentation rate etc. as a means of increasing predictive accuracy. An abnormality in at least two of these parameters was considered to be diagnostic for sepsis.

In general, the evaluation of the according investigations has not led to the establishment of an absolutely unfailing screening test, although the negative predictive value has improved. The latter may result in a significant decrease in the use of antibiotics and/or in earlier discontinuation from treatment in an intensive care nursery.

Thus the history, the physical examination and careful longitudinal evaluation of the infants status remain the main determinants for use of antimicrobial agents. The results of laboratory tests are only used to support the initial clinical diagnosis of neonatal sepsis. In case of doubt antibiotic therapy should be initiated.

Therapy

Antimicrobial Therapy [1, 2, 7]

If the history of perinatal risk factors and clinical signs lead the physician to suspect neonatal sepsis, appropriate laboratory studies and cultures of blood, urine and cerebral spinal fluid (if appropriate) should be obtained, a chest film should be considered and antibiotic therapy should be initiated.

This approach has to be chosen because of the subtlety of nonspecific clinical manifestations of sepsis, the rapid progression of the disease and the still high mortality and morbidity associated with delayed begin of therapy. Consequently, one has to accept that the relatively low incidence of neonatal sepsis, coupled with the uncertainties in making a definitive diagnosis results in a majority of infants treated for sepsis not having this condition, as defined by documentation of bacterial disease (i.e.positive blood, urine or spinal fluid culture results) (e.g. 1:15 or 1:28 within the first few days).

Initial Antibiotic Therapy

The choice of antibiotics for the initial therapy must be based on the historical experience of the nursery, the antimicrobial susceptibility of bacteria recently isolated from both sick and healthy newborns and the maternal history.

Initial antibiotic therapy in early-onset sepsis must include coverage of gram-positive cocci, particularly group B streptococci, and gram-negative enteric organisms.

Treatment of the infant with late-onset sepsis may need to include coverage for hospital-acquired organisms such as Staphylococcus aureus, Staphylococcus epidermidis and gram-negative enteric organisms such as Pseudomonas sp.

Group B streptococci are uniformly sensitive to penicillin. Ampicillin and third generation cephalosporins are also highly active. Most strains of Staphylococcus aureus and Staphylococcus epidermidis produce beta-lactamase and are in principle sensitive to the penicillinase-resistant penicillins and selected cephalosporins. Nevertheless, many strains are already resistant to penicillin and are only sensitive to vancomycin. Enterococci (group D streptococci) vary in susceptibility to penicillin. The most promising therapy includes a combination of ampicillin and an aminoglycoside.

Ampicillin is the drug of choice for Listeria monocytogenes.

The initial choice of antibiotics for infections with gram- negative bacteria depends on the particular pattern of susceptibility of the flora of the neonatal intensive care unit. These patterns vary from institution to institution.

The aminoglycosides are highly effective against most gram-negative bacteria like Escherichia coli, Enterobacter, Klebsiella, Proteus sp. and Pseudomonas aeruginosa.

It follows from the preceding discussion that the initial treatment for early-onset neonatal sepsis consists of a penicillin, usually ampicillin plus an aminoglycoside such as gentamicin or netilmicin.

When the historical experience of the nursery suggests staphylococcus infection the initial treatment of late-onset sepsis should include a penicillinase-resistant penicillin or vancomycin (if resistance to penicillinase-resistant penicillin has been documented) (e.g. vancomycin plus aminoglycoside). Third generation cephalosporins coupled with aminoglycoside provide therapy against Pseudomonas aeruginosa.

The extensive use of broad-spectrum antibiotics should be avoided since it may lead to alteration of the microbial flora in nurseries. This also holds true for the routine use of third-generation cephalosporins (e.g. cefotaxime, ceftazidime, ceftriaxone) for treatment of neonatal sepsis or even suspected sepsis. These antibiotics have excellent in vitro activity against group B streptococci,

Escherichia coli and other gram-negative organisms (not against Listeria monocytogenes and enterococci), provide high concentrations in the cerebral spinal fluid, and lack dose-related toxicity. Because of the before mentioned risk of rapid emergence of drug resistant organisms, it is frequently recommended to use cephalosporins only selectively in infants with severe disease such as meningitis.

Definitive Therapy

Continuous antibiotic therapy (7–10–(14) days in most infants with sepsis and minimal or absent focal infection; at least 21 days for infants with meningitis caused by group B streptococci or gram-negative enteric organisms) is, of course, based on culture and sensitivity results. In case of negative bacterial cultures the subsequent course of therapy depends on the clinical condition of the newborn. If the neonate appears to be well after approximately three days, if the laboratory tests are normal and if there is reason to believe that another diagnosis was responsible for the early signs, antibiotic treatment can and should be discontinued. This is important since many newborns still receive initial antibiotic treatment for suspected sepsis. If the newborn's clinical condition remains precarious and if there is still suspicion of an infectious process, antibiotic therapy has to be continued in spite of negative bacterial cultures.

Treatment after Discharge

In case of late-onset sepsis, the following treatment plan is recommended:
- term newborns younger than two weeks: ampicillin plus an aminoglycoside
- preterm babies during the first two months of life: ampicillin plus aminoglycoside or cefotaxime
- term newborns after the second week: ampicillin plus third generation cephalosporin
- if there is concern of an infection caused by Staphylococcus aureus: penicillinase-resistant penicillin or vancomycin

Supportive Care

In addition to antibiotic therapy, supportive care of the infected neonate is essential. Close attention to respiratory, cardiovascular, fluid and electrolyte and hematologic support is essential to optimize outcome [8, 9]. This is of utmost importance if the newborn shows signs of septic shock. Once septic shock is recognized, support of circulation is the most important part of therapy. The primary goal is to restore the circulating blood volume to normal. Since shock exists when there is an imbalance between oxygen demand and oxygen utilization within the tissues, efforts must be made to reduce oxygen

consumption (ventilatory support; sedation; anticonvulsive therapy; avoidance of external stimuli) and to increase oxygen delivery (increase of cardiac output and of oxygen-carrying capacity of the blood). The latter may be reached by:
- early use of ventilatory support
- adequate volume replacement
- early use of catecholamines as the situation requires

This aggressive management approach also always needs close clinical observation and monitoring of the newborn.

Adjunctive Therapy

In addition to appropriate antibiotic and optimal supportive therapy, potential adjunctive modes of treatment have been developed and partially evaluated.

These therapies aim at
- the improvement of cellular host defense mechanisms
- the binding or neutralization of mediators
- and the binding and neutralization of bacterial cell wall components (e.g. endotoxin).

Measures to overcome deficits in the host defense of the neonate include granulocyte-transfusions, infusions of fresh frozen plasma or use of intravenous immunoglobulins [10, 11] or monoclonal antibodies [12]. Clear evidence of benefit by using these modes of treatment has not been shown yet.

The immediate host response to the inciting organisms is the sequential production of several inflammatory cytokines like tumor necrosis factor or interleukin-1. Once these primary mediators are produced, only agents directed to bind and neutralize them or to prevent their action on specific receptors are likely to be beneficial. But again, first clinical evaluations of these agents have been inconclusive or disappointing. The latter also holds true for the use of corticosteroids in patients with sepsis.

Fresh frozen plasma or monoclonal IgM antibodies should be able to neutralize or bind endotoxin of gram-negative bacteria. Convincing results of adequate trials are still lacking.

Prognosis

The mortality rate in neonatal sepsis decreased from almost 100% before the availability of antibiotics to about 25% in 1980. Today it is approximately 2–10%. Higher mortality rates are still found in fulminant sepsis within the first 24 hours of life and in meningitis. Mortality is also higher in preterm babies than term babies and higher in early-onset sepsis than in late-onset disease. The latter has a much better prognosis if Staphylococcus epidermidis is the cause of the infection. Few data are available about sequelae from neonatal sepsis without meningitis. Significant neurologic sequelae develop in infants who survive sepsis with meningitis caused by gram-negative enteric organisms or group B streptococci.

Prevention

In principle it seems reasonable to assume that measures to decrease the rate of prematurity and a more appropriate management of prolonged interval after rupture of maternal membranes, of maternal peripartum infections and of fetal distress should lower the rate of systemic infection in the neonate.

Antepartum treatment of pregnant women colonized with group B streptococci in the third trimester achieves a marked but transient reduction in colonization, but by term the colonization rate returns to pretreatment levels. However, intrapartum treatment of colonized women with ampicillin has been shown to reduce significantly and consistently early-onset group B streptococci infections and mortality [13, 14].

On the other hand, prophylactic treatment of all exposed neonates shortly after birth has produced mixed results. In addition, infection with penicillin-resistant organisms increased among treated infants. Therefore, routine use of penicillin/ampicillin prophylaxis is currently not recommended for exposed but asymptomatic neonates.

In order to reduce nosocomial infections in preterm infants who have low serum Ig G levels at birth, intravenous immunoglobulin prophylaxis has been considered. The available results of clinical trials are contradictory and do not allow a general recommendation [15].

Since the incidence of nosocomial sepsis especially in low birth weight infants is related to indwelling catheters, there should be strong indications for the use of central venous catheters, and the catheter should remain indwelling for as short a period as possible. Though it has been demonstrated that vancomycin added to nutritional solutions, including lipids, virtually eliminated the incidence of gram-positive bacteremia in at-risk populations of very low birth weight infants, the adoption of this prophylaxis strategy is not recommended because of safety concerns (e.g. emergence of vancomycin-resistant organisms) [16]. Prevention of nosocomial infection in nurseries and NICUs requires establishment of and rigorous adherence to at least some well defined policies and basic procedures. Though some nursery routines have evolved by custom or consensus and represent compromises between the ideal and the practical, many infection control policies have been evaluated and validated by epidemiologic studies. The latter include surveillance of nosocomial infections, adequate nursery design and environment, appropriate hand-washing by nurses and physicians, medical evaluation of the nursery personnel, frequent use of one way instruments, effective decontamination of e.g. floors, walls and incubators.

References

1. Roberton NRC (1992) Infection in the newborn. In: Roberton NRC (ed) Textbook of Neonatology, 2nd edn. Churchill Livingstone, Edinburgh, pp 943–1006.
2. Klein JO, Marcy SM (1990) Bacterial sepsis and meningitis. In: Remington JS, Klein JO (eds) Infectious Diseases of the Fetus and Newborn Infant, 3rd edn. Saunders, Philadelphia, pp 601–644.
3. Ascher DP, Wilson S, Mendiola J, Fischer GW (1991) Group B streptococcal latex agglutination testing in neonates. J Pediatr 119:458.
4. Lloyd BW, Oto A (1982) Normal values for mature and immature neutrophils in very preterm babies. Arch Dis Child 57:233.
5. Manroe BL, Weinberg AG, Rosenfeld ChR, Browne R (1979) The neonatal blood count in health and disease. I.Reference values for neutrophilic cells. J Pediatr 95:89.
6. Buck C, Bundschu J, Gallati H, Bartmann P., Pohlandt F (1994) Interleukin-6: A sensitive parameter for the early diagnosis of neonatal bacterial infection. Pediatrics 93:54.
7. Starr SE (1985) Antimicrobial therapy of bacterial sepsis in the newborn infant. J Pediatr 106:1043.
8. Stopfkuchen H (1985) Pathophysiologie der Hämodynamik im Schock. Monatsschr Kinderheilkd 133:391.
9. Schreiber MD, Covert RF, Torgerson LJ (1992) Hemodynamic effects of heat killed group B beta-hemolytic Streptococcus in newborn lambs: Role of leukotriene D4. Pediatr Res 31:121.
10. Haque KN, Zaidi MH, Bahakim H (1988) IgM-enriched intravenous immunoglobulin therapy in neonatal sepsis. AJDC 142:1293.
11. Harper TE, Christensen RD, Rothstein G (1987) The effect of administration of immunoglobulin to newborn rats with escherichia coli sepsis and meningitis. Pediatr Res 22:455.
12. Teng NNH, Kaplan HS, Herbert JM, Moore C, Douglas H, Wunderlich A, Braude AI (1985) Protection against Gram-negative bacteremia and endotoxemia with human monoclonal IgM antibodies. Med Sci 82:1790.
13. Pylipow M, Gaddis M, Kinney JS (1994) Selective intrapartum prophylaxis for group B Streptococcus colonization: Management and outcome of newborns. Pediatrics 93:631.
14. Strickland DM, Yeomans ER, Hankins GDV (1990) Cost-effectiveness of intrapartum screening and treatment for maternal group B streptococci colonization. Am J Obstet Gynecol 163:4.
15. Baker CJ et al (1992) Intravenous immune globulin for the prevention of nosocomial infection in low-birth weight neonates. N Engl J Med 327:213.
16. Spafford PS et al (1994) Prevention of central venous catheter-related coagulase-negative staphylococcal sepsis in neonates. J Pediatr 125:259.

Definitions, Risk Factors, and Outcome of Sepsis in Children

F. Leclerc, A. Martinot and C. Fourier

Introduction

Septicemia is the most common cause of death in medical and surgical intensive care units (ICUs). Statistics including persons ≥ 1 year of age indicate that the incidence of this disease has increased by 139% from 1979 to 1987 [1]. Morbidity and mortality of sepsis are increasing because we are treating more severely ill patients at more advanced stages of disease [2, 3]. For children one to four years of age, septicemia represents the 9th leading cause of death with an estimated annual mortality rate of 0.5/100,000 population ; in infants younger than 1 year the incidence of sepsis and associated mortality is higher peaking in premature infants in whom mortality rates approach 50% [4].

Definitions

Signs and symptoms of sepsis are highly variable. Table 1 presents the most important signs of sepsis in adults and children.

Clearly none is either sensitive or specific, especially in critically ill patients [5]. Furthermore, there really is not any "typical" patient with sepsis; in other words, the term sepsis is not sufficient to describe either patient.

In neonates, sepsis may especially start with minimal or non-specific symptoms, and approximately one third of cases are associated with concurrent me-

Table 1. Signs of sepsis in adults and children. (Adapted from Zimmerman [2] and Vincent [5])

Clinical signs	Other markers
- Hyper or hypothermia	- Hyperleukocytosis or leukopenia
- Tachycardia	- Respiratory alkalosis
- Tachypnea	- Increased O_2 consumption
- Cutaneous, ophthalmic manifestations	- Elevated CO, low SVR
- Organ dysfunction	- Inflammatory signs
	- Elevated cytokines levels

CO: cardiac output; SVR: systemic vascular resistances

Table 2. Signs of sepsis in neonates. (From Zimmerman [2], Dashefsky [6], Gerdes [7], Gladstone [8], and Buck [9])

- Fever or hypothermia, "not looking well"
- Tachycardia, bradycardia, shock, or poor perfusion
- Respiratory distress, apnea, grunting, cyanotic spells
- Lethargy, irritability, seizures, full fontanelle, hypotonia
- Feeding difficulties, vomiting, abdominal distension
- Diarrhea, jaundice, hepatosplenomegaly
- Rash, localized infection

ningitis which is clinically indistinguishable from sepsis [6]. Sepsis must be considered in any neonate with fever and signs of illness (Table 2) in the presence of risk factors (see below).

As in adults, lactic acidosis [10], elevated serum cytokines [9, 11, 12] and plasma nitric oxide [13] may be early indicators of sepsis and septic shock in neonates [9–13]; unfortunately, most of them are not rapidly available. Procalcitonin, that is released into circulation simultaneously to cytokines and has a long plasma half-life, may be of value in the early diagnosis of neonatal sepsis [14]; furthermore, it can be assessed within one hour.

Septic shock has no universal definition [5, 15, 16] and may present dramatically (as in fulminant meningococcemia) or insidiously, (such as candidemia in an immunosuppressed patient) [2]. In order to propose a set of definitions, which should assist clinicians who deal with sepsis and conduct therapeutic trials, a consensus conference was organized in August 1991 by the American College of Chest Physicians (ACCP) and the Society of Critical Care Medicine (SCCM) [17]. This terminology, adapted to children, is given in Table 3.

The terms septicemia, "septic syndrome", and refractory shock [4, 19] have been eliminated. Sepsis can be diagnosed only when infection is confirmed [20]. In adults series, only 25 to 40% of patients with bacteremia will develop sepsis [21], shock develops in approximately 40% of patients with sepsis [21], and about 50% of patients with severe sepsis have documented bacteremia [15].

The problems in applying this system to adults have been extensively discussed, in particular the heterogeneity of population : various sources of infection, medical surgical and traumatized patients, various degrees of underlying impairment [5, 15, 20]. It has also been recently proposed to categorize patients with sepsis related diseases into three groups: proven, possible, or absent infection [5, 15], and to use the term "bacteremic sepsis" to better discriminate sepsis with or without positive blood culture [22].

Recently, Hayden has recommended the use of the SCCM/ACCP system in children to allow comparison of data from studies of adults and children [18]. The first problem in applying the SCCM/ACCP system to children concerns age related normal values for arterial pressure, heart rate, respiratory rate, oliguria, and leukocyte count. Several authors have suggested alterations for children [3, 4, 18, 23, 24]; they are presented in Table 4 and 5, including diastolic arterial

Table 3. ACCP/SCCM Sepsis terminology [17]. (Adapted to children by Hayden [18])

Infection: microbial phenomenon characterized by an inflammatory response to the presence of microorganisms (bacteria, viruses, parasites) or the invasion of normally sterile host tissue by those organisms.

Bacteremia: the presence of viable bacteria in the blood.

Systemic inflammatory response syndrome (SIRS): the systemic response to a variety of severe clinical insults (infection, trauma, burns). The response is manifested by two or more of the following:
- Temperature $>38°$ or $<36\,°C$
- Heart rate >2 standard deviations above age normal
- Respiratory rate >2 standard deviations above age normal
- Leukocyte count >12000 cells/mm^3, <4000 cells/mm^3, or $>10\%$ band forms

Sepsis (SIRS plus infection): the systemic response to infection.

Severe sepsis: sepsis associated with organ dysfunction, hypoperfusion, or hypotension. Hyperperfusion and perfusion abnormalities may include, but are not limited to, lactic acidosis, oliguria, or an acute alteration in mental status.

Septic shock: sepsis associated with hypotension despite adequate fluid resuscitation, in addition to the persence of perfusion abnormalities that may include, but are not limited to, lactic acidosis, oliguria, or an acute alteration in mental status. Patients who are receiving inotropic or vasopressor agents may not have hypotension when perfusion abnormalities are measured.

Hypotension: a systolic blood pressure reading more than 2 standard deviations below the mean for age.

Multiple organ dysfunction syndrome: the presence of altered organ function in an acutely ill patient so severe that homeostatis cannot be maintained without intervention.

pressure (DAP) as suggested by some authors [3, 15]. In the SCCM/ACCP system systolic arterial pressure (SAP) is used to define hypotension. Mean arterial pressure (MAP), that represents the organ perfusion pressure, should be routinely used to define hypotension.

In adults, circulation failure is defined as a MAP $<$ 70 mmHg and a MAP $\geq$ 80–85 mmHg is a main goal of treatment. In children circulation failure has been defined as a MAP value $<$ 65 mmhg between 14 and 18 years, $<$ 60 mmHg between 10 and 14 years, $<$ 55 mmHg between 4 and 10 years, $<$ 50 mmHg between 1 and 4 years, $<$ 45 mmHg between 6 months and 1 year, and $<$ 40 mmHg between 3 and 6 months (unpublished data). MAP can be measured or calculated with the following formula : $MAP = (SAP + 2\ DAP)/3$.

As in adults, only 25 to 35% of children with bacteremia will develop sepsis [2]. The introduction of SIRS is also questionable because a large number of ICU patients, for example dehydrated children, meet the SIRS criteria [15]. Furthermore, many children with a diagnosis of streptococcus throat infection may meet the sepsis criteria [25]. Finally, several syndromes mimic septic shock: toxic shock syndrome, necrotizing enterocolitis, hemorrhagic shock and encephalopathy syndrome [2, 3]. The definition of organ dysfunction is another problem. Several systems have been proposed for adults [5, 15]. Wilkinson et al. [26] have defined criteria for organ system failure (OSF) in infants

Table 4. Suggested alterations for children

	Jafari [4] (PRISM score)	Hayden [18]	Hazelzet [3]	Wong [23]
Tachycardia (/mn)	Infants >160 Children >150	>2 SD	>2 SD	>2 SD
Tachypnea (/mn)	Infants >60 Children >50	>2 SD	>2 SD	>2 SD
Hyperthermia (°C)	>38	>38	>38.5	>38.5
Hypothermia (°C)	<36	<36	<36	<35
Hypotension	SAP<2 SD	SAP<2 SD	S or DAP<SD	MAP<5th p. or vasopressors.
Oliguria (ml/kg/h)	ND	ND	<0.8	<0.5

S: systolic, D: diastolic, M: mean; AP: arterial pressure; ND: not defined

Table 5. Alterations proposed by a French expert panel [24]

	Newborns day 1	Infants ≤1 month	Children ≤2 years	Children ≤10 years
Respiratory rate/mn>90th p.	> 60	> 40	> 30	> 20
Heart rate/mn>90th p.	>180	>160	>130	>120
Systolic blood pressure (mmHg)* <10th p.	< 50	< 65	< 70	< 80
Diastolic blood pressure (mmHg) <10th p.	< 30	< 35	< 40	< 50
Urine output (ml/kg/h)<10th p.		<0.5		
PaO_2 (mmHg)<10th p.	< 40	< 70	< 80	< 90
$PaCO_2$ (mmHg)>90th p.	> 50	> 45	> 45	> 45
pH<10th p.	< 7.20	< 7.30	< 7.35	< 7.35

p: percentile. * systolic BP for premature neonates: <40 mmHg<36 weeks gestation, <30 mmHg<32 weeks gestation

and children, and higher mortality rate has been observed with an increased number of simultaneous OSF. However, this system cannot be used in neonates weighing less than 2000 g and/or of less than 36-weeks gestation who were excluded from the study of Wilkinson et al. [26].

It is time to organize a pediatric expert conference to develop definitions applicable to children of all ages (including premature neonates). Only then can systematic evaluation of a child-adapted SCCM/ACCP system be achieved [18].

During the SCCM/ACCP conference, it was also recommended to combine the proposed definitions with an evaluation of the severity [17]. In infants and children the pediatric risk of mortality (PRISM) score [27] is predictive of mortality risk and can be used [3, 15]. In fact, sepsis syndrome children with hypotension had greater PRISM scores than sepsis syndrome children without hypotension [23]. The PRISM III has recently been presented [28] : its advantages over the PRISM include superior predictor performance and two time periods (first 12 hours and first 24 hours). In premature newborns the PRISM score cannot be used and two other scores have been developed : the clinical risk index for babies (CRIB) [29] and the score for neonatal acute physiology (SNAP) [30]. The CRIB, which consists of 6 items, is more simple for routine use than the SNAP which consists of 26 items. However, these scores have been developed to evaluate the risk of death 12 (CRIB) or 24 h (PRISM score and SNAP) after ICU admission; they cannot theoretically be used in patients who develop sepsis while they are treated in the ICU; furthermore, an important limitation of severity indexes is that the influence of therapy is not taken into account [5, 15].

Risk Factors

The incidence of sepsis shows a bimodal distribution : a first peak in the neonatal period and a second one around the age of two years. The incidence of sepsis for all PICU admissions may be up to 24% [26, 33]. In a recent French collaborative study (from 4/1 to 28/2/93), the incidence of sepsis syndrome in 36 NICUs and PICUs was 3% (three times less than in adult ICUs) with a mortality rate of 40%. The incidence was not related to age, sex, and disease (medical/surgical), but increased with the length of ICU stay. The origin was nosocomial in 19%; a bacteremia was associated in 49% of cases (Gram negative : 58%, Gram positive : 42%) [24]. Epidemiological studies have shown a decreasing incidence of *Haemophilus influenzae*, coincident with the use of Hib vaccine, and an increasing incidence of coagulase negative staphylococci (especially in infants receiving lipids through central venous lines), enterococci (especially in children with underlying diseases and central venous lines), and *Enterobacter cloacae* [34]. The most common infection in nosocomial bloodstream infections is coagulase negative staphylococci, followed by *Staphylococcus aureus* and enterococci [35]; the frequency of fungal infections is increasing, accounting for 20% of all pediatric intensive care-related nosocomial infections [35]. The majority of nosocomial infections are primary bacteremias (two thirds occurring in association with intravascular catheters) and lower respiratory tract infections [33, 35]. In one study, 90% of the children with nosocomial infection developed the infection after the beginning of their second week of hospitalization [35].

Table 6. Risk factors for neonatal sepsis. (Adapted from Dashefsky [6] and Gerdes [7])

- Male gender
- Prematurity
- Low birth weight
- Prolonged rupture of membranes
- Peripartum maternal fever or infection
- Fetal distress or hypoxia
- Obstetric or perinatal complications

Table 7. Risk factors for sepsis. (Adapted from Zimmerman [2] and Bone [21])

Host related	Treatment related
- Malnutrition	- Surgical, invasive procedures
- Debilitation	- Invasive devices
- Immunodeficiency	- Antibiotics
- Chronic health problems	- Immunosuppression
- Traumatic/thermal wounds	- Length of stay
- Severity of illness	- Hospital environment

Risk factors for neonatal sepsis are presented in Table 6 [6, 7]. Recent studies have documented more early-onset sepsis in newborns with neutropenia who were born to mothers with preeclampsia. Other factors increase the risk of sepsis especially of nosocomial origin (Table 7) [2, 35], and the risk of death [21].

Pollock et al., observed that children with a PRISM score $\geq$ 10 on PICU admission were at increased risk of infection (x 3); however the positive predictive value was only 11 %, and when length of stay was taken into account, illness severity was not associated with infection rates [33]. Gray et al. observed among very low birth weight infants that assessment of illness severity with SNAP provided information regarding nosocomial infection risk (coagulase-negative staphylococcal bacteremia) beyond that available from birth weight alone [36].

Outcome

Mortality rates depend on definitions, and the presence of shock and underlying diseases. For neonates, the risk of mortality of sepsis is approximately 15 to 30% [7, 8]; for older children mortality rate of sepsis and septic shock ranges from 10 to 50% [31, 32, 34, 37] (Table 8).

The overall mortality attributable to nosocomial infections is approximately 11% for both pediatric and neonatal nosocomial infections [35]. In children, mortality of sepsis is mainly confined to the first 48 h of the disease [3].

Table 8. Mortality rates of sepsis shock in infants and children

	Jacobs [31] septic shock	Carcillo [37] septic shock	Romano [34] sepsis + Gram neg. bacteremia treated with HA-1A	Storgion [32] "clinical sepsis"
No. of patients	143	34	23	55
Mortality rate (%)	10	47*	26	25

* Death rate of 73% in children with a chronic disease

In adults and children, outcome of sepsis is determined by a long list of factors : co-morbidities, physiologic dysfunctions (including the degree of tachycardia, and hypothermia), shock, organ failure, neutropenia, lactic acidosis, disseminated intravascular coagulation, and low gastric mucosal pH; origin of sepsis, causative pathogen, nosocomial infection, multiple bacteremia, and inadequacy of treatment also affect outcome [4, 5, 21, 22, 38, 39]. In adults, there is a clear relationship between the number of co-morbidities and increased mortality; patients are classified according to their underlying disease as being rapidly fatal (one year), ultimately fatal (five years), and non fatal [21, 22]. For children, Pollack et al. have proposed a chronic-disease (> 30 days) classification used for all chronic conditions present on admission to the ICU consisted of two qualitative categories : 1) serious underlying disease expected to limit life expectancy to a period not extending into adulthood or to prevent independent functioning as an adult, 2) no such serious underlying chronic disease [40]. This classification is not enough precise and has not been validated in terms of mortality rate. The PRISM III score, that includes new definitions of co-morbidities (non operative cardiovascular disease, chromosomal anomaly, cancer), may be more accurate [28].

In adults and children the best clinical indicator of sepsis and poor outcome is the presence of shock. Meningococcemia is a good example : in a recent review of 30 series from the literature [16], 988 patients were in shock and 38.1% died, 1378 were not in shock and 3.7% died ($p < 0.000001$). Early recognition and appropriate treatment of shock are important factors of prognosis : among 42 children with meningococcal septicemia, only 12 received appropriate treatment : 13 died and there was a significant correlation between delay of institution of therapy and outcome (unpublished data). In a recent study including 242 episodes of bacteremia and fungemia in children, seven variables that independently and significantly affected mortality were identified : shock, polymicrobial, recurrent, hospital acquired bacteremia, candidemia, and inappropriate antibiotic therapy [41]. Biological abnormalities, such as disseminated intravascular coagulation [16], lactic acidosis [3], high procalcitonin level [14], and low gastric intramucosal pH [42] adversely influence survival. Mortality prediction has also been carried out from the assessments of mediators (endotoxin, cytokines, and others) and coagulation factors (extrinsic pathway inhibitor, plasminogen activator inhibitor I, protein C, protein S, and antithrombin III) [3, 11, 16, 21, 39]. These determinations are expensive and unavailable on a routine basis, but may be useful for stratification of patients to evaluate the effectiveness of treatment strategies [9, 11, 12].

Numerous sepsis scoring systems have been developed either in adults [39] or children, particularly for meningococcemia [16]. The purpose is to stratify patient populations for evaluation of various interventions, not for clinical decision-making. The severity scores for meningococcemia are usually determined at admission. Although it is calculated after 24 hours, the "generic" PRISM score, that is easy to use and validated on large populations of different countries, should be used in place of "specific" scores. As an example, mortality rates for patients with acute meningococcal infection have been demonstrated to be accurately predicted by the PRISM score [43]. For premature newborns, the CRIB or the SNAP should be recommended.

Conclusion

There is a need for universal definitions of sepsis related diseases, including definitions of shock and organ failure based on quantifiable measurements. In combination with a classification of co-morbidities (which has yet to be defined), and an evaluation of the severity, this should assist clinicians to recognize the "at risk" patients. In fact, clinical trials should focus first on critically ill septic patients with documented infections, excluding not only patients with minor severity of illness but also those with terminal disease.

References

1. Increase in National hospital discharge survey rates for septicemia – United States, 1979–1987 (1990) From the Centers for Disease Control. JAMA 263:937–938.
2. Zimmerman JJ, Dietrich KA (1987) Current perspectives on septic shock. Pediatr Clin North Am 34:131–163.
3. Hazelzet JA, De Groot R. Sepsis-related problems in pediatric patients (1994) In : Reinhart K, Eyrich K, Sprung C (eds) Update in intensive care and emergency medicine 18. Sepsis. Current perspectives in pathology and therapy. Springer-Verlag. Berlin, Heidelberg, pp 217–227.
4. Jafari HS, McCracken GH (1992) Sepsis and septic shock : a review for clinicians. Pediatr Infect Dis J 11:739–748.
5. Vincent JL (1995) The "At Risk" patient population. In : Sibbald WJ, Vincent JL (eds) Update in intensive care and emergency medicine 19. Clinical trials for the treatment of sepsis. Springer-Verlag. Berlin, Heidelberg, pp 13–34.
6. Dashefsky B (1991) Life-threatening infections. Pediatr Emerg Med Care 7:244–253.
7. Gerdes JS (1991) Clinicopathologic approach to the diagnosis of neonatal sepsis. Clin Perinatol 18:361–381.
8. Gladstone IM, Ehrenkranz RA, Edberg SC, Baltimore RS (1990) A ten-year review of neonatal sepsis and comparison with the previous fifty-year experience. Pediatr Infect Dis J 9:819–825.

9. Buck C, Bundschu J, Gallati H, et al (1994) Interleukin-6 : a sensitive parameter for the early diagnosis of neonatal bacterial infection. Pediatrics 93:54–58.
10. Fitzgerald MJ, Goto M, Myers TF, Zeller PW (1992) Early metabolic effects of sepsis in the preterm infant : lactic acidosis and increased glucose requirement. J Pediatr 121:951–955.
11. Harris MC, Costarino AT, Sullivan JS, et al (1994) Cytokine elevations in critically ill infants with sepsis and necrotizing enterocolitis. J Pediatr 124:105–111.
12. Roman J, Fernandez F, Velasco F, et al (1993) Serum TNF levels in neonatal sepsis and septic shock. Acta Paediatr 82:352–354.
13. Shi Y, Li HQ, Shen CK, et al (1993) Plasma nitric oxide levels in newborn infants with sepsis. J Pediatr 123:435–438.
14. Assicot M, Gendrel D, Carsin H, et al (1993) High serum procalcitonin concentrations in patients with sepsis and infection. Lancet 341:515–518.
15. An expert report of the European Society of Intensive Care Medicine. The problem of sepsis. (1994) Intensive Care Med 20:300–304.
16. Leclerc F, Giraud T, Delepoulle F, et al (1993) Facteurs de gravité des méningococcémies. In : Actualités en réanimation et urgences. Arnette Paris, pp 105–122.
17. American College of Chest Physicians/Society of Critical Care Medicine consensus conference (1992) Definitions for sepsis and organ failure and guidelines for the use of innovative therapies in sepsis. Crit Care Med 20:864–874.
18. Hayden WR (1994) Sepsis terminology in pediatrics. J Pediatr 124:657–658.
19. Sáez-Llorens X, McCracken GH (1993) Sepsis syndrome and septic shock in pediatrics : current concepts of terminology, pathophysiology, and management. J Pediatr 123:497–508.
20. Sibbald WJ, Doig G, Inman KJ (1995) Sepsis, SIRS and infection. Intensive Care Med 21:299–301.
21. Bone RC (1994) Clinical manifestations and prognostic indicators in sepsis. In : Reinhart K, Eyrich K, Sprung C (eds) Update in intensive care and emergency medicine 18. Sepsis. Current perspectives in pathology and therapy. Springer-Verlag. Berlin, Heidelberg, pp 16–22.
22. Gasche Y, Pittet D, Suter PM (1995) Outcome and prognostic factors in bacteremic sepsis. In : Sibbald WJ, Vincent JL (eds) Update in intensive care and emergency medicine 19. Clinical trials for the treatment of sepsis. Springer-Verlag. Berlin, Heidelberg, pp 35–51.
23. Wong HR, Carcillo JA, Burckart G, et al (1995) Increased serum nitrite and nitrate concentrations in children with the sepsis syndrome. Crit Care Med 23:835–842.
24. Mercier JC, Doyon F, Brun-Buisson C, et le Groupe francophone de Réanimation Pédiatrique (1995) Epidémiologie des syndromes septiques et bactériémies chez l'enfant et le nouveau-né. In : Etats septiques graves. XXIIIe Congres de la Société de Réanimation de Langue Française. Paris, pp 17–20.
25. Hayden WR (1993) . Sepsis and organ failure. Definitions and guidelines. Crit Care Med 21:1612–1613.
26. Wilkinson JD, Pollack MM, Glass NL, et al (1987) Mortality associated with multiple organ system failure and sepsis in pediatric intensive care unit. J Pediatr 111; 324–328.
27. Pollack MM, Ruttimann UE, Getson PR (1988) Pediatric risk of mortality (PRISM) score. Crit Care Med 16:1110–1116.
28. Pollack MM, Patel KM, Ruttimann UE (1995) PRISM III. Crit Care Med 23:A223 (Abst).
29. The International neonatal network (1993) The CRIB (clinical risk index for babies) score : a tool for assessing initial neonatal risk and comparing performance of neonatal intensive care units. Lancet 342:193–198.
30. Richardson DK, Gray JE, McCormick MC, et al (1993) Score for neonatal acute physiology : a physiologic severity index for neonatal intensive care. Pediatrics 91:617–623.
31. Jacobs RF, Sowell MK, Moss M, Fiser DH (1990) Septic shock in children : bacterial etiologies and temporal relationships. Pediatr Infect Dis J 9:196–200.
32. Storgion SA, Beck RJ, Leggiadro RJ (1994) Frequency and outcome of infectious disease admissions to a pediatric intensive care unit. South Med J 87:1121–1124.

33. Pollock E, Ford-Jones EL, Corey M, et al (1991) Use of the pediatric risk of mortality score to predict nosocomial infection in a pediatric intensive care unit. Crit Care Med 19:160–165.
34. Romano MJ, Kearns GL, Kaplan SL (1993) Single-dose pharmacokinetics and safety of HA-1A, a human IgM anti-lipid-A monoclonal antibody, in pediatric patients with sepsis syndrome. J Pediatr 122:974–981.
35. Stein F, Trevino R (1994) Nosocomial infections in the pediatric intensive care unit. Pediatr Clin North Am 41:1245–1257.
36. Gray JE, Richardson DK, Mc Cormick MC, Goldmann DA (1995) Coagulase-negative staphylococcal bacteremia among very low birth weight infants : relation to admission illness severity, resource use, and outcome. Pediatrics 95:225–230.
37. Carcillo JA, Davis AL, Zaritsky A (1991) Role of early fluid resuscitation in pediatric septic shock. JAMA 266:1242–1245.
38. Balk RA, Parrillo JE (1992) Prognostic factors in sepsis : the cold facts. Crit Care Med 20:1373–1374.
39. Barriere SL, Lowry SF (1995) An overview of mortality risk prediction in sepsis. Crit Care Med 23:376–393.
40. Pollack MM, Ruttimann UE, Getson PR, and members of the multi-institutional study group (1987) Accurate prediction of the outcome of pediatric intensive care. A new quantitative method. N Engl J Med 316:134–139.
41. Ashkenazi S, Leibovici L, Samra Z, et al (1992) Risk factors for mortality due to bacteremia and fungemia in childhood. Clin Infect Dis 14:949–951.
42. Krafte-Jacobs B, Carver J, Wilkinson JD (1995) Comparison of gastric intramucosal pH and standard perfusional measurements in pediatric septic shock. Chest 108:220–225.
43. Algren JT, Lal S, Cutliff SA, Richman BJ (1993) Predictors of outcome in acute meningococcal infection in children. Crit Care Med 21:447–452.

Systemic Inflammatory Response Syndrome (SIRS) in Pediatric Patients

J. Fischer and S. Fanconi

Introduction

Sepsis is an important cause of morbidity and mortality both in neonates and children. Septic episodes caused by bacteria may rapidly progress from mild to severe illness with shock and multiorgan failure. Early recognition of bacterial infection and initiation of appropriate antimicrobial treatment decreases morbidity and mortality [1]. However, other non-bacterial pathologies like burns, trauma, major surgery, reperfusion after ischemia or Addisonian crisis can elicit a systemic inflammatory response syndrome (SIRS) clinically similar to bacterial sepsis [2]. Careful evaluation of history and clinical circumstances helps but does not resolve the inaccuracy of presumptive diagnosis. Despite maximized efforts to isolate bacteria, about half of the septic episodes in adult [3] and pediatric patients [4] remain culture-negative.

The immune response causing the clinical symptoms of sepsis is not a simple cascade of events, but requires organized coordination of pro- and anti-inflammatory processes. Cytokines are involved in the activation of major immunogenic cell lines [5], and alterations of neuro-endocrine feedback circuits play an important role [6]. A certain proportion of episodes with systemic inflammatory response will, regardless of bacterial or non-bacterial cause, progress to more severe stages of illness with shock and severe organ dysfunction. Most of these disturbances are not caused by invading organisms but by the hosts' defense mechanisms [7]. The primary site of damage is the endothelial layer of the vascular bed [8, 9].

Most of the published clinical trials on immunomodulatory treatment of sepsis used clinical criteria to define the "sepsis syndrome" [10]. These were clinical evidence of infection associated with tachypnea, tachycardia, hyperthermia or hypothermia as well as altered organ perfusion (hypotension, altered mental status, decreased PaO_2/FiO_2, increased lactate or oliguria) [11]. This definition [12] led to the inclusion of patients with varying severity of illness and different underlying disorders, which was subsequently viewed as one of the reasons why human trials were not able to reproduce the benefits of immunomodulation observed in animal studies. From these data and from recent animal experiments it appears that almost contradictory immunomodulatory strategies may be necessary depending on the presence or absence of bacteria, underlying pathology and time-course of the disease [12].

Because prophylactic measures failed to reduce morbidity and mortality from systemic bacterial infection in premature infants and neonates [13], immunomodulatory prophylaxis or treatment of neonatal sepsis has been advocated. But before starting clinical trials subject to the same problems as the early trials in septic adult patients, a classification system is necessary addressing the different pathologies leading to clinical sepsis [14]. This classification should be able to describe course over time and to assess severity of illness. In this chapter we suggest a pediatric adaptation of the definitions of sepsis and multiorgan failure of the Consensus Conference of the American College of Chest Physicians and the Society of Critical Care Medicine [15] for adult patients.

Pathogenesis

Many reviews have appeared over the past five years dealing in detail with cells and cytokines involved in the systemic inflammatory response [7, 16]. Here we can only summarize the key mechanisms of SIRS. A systemic inflammatory response is now understood as a general reaction of the organism against a great variety of stimuli, one of them being systemic bacterial infection [15].

Figure 1 presents the most important causes encountered in pediatric intensive care. Cytokines play a major role in activating this immune response [5]. They exert effects both locally and systemically. Over short distances they regulate interactions between immunogenic cells or leukocytes and endothelium in a paracrine fashion. Systemic effects of cytokines include readjustment of insulin sensitivity or activation of the hypopituitary-adrenal axis. The latter

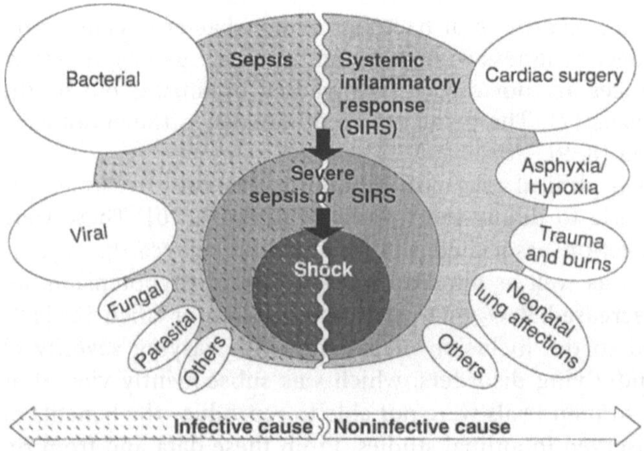

Fig. 1. Systemic inflammatory response syndrome (SIRS) in pediatric patients. Infectious and non-infectious conditions may resolve without systemic inflammatory response or can trigger SIRS with potential progress to severe illness.

results in increased blood levels of glucocorticoids, an important inhibitor of further cytokine production [6].

Of the various cytokines appearing in the bloodstream in measurable quantities in patients with sepsis [5] and after experimental endotoxin challenge [17], three deserve special mention. The primary cytokine initiating a systemic immune response is tumor necrosis factor (TNFa) observed 1.5–2 hours after injection. Besides stimulation of immunogenic cells this cytokine accounts for myocardial depression, inhibition of oxygen radical scavengers in the endothelium and dilatation of vascular smooth muscles [7]. About two hours later, interleukin-6 (IL-6) and granulocyte-colony stimulating factor (G-CSF) among other cytokines become markedly elevated [17]. IL-6 has several functions: it is a strong activator of the pituitary gland, it promotes differentiation of T-lymphocytes, it increases production of IgG by B-lymphocytes and induces hepatocytic acute phase protein synthesis. IL-6 can also activate neutrophile granulocytes. In contrast to TNFa, G-CSF can be injected into healthy subjects in high dosages with few side effects [18]. The predominant action of this cytokine is activation of neutrophile granulocytes and augmentation of their numbers. The latter is achieved by delaying apoptosis (prolonged survival in circulation from the usual 6–8 hours to 72–96 hours) [18] and by increasing production from the bone marrow. G-CSF also enhances neutrophile degranulation, adherence to endothelium, and oxidative burst. This cytokine is chemotactic for granulocytes and is found in very high concentrations (>5000 pg/ml) together with IL-6 at sites of infection [18].

Activated neutrophile granulocytes are believed to contribute to septic shock and ARDS by endothelial damage. This occurs particularly if TNFa is elevated. TNFa inhibits oxygen radical scavenger enzymes in endothelial cells. After priming with TNFa, endothelial cells are much more vulnerable to the oxidative disgorge of activated and adhering neutrophiles [8].

If the immune response is down regulated in time, the host may survive after endothelial recovery. If the process continues, endothelial damage will trigger disseminated intravascular coagulation, and will later cause myocardial depression [19]. Further consequences are abnormal microcirculation with impaired oxygen delivery and subsequent organ failure.

Terminology

The term "sepsis syndrome" emerged from the literature of the 1980s. This rather broad definition served as inclusion criterium for multicenter trials on the benefits of glucocorticoids in early treatment of sepsis. The terminology for description of septic episodes in pediatric patients was derived from this concept. Sepsis was viewed as a cascade of subsequent stages of illness, namely bacteremia, sepsis, compensated septic shock, irreversible shock and multiple organ failure [16].

Several authors in the early 1990s addressed the urgent need to agree on commonly used definitions for sepsis. In 1992 the suggestions from a consensus conference held by the American College of Chest Physicians and the Society of Critical Care Medicine were published [15]. The Consensus Conference agreed upon the term "systemic inflammatory response syndrome" (SIRS) to provide a conceptual framework including all bacterial and non-bacterial causes of clinical sepsis. It was suggested that multiple organ failure be viewed as the ultimate end point on a continuous scale of increasing organ dysfunction.

Although the conference agreed that non-bacterial SIRS might also progress to shock, no terminology was provided to address this assumption correctly. Subsequent epidemiological studies used the terms culture-positive and culture-negative septic shock [3].

Table 1. Definitions of systemic inflammatory response syndrome (SIRS)

Age	Breath rate	Heart rate	Temperature	Leucocyte count or immature (band) count[b]
Adults[a] >15 years	>20/min	> 90/min	>380C or <360C	>12×109/l, or <4×109/l or >0.1 bands
12–15 years	>25/min	>100/min	>38.50C or <360C	>12×109/l, or <4×109/l or >0.1 bands
5–12 years	>30/min	>120/min	>38.70C or <360C	>12×109/l, or <4×109/l or >0.15 bands
2–5 years	>35/min	>130/min	>390C or <360C	>15×109/l, or <4×109/l or >0.15 bands
1–2 years	>40/min	>140/min	>390C or <360C	>15×109/l, or <4×109/l or >0.15 bands
1–12 months[c]	>45/min	>160/min	>38.50C or <360C	>15×109/l, or <4×109/l or >0.20 bands
<1 month[c]	>60/min	>190/min	>380C or <35.50C	>20×109/l, or <4×109/l >0.25 bands
>5 days[c]	>60/min	>190/min	>380C or <35.50C	>35×109/l, or <4×109/l or >0.30 bands

Diagnosis of SIRS requires two of the above four criteria. For leucocyte count either criterium (leukocytosis or leukopenia or increased band count) must be met.

[a] Consensus Conference definitions [15]

[b] Has to be adjusted to individual laboratory values

[c] Breath rate, heart rate, temperature: gestational age. Leucocyte and band count: postnatal age

However, there are no reports of further attempts to differentiate between the various causes of "culture-negative" shock: sepsis with failure to grow viable bacteria, advanced localized infection, systemic viral infection or shock after runaway immune response to hypoxia, trauma, or burns. For moderate illness the concept of SIRS has been recognized as being a definition of high sensitivity with little prognostic properties [3]. Despite these limitations, adaptation of the Consensus Conference definitions was suggested for pediatric patients [14]. The benefit of a uniform classification was seen in the possibility of comparing pediatric studies with trials in adults. Table 1 presents the Consensus Conference definitions and our proposed adaptations, derived from Hayden [14].

Epidemiology

Two recently published studies evaluated prevalence, incidence and evolution of SIRS in adult intensive care. Rangel-Frausto [3] investigated the epidemiology of SIRS, sepsis, severe sepsis and shock for a period of 9 months in three general wards and three ICUs of a 900-bed Iowa teaching hospital. Salvo and coworkers [20] examined the incidence of SIRS and progression to more severe illness in 99 Italian ICUs over a period of one year. The Iowa study included a total of 3708 patients, the Italian investigation presented data from 1101 patients. Upon admission to the ICU in the Italian study, 61.8% of patients fulfilled the criteria for SIRS; of these 7.3% had sepsis, 3.4% severe sepsis, and 4.9% were admitted in septic shock. Progress of illness to more severe stages was observed in approximately 30% of patients. The Iowa study reported a comparable incidence of SIRS ranging from 542 to 857 per 1000 patient days for the three ICUs studied (cardiovascular, medical, surgical). 68% of the patients met the criteria for SIRS.

The Iowa study also assessed the progression of illness from SIRS to shock. Of those patients who finally developed culture-proven septic shock, 71% had been previously classified as having severe sepsis, sepsis or SIRS. The remaining 29% fulfilled the criteria for shock within the first day of admission. Mortality was 46% in patients with septic shock, 20% in patients with severe sepsis, 16% in patients with sepsis and 7% in patients with SIRS, compared to 3% in the population without SIRS. 62% of the patients with SIRS fulfilled clinical criteria for sepsis and were prescribed antibiotics. In 42% of these infection could be documented, in 58% cultures remained negative. Patients with a culture-negative shock had a similar crude mortality and rate of organ failure (ARDS, acute renal failure, DIC) as those with culture-positive shock. In patients whose condition did not exceed severe sepsis, mortality was slightly lower in culture-negative episodes than in culture-positive ones. In both studies the diagnosis of SIRS alone did not have any prognostic implications.

We performed an 11-month study on early markers of sepsis in an 18-bed neonatal and pediatric intensive care unit of a tertiary teaching hospital [4]. In 127 episodes sepsis was clinically suspected and antimicrobial treatment ini-

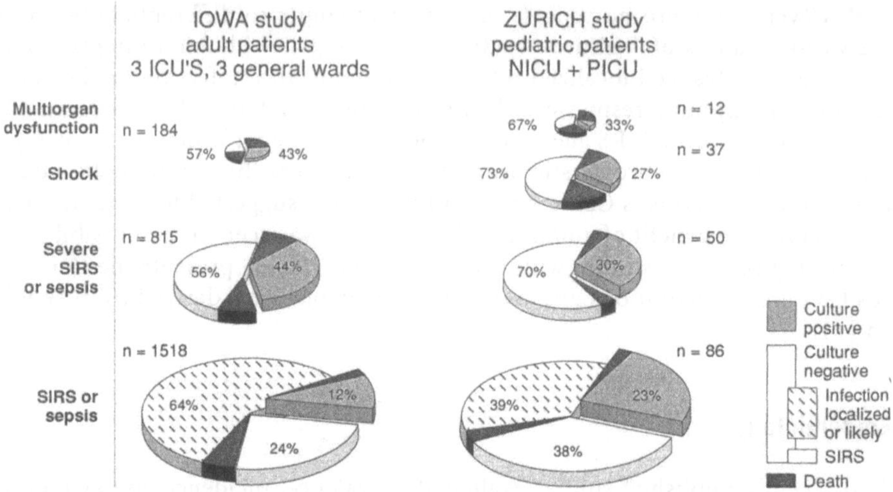

Fig. 2. Mortality and distribution of SIRS, sepsis, severe sepsis, septic shock and multiorgan dysfunction in pediatric and adult patients. Area of circles represents relative proportion of the different subgroups. No data for further differentiation of episodes with culture-negative severe sepsis or shock were reported from the Iowa study [3].

tiated. In 38% of episodes systemic infection could be documented. Cultures remained negative in 62% of the cases. Culture-negative episodes included inflammatory response with no or unlikely bacterial infection (defined as SIRS, 20%), episodes due to localized bacterial focus (20%) and septic episodes with undocumented but very likely systemic bacterial infection (defined as culture-negative sepsis). The latter accounted for 22% of the episodes of suspected sepsis. Two hypotheses may explain this relatively large percentage. First, at the time when blood cultures were taken, neutrophile defense had successfully cleared viable bacteria from the blood stream. Second, the restricted sampling size in premature infants and neonates (0,5–1ml per bottle) reduced the chance of isolating viable bacteria. 57% of patients with suspected sepsis progressed to severe illness. Mortality was 75% for patients with multiorgan failure and documented systemic bacterial infection, 33% for patients with septic shock, 16% for patients with severe sepsis and 7.5% for patients with sepsis (Figure 2).

In order to study SIRS in absence of bacteria, a control group was recruited from patients at risk of developing SIRS. 78 consecutive admissions after cardiac surgery, asphyxia, resuscitation, respiratory distress and trauma were enrolled. 54 out of 78 of patients (74%) developed SIRS within 24 hours of admission, of these 46% progressed to severe illness. Mortality was significantly lower than in patients with documented systemic infection. Severity of illness was classified according to the Consensus Conference definitions. Table 2 presents the pediatric adaptations used in our study compared to the definitions used by the Iowa group. Interestingly, distribution of stages of illness is similar for adult and pediatric patients with the possible exception that mortality is lower in pediatric SIRS/sepsis and severe SIRS/sepsis, and that there are more positive blood cultures in pediatric SIRS/sepsis than in adults.

Severity of Illness

Most published scores attempt to predict mortality by assessing physiological abnormalities observed at admission or over the first 24 hours of hospitalization. Because in sepsis prediction is poor, Le Gall and Lemeshov suggested a remodelled scoring system for adults [21]. Although this system is elaborate and refined to meet the particular derangements observed in sepsis, some problems were not resolved: Scoring systems focus on prediction of death, not on organ dysfunction or quality of life. The scores are usually established within 24 hours of admission, but severe sepsis or shock may develop later [22]. Almost all scoring systems are affected by therapeutic efforts: sedation and analgesia will alter mental status, and oscillators, nitric oxide and kinetic treatment may improve oxygenation. Mortality, particularly in pediatric patients, is not a stable outcome measure in itself: some institutions sustain intensive care therapy despite major brain damage, while others decide to withdraw further treatment in the same situation. In our unit the decision to withdraw intensive care treatment led to death in more than half of the septic episodes with lethal outcome. Some patients might have survived if maximum treatment had been pursued but would have been severely handicapped.

A further problem of scoring systems is rapid progression of illness over time, like in meningococcemia, gram-negative sepsis in premature infants or β-hemolytic streptococcal sepsis in neonates. Shock may develop within a few hours, preceding major changes in mental status, pulmonary, renal or liver function in the following 24 to 48 hours. If pathology is recognized early, admission scores underestimate severity of illness. The resulting difficulty in predicting mortality of neonatal sepsis was reported from a study on the applicability of the "score for neonatal acute physiology" (SNAP) [23].

Recent comments on the concept and definitions of SIRS suggested that circulatory criteria may be better in identifying patients "at risk" [22]. It was argued that shock or impaired oxygen delivery to vital organs is strongly associated with higher risk of morbidity and mortality. In pediatric patients hypotonia is a late sign of shock. Determinations of cardiac output are not used routinely. In clinical practice, assessment of shock or impaired circulation is derived from heart rate, blood pressure, peripheral perfusion, urinary production, base excess, and mixed venous saturation. Attempts to operationalize these parameters into one summarizing score require computational effort, which is not practical for bedside use. In the absence of cardiac output measurements we prefer to accept the rather broad definition of "adequate circulation" and to rely on interventional requirements for staging of illness. If cardiac output measurements are performed, a cardiac index exceeding 3 l/m2 is regarded as "adequate". The resulting and suggested assessment system (Table 2 and 3) is simple, corresponds to the classification system of the Consensus

Table 2. Definitions of severity of illness in SIRS and sepsis (primary parameters)

Severity of illness	Consensus Conference [15]	Iowa study [3]	Proposed pediatric definitions
SIRS/sepsis[a]	Two of four criteria		Two of four criteria, adequate perfusion with intravenous fluid additional to maintenance: <20 ml/kg/8 h
Severe SIRS/sepsis	Sepsis associated with organ dysfunction, hypoperfusion, or hypotension. Hypoperfusion[b] and perfusion abnormalities may include but are not limited to, lactic acidosis, oliguria, or acute alterations in mental status		SIRS/sepsis, adequate perfusion with intravenous fluid additional to maintenance: >20 ml/kg/8 h Vasopressors (≥8 hours): dopamine plus dobutamine ≤10 μg/kg/min, epinephrine ≤0.05 μg/kg/min or SIRS/sepsis, adequate perfusion but organ dysfunction in >3 organs
SIRS/sepsis with shock	Sepsis with hypotension despite adequate fluid resuscitation, along with the presence of perfusion abnormalities that may include but are not limited to lactic acidosis, oliguria, or acute alterations in mental status. Patients who are on inotropic or vasopressor agents may not be hypotensive at the time that perfusion abnormalities are measured	Hypotension not responsive to a 500-ml intravenous fluid challenge plus manifestations of peripheral hypoperfusion. Patients without hypotension but receiving more than 5 μg/kg per minute of dopamine or any other vasopressor agent	SIRS/sepsis plus adequate perfusion with vasopressors (more than 8 hours): dopamine plus dobutamine dose ≥10 μg/kg/min, and/or epinephrine/norepinephrine ≥0.05 μg/kg/min, or SIRS/sepsis with serum lactate 2–10 mmol/l (more than 8 hours) or SIRS/sepsis plus severe organ dysfunction in ≥3 organs

[a] Sepsis: is SIRS plus documented infection (positive blood cultures). Culture-negative sepsis is SIRS with clinical course, laboratory data and cytokine studies highly suggestive of sepsis. All other conditions are SIRS.

[b] Hypotension [3]: Adults (systolic pressure): <90 mmHg or 50% reduction in hypertensive patients. Children (mean arterial pressure [14]): 50% reduction in hypertensive children or <60 mmHg (12–16 years), <55 mmHg (5–12 years), <50 mmHg (1–5 years), <45 mmHg (1–12 months), <40 mmHg (term newborns to 1 month), <35 mmHg (32–38 gestational weeks), <30 mmHg (<32 gestational weeks).

[c] Adequate perfusion: If cardiac output is measured: cardiac index >3 l/m². Otherwise restore blood pressure above hypotension.

[d] Criteria for organ dysfunction see Table 3

Conference and correlates with the risk of mortality in a clinically relevant manner [4].

Likelihood of Bacterial Infection

Staging of severity of illness does not yield information about the presence or absence of invading microorganisms. In contrast to adult patients, children are more likely to develop systemic illness in response to localized infections. With respect to bacterial infection, four possible states must be considered: First, the infection is systemic and can be documented by cultures (38% of episodes in our study). Second, the patient has systemic bacterial infection but all microbial studies fail to grow microorganisms (22%). Third, the child suffers from localized bacterial infection (20%). Fourth, both localized and systemic bacterial infection is absent (20%). The first two groups will benefit from early initiation of appropriate antimicrobial medication, the third from surgical elimination of focus and/or antibiotic treatment. The last group will not profit from antimicrobial treatment and is at risk of being exposed to several broad spectrum antibiotics with the potency of acquiring antibiotic resistant infections, fungal superinfection or serious side effects.

As long as treatment of severe illness consists of antimicrobial therapy and supportive measures, early identification of episodes before results of blood cultures become available may only be vitally important in those rare pediatric patients with other rapidly progressing nonbacterial conditions, like adrenal insufficiency. However, if immunomodulatory treatments are considered, early and correct assessment of the likelihood of bacterial infection is critical. Presence or absence of bacteria in the bloodstream may require entirely different interventional approaches [12, 24].

Current literature uses the terms sepsis, SIRS and culture-negative sepsis [3]. We propose to restrict the term sepsis to episodes of blood borne bacterial or fungal infection. A differentiation should be made between culture-positive sepsis and culture-negative sepsis. The latter should be defined as a septic episode if the clinical course, laboratory data and relevant cytokine studies are highly suggestive of a systemic bacterial or fungal infection. All other conditions with systemic inflammatory response should be named SIRS. The various underlying pathologies or treatment modes can be further differentiated with the help of appropriate specifications, for example: SIRS with documented localized infection, SIRS with antibiotic treatment, SIRS without antibiotic treatment, SIRS with absent or unlikely infection.

Crude and Attributable Mortality

Mortality depends on previous state of health. Patients already requiring vasopressors for circulatory support due to an underlying disorder, for example low output after cardiac surgery, run a higher risk of mortality than previously healthy subjects when threatened by gram-negative sepsis. This may explain the differences between the crude mortalities in the three studies. The mortality of patients with documented bacterial sepsis and septic shock was 82% in the Italian study, 52% for patients with severe sepsis and 36% for patients with sepsis [20], The mortality in our study was 37% for patients with septic shock, 9% in episodes of severe sepsis, and 5% for patients with sepsis. From the Italian study a mortality of 25% was reported for patients never developing SIRS, compared to 0% in our study population. Data from the Iowa study are presented in Figure 2. Indications for attributable mortality can be derived from assessing severity of underlying illness and its associated risk of mortality during a stable baseline period immediately before onset of symptoms of a septic episode. For these conditions the prognostic value of SNAP and pediatric risk of mortality (PRISM) is well established [25, 26].

Proposed Adaptation to Pediatric Patients

The definitions suggested by the Consensus Conference require adaptation to the pediatric population. Breath rate, heart rate, temperature control, leukocyte and differential counts change over time reflecting the development of the growing organism [14]. In a first step the criteria for SIRS therefore need age-adjustment: It appears logical to use the age-appropriate percentiles. For reasons of practicability we suggest a simplification by using the following age groups: newborns under five days of age, newborns five days to one month, infants aged one month to one year, one to two years and children aged two to five and five to twelve years (Table 1).

Definitions for organ dysfunction are derived from published trials in adult patients [3, 20]. The Glasgow coma scale is used to assess brain function in infants older than six months. Function of kidney, lung, liver and hemostasis can be judged by the same parameters used in adult patients. Neonatal adjustments are necessary for clotting parameters. Cardiovascular function is assessed by parameters similar to those used for adult patients, however, with differing interventional requirements in each category (Table 2). In consideration of recent suggestions for identifying populations "at risk" to develop severe sepsis or shock, we designed criteria to discriminate between four distinct stages: a) circulation is stable, b) circulation can be stabilized with fluid resuscitation or moderate vasopressor support, c) circulation can only be stabilized with significant vasopressor support, d) circulatory failure. In order to stabilize the classification against short-term perturbations, interventional requirements have to fulfill the criteria for a period of more than eight hours. Circulatory criteria serve as primary stratification parameter (Table 2), organ dysfunction as secondary parameter (Table 3). This results in a straightforward, simple assessment of severity for most patients. In our experience [4] secondary reassessment has to be performed in a minority of patients, whose circulation is stable with little intervention, but who show severe dysfunction of other organ systems (e.g. DIC, ARDS and kidney failure). A higher severity of illness than

Table 3. Organ dysfunction (secondary criteria)

Organ system	Organ dysfunction	Severe organ dysfunction	Organ failure
Lung	Spontaneous breathing: $FiO_2 \geq 0.5$ Ventilated: FiO_2 0.35–0.7	Spontaneous breathing: Ventilation required to maintain arterial saturation >90% or pH >7.25 Ventilated: $FiO_2 \geq 0.7$ or increase in FiO_2 by >0.4 for more than 12 hours	X-ray findings of ARDS and alveolar/art. difference >35 kPa (>280 mmHg) and/or art saturation cannot be maintained above 90% despite $FiO_2 \geq 0.7$ without application of nitric oxide, high frequency oscillation or ECMO
Renal	Oliguria <1.0 ml/kg/h (<5 years); <0.5 ml/kg/h (>5 years), creatinine elevated but <120 mmol/l (1.4 mg/dl). Urinary output restored with fluid, inotropic support and/or furosemide i.v. <3 mg/kg/d	Oliguria <1.0 ml/kg/h (<5 years); <0.5 ml/kg/h (>5 years) and/or creatinine 120–250 mmol/l (1.4 mg/dl). Urinary output restored with fluid, inotropic support and furosemide i.v. 3–12 mg/kg/d	Anuria or oliguria <1.0 ml/kg/h (<5 years); <0.5 ml/kg/h (>5 years) despite maximum diuretic support (furosemide i.v. ≥12 mg/kd/d) and/or creatinine >250 mmol/l (>2.8 mg/dl), and/or renal support required to keep potassium <6 mmol/l
Hemostasis	Thrombocytes <100 000, and/or prothrombin time (Quick) or partial thromboplastin time (PTT) >1.5 times age-appropriate normal value	Moderate DIC requiring one replacement over 12 hours with Thrombocytes <50 000, and/or prothrombin time (Quick) or partial thromboplastin time (PTT) 1.5–2 times above age-appropriate normal values, Fibrinogen <1.3 g/l	Severe DIC requiring repetitive replacements of thrombocytes and clotting factors with thrombocytes <30 000, and/or prothrombin time (Quick) or partial thromboplastin time (PTT) >2 times age-appropriate normal values, or fibrinogen <1.0 g/l

resulting from circulatory criteria should be assigned if the patient fulfills criteria of increased severity of dysfunction in three or more organ systems. Thus the classification is not influenced by non-circulatory single organ failure.

Obviously, the proposed definitions require further validation by prospective studies in different institutions. If the concept proves valid, it offers a two-dimensional matrix allowing differentiation between a variety of clinical situations, previously pooled under the term sepsis (Figure 3): Thereby addressing severity of illness (vertical axis in Figure 3) and likelihood of systemic bacterial

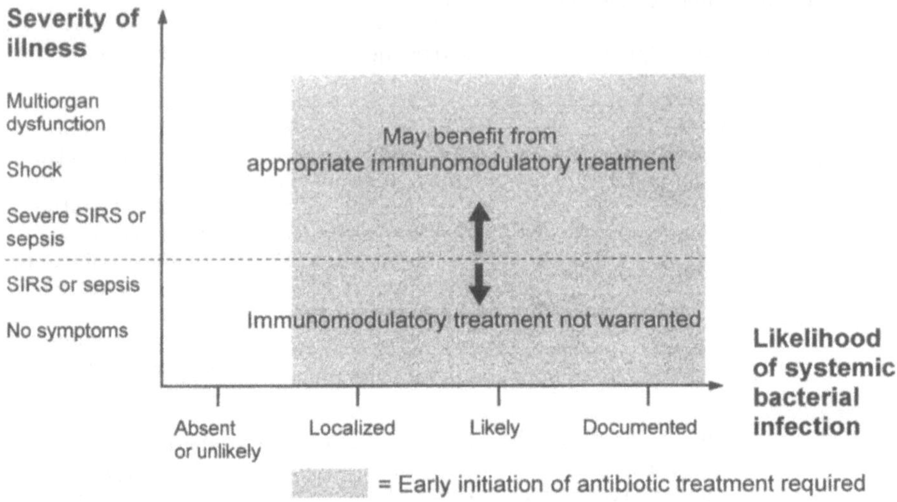

Fig. 3. Classification matrix for septic episodes. Vertical axis assesses severity of illness, horizontal axis likelihood and site of bacterial infection.

infection (horizontal axis in Figure 3). This differentiation appears to be an important prerequisite when evaluating new therapeutic strategies.

Diagnosis

If the matrix is used to stratify "septic episodes" it allows simple graphic orientation (Figure 3). To the top of the matrix are those patients progressing to severe illness, to the bottom those with a clinical course which does not exceed moderate illness. To the right are those patients with a high likelihood of systemic bacterial infection, to the left those with a low likelihood of bacterial infection.

In clinical routine early discrimination of bacterial and non-bacterial cause is a major diagnostic problem. Only a few conditions like purpura fulminans associated with fever and signs of impaired circulation offer pathognomonic patterns that immediately allow initiation of therapy even without performing further diagnostic tests. In the majority of cases however, at presentation there is uncertainty about the underlying pathology. This results in two almost inevitable potential errors: the first is unwarranted initiation of antimicrobial treatment with associated side effects, the second unwarranted delay of medication with resulting increase in morbidity and mortality.

We found that in critically ill children with progressing severity of illness, routine laboratory parameters like leukocyte count, differential count and C-reactive protein are of limited specificity and sensitivity in the early sepsis workup [4]. Although elevations in CRP finally occurred in all patients with sepsis, reflecting activation of the immune response, in half of the episodes levels were below 30 mg/l at intention to treat.

As mentioned earlier, cytokines rise very early during the immune response, whereby IL-6 elevations reflect the general activation of the immune system, while G-CSF indicates activation of neutrophiles in the bloodstream [18]. In severe illness levels of both cytokines rise to levels more than 100 fold above those obtained from healthy subjects [5, 27]. In our study over 80% of patients with likely or documented systemic bacterial infection had markedly elevated levels of G-CSF (>750 pg/ml). In patients with SIRS, severe SIRS or shock but localized bacterial processes or unlikely or no infection G-CSF rarely exceeded 500 pg/ml. G-CSF levels above 1500 pg/ml practically proved severe bacterial sepsis. If G-CSF measurements become available for routine laboratory determinations, this parameter should be included in sepsis workup of symptomatic neonates and critically ill children. G-CSF measurements allow differentiation between severe sepsis / SIRS, shock and multiorgan dysfunction of bacterial and nonbacterial origin.

Consequences for Future Clinical Trials

Although incidence of infections and systemic inflammatory response to various stimuli is high in the pediatric population, progress to severe illness with increased mortality is confined to few clinical settings and a small number of conditions. Only the subgroup of patients who progress to severe illness with a high risk of mortality should be included in clinical studies evaluating the benefit or harm of immunomodulatory treatments for sepsis. The broad definition of sepsis / SIRS needs clarification with respect to severity of illness and likelihood of systemic bacterial infection. It is very unlikely that a "magic bullet" will be found as a remedy against runaway inflammation due to differing underlying pathologies. The best we can offer to pediatric patients still is early recognition of the underlying pathology and rapid initiation of appropriate treatment. Immunomodulatory interventions like anticytokine antibodies or application of G-CSF in non-neutropenic patients must carefully be assessed for their potential harm. For comparison of study results authors should provide information about the likelihood of bacterial infection, the maximum severity of illness and the time elapsed between onset of significant symptoms, peak of severity and therapeutic interventions. Recent animal experiments underscore the importance of timing of an immunotherapeutic intervention: In a canine model of sepsis, mortality was decreased if G-CSF was applied prophylactically. The same cytokine applied after onset of symptoms resulted in increased mortality [28].

Conclusion

The proposed definitions of SIRS and of multiple organ dysfunction provide a conceptual framework applicable to pediatric patients. The concept adds to the understanding of pathogenesis of sepsis in absence of bacteria. The unmodified concept however is of little aid to clinical decision making. In non-ICU patients currently available routine measures suffice for evaluation [29]. In critical care, the majority of patients fulfill SIRS criteria. From a moderate inflammatory response to different stimuli an uncontrolled systemic process may result, progressing to severe illness or even death. The sequence of events in this process is similar for a variety of underlying pathologies both in pediatric and adult patients. Key cytokines involved in the immune response may serve to identify patients with high likelihood of systemic bacterial infection and severe course of disease. If measured at presentation, these parameters appear to exceed the diagnostic value of all other routine laboratory parameters.

Definitions of SIRS, sepsis and multiorgan dysfunction adapted for pediatric patients provide an easy-to-perform staging system. It allows assessment of the progress of disease over time which is independent of interactions between physiological derangements and interventions. If this classification is complemented by assessment of likelihood of bacterial infection, a two-dimensional matrix results in which one axis defines severity of illness, the other likelihood of systemic bacterial infection. This allows identification of the subgroups of septic patients that may benefit from entirely different immunomodulatory strategies.

Recommendations

- The term sepsis should be reserved to episodes of systemic bacterial or fungal infection. If an organism can be documented by cultures, the episode should be named culture-positive sepsis.
- Culture-negative episodes should only be named culture-negative sepsis if cytokine studies, clinical course and routine laboratory data are highly suggestive of systemic bacterial or fungal infection.
- The term SIRS should be applied to the remaining conditions. Appropriate specifications further differentiate SIRS with localized infection, SIRS with absent or unlikely infection, SIRS with or without antibiotic treatment.
- Severity of illness should be assessed by a pediatric adaptation of the staging system suggested by the Consensus Conference for adult patients.

References

1. Kreger BE, Craven DE, McCabe WR (1980) Gram-negative bacteremia. IV. Re-evaluation of clinical features and treatment in 612 patients. Am J Med 68:344–355.
2. Bone RC (1992) Toward an epidemiology and natural history of SIRS (systemic inflammatory response syndrome) Jama 268:3452–3455.
3. Rangel-Frausto MS, Pittet D, Costigan M, Hwang T, Davis CS, Wenzel RP (1995) The natural history of the systemic inflammatory response syndrome (SIRS). A prospective study. Jama 273:117–123.

4. Fischer JE, Fischer JC, Printzen G, Nadal D, Schmid E, Fanconi S (1996) Endogenous granulocyte-colony stimulating factor in the early diagnosis of sepsis. (in preparation) .
5. Thijs L,Hack C (1995) Time course of cytokine levels in sepsis. Intensive Care Med 21:S258-S263.
6. Besedovsky H,Del Rey A (1996) Immune-Neuro-Endocrine Interactions: Facts and Hypotheses. Endocrine Rev 17:1-39.
7. Parrillo J (1993) Pathogenetic mechanisms of septic shock. New Eng J Med 328:1471-1477.
8. Ward P (1991) Mechanisms of endothelial cell killing by H_2O_2 or products of activated neutrophiles. Am J Med 91:3C-89S-94S.
9. Weiss J (1989) Tissue destruction by neutrophiles. N Engl J Med 320:365-376.
10. Fisher CJ, Jr., Slotman GJ, Opal SM, et al (1994) Initial evaluation of human recombinant interleukin-1 receptor antagonist in the treatment of sepsis syndrome: a randomized, open-label, placebo-controlled multicenter trial. Crit Care Med 22:12-21.
11. Bone R, Fischer CJ, Clemmer T, et al (1987) A controlled clinical trial of high-dose methylprednisolone in the treatment of severe sepsis and septic shock. N Engl J Med 317:653-658.
12. Natanson C, Hoffman WD, Suffredini AF, Eichacker PQ, Danner RL (1994) Selected treatment strategies for septic shock based on proposed mechanisms of pathogenesis. Ann Intern Med 120:771-783.
13. Fanaroff AA, Korones SB, Wright LL, et al (1994) A controlled trial of intravenous immune globulin to reduce nosocomial infections in very-low-birth-weight infants. N Engl J Med 330:1107-1113.
14. Hayden W (1994) Sepsis terminology in pediatrics. J Pediatrics 124:657-658.
15. Bone RC, Balk RA, Cerra FB, et al (1992) Definitions for sepsis and organ failure and guidelines for the use of innovative therapies in sepsis. The ACCP/SCCM Consensus Conference Committee. American College of Chest Physicians/Society of Critical Care Medicine. Chest 101:1644-1655.
16. Saez Llorens X, McCracken GH, Jr. (1993) Sepsis syndrome and septic shock in pediatrics: current concepts of terminology, pathophysiology, and management. J Pediatr 123:497-508.
17. Kuhns DB, Alvord WG, Gallin JI (1995) Increased circulating cytokines, cytokine antagonists, and E-selectin after intravenous administration of endotoxin in humans. J Infect Dis 171:145-152
18. Dale D, Liles W, Summer W, Nelson S (1995) Review: Granulocyte Colony Stimulating Factor-Role and Relationships in Infectious Diseases. J Infect Dis 172:1061-1075.
19. Walley K (1995) Ventricular dysfunction during sepsis. In Vincent J (ed) 1995 Yearbook of intensive care and emergency medicine. Springer, Berlin, Heidelberg, pp 505-517.
20. Salvo I, de Cian W, Musicco M, et al (1995) The Italian SEPSIS study: preliminary results on the incidence and evolution of SIRS, sepis, severe sepsis and septic shock. Intensive Care Med 21:S244-S249.
21. Le Gall J, Lemeshov S (1995) SAPS II and MPM II models for early severe sepsis. In Sibbald W, Vincent J (ed) Clinical trials for the treatment of sepsis. Springer, Berlin Heidelberg, pp 13-34.
22. Vincent J (1995) The „at risk“ patient population. Sibbald W, Vincent J (ed) Clinical trials for the treatment of sepsis. Springer, Berlin Heidelberg, pp 13-34.
23. Escobar G, Fischer A, De Kun L, Kremers R, Armstrong M (1995) Score for neonatal acute physiology: validation in three Kaiser Permanente neonatal intensive care units. Pediatrics 98:918-922.
24. Eidelman L, Sprung C (1994) Why have new effective therapies for sepsis not been developed. Crit Care 22:1330-1334.
25. Richardson DK, Gray JE, McCormick MC, Workman K, Goldmann DA (1993) Score for Neonatal Acute Physiology: a physiologic severity index for neonatal intensive care. Pediatrics 91:617-623.
26. Pollack M, Ruttimann U, Getson P (1988) Pediatric risk of mortality (PRISM) score. Crit Care 16:1110-1116.

27. Gessler P, Kirchmann N, Kientsch ER, Haas N, Lasch P, Kachel W (1993) Serum concentrations of granulocyte colony-stimulating factor in healthy term and preterm neonates and in those with various diseases including bacterial infections. Blood 82:3177–3182.
28. Eichacker P (1995) Neutrophile directed therapies in sepsis, 24th Annual Meeting of the International Society for Experimental Hematology. Düsseldorf.
29. Baraff LJ, Bass JW, Fleisher GR, et al (1993) Practice guideline for the management of infants and children 0 to 36 months of age with fever without source. Ann Emerg Med 22:1198–1210.

Septic Shock: Cardiovascular Function and Management

M. M. Parker

Introduction

Septic shock is one of the most common causes of morbidity and mortality in patients in intensive care units. Despite the great advances in antibiotic therapy over the past two decades, the mortality from septic shock has not decreased appreciably. Our understanding of the pathophysiology of sepsis and septic shock has evolved rapidly over this time. As we understand the pathophysiology of the syndrome better, our treatment of patients will become more focussed and, we hope, more effective. The acute event that brings the patient to the intensive care unit is often the development of shock. This article will discuss the changes in cardiovascular function that occur in the patient with septic shock and the current approaches to hemodynamic management.

Cardiovascular Function

It is well-recognized that the characteristic hemodynamic profile which is seen in septic shock is a hyperdynamic state manifested as tachycardia, an increased cardiac output, and a decreased systemic vascular resistance [1, 2]. A wide variety of organisms can cause septic shock, including gram positive, gram negative, fungal, viral, and rickettsial organisms. The hemodynamic profile does not vary with different types of organisms [1]. Parker et al studied serial hemodynamic parameters in survivors and nonsurvivors of septic shock to look for prognostic indices [2]. On initial presentation, both survivors and nonsurvivors presented with a hyperdynamic hemodynamic profile. Those patients who had a relatively low heart rate, or in whom the heart rate or cardiac output decreased toward normal over the first 24 hours had a more favorable prognosis, as did those whose systemic vascular resistance had risen toward normal by 24 hours. Most patients who die of septic shock have a persistently low systemic vascular resistance and refractory hypotension. A small number of patients develop a cardiogenic shock-like state, with a low cardiac output and high systemic vascular resistance. A substantial minority of patients recover from the initial hypotensive event only to go on and develop multiple organ failure, which then leads to their death [2, 3]. Patients who die of multiple organ failure typically linger over a longer time course than do those patients who die of refractory hypotension or myocardial depression.

Patients with septic shock also demonstrate abnormalities of oxygen utilization [4, 5]. Oxygen consumption is frequently dependent upon oxygen delivery at a much higher level than in normal people, so that increasing the oxygen delivery above normal often results in an increase in oxygen consumption. Oxygen extraction is also impaired, possibly because of peripheral arterial-venous shunting, maldistribution of blood flow because of impaired autoregulation, or cellular damage which disrupts oxidative phosphorylation and oxygen utilization. A higher level of oxygen delivery than normal may be needed to maintain aerobic metabolism. Some investigators, however, have questioned the concept of supply-dependent oxygen consumption in children because of methodologic concerns, and caution against using this relationship as a rationale for increasing oxygen delivery as a therapeutic goal in critically ill children [6]. Nonetheless, many critical care physicians believe that optimizing oxygen delivery is important in patients with septic shock because oxygen supply-dependency can frequently be demonstrated and because survivors have a higher oxygen delivery than nonsurvivors [4].

Myocardial Depression

Even though patients with septic shock usually demonstrate a hyperdynamic hemodynamic profile, depression of myocardial function can be demonstrated in a variety of ways. Radionuclide cineangiography with simultaneous thermodilution cardiac output measurements has been used to study myocardial function in critically ill patients with septic shock [7, 8]. Survivors of septic shock demonstrate a marked decrease in left and right ventricular ejection fraction, associated with an increased end diastolic volume index. These changes occur during the first few days following the onset of shock. Ventricular size and function return toward normal over 1–2 weeks as the patient recovers. Nonsurvivors do not demonstrate significant changes in ejection fraction or ventricular size. The reasons for this apparent paradox are not clear. Patients with sepsis without shock have been shown to have a relative depression of myocardial depression compared to critically ill hyperdynamic patients without sepsis [9]. Echocardiography can also be used to demonstrate a decrease in left ventricular ejection fraction in hyperdynamic patients with septic shock.

There has been an ongoing debate regarding the mechanism by which myocardial depression is produced in septic shock. There are two major theories to explain this phenomenon. Some investigators have proposed that inadequate coronary blood flow produces a global myocardial ischemia with resultant depression of myocardial function. Others have presented data supporting the concept that a circulating humoral substance is responsible for the decrease in myocardial function which can be seen in septic shock. To investigate the first mechanism, Cunnion et al placed thermodilution coronary sinus catheters in 7 adults with septic shock to measure coronary blood flow [10]. Coronary blood flow was found to be normal or increased in all 7 patients, and none had net myocardial lactate production. The fractional extraction of arterial oxygen was decreased, analogous to the global decrease in oxygen utilization seen in patients with septic shock. These data argue against inadequate coronary blood flow with global ischemia as the cause of myocardial depression in septic shock.

An in vitro system using spontaneously contracting rat myocardial cells was developed by Parrillo et al to investigate the presence of a circulating humoral myocardial depressant substance as the mechanism of myocardial depression in humans with septic shock [11]. By measuring the area covered by an individual cell during systole and during diastole, the contraction of the cell was quantified. Serum from normal laboratory personnel, patients with structural heart disease, or critically ill nonseptic patients had no effect on the contraction of the rat myocardial cells in vitro. In contrast, serum from patients with septic shock produced a significant decrease in the extent and velocity of myocardial cell contraction. Serum from some of these same patients before shock or after recovery did not decrease myocardial cell contraction. The decrease in ejection fraction of the patients with septic shock correlated with the decrease in myocardial cell contraction in vitro. The results of these studies strongly support the presence of a circulating humoral substance as the cause of myocardial depression in septic shock.

The identity of the circulating myocardial depressant substance(s) has not been completely determined. Endotoxin has been strongly implicated in the pathophysiology of septic shock, although it has not consistently been shown to depress myocardial cell contraction in vitro. Endotoxin has been found commonly in the serum of patient with septic shock [12]. On serial determinations in 100 patients with clinical septic shock, Danner and colleagues found detectable endotoxin in 43%. In patients with positive blood cultures, the presence of endotoxin in the blood was associated with cardiac depression, multiple organ failure and death, suggesting that endotoxin is an important mediator of septic shock. Further evidence that endotoxin is important in septic shock came from Suffredini et al in their studies of the effects of endotoxin administered to normal humans [13]. Following a small dose of intravenously administered endotoxin, serial hemodynamic parameters and left ventricular ejection fraction were measured. The subjects developed a hyperdynamic state, with tachycardia, increased cardiac index, and reduced systemic vascular resistance index. The left ventricular ejection fraction decreased 5 hours after endotoxin, and the end diastolic volume index increased. These changes are qualitatively similar to those observed in patients with septic shock.

Tumor necrosis factor (TNF) has been widely implicated as an important cytokine in septic shock. Following the administration of endotoxin in normal volunteers, there is an abrupt rise in serum TNF levels, preceding the hemodynamic changes that occur [13]. TNF can also depress myocardial contractility in vitro, as can other cytokines including interleukin-2 (IL-2) and interleukin-6 (IL-6) [14].

Nitric oxide (NO) has recently emerged as an important molecule in the regulation of vascular tone. It is synthesized in endothelial cells from the amino acid L-arginine by the enzyme NO synthase; its synthesis can be inhibited by analogues of L-arginine. In nonseptic sheep, inhibition of NO synthase increases blood pressure and systemic and pulmonary vascular resistance, decreasing cardiac index [15]. In septic animals, NO synthase inhibition produces a less marked increase in blood pressure and systemic vascular resistance; the administration of L-arginine produces systemic and pulmonary vasodilation. In vitro depression of contractility of mammalian heart cells by the cytokines TNF, IL-2, and IL-6 can be blocked by the inhibition of NO synthase, demonstrating that the myocardial depression caused by these cytokines is mediated through nitric oxide [14]. An increasing body of evidence implicates nitric oxide as an important factor in the pathophysiology of septic shock.

Management of Septic Shock

The initial approach to the management of septic shock is aggressive fluid resuscitation. Basic measures including antibiotics, removal (if possible) of the source of infection, and support of airway and breathing are, of course, essential. There are no convincing data as to which type of fluid is the best; most clinicians use either normal saline or Ringers lactate initially. The decision whether to use colloids must be made at the bedside; packed red blood cells should be used only if the patient is known to be anemic or bleeding. Fresh frozen plasma may be used if the patient is known to have a clotting factor deficiency. The amount of fluid to use is sometimes difficult to determine. Data in adults suggests that giving fluids to maintain a pulmonary artery occlusion pressure of approximately 12 mmHg provides maximal improvement in cardiac function [1]. Carcillo and colleagues retrospectively studied 34 children who presented with septic shock to evaluate the association of fluid resuscitation with outcome [16]. They divided the children into three groups; group 1 received <20 ml/kg fluid in the first hour, group 2 received 20–40 ml/kg, and group 3 received >40 ml/kg. Survival in group 3 was significantly better than that in either of the other two groups. There was no difference in the incidence of adult respiratory distress syndrome or cardiogenic pulmonary edema between the three groups. It is of particular note that all 8 patients (6 in group 1 and 2 in group 2) who were hypovolemic at 6 hours (defined as hypotension, oliguria, and a pulmonary artery occlusion pressure <8 mmHg) subsequently expired. This study underscores the importance of aggressive fluid resuscitation early in the management of septic shock in children.

While it is clear that early fluid resuscitation is important, it must also be remembered that cardiac function is not normal in septic shock. The response to volume loading may differ in the patient with sepsis or septic shock from what would be expected in a normal person. Ognibene et al studied the response to volume infusion in patients with sepsis or septic shock compared to critically ill nonseptic patients using radionuclide cineangiography and simultaneous thermodilution cardiac output measurements [17]. Patients with sepsis or septic shock had less of an increase in left ventricular stroke work index following volume infusion than did nonseptic patients, demonstrating altered ventricular performance. Given the abnormalities of cardiac function that are common in septic shock, it is incumbent upon the physician to observe the patient closely and reassess frequently during aggressive fluid resuscitation.

When a patient with septic shock does not respond adequately to fluid resuscitation, then inotropic/vasopressor agents must be considered. Dopamine is the initial drug chosen by most clinicians. At low doses (1–5 mcg/kg/min), it is a modest inotrope as well as activating the dopaminergic receptors in the kidney, potentially having a beneficial effect on renal blood flow. At higher doses, dopamine has primarily alpha-adrenergic effects, which may help to support the blood pressure; but the effects on renal blood flow are lost at higher doses.

Norepinephrine is an alpha-adrenergic agonist which is commonly used to increase systemic vascular resistance and hence blood pressure in patients with septic shock who are persistently hypotensive despite adequate fluid resuscitation and dopamine support. Many clinicians are reluctant to use norepinephrine, however, because of concern that vasoconstriction of the renal arteries will increase the risk of renal failure. Several recent studies, however, have demonstrated that norepinephrine can be used safely in patients with septic shock [18]. It must be used with care in patients who have an elevated serum lactate, as those patients may be at higher risk of an adverse response to norepinephrine. The combination of a norepinephrine infusion with a low dose infusion of dopamine is often recommended to provide cardiovascular support while protecting renal blood flow.

Dobutamine is a beta-adrenergic agent which has been recommended in septic shock to improve cardiac function. There is concern, however, that the vasodilating effects of dobutamine may further exacerbate hypotension in the setting of an already vasodilated patient. Vincent et al added dobutamine to the treatment of 18 patients with septic shock who had already been treated with fluid resuscitation. Four of the patients were receiving high-dose dopamine or norepinephrine [19]. They found that dobutamine was well tolerated and increased oxygen delivery and consumption. A subgroup of the patients had a modest decrease in mean arterial pressure; most had an increase in blood pressure. Dobutamine may be beneficial in supporting cardiac function and improving oxygen delivery in patients with septic shock, but care must be taken to ensure that the patient has received adequate fluid resuscitation prior to adding this drug.

Epinephrine has both alpha- and beta-adrenergic properties and has been used for inotropic support in septic shock. After adequate volume loading, the administration of epinephrine can produce a dose related increase in heart rate, mean arterial pressure, cardiac index, left ventricular stroke work index, and oxygen delivery and consumption [20]. The increase in heart rate produces a marked increase in myocardial oxygen demand, which raises concerns about the safety of the use of epinephrine in adults, who may have unrecognized coronary artery disease. This concern is minimal in children; epinephrine is a very effective and safe inotropic agent for children with septic shock who have not responded to fluid resuscitation and support with dopamine.

The findings of an altered oxygen supply/demand relationship and the observation that survivors demonstrate a higher level of oxygen delivery than do nonsurvivors of septic shock has led to the theory that increasing the cardiac output and oxygen delivery to supranormal levels will improve outcome from septic shock. Tuchschmidt et al randomized 25 patients with septic shock to normal treatment (NT group) and 26 to treatment designed to increase the cardiac index to 6 L/min/m^2 or more (OT group), both groups treated to maintain a systolic blood pressure of at least 90 mmHg [21]. To accomplish these goals, 5% albumin was administered until the pulmonary artery occlusion pressure was 15 mm Hg. If the patient remained hypotensive, dopamine was added and titrated to maintain the blood pressure at the desired level. If the patient was not hypotensive and the cardiac index was below the assigned goal, dobutamine was added and titrated to maintain the cardiac index at the desired goal. Cardiac index and oxygen delivery were significantly higher in the OT group. Overall there was no significant difference in mortality between the two groups. Within the NT group were some patients who spontaneously met OT goals, and within the OT group were some patients who did not meet the OT goals. The mortality of the OT patients who met the OT goals (40%) was significantly lower than the mortality of the NT patients who did not meet OT goals (74%). The study suggests but does not prove that increasing cardiac index (and hence oxygen delivery) may be beneficial in septic shock. In a large multicenter study in critically ill patients, Gattinoni and colleagues randomized 252 patients to standard treatment, 253 to treatment designed to increase the cardiac index to a supranormal level, and 257 to treatment designed to increase the mixed venous oxygen saturation to a normal level [22]. There was no significant difference in morbidity or mortality between the three groups, either at the time of discharge from the intensive care unit or six months later. A subgroup analysis of the patients in whom the preset hemodynamic goals were reached also did not show any difference in mortality. Further subgroup analysis of the patients with sepsis or septic shock also did not show any decrease in mortality by increasing cardiac index or mixed venous oxygen saturation. This study clearly does not support the theory that therapeutically increasing cardiac output and oxygen delivery to arbitrary preset goals is of benefit in septic shock. Give the lack of supporting data, as well as the concerns raised about the validity of oxygen transport measurements in children, [6] pursuing specific hemodynamic goals in children with septic shock cannot be strongly recommended. Each patient should be managed with a goal of optimizing both the hemodynamic state and organ function, as well as ensuring the adequacy of overall perfusion.

Conclusion

Septic shock is a common life-threatening problem with a characteristic hemodynamic profile. The hyperdynamic state is characterized by tachycardia, an increased cardiac index, and a decreased systemic vascular resistance index. Myocardial depression is common and is manifested by a decreased right and left ventricular ejection fraction with dilation of the ventricles. These changes are reversible over one to two weeks as the patient recovers. There is strong evidence that myocardial depression is caused by a circulating myocardial depressant substance(s), although a specific agent (or agents) have not been clearly identified. Aggressive fluid resuscitation early in the management of septic shock is important to decrease mortality. In patients who do not respond adequately to volume, inotropic support may be necessary. Managing patients with a goal of reaching preset hemodynamic parameters has not convincingly been shown to improve outcome.

References

1. Parker MM, Fink MP (1992) Septic shock. J Intensive Care Med 7:90–100.
2. Parker MM, Shelhamer JH, Natanson C, Alling DW, Parrillo JE (1987) Serial cardiovascular variables in survivors and nonsurvivors of human septic shock: Heart rate as an early predictor of prognosis. Crit Care Med 15:923–929.
3. Groeneveld ABJ, Nauta JJP, Thijs LG (1988) Peripheral vascular resistance in septic shock: its relation to outcome. Intensive Care Med 14:141–147.
4. Tuchschmidt J, Oblitas D, Fried JC (1991) Oxygen consumption in sepsis and septic shock. Crit Care Med 19:664–671.
5. Pollack MM, Fields AI, Ruttimann UE (1984) Sequential cardiopulmonary variables of infants and children in septic shock. Crit Care Med 12:554–559.
6. Seear M, Wensley D, MacNab A (1993) Oxygen consumption-oxygen delivery relationship in children. J Pediatr 123:208–214.
7. Parker MM, Shelhamer JH, Bacharach SL, et al (1984) Profound but reversible myocardial depression in patients with septic shock. Ann Intern Med 100:483–490.
8. Parker MM, McCarthy KE, Ognibene FP, Parrillo JE (1990) Right ventricular dysfunction and dilatation, similar to left ventricular changes, characterize the cardiac depression of septic shock in humans. Chest 97:126–131.
9. Raper R, Sibbald WJ, Driedger AA, Gerow K (1989) Relative myocardial depression in normotensive sepsis. J Crit Care 4:9–18.
10. Cunnion RE, Schaer GL, Parker MM, Natanson C, Parrillo JE (1986) Circulation 73:637–644.
11. Parrillo JE, Burch C, Shelhamer JH, Parker MM, Natanson C, Schuette W (1985) A circulating myocardial depressant substance in humans with septic shock. J Clin Invest 76:1539–1553.
12. Danner RL, Elin RJ, Hosseini JM, Wesley RA, Reilly JM, Parrillo JE (1991) Endotoxemia in human septic shock. Chest 99:169–175.
13. Suffredini AF, Fromm RE, Parker MM, et al (1989) The cardiovascular response of normal humans to the administration of endotoxin. N Engl J Med 321:280-287.
14. Finkel MS, Oddis CV, Jacob TD, Watkins SC, Hattler BG, Simmons RL (1992) Negative inotropic effects of cytokines on the heart mediated by nitric oxide. Science 257:387-389.
15. Lorente JA, Landin L, Renes E, et al (1993) Role of nitric oxide in the hemodynamic changes of sepsis. Crit Care Med 21:759-767.

16. Carcillo JA, Davis AL, Zaritsky A (1991) Role of early fluid resuscitation in pediatric septic shock. JAMA 266:1242-1245.
17. Ognibene FP, Parker MM, Natanson C, Shelhamer JH, Parrillo JE (1988) Depressed left ventricular performance: Response to volume infusion in patients with sepsis and septic shock. Chest 93:903-910.
18. Martin C, Eon B, Saux P, Aknin P, Gouin F (1990) Renal effects of norepinephrine used to treat septic shock patients. Crit Care Med 18:282-285.
19. Vincent JL, Roman A, Kahn RJ (1990) Dobutamine administration in septic shock: Addition to a standard protocol. Crit Care Med 18:689-693.
20. Moran JL, O'Fathartaigh MS, Peisach AR, Chapman MJ, Leppard P (1993) Epinephrine as an inotropic agent in septic shock: A dose-profile analysis. Crit Care Med 21:70-77.
21. Tuchschmidt J, Fried J, Astiz M, Rackow E (1992) Elevation of cardiac output and oxygen delivery improves outcome in septic shock. Chest 102:216-220.
22. Gattinoni L, Brazzi L, Pelosi P, et al (1995) A trial of goal-oriented hemodynamic therapy in critically ill patients. N Engl J Med 333:1025–1032.

Plasma Concentrations of Fibronectin in Critically Ill Children

L. Shao, D. Guo and J. Huang

Introduction

The morbidity and mortality of severe infection, disseminated intravascular coagulation (DIC), septic shock, respiratory failure (RF) and severe diseases of central nervous system (CNS) are very high in children. Under these conditions, the defensive function of the reticuloendothelial system (RES) is markedly depressed [1]. It was demonstrated that an immuno-opsonic substance was obviously reduced in severe infection, the reduction of this substance could not be corrected by the administration of IgG or C3, and a significant depress of immuno-opsonic function could also be found in some patients with normal IgG and C3 levels [2]. This indicates that there is an opsonin which is different from IgG or C3. Currently, it is established that this opsonin is fibronectin (Fn).

Fibronectins are a family of high-molecular-weight glycoproteins found in plasma (plasma Fn) and tissues (cellular Fn) that are involved in cell motility and adhesion, embryonic development, regulation of cell morphology, phagocytic function, wound healing, and inflammatory response and host defense and may contribute to the maintenance of microvascular integrity during septic episodes [3–6]. Cellular fibronectin can be converted into plasma Fn (PFn) and vice versa [7]. Fn produced by fibroblasts enters the blood stream through lymph, while that produced by vascular endothelial cells enters the blood stream directly [8]. Thus a dynamic Fn equilibrium is maintained despite its uninterrupted consumption in the body.

Plasma Fn (PFn) is a main opsonin in the mononuclear macrophage system. It has the opsonic effects on the fibrin, fibrinogen-fibrin compound, collagen debris, altered platelets, damaged cell debris, hyaluronic acid, Staphylococcus aureus and non-bacterial toxic substances, and has the function to promote RES to remove them [9]. Dysfunction of RES results in the formation of protein microaggregates and the aggregation of collagen debris and immunocomplex, which exacerbates the damage of the microcirculation and vital organs.

PFn is very important in maintaining the body resistance against infection. It has the action of chemotaxis, the function to attract macrophages and stimulate their phagocytosis at the site of inflammation [10]. Fn has been implicated not only in the adhesive interactions between cells and extracellular matrices but also in the adhesive interactions between cells [11–13]. Thus it plays an important role of adhesion in maintaining the integrity of cells and tissues.

The present study population consisted of 75 patients who were admitted to the PICU of Tianjin Children's Hospital during the period of 1991–1994, and 22 patients seen in the out-patient department (OPD) of the hospital in 1992. The patients studied in the PICU included those with severe bacterial infection, RF due to different underlying diseases, and CNS diseases, ranging in age from 40 days to 12 years, while those studied in the OPD aged from 7 months to 10 years, suffering from bronchitis and mild bronchopneumonia. Table 1 shows the diagnosis, the number of the patients and the pathogens of the diseases.

The patients listed in table 1 were all in accordance with the diagnostic criteria for respiratory failure (irregular respiratory rhythm or respiratory distress, tachypnea (>50/min) or bradypnea (<5/min), tachycardia (>160–180/min), obvious retractions of supraclavicular, intercostal and subcostal areas and cyanosis. Most patients were associated with disturbance of consciousness of various degree. In the 33 patients with RF, PaO_2 was <6.69 Kpa, $PaCO_2$ >6.67 Kpa, and, the oxygenation index and PAO_2-PaO_2 were decreased. 18 of the 33 patients were symptomatically improved after airway clearance, oxygen inhalation with mask or hood (FiO_2=30–60%), correction of metabolic acidosis, amelioration of blood circulation and antishock treatment. However in the other 15 patients, some were not found to have any significant improvement after the same treatments, and some already had severe RF and were put on intubation and mechanical ventilation at the time of admission. Of the 75 patients admitted to the PICU, 32 had clinical manifestations of systemic bacterial infections. Among the 32 patients, 10 had positive cultures which were revealed to be Staphylococcus aureus in 3, Pseudomonas aeruginosa in 1, Salmonella typhimurium in 1, and Diplococcus meningitidis in 5. Among the patients with

Table 1. Diagnosis of the patients with respiratory failure in whom Fn was determined

Diagnosis	No of Patients	Pathogens
Severe pneumonia	4	Syncytial virus
	3	Influenza virus
	5	Unknown
	1	
Hemosiderosis	1	
Acute lymphatic leukemia associated with infection	1	Pneumocystis carinii
Bacterial meningitis	4	Neisseria meningitidis
	2	Diplococcus pneumoniae
	1	Gram-negative bacilli
Non-bacterial encephalitis	3	Positive EB virus antibody
	3	Unknown
Septic shock	3	Gram negative bacteria
Cardiogenic shock		
Endocardial fibroelastosis	2	
Myocarditis	1	

Table 2. Numbers of patients with different CNS diseases

Diagnosis	No.
Purulent meningitis	7
Epidemic cerebrosopinal meningitis	5
Intracranial hemorrhage	6
Non-bacterial encephalitis	9

negative cultures, 5 had clinical manifestations of septicemia with positive endotoxin test results. Of the 75 patients, 27 were found to have CNS diseases as shown in Table 2.

Blood samples were obtained from the out-patients when they were first seen before treatment, and collected from the PICU patients within one hour after their admission. 0.9 ml of venous blood drawn was immediately put in a test tube containing 0.1 ml of 3.8% sodium citrate and centrifuged at 3,000 rpm for 10 minutes. 10 μl of the plasma separated was tested for Fn at a room temperature of 20–22 C by rocket immunoelectrophoresis (Human Fn antiserum and standard antigen were from Shanghai Institute of Biologicals). PFn in the out-patients with bronchitis and mild pneumonia was 237.27±29.86 mg/L which was not significantly different from that in normal children (259±34.68mg/L, $t=1.871$, $P>0.05$). In the 75 PICU patients studied, PFn was 160.42±78.18 mg/L (X+SD) which showed a very significant difference as compared with normal children ($t=5.111$, $p<0.01$). In the 33 RF patients, PFn was 152.49±67.17 mg/L which is very significantly different from that in normal children ($t=7.190$, $P<0.01$). Table 3 showed there was a significant difference in PFn between the patients who required mechanical ventilation and those who did not require it ($t=3.152$, $0.05>p>0.01$).

The patients with CNS diseases were found to have a significantly decreased PFn (181.87±69.25 mg/L) as compared with normal children ($t=3.669$, $0.05>p>0.01$). Very significant difference in PFn was also found between the patients with systemic infections (128.39+51.21 mg/L) and normal children ($t=8.360$, $p<0.01$). As seen in Table 4, significant difference in Pfn was found between the patients with septic shock and the patients with infection but without shock ($t=3.105$, $0.05>p>0.01$).

Fn is an opsonin with multiple bioactivity. It differs antigenically from fibrinogen and other plasma proteins. In critically ill patients, particularly in patients with severe infection, shock, trauma, leukemia, RF, circulatory failure

Table 3. PFn concentrations in patients with different degree of RF

Patient	N	X+SD (mg/L)
Severe RF patients who required MV	15	122.92+56.15
RF patients who did not require MV	18	176.80+77.15

Table 4. PFn concentrations in patients with infections of different severity

Patient	N	X+SD (mg/L)
Patients with septic shock	13	98.01+46.22
Patients with infection but without shock	19	149.18+61.31

and CNS diseases, Fn decreases significantly. Reduction in PFn may result from its inadequate synthesis and release, and excessive exhaustion caused by various clinical entities, and may decrease the body resistance against infection. As a consequence of infection, Fn is further reduced, which leads to a vicious cycle [7].

The PFn value of the 75 PICU patients was obviously lower than that in normal children, which showed a statistically significant difference ($t=5.111$, $p<0.01$). Also we compared PFn in the critically ill patients with different severity of disease and found that the decreased PFn in RF patients was significantly different from that in normal children. Particularly the decrease of PFn in severe RF patients who required mechanical ventilation was more obvious than RF patients who did not require it. Many investigators have found that the vascular permeability was increased with decreased Fn in the presence of hypoxia with hypercapnia [15], and that the increased vascular permeability was improved after reversal of Fn deficiency [16]. Fn involves in cell-cell adhesion, cell migration and chemotaxis. Hence, Fn decrease may lead to the accumulation of fibrin in the lungs and the peripheral blood vessels, resulting in the exacerbation of pulmonary dysfunction. The fact that Fn decrease depends on the severity of RF indicates its importance as a nonspecific opsonin in pulmonary infection, and as an index of the severity of the disease. Meanwhile, the study of Fn gave a clue to improving the survival rate of RF patients in terms of enhancing the opsonic function. It was also found that PFn was significantly decreased in patients with systemic infection as compared with normal children. This showed that decreased Fn concentration resulted in decreased body resistance against the infection.

Mononuclear-macrophages play an important role in the clearance of dead cells and tissue debris to maintain homeostasis. The function of RES is closely related to Fn levels, hence, the change of Fn reflects the functional status of the body against infection. Further exacerbation of the infection occurs with the reduction of Fn. Among the children with infection, the most obvious Fn reduction was found in those with septic shock. In two leukemic children with infection (septic shock), Fn contents were 2 and 16 mg/L respectively at the time of admission, and both became 0 about 1–2 hr before death, Thus, PFn may be used as an index of the severity of the disease and as a predictor for the prognosis of the patient.

Conclusion

To investigate the change of PFn and its clinical significance in sick children of different severity, we determined PFn values in 22 out-patients with mild or moderate respiratory tract infection and 75 critically ill patients admitted to the PICU. PFn values in the 22 out-patients were not found to have any abnormal changes, but were markedly reduced in the 75 critically ill patients, as compared with normal children. Significant decrease of PFn was seen in the patients with RF, systemic infection and CNS infection, and very significant decrease was seen in the patients with septic shock. In two leukemic patients with associated infection, PFn became undetectable before death. Persistent PFn reduction without improvement after treatments predicts a poor diagnosis. The results indicate that low PFn concentration is of prognostic value, and may be considered as an index of exogenous Fn replacement therapy.

References

1. Loegering DJ (1979) Humoral factor depletion and reticuloendothelial depression during hemorrhagic shock. Am J Physiol 232:H283.
2. Jin H (1986) Fibronectin levels in septic shock and disseminated coagulation. Chinese J Pathophysiol 3:164.
3. Godfrey HP, Feng Z, Mandy S, et al (1992) Modulation of expression of delayed hypersensitivity by mycobacterial antigen 85 fibronectin-binding proteins. Infection and Immunity 60:2522.
4. Yamada KM, Olden K (1978) Fibronectins-adhesive glycoproteins of cell surface and blood. Nature 275:179.
5. Hynes RO, Yamada KM (1982) Fibronectins: Multifunctional modular glycoproteins. J cell Biol 95:369.
6. Chijiiwa K, Nakano K, Kameoka N, et al (1994) Proliferating cell nuclear antigen, plasma fibronectin, and liver regeneration rate after seventy percent hepatectomy in normal and cirrhotic rats. Surgery 116:544.
7. Jin H (1993) Fibronectin. In: Cui N (ed) Critical care medicine, 1st edn. Tianjin Translating and Publishing Corporation, Tianjin, pp 93–100.
8. Ye Y, Ding W, Su Z (1985) Plasma fibronectin level in normal children. Chinese J Surgery 6:205.
9. Gomez-Lectin MJ, Costed JV (1986) Measurement of fibronectin in human body fluid. J Clin Chem Clin Biochem 24:333.
10. Mosher DF, Furcht LT(1981) Fibronectin: Review of its structure and possible functions. J Invest Dermatol 77:175.
11. Marino JA, Pensky J, Culp LA, Spagnuolo PJ (1985) Fibronectin mediates chemotactic factor stimulated neutrophil-substrate adhesion. J Lab Clin Med 105:725.
12. Plow EF, Ginsberg MH (1981) Specific and saturable binding of plasma fibronectin to thrombin-stimulated human platelets. J Biol Chem 256:9477.
13. Spagnuolo PJ, Donofrio B, Litzenberg WE, Fratianne RB, Manno JA (1992) Fibronectin binding and neutrophil aggregation in burn injury. J Surg Res 53:211.
14. Chen D, Zhu Y, Jin H (1987) Relationship between fibronectin and change of cerebral microvascular permeability of rats with hypoxia and hypercapnia. Chinese J Med 5:261.
15. Saba TM, Lanser ME (1983) Lung vascular permeability after reversal of fibronectin deficiency in septic sheep. Ann Surg 198:654.
16. Zhao J, Zhuang W, Zhu X, Shao N, Ouyang R, Pan R (1985) Fibronectin determination in acute and chronic leukemia, Shanghai Med 8:311.

Pulmonary

Mechanisms of Respiratory Failure and New Management Strategies

B. Lachmann, D. Gommers and S. Böhm

Introduction

Acute Respiratory Distress Syndrome (ARDS) has become a well-recognized condition that can result from a number of different causes, e.g. sepsis, shock, pneumonia, trauma, liquid aspiration, hematologic disorders, smoke inhalation, and many others [1]. Despite diverse etiologies, the final pathway results in damage of the alveolar epithelium and endothelium, resulting in high-permeability pulmonary edema. The permeability changes, along with the inflammatory response, result in influx of proteins and inflammatory cells into the airspace with loss of functional active surfactant [2]. Surfactant normally present in the lung has the unique property of lowering surface tension at the air-liquid interface in parallel with the decrease in alveolar radius, thus keeping the ratio of surface tension divided by radius constant and guaranteeing end-expiratory alveolar stability. Surfactant normally present in the lung has the unique property of lowering surface tension at the air-liquid interface in parallel with the decrease in alveolar radius, thus keeping the ratio of surface tension divided by radius constant and guaranteeing end-expiratory alveolar stability.

Diminished active surfactant has far-reaching consequences for lung function and the lung finally 'fails' as a gas exchange organ (Fig. 1).

The exact mechanisms responsible for injury of the alveolar-capillary membrane are complex and are still under discussion [3]. The failure of the lung as a gas exchange organ results in peripheral tissue hypoxia, which appears to be related to the development of multiple organ failure (MOF). Since MOF is the predominant cause of death in ARDS, therapeutic efforts in ARDS are aimed at improving oxygen delivery to the tissues.

ARDS is characterized by non-cardiogenic pulmonary edema, hypoxemia, decreased lung compliance, increased pulmonary arterial pressures, and the requirement need for mechanical ventilation. Despite advances in the understanding of mechanical ventilation, morbidity and mortality remain unacceptably high. Available treatments include high inspired oxygen concentration and high peak alveolar pressures in association with large distending tidal volumes, but these are known to induce lung damage [4]. Therefore, management strategies aiming to reduce the mechanical ventilator's contribution to lung damage are currently under investigation with the aim to reduce morbidity and

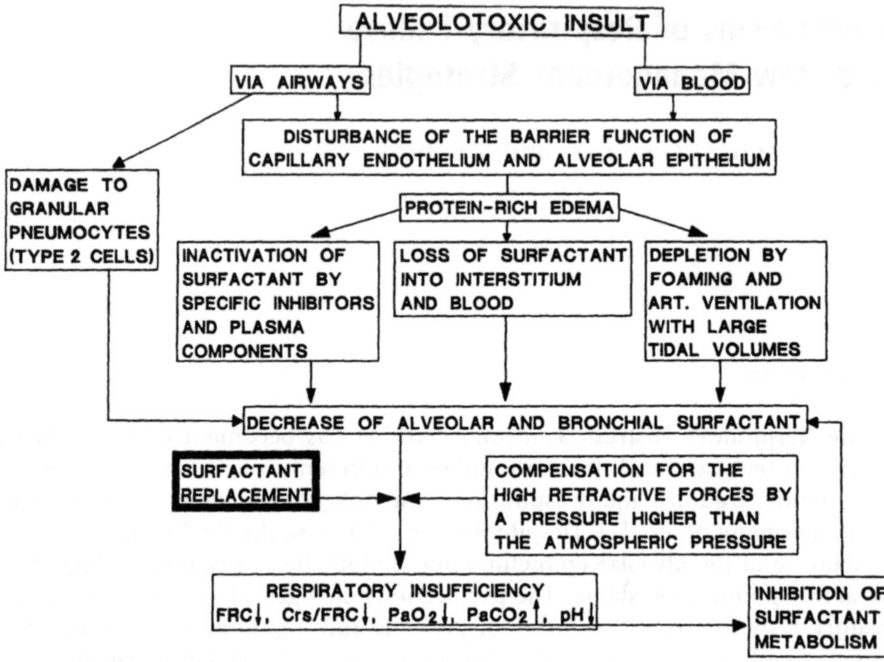

Fig. 1. Pathogenesis of ARDS with special reference to the surfactant system, including suggestions to compensate for a damaged surfactant system.

mortality. These strategies of improving gas exchange based on physiological rationale consist of:

- Balancing the increased collapsive tendency of the lung by applying optimal modes of ventilation with minimal pressure swings to reduce shear forces [5],
- Elimination of the air-liquid interface by filling the lung with perfluorocarbon that is capable to maintain gas exchange at the alveolar capillary membrane to reduce the high retractive forces due to a diminished surfactant system [6],
- Instillation of exogenous surfactant to re-establish a physiological low surface tension at the air-liquid interface as a prerequisite for normal lung function [7].

In this article, we describe the above-mentioned new rationales for improving lung function in ARDS which are currently under evaluation.

Improving Gas Exchange by Optimal Ventilator Settings

Ventilator-induced lung injury does not only consist of pulmonary air leaks but also compromises damage to the alveolar capillary membrane. The two major contributors to this ventilator-induced injury are large volume and big pressure swings explaining the terms volume- and barotrauma, respectively.

More than twenty years ago Mead et al. [8] have stated: "at a transpulmonary pressure of 30 cmH_2O, the pressure tending to expand an atelectatic region surrounded by a fully expanded lung would be approximately 140 cmH_2O". Such forces may well be the major cause of structural damage especially to bronchiolar epithelium, alveolar epithelium and capillary endothelium and may not only be the basis for formation of hyaline membranes but may also cause the release of mediators from the disrupted parenchyma – triggering the pathophysiological mechanisms of ARDS [4]. During ventilation of patients with ARDS, who generally have atelectatic lung regions, pressure differences of 30 cmH_2O or higher are quite common. However, it is not the 30 cmH_2O pressure difference that damages the lungs but rather the resulting shear forces of more than 140 cmH_2O which are responsible for the barotrauma. Hence, to prevent lung damage due to high shear forces between open and closed lung units only ventilation modes which result in the smallest possible pressure amplitude should be used.

The principle of volume trauma lies in the continuous mechanical consumption of alveolar surfactant. Studies have shown that, ventilator modes with large tidal volumes and high peak inspiratory pressures during artificial ventilation affect the pulmonary surfactant system [4]. Moreover, these changes are directly related to the tidal volume used and the duration of the mechanical ventilation. The exact mechanism by which the surfactant system is affected by artificial ventilation is not yet entirely clear. One factor is that the surfactant in the alveolar lining is actively removed from the alveolus towards the larger airways; this can lead to a shortage of surfactant at the alveolar level causing changes in surface tension characteristics in the lung, seen during or after prolonged periods of mechanical ventilation [4].

In normal spontaneous breathing, during end-expiration the surfactant molecules covering the alveolar epithelium are compressed on the small alveolar areas leading to low surface tension or a high surface pressure thus preventing the alveoli from collapse. If the surface of the alveolus is smaller than the surface occupied by the surfactant molecules, the molecules are squeezed out of the surface and forced towards the airways. These surfactant molecules are then 'lost' for the alveoli and are eventually cleared from the lungs. During the following inflation of the alveoli, the surface is replenished with surfactant molecules coming from the underlying hypophase where surfactant molecules in micelles are 'stored' for later use. During the next expiration, the mechanism repeats itself and again surfactant molecules are forced out of the alveolus and subsequently replenished from the hypophase; this is a continuing cycle (Fig. 2) [4].

The amount of surfactant that must be produced and subsequently secreted by the alveolar type II cells is proportional to the loss of surface active molecules during the breathing cycle. When production and secretion of new surfactant molecules keep pace with consumption, no surfactant deficiency can occur, as in a normal healthy lung.

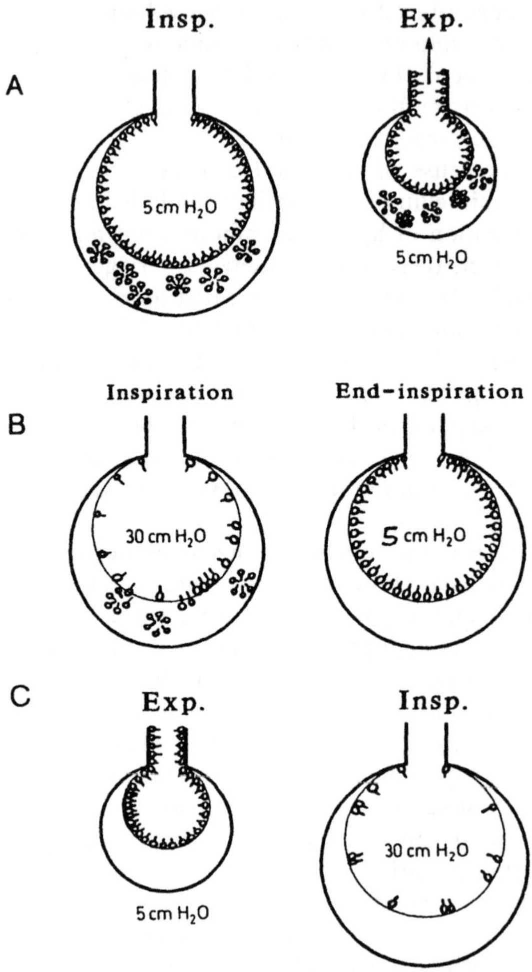

Fig. 2. (**A**) Balance between synthesis, release and consumption of surfactant in the healthy lung. The pressure values given represent the intrapulmonary pressure needed to open up the alveolus. At the surface and the hypophase (micelles), there are sufficient molecules of surfactant. These micelles deliver the surfactant necessary to replace the molecules squeezed out during expiration (Exp). (**B**) Imbalance between synthesis, release and consumption of surfactant due to artificial ventilation. At the beginning of inspiration, there exists an apparent deficiency of surfactant molecules but there is a respreading of molecules stored in the hypophase to the surfactant layer. At the end of inspiration there is, in principle, enough surfactant on the surface. (**C**) With the next expiration (Exp), surface active molecules are squeezed out and no surface active molecules are left in the hypophase for respreading, creating the situation where a serious surfactant deficiency follows. Insp = inspiration.

It becomes clear that the rate of loss of surfactant is greater when the phasic volume changes of the alveolus are larger during the breathing cycle. When the alveoli are collapsed, for instance in atelectatic lung areas, the surfactant molecules are highly compressed on the surface and a significant part is forced out of the alveolus. The smaller the airspace, the lower the surface tension must be to retain airspace stability. If the collapsed alveolus is subsequently highly inflated, replenishment from the hypophase must accordingly be larger than normal; even more so when a combination of high peak inspiratory pressures and large tidal volumes is used to open up collapsed airspaces. In these situations, consumption is greater than normal and production and secretion of surfactant must increase to prevent a surfactant-deficient state.

Thus optimal ventilator mode should produce minimal pressure swings during the ventilatory cycle and keep the lung volume at end-expiration equal to or just above the FRC level and PEEP therefore prevents a significant depletion

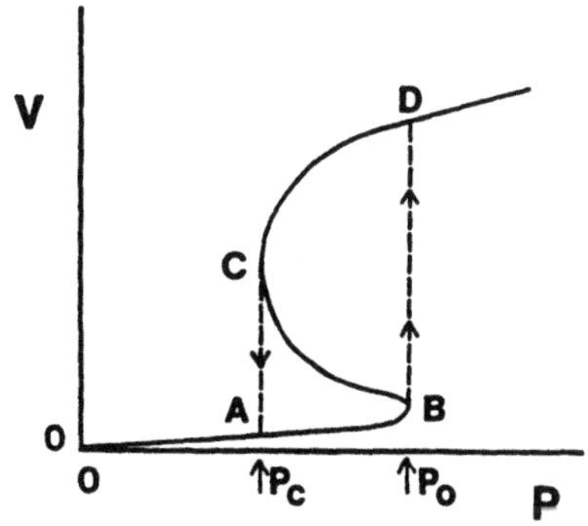

Fig. 3. Theoretical pressure-volume characteristics of alveolus showing region of negative compliance from B to C, causing an alveolus when inflated to critical opening pressure (Po) to jump from B to D and when deflated to critical closing pressure (Pc) to jump from C to A.

of surface active material. As shown in Figure 3, the pressure needed to keep the alveoli open is smaller at a high FRC level.

But to reach this level, an initial opening pressure is required. Since the critical opening pressure is inversely proportional to alveolar unit size, it follows that progressive recruitment of air spaces requires a continuously increasing pressure during inflation which translates to high peak inspiratory pressure. The pressure necessary to induce volume changes depends on the initial radius. In other words, to get a certain volume change in large alveoli, the necessary pressure changes are much smaller compared to alveoli which are collapsed or have a lower volume. Therefore, the PEEP necessary to stabilize the end-expiratory volume can be minimized if the lungs are totally opened to the FRC level of a healthy lung [5].

In practice, this means that at pressure controlled ventilation after the whole lung is re-aerated the pre-set peak inspiratory pressure has to be set to a value which just compensates for the retractive forces of the whole lung. If one then either increases the I/E ratio at a constant frequency, or increases the frequency at a constant I/E ratio (or both) to establish an expiratory time which will be too short to allow emptying of the lung to the ambient pressure, an intrinsic PEEP will be created. If one chooses the absolute time of the expiratory phase so short that also the stiffest parts of the lung have no time for collapse, the lungs will be kept open and can then be ventilated with a significantly smaller pressure amplitude compared to volume controlled PEEP ventilation. This concept of 'open up the lung and keep the lung open' maintains sufficient gas exchange with the smallest possible pressure amplitude and was successfully applied for the first time in ARDS patients in 1978/1982 [9, 10] and confirmed by two recent studies [11, 12].

Improving Gas Exchange by Perfluorocarbons

In 1929 von Neergard [13] noticed that when filling up a healthy lung with fluid, much lower pressures were needed to fill the lung to a certain volume when compared to filling it with gas. He deduced that each alveolus has a liquid-air interface, which tends to retract and is abolished when filling the lung up with fluid (Fig. 4). Thus, there is a possibility for providing normal tidal volumes in surfactant deficient lungs at low airway pressures by filling up these lungs with fluid. This shifts the pressure-volume relationship of these lungs to the left and provides normal tidal volumes changes at lower pressures amplitude.

Therefore, Shaffer and colleagues [14] investigated in 1976 whether perfluorocarbons (PFCs), which are known to decrease surface tension and have the ability to dissolve high amounts of oxygen, would eliminate the surface forces in 'stiff' lungs and could improve oxygenation; since then PFCs have been investigated intensively as an alternative means of respiratory support. This alternative respiratory support was originally performed by totally filling the lungs with PFC using a modified ventilator, which oxygenates the perfluorocarbon extra corporeally; this was called total liquid ventilation. This technology is not encouraging as it requires sophisticated equipment; thus the search began for a simpler technique of liquid ventilation to support pulmonary gas exchange.

Perfluorocarbons (PFCs)

The physical properties that make PFC fluids suitable for liquid ventilation are their low surface tension and their ability to dissolve high amounts of oxygen (O_2) and carbon dioxide (CO_2) (Table 1). The total amount of O_2 solved in PFC is about three times as much as the same amount of blood can chemically bind. PFCs are colorless, clear and odorless liquids with a high density. They are chemically very stable, biologically inert liquids and can not be metabolized in biological systems due to the strong bond between carbon and fluorine atoms present. PFCs can be derived from simple organic compounds (such as benzene) and can be produced cheaply and in large quantity.

Animal Experiments with Partial Liquid Ventilation (PLV)

Fuhrman et al. [15] demonstrated that it was possible to install PFCs (30 ml/kg) in healthy piglets during mechanical ventilation without deterioration of gas

Table 1. Physical properties of a PFC liquid (Perflubron)

Density (g/ml)	1.92
Vapor Pressure (mmHg at 37 °C)	10.5
Surface tension (dynes/cm)	18
O_2 Solubility (ml/100 ml)	53
CO_2 Solubility (ml/100 ml)	210

exchange. The adequate gas exchange was achieved at tidal volumes and airway pressures comparable with mechanically gas ventilated animals. After these experiments, our group applied this concept to acute respiratory failure in surfactant-depleted animals. Lung-lavaged rabbits were mechanical ventilated and treated with incremental doses of 3 ml/kg bodyweight PFC up to a total volume of 15 ml/kg body weight (BW) [16]. Oxygenation in the PFC treated animals improved significantly with each subsequent dose of PFC to values that did not significantly differ from the values pre-lavage. $PaCO_2$ and peak airway pressures decreased significantly after instillation of 3 ml/kg PFC and remained stable with the subsequent treatment doses. To see if these effects were longer lasting, we conducted three-hour experiments in the same model [17]. Oxygenation restored almost to 'healthy' state after instillation of PFC (18 ml/kg BW) within 30 min and remained stable during the three-hour observation period. The PFC treated animals showed a persistent and significant decrease in respiratory resistance at inspiration, peak and mean airway pressure from post-lavage data and respiratory system compliance consequently improved. Microscopic examination of the lungs from PFC treated animals did not reveal any morphological abnormalities while the lungs of the conventionally ventilated group had alveolar damage, including distension and rupture of alveoli. In the next study [18], the effect of four different doses of intratracheal PFC (3–12 ml/kg bodyweight) in lung-lavaged rabbits was evaluated for a six-hour period. It was shown that the beneficial effects on oxygenation were dose-dependent, and oxygenation showed a time-dependency for each dose with decreasing oxygenation over time. The relationship between the dose of PFC administered and the time at which impairment of lung function was seen, strongly supports the suggestion that evaporation of PFC over time would cause the affected alveoli to collapse and, therefore, limit the efficacy of pulmonary gas exchange, which will occur sooner with small doses of PFC. Moreover, in the same study it was shown that at increasing doses of PFC in doses up to 40 ml/kg, gas ventilation with constant tidal volumes resulted in higher peak airway pressures. This effect was attributed to tissue elasticity becoming the predominant component of alveolar retractive forces.

The above-mentioned studies were conducted in rabbits with a small thoracic diameter. Because PFC has a high specific gravity, we hypothesized that PFC could lead to hemodynamic compression in which PFC might block pulmonary capillary perfusion in the lower parts of the lung of an adult person with a large thoracic diameter. Therefore, the dose-related effect of PFC administration on hemodynamics and gas exchange was investigated in lung-lavaged pigs with a thoracic diameter of 24 cm [19]. It was found that increasing doses of PFC have no deleterious effect on any hemodynamic parameter and mean pulmonary artery pressure even showed a persistent decrease after the first 5 ml/kg bodyweight of PFC. This can be explained by the effect of abolishment of hypoxic pulmonary vasoconstriction on mean pulmonary artery pressure. From all above-mentioned studies in RDS models it can be concluded that a volume of intratracheal PFC equalling FRC is the ideal dose for PLV, giving a long-lasting maximal effect on oxygenation and lung mechanics without negative effects on peak inspiratory pressure, hemodynamics or the endogenous surfactant system.

These beneficial effects of PLV were shown not to be solely related to the broncho-alveolar lavage model, but were also confirmed in other animal models of respiratory insufficiency [20].

Mechanics of PLV in the Lung

The hypothetical mechanism of PLV is explained in Figure 4. Figure 4A shows the atelectatic RDS lung. After a small dose of PFC (3 ml/kg) a thin film of PFC with a low surface tension would probably be formed at the air-liquid interface due to evaporation of PFC (Fig. 4B) and covers the alveoli of the whole lung.

Due to this film the increased surface tension in the diseased lung is reduced to a low and constant value, which leads to improved compliance which does not further improve with additional doses of PFC. The dose-dependent improvement in oxygenation may be due to the filling of the most dependent alveoli with PFC. The more PFC is applied the more collapsed atelectatic alveoli can be opened by the non-compressible, high density PFC, and prevented from end-expiratory collapse (Fig. 4B vs 4C) thus eliminating intrapulmonary shunt. This mechanism was supported recently by computed tomographic scans from Quintel et al. [21] who showed that PFC distributed predominantly to the lower lung regions, while gas distributed to the upper lung regions during partial liquid ventilation. Moreover, the low surface tension PFC will allow formation

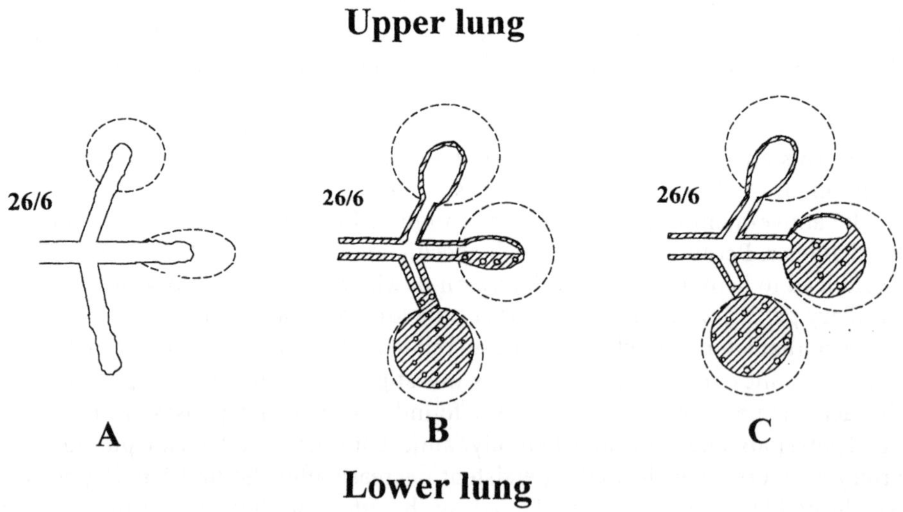

Fig. 4. The lining of the air-liquid barrier in the alveoli and the dose-dependent improvement in oxygenation after instillation of perfluorocarbon. (A) Shows the atelectatic RDS lung. (B) Shows the partially perfluorocarbon-filled lung. (C) Shows the effect of instilling additional perfluorocarbon. See text for details (solid line = end expiration; dashed line = end inspiration)

of air bubbles with the superimposed tidal gas volumes and gas diffusion from PFC to alveolar vessels will contribute to effective gas exchange.

Surfactant normally present in the lung has the unique property of lowering surface tension at the air-liquid interface in parallel with the decrease in alveolar radius, thus keeping the ratio of surface tension divided by radius constant and guaranteeing end-expiratory alveolar stability. Perfluorocarbons do not have this property and when the alveoli are not fully filled with PFC (in contrast to total liquid ventilation) end-expiratory collapse can occur in these alveoli during expiration. To prevent such collapse during PLV, one needs a certain level of PEEP which compensates for the retractive forces of a surface tension of 18 dynes/cm of the PFC (Table 1).

Further on, the use of PEEP is important because it prevents the bulk movement of the fluid being present in the alveoli when instituting the next inspiration and due to this movement the resistance increase and would lead to high peak pressures during partial liquid ventilation [16]. PEEP prevents this movement by pressing the fluid distally, keeping it in the alveoli.

Clinical Trials with PLV

Following these positive results in animal experiments, PLV is currently used in human trials in neonates and adults with RDS. Leach et al. reported a pilot safety and efficacy study in seven premature newborns with RDS who failed to respond to conventional therapy and exogenous surfactant treatment [22]. All patients showed improved PaO_2 and five of seven patients showed improved $PaCO_2$ and lung compliance. Two infants who became hypercapnic were resumed to high frequency ventilation. There were no serious adverse effects associated with PLV and three of these patients survived.

Recently, Hirschl et al. [23] evaluated the safety and efficacy of PLV in a series of 19 adults, children, and neonates who were in respiratory failure and on extracorporeal life support. During PLV, the alveolar arterial oxygen difference decreased from 590 to 471 mmHg and static compliance increased from 0.18 to 0.29 ml/cmH_2O/kg. Mean initial dose of PFC was 13.9 ± 2.2 ml/kg and the patients were redosed with a mean cumulative dose of 36.3 ± 3.6 ml/kg over the next 1–7 days. All patients tolerated administration of PFC without hemodynamic compromise but pneumothoraces re-accumulated in six patients with previous ipsilateral pneumothoraces and new pneumothoraces occurred in three patients. This study was without a control group and therefore Hirschl and colleagues concluded that they were unable to ascertain whether the improvements in gas exchange and pulmonary compliance were due to management with PLV.

Improving Gas Exchange by Exogenous Surfactant

The morbidity and mortality rates of premature infants suffering from the respiratory distress syndrome (RDS) have been decreased by exogenous surfactant therapy and this treatment is now routinely used in most neonatal intensive care units [24]. The clinical and pathological features in neonatal RDS are very similar to those seen in patients with ARDS. Neonatal RDS, however, is characterized by primary surfactant deficiency due to immaturity of the lungs, whereas in ARDS surfactant deficiency is a complication of lung injury. The value of surfactant therapy in this concept is that the functional impairment of surfactant in ARDS may be reversed by instillation of an excess of exogenous surfactant [25]. Furthermore, there is evidence that treatment with exogenous surfactant may stimulate synthesis and secretion of the endogenous surfactant in these patients [26].

From clinical experience of surfactant therapy in neonates with RDS, we have learned that the response after exogenous surfactant therapy depends not only on the course of the injury, but also on the timing of surfactant therapy, the used dose of exogenous surfactant, the type of surfactant preparation, and the ventilator settings of the mechanical ventilation [24]. In particular the level of PEEP used, and the method of administration of exogenous surfactant (which is important for the distribution of the instilled surfactant) play an important role.

Clinical Experience

Evidently, it is rational to administer exogenous surfactant in ARDS patients, but the question then arises why is this not yet a reality. At this moment, only a few case reports and results of limited clinical studies are available in which adult patients with ARDS are treated with exogenous surfactant [27]. Although these reports showed that some patients did not respond to, or had an only transient improvement after a single dose of surfactant, better results were seen with higher or multiple surfactant doses. The reason for lack of response, or only transient improvement after exogenous surfactant application, is attributed to the inhibition of the instilled surfactant by plasma components filling the alveolar space. Thus, the therapeutic goal must be to overcome the inhibitor capacity by exogenous surfactant. This implies that, if after surfactant instillation there is no, or only transient, improvement of blood gases in these patients (fibrotic lungs excluded) this does not mean that surfactant treatment does not work, it only means that the concentration of the exogenous surfactant used is too low in relation to the amount of surfactant inhibitors in the lung [25]. Thus, for treatment of ARDS, a high concentration of surfactant is required to overcome the inhibitory effect of plasma components. This is confirmed by the results of Gregory and colleagues [28] in a multicenter, randomized pilot study in 59 ARDS patients of different etiologies. In this study, four different dosing strategies were tested and the results showed that maximum improvement in oxygenation, minimum ventilatory requirements, and lowest mortality rate were obtained following treatment with 400 mg surfactant per kg body weight. The surfactant used in Gregory's study was a natural surfactant, as already used in neonates, and it was given as a bolus. This study is, to our knowledge, the first controlled trial in which the mortality of ARDS could be decreased (from 43.8% to 17.6%) by a therapeutic intervention. However, a relative small group of patients were treated and further clinical trials are required to confirm these results.

Various surfactant preparations are available on the market, and have been used successfully in worldwide clinical trials in neonates with RDS [24]. The natural surfactants (derived from animal lungs) contain surfactant proteins B and C while the artificial surfactant preparations are protein-free. From animal studies and studies in neonates with RDS, it has been demonstrated that natural surfactant preparations are more effective in improving lung function immediately after instillation than the artificial surfactant preparations, due to the lack of surfactant proteins [24]. Also, different studies have demonstrated that surfactant proteins reduce the surfactant inactivation that may be caused by plasma constituents which is of special importance in ARDS [29]. This could explain the results of Anzueto et al. [30] who reported currently available data of the first 498 patients of a multicenter, randomized placebo-controlled trial in 725 patients with sepsis-induced ARDS. The preliminary results of this study show that artificial surfactant (without surfactant proteins) has no effect on 30-day mortality and little effect on physiologic measurements during the 5 days of treatment, compared with the control group. The surfactant was delivered as an aerosol which may also play an important role [27].

Another important issue is that the ventilator pattern strongly influences exogenous surfactant therapy. Several studies have demonstrated that surfactant therapy and PEEP ventilation produces the largest and most sustained therapeutic effect [31]. Surfactant administration does not permit immediate withdrawal of PEEP, but it is usually possible to reduce the peak inspiratory pressures as lung function improves. This avoids over distension of the alveoli and increased perfusion of the lung. It also reduces the number of pneumothoraces.

Conclusion

In ARDS, available treatments include mechanical ventilation with high oxygen concentrations but still remain inadequate, and mortality rates have not improved on those reported on 1967 [32]. Now, there is evidence that some ventilatory strategies contribute to lung injury and that an optimal ventilatory mode should open up the lung and keep it open during the ventilatory cycle. This 'open the lung concept' minimizes the shear forces during ventilation leading to less damage of the epithelium and the surfactant system.

Partial liquid ventilation is a new promising technique and which shows improvement of gas exchange and lung mechanics and has no adverse effects on the cardiovascular system. PFC is readily available and there are no problems with distribution of this material in the lung. At this moment, only results of two pilot studies, without a control group, are available which show no serious side-effects in patients.

Convincing results of surfactant replacement studies in different animal models, a few case reports in human ARDS, and randomized clinical pilot studies strongly support the central role of surfactant in the pathophysiology of ARDS. This indicates the potential of exogenous surfactant therapy as an important therapeutic measure for treatment of ARDS. However, the prohibitive price and the non-availability of large amounts of surfactant, make surfactant therapy not yet feasible in ARDS.

In conclusion, it should be realized that the first two mentioned therapies are a supportive therapy and that exogenous surfactant therapy could be a merely curative intervention.

References

1. Bernard GR, Artigas A, Brigham KL, et al. (1994) The American-European concensus conference on ARDS: definitions, mechanics, relevant outcomes, and clinical trial coordination. Am J Respir Crit Care Med 149:818–824.
2. Seeger W, Günther A, Walmrath HD, Grimminger F, Lasch HG (1993) Alveolar surfactant and adult respiratory distress syndrome. Clin Investig 71:177–190.
3. Rinaldo JE, Rogers RM (1982) Adult respiratory distress syndrome: changing concepts of lung injury and repair. N Eng J Med 306:900–909.
4. Houmes RJ, Bos JAH, Lachmann B (1994) Effects of different ventilator settings on lung mechanics: with special reference to the surfactant system. Appl Cardiopulm Pathophysiol 5:117–127.
5. Lachmann B (1992) Open up the lung and keep the lung open. Intensive Care Med 118:319–321.
6. Verbrugge S, Gommers D, Lachmann B (1995) Liquid ventilation as an alternative ventilatory support. Current Opinion Anaesthesiol 8:551–556.
7. Gommers D, Lachmann B (1995) Surfactant therapy in the adult patient. Current Opinion Crit Care 1:57–61.
8. Mead J, Takashima T, Leith D (1970) Stress distribution in lungs: a model of pulmonary elasticity. J Appl Physiol 28:596–608.
9. Haendly B, Lachmann B, Schulz H, Jonson B (1978) Der Einflußverschiedener Beatmungsmuster auf Lungenmechanik ung Gasaustausch bei Patienten wahrend Respiratorbehandlung. Kongreßbericht Anaesthesie 1:665–678.
10. Lachmann B. Danzmann E, Haendly B, Jonson B (1982) Ventilator settings and gas exchange in respiratory distress syndrome. In Prakash O (ed) Applied physiology in clinical respiratory care. Nijhoff, The Hague, pp 141–176.
11. Kesecioglu J, Tibboel D, Lachmann B (1994) Advantages and rationale for pressure controlled ventilation. In: Vincent JL (ed) Yearbook of intensive care and emergency medicine. Berlin, Heidelberg, New York, pp 524–533.
12. Amato MBP, Barbas CSV, Medeiros DM, Schettino GPP, Filho GL, Kairalla RA et al. (1995) Beneficial effects of the "open lung approach" with low distending pressures in acute respiratory distress syndrome. Am J Respir Crit Care Med 152:1835–1846.
13. Von Neergaard K (1929) Neue Auffassungen über einen Grundbegriff der Atemmechanik; Die Retraktionskraft der Lunge, abhängig von der Oberflächenspannung in den Alveolen. Z Ges Exp Med 66:373–394.
14. Shaffer TH, Rubenstein D, Moskowitz GD, Delivoria-Papadopoulos M (1976) Gaseous exchange and acid-base balance in premature lambs during liquid ventilation since birth. Pediat Res 10:227–231.
15. Fuhrman BP, Paczan PR, DeFrancis M (1991) Perfluorocarbon-associated gas exchange. Crit Care Med 19:712–722.

16. Tütüncu AS, Faithfull NS, Lachmann B (1993) Intratracheal perfluorocarbon administration combined with artificial ventilation in experimental respiratory distress syndrome: dose dependent improvement of gas exchange. Crit Care Med 21:962–969.
17. Tütüncu AS, Faithfull NS, Lachmann B (1993) Comparison of ventilatory support with intratracheal perfluorocarbon administration and conventional mechanical ventilation in animals with acute respiratory failure. Am Rev Respir Dis 148:785–792.
18. Tütüncu AS, Faithfull NS, Lachmann B (1993) Intratracheal perfluorocarbon administration as an aid in the ventilatory management of respiratory distress syndrome. Anesthesiology 79:1083–1093.
19. Houmes RJM, Verbrugge S, Hendrik ER, Lachmann B (1995) Hemodynamic effects of partial liquid ventilation with perfluorocarbon in acute lung injury. Intensive Care Med 21:966–972.
20. Lachmann B, Verbrugge S (1996) Liquid ventilation. Current Opinion Crit Care; In press.
21. Quintel M, Hirschl RB, Roth H, et al. (1995) Assessment of perfluorocarbon (PFC) distribution during partial liquid ventilation (PLV) in the setting of acute respiratory failure. Am Rev Resp Crit Care Med 151(4):A446 (Abst).
22. Leach CL, Greenspan JS, Rubenstein SD, et al. (1994) Partial liquid ventilation with Perflubron (LiquiVent™): a pilot safety and efficacy study in premature newborns with severe RDS who have failed conventional therapy and exogenous surfactant. In: Lucey JF (ed) ROSS Special Conference, Hot Topics '94 in Neonatology, Washington DC, pp 161.
23. Hirschl RB, Pranikoff T, Gauger P, Schreiner RJ, Dechert R, Bartlett RH (1995) Liquid ventilation in adults, children, and full-term neonates. Lancet 346:1201–1202.
24. Jobe AH (1993) Pulmonary surfactant therapy. N Eng J Med 328:861–868.
25. Lachmann B, Eijking EP, So KL, Gommers D (1994) In vivo evaluation of the inhibitory capacity of human plasma on exogenous surfactant function. Intensive Care Med 20:6–11.
26. Pinkerton KE, Lewis J, Mulder AM, Ikegami M, Jobe AH (1993) Surfactant treatment effects on alveolar type II cell morphology in rabbit lungs. J Appl Physiol 74:1240–1247.
27. Gommers D, Lachmann B (1993) Surfactant therapy: does it have a role in adults? Clin Intensive Care 4:284–295.
28. Gregory TJ, Gadek JE, Weiland JE, et al. (1994) Survanta supplementation in patients with acute respiratory distress syndrome (ARDS) Am J Respir Crit Care Med 149:A567 (Abst).
29. Seeger W, Grube C, Günther A, Schmidt R (1993) Surfactant inhibition by plasma proteins: differential sensitivity of various surfactant preparations. Eur Resp J 6:971-977.
30. Anzueto A, Baughman R, Guntupalli K, et al. (1994) An international, randomized, placebo-controlled trial evaluating the safety and efficacy of aerosolized surfactant in patients with sepsis-induced ARDS. Am J Respir Crit Care Med 149:A567 (Abst).
31. Froese AB, McCulloch PR, Sugiura M, Vaclavik S, Possmayer F, Moller F (1993) Optimizing alveolar expansion prolongs the effectiveness of exogenous surfactant therapy in the adult rabbit. Am Rev Respir Dis 148:569–577.
32. Asbaugh DG, Bingelow DB, Petty TL, Levine BE (1967) Acute respiratory distress in adults. Lancet 2:319–323.

High-Frequency Jet Ventilation or Oscillation?

A. J. van Vught, D. G. Markhorst and R. J. B. J. Gemke

Introduction

The development of artificial ventilation at the beginning of this century constituted a major progress in medical care. Initially, mechanical ventilation was mainly applied during surgery. Later, during the poliomyelitis epidemics in the fifties large numbers of patients were ventilated outside the operation room, at first by hand and subsequently by mechanical ventilators. Nowadays, mechanical ventilation is a standard technique to combat imminent or overt respiratory insufficiency.

However, mechanical ventilation does have adverse side effects and therefore has its limitations. For an adequate gas exchange, especially under pathological pulmonary conditions, insufflation of large volumes of gas with high inspiratory airway pressures, sustained expansion of the lungs by a positive end-expiratory pressure (PEEP) and long inspiratory times may sometimes be necessary. This may lead to overstretch and shear stress of lung tissue and to lung damage (barotrauma). An elevated intrathoracic pressure will decrease venous return, leading to a decrease in cardiac output and thus oxygen delivery to the organs. The imposed respiratory pattern of the ventilator may interfere with the patient's own breathing pattern, leading to large and unpredictable changes in airway pressure and intrathoracic pressure and therefore, to hemodynamic instability. This often necessitates sedation or even complete induced paralysis of the patient, which entails new complications in the treatment.

An ideal ventilatory pattern should result in an adequate gas exchange in the lungs without causing lung damage and without impairment of the circulation or other organ functions. Unfortunately, the conditions that minimize the side effects are often opposed to conditions that promote gas exchange in the lungs. Thus, the ventilatory pattern for a given patient will usually be a compromise between benefits and adverse effects. When an acceptable compromise cannot be attained, the consequence is a failure of conventional mechanical ventilation to support life. Other modes of ventilation are then needed. One of these may be high-frequency ventilation.

In this paper we will give a short overview of the history of, and rationale behind high–frequency ventilation and summarize the concepts of gas exchange during high-frequency ventilation. Subsequently, we will discuss the main features of high-frequency jet ventilation and high-frequency oscillation, as the two dominant modes of high-frequency ventilation, and review the very few comparative data about these methods. And finally, we will try to formulate some conclusions regarding the current application of the two modes.

A Short History of High-Frequency Ventilation

At the end of the sixties Öberg and Sjöstrand [1, 2] while studying blood pressure regulation and the carotid sinus reflex in ventilated animals, found their measurements disturbed by respiratory synchronous variations in blood pressure. Therefore, they needed a method of artificial ventilation without this effect. Insufflation of the ventilating gas deep into the trachea via an endotracheal catheter reduced the anatomical dead space and consequently smaller tidal volumes at higher frequencies, 60–120 min^{-1}, could be used. This reduced pressure variations in the airways and in the intrathoracic space and diminished the circulatory effects of ventilation. Short insufflation times, less than 0.3 of the ventilatory cycle, reduced the circulatory effects even further by the inertia characteristics of the respiratory system. The circulation remained stable and adequate gas exchange was obtained at lower inspiratory peak pressures, lower mean airway pressures and lower transpulmonary pressures. In addition, spontaneous breathing movements disappeared. Experimental animals and later on patients accepted these ventilatory conditions without breathing against the ventilator. For this mode of ventilation Sjöstrand and co-workers introduced the term high-frequency positive pressure ventilation (HFPPV) [1]. Although originally designed for experimental physiological studies HFPPV was recognized to have important clinical advantages and the method has since been developed for clinical application.

In 1977 Klain et al. [3] described the insufflation of small volumes of gas under high pressures (jets) with frequencies up to 200 min^{-1}, later up to 600 min^{-1}, into the trachea of dogs via a percutaneously introduced catheter. Adequate gas exchange was achieved at low airway pressures, while the circulation remained stable. This method was called high-frequency jet ventilation (HFJV). For clinical use the insufflation catheter can be placed either directly into the trachea via the nasotracheal route or into an endotracheal tube (Figure 1).

In 1980 Bohn et al. [4] and Butler et al. [5] demonstrated that adequate gas exchange was also possible by generating oscillations in the airways at a frequency of 15 Hz. Originally, they used a loudspeaker to evoke the oscillations, later on an electronically driven piston pump. Earlier, Lunkenheimer et al. [6] had found adequate CO_2 elimination by comparable methods with frequencies between 20–40 Hz. This method, high-frequency oscillation (HFO), is characterized by the generation of pressure swings with, in contrast to HFPPV and HFJV, an active withdrawal of air from the airways. Refreshment of gas takes place via a fresh gas flow (bias flow) in the upper part of the ventilatory circuit (Figure 2).

Several modifications of HFJV and HFO have been tested since, both experimentally and clinically. Extensive clinical experience has been gathered to date

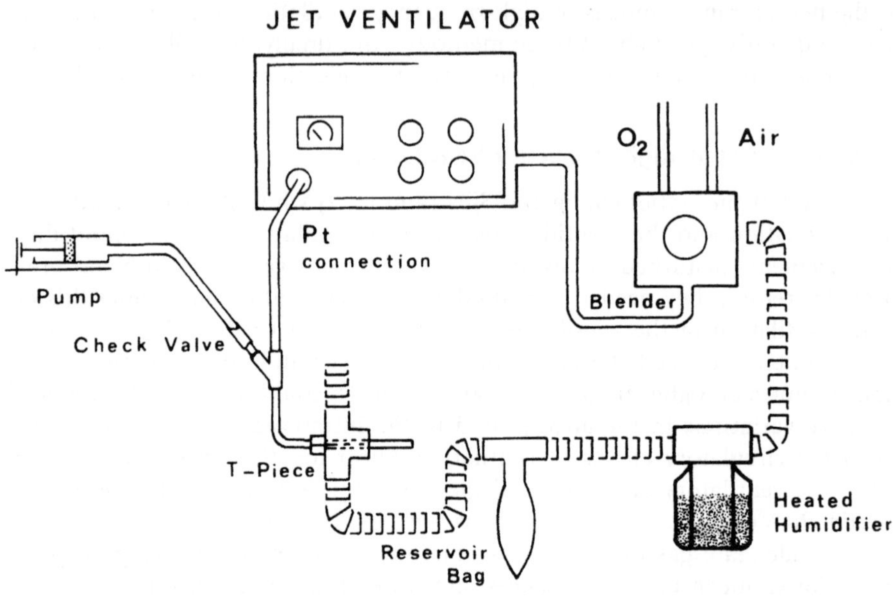
JET VENTILATOR
O2
Air
Pt
connection
Pump
Blender
Check Valve
T-Piece
Heated
Humidifier
Reservoir
Bag

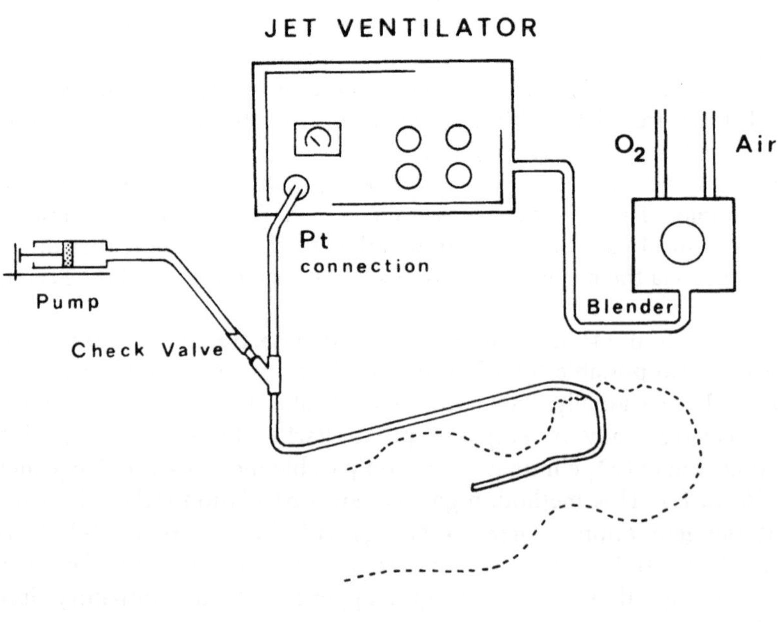
JET VENTILATOR
O2
Air
Pt
connection
Pump
Blender
Check Valve

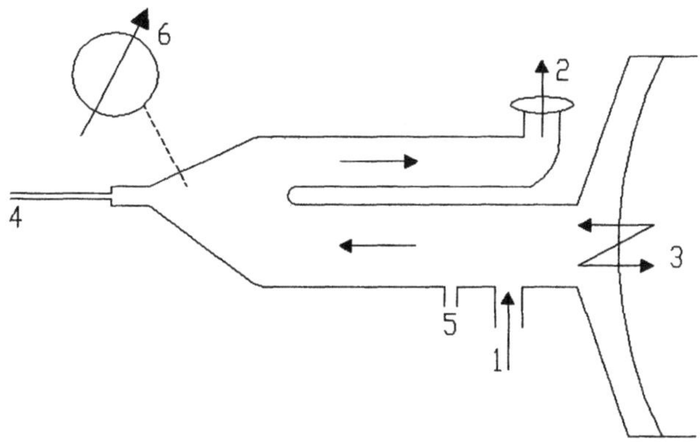

Fig. 2. High-frequency oscillator. Oscillations are generated by a vibrating membrane (3) and propagated to the endotracheal tube (4). Frequency and amplitude of the oscillations can be controlled electronically. Humidified gas is led into the respiratory circuit (1). Mean airway pressure can be regulated by adapting the inflow of gas into the system and/or the outflow resistance (2). At point 6 pressure and temperature are measured. Inlet port 5 can be used for adding nitric oxide to the ventilating gas

with HFPPV, HFJV and HFO. High-frequency ventilation has gained a definite place in the treatment of severe respiratory insufficiency, although its position between conventional mechanical ventilation and extra corporeal membrane oxygenation (ECMO) [7] is still under discussion, particularly after the introduction of nitric oxide and its combination with HFO [8-10].

Methodologically, HFPPV closely resembles conventional mechanical ventilation. However, tidal volumes and accordingly inspiratory peak pressures are smaller. In HFJV tidal volumes approximate the volume of the anatomical dead space. With HFO tidal volumes are even smaller. Alveolar ventilation under these conditions cannot be explained by the classical concepts of gas exchange and other mechanisms must be involved.

Gas Exchange in High-Frequency Ventilation

Classical concepts of gas exchange, i.e. bulk flow and mass transport up and down the airways and gas mixing and molecular diffusion in the alveolar space, are inadequate to explain alveolar ventilation in high-frequency ventilation in

Fig. 1. Clinical set-up of high-frequency jet ventilation. The upper panel shows the jet cannula placed into a T-piece which can be connected to the endotracheal tube. The high inspiratory gas velocity entrains air from outside into the tube. The actual tidal volume is the sum of jet volume (V_{jet}) and volume of entrained air ($V_{entrained}$). To assure that the composition of the ventilating gas is independent of the ratio between V_{jet} and $V_{entrained}$ a bias flow with the same composition as the jet gas is led past the tube. In the lower panel the gas is insufflated directly into the trachea via an endotracheally placed jet catheter. In this set-up there is no entrainment of air. Humidification is effectuated by infusion pumps.

which tidal volumes are smaller than the volume of the airways. Other or at least additional mechanisms must be assumed. In 1984 Chang [11] summarized these mechanisms. Since his paper appeared the discussions have been focused on the relative contribution of each mechanism and their interrelations, without changing the overall concepts.

Five mechanisms are distinguished. At first, direct alveolar ventilation of proximally situated alveoli. Small volumes of insufflated gas may reach these alveoli situated high up at the bronchial tree. The contribution of direct alveolar ventilation is dependent on tidal volume and on the distribution of pathway lengths from the airway opening to the alveoli. A second mechanism is gas mixing by high-frequency "pendelluft". Because of the inhomogeneity of time constants of different lung units there will be inspiratory and expiratory phase lags between adjacent units, which are greatly exaggerated during high-frequency ventilation. In this way lung units can ventilate each other and gas transport can take place even over long distances between lung units with different compliances and resistances. A third mechanism is convective dispersion due to asymmetric inspiratory and expiratory flow profiles, especially at airway bifurcations. Molecules near the center of the airways are displaced towards the alveoli, while molecules near the walls are displaced towards the airway opening. This mechanism is closely related to the Taylor type of dispersion, the fourth mechanism. In Taylor type dispersion there is a combination between axial convection and radial diffusion. Convection of gas in the central parts of the airways gives rise to axial concentration gradients, resulting in diffusion over these gradients. The fifth and last mechanism is molecular diffusion, but it seems unlikely that this mechanism which takes place in the alveoli is a leading mechanism distinguishing gas exchange in high-frequency ventilation from that in conventional mechanical ventilation.

It is probable that at distinct levels in the respiratory system, from trachea to alveoli, one or another of the above mentioned mechanisms of gas transport is more dominant than the others. In addition, it is likely that the relative contribution of each mechanism to gas exchange in high-frequency ventilation is dependent on the mode of ventilation and the design of the ventilatory circuit. This is important in comparing the effects of different types of ventilation.

High-Frequency Jet Ventilation

Characteristic for HFJV is the intermittent insufflation of air under high pressure at high rates, usually from 150 to 300 min^{-1}. Expiration is passive, the air leaving the respiratory system along the insufflation catheter or nozzle via the free upper airways. The difference between the alveolar pressure, which depends on lung volume and the combined recoil forces of lung and thoracic cage, and the pressure at the airway opening is the driving force for expiration. Tidal volume in HFJV depends on the driving pressure for jet generation, inspiratory time, cannula resistance and back-pressure in the respiratory system, and on the volume of environmental air entrained by the jet stream. Lung volume during HFJV depends on delivered tidal volume, which is the sum of insufflated and entrained volume, and on compliance and resistance of the respiratory system. Consequently, delivered tidal volume and the resulting lung volume are determined by mechanical properties of the lung and airways and are distinctly influenced by changes in these mechanical characteristics. This makes control of gas exchange in instable airways unpredictable.

High-frequency flow interruption (HFFI) is a modification of HFJV. In HFFI pulses of gas are released from a high pressure source by some control mechanism, often a rotating ball valve. The pulses of gas are delivered in the inspiratory circuit rather than directly into the trachea. There is no entrainment of environmental air, operating frequencies are usually higher and range from 300 to 900 min^{-1}, peak flow rates are usually lower. Expiration remains passive. HFFI is sometimes incorrectly classified as high-frequency oscillation.

The first use of HFJV in pediatrics has been reported by Pokora et al. [12] in 10 neonates. In their report they already pointed to fatal tracheal obstruction and necrotizing tracheobronchitis (NTB) as important side effects. In a later report of the same group [13] 10 out of 12 patients who died after more than 8 hours of jet ventilation revealed tracheal injury of varying degrees at autopsy. High flow rates and inadequate humidification are main initiating elements in the pathogenesis of NTB, but other factors, such as oxygen toxicity and epithelial ischemia, may be involved too [14-16]. There are only a few randomized trials comparing HFJV with conventional mechanical ventilation in infants and children, comprising, moreover, only small numbers of patients [17-19]. Complications, such as NTB, bronchospasms, tube obstruction and airway blockade, overdistension by inadvertent PEEP and unpredictable changes in lung volume, have limited widespread use of HFJV in pediatrics. The more so as new modalities of high-frequency ventilation appeared to be equally effective in gas exchange, but with fewer side effects. Because in HFFI inspiratory flows are lower and humidification is easier to achieve the incidence of NTB may be lower. However, also with HFFI local air trapping with the formation of pseudocysts in the lungs of premature baboons have been reported [20].

Nowadays, the use of HFJV is limited to adult patients, in which this is the only mode of high-frequency ventilation able to maintain adequate gas exchange, and to a limited number of special indications, such as laryngeal and airway surgery and emergency transtracheal ventilation when immediate laryngeal intubation is difficult or impossible.

High-Frequency Oscillation

In HFO oscillations of air are generated either by a piston pump or by an electronically driven and powerful vibrating diaphragm. The oscillations are propagated to the airways via an endotracheal tube. Oxygen enters the system and carbon dioxide is removed by a bias flow of fresh gas. The exit port of the bias flow serves as a low pass filter preventing loss of oscillatory volume. Oscillatory volume can be adjusted by changing the amplitude of the piston or diaphragm displacements, mean airway pressure can be regulated by adapting the inflow of fresh gas and/or the outflow resistance (Figure 2). With a piston pump type of oscillator pressure wave form is always sinusoidal. With an electronically driven diaphragm pressure wave forms can also have a more block form configuration and inspiratory to expiratory ratio may be altered. Theoretically, a block wave may have advantages, but this has to be confirmed experimentally and clinically. An essential feature of HFO is the biphasic pressure wave form with an active expiratory phase. This reduces inadvertent air trapping [21]. By decreasing the inspiratory fraction of the oscillatory cycle air trapping can be reduced still further [22].

In HFO mean airway pressure and therefore lung volume, alveolar recruitment and oxygenation can be regulated independent from CO_2 elimination. Empirically, CO_2 removal (V'_{co2}) follows the relation $V'_{co2} = f^a \times TV^b$, where f represents ventilatory frequency and TV tidal volume and where a in most studies reaches values around 1 and b around 2 [11]. Due to the relatively small tidal volumes delivered by the presently available oscillators, HFO is up till now not feasible for patients weighing more than 40 kg.

After the preliminary observations of Lunkenheimer [6], Bohn et al. [4] demonstrated in 1980 for the first time adequate gas exchange in dogs weighing 11 kg, with an oscillatory frequency of 15 Hz and a volume of 15 ml. Also in 1980, Butler et al. [5] reported for the first time the effective use of HFO with a piston pump in human patients. In 1981 the first preliminary report was published on HFO in neonates with RDS [23]. After several promising reports, the results of the first randomized multicenter trial, comparing HFO and conventional mechanical ventilation in 673 preterm infants, published in 1989 [24], were disappointing and led to an in depth discussion regarding the advantages and disadvantages of different HFO strategies [25]. Optimal alveolar recruitment, achieved by the so called high volume strategy, and early onset, that is to say before barotrauma has been induced by conventional mechanical ventilation, turned out to be the major prerequisites for optimal results of HFO [26, 27]. This appeared to be confirmed again by studies on the application of exogenous surfactant during HFO as compared to conventional mechanical ventilation [28].

High mean airway pressures, when resulting in high intrathoracic pressures, impede venous return and thus depress cardiac output. Appropriate filling of the circulatory system prevents the negative circulatory effect of the high volume strategy. In addition, optimal pulmonary blood volume improves oxygenation, possibly by stretching alveolar capillaries and with them the alveolar septa, thus improving the diffusion characteristics.

Inhalation of nitric oxide (NO) has been shown to decrease pulmonary hypertension and to improve ventilation perfusion distribution throughout the lungs. The beneficial effect of NO inhalational therapy appears to be dependent on optimal alveolar recruitment [8-10]. Therefore, the combination of HFO and NO inhalational therapy has been shown to be successful in the treatment of persistent pulmonary hypertension of the neonate and in severe respiratory failure, making this treatment a serious alternative to ECMO [7, 9].

Although the major indications and advantages for HFO are in neonates, HFO has been shown to offer significant benefits also in respiratory failure of older children, improving outcome where conventional mechanical ventilation has failed [29–31].

Complications of HFO are mainly caused by inappropriate initial settings of the oscillator and large swings in airway pressure and oscillatory volume resulting in inadvertent variations in ph and blood gases and in cardiac output. As with many new technologies the complication rate decreases as experience increases [25]. Although less frequent than in HFJV tracheal lesions and overdistension of lung segments have been reported in HFO too [32].

Comparative Studies

Comparative studies are mainly confined to conventional mechanical ventilation versus different modes of high-frequency ventilation. There are no clinical studies comparing the impact and outcome of different modes of high-frequency ventilation. There are only a few comparative studies in experimental animals such as baboons [33], rabbits [21], cats [32,34,35] and piglets [36]. These studies reflect the difficulties and pitfalls encountered when evaluating the differences between the distinct modes of high-frequency ventilation. In HFJV the venturi effect near the jet entry point and entrainment of air can profoundly influence the delivery of tidal volume and pressure measurements. The position of the measurement sites in the circuit is essential for correct interpretation of the values. Passive versus active expiration will entail dissimilar effects of distinct respiratory patterns on lung volume. In fact, jet ventilators and oscillators are completely different machines and seemingly subtle differences in design may have major differences in impact [35].

Conclusions

There are at present no comparative clinical studies between HFJV and HFO. Comparative experimental studies often deal with different ventilator designs and different ventilatory patterns rather than the jet versus oscillatory pattern by itself and therefore, are inconclusive or at least difficult to interpret. Nonetheless, some conclusions may be warranted. Lung volume, alveolar recruitment and gas exchange are more easily controlled in HFO. There are fewer side effects and complications in HFO than in HFJV. Although there still are some distinct indications for HFJV, such as ventilation during airway surgery and emergency onset of ventilation in cases of difficult airway management, HFO is now by far preferred in neonatal and pediatric patients. Surfactant replacement therapy and NO inhalational therapy in combination with HFO may serve as an early step between conventional mechanical ventilation and ECMO and finally may turn out to be a satisfactory alternative in severe respiratory failure.

Acknowledgements. The authors express their gratitude to Mr. T. Leenhoven, Professor J. Huber and Dr. E.L.I.M. Duval for their critical remarks and to Elmer van Vught for designing Figure 2.

References

1. Jonzon A, Oberg PA, Sedin G, Sjostrand U (1971) Highfrequency positive-pressure ventilation by endotracheal insufflation. Acta Anaesth Scand 43 Suppl: 1–43
2. Sjostrand U (1977) Review of the physiological rationale for and development of high-frequency positive-pressure ventilation- HFPPV. Acta Anaesth Scand 64 Suppl: 7–27
3. Klain M, Smith RB (1977) High frequency percutaneous transtracheal jet ventilation. Crit Care Med 6:280–287
4. Bohn DJ, Miyasaka K, Marchak BE, Thompson WK, Froese AB, Bryan AC (1980) Ventilation by high-frequency oscillation. J Appl Physiol 48:710–716
5. Butler WJ, Bohn DJ, Bryan AC, Froese AB (1980) Ventilation by high-frequency oscilation in humans. Anesth Analg 59:577–584
6. Lunkenheimer PP, Rafflenbeul W, Keller H, Frank I, Dickhut HH, Fuhrmann C (1972) Application of transtracheal pressure oscillations as a modification of "diffusive respiration". Brit J Anaesth 44:627
7. Carter JM, Gerstmann DR, Clark RH, Snyder G, Cornish JD, Null DM, deLemos RA (1990) High-frequency oscillatory ventilation and extracorporeal membrane oxygenation for the treatment of acute neonatal respiratory failure. Pediatrics 85:159–164
8. Kinsella JP, Neish SR, Ivy DD, Shaffer E, Abman SH (1993) Clinical responses to prolonged treatment of persistent pulmonary hypertension of the newborn with low doses of inhaled nitric oxide. J Pediatr 123:103–108
9. Kinsella JP, Abman SH (1993) Inhalational nitric oxide therapy for persistent pulmonary hypertension of the newborn. Pediatrics 91:997–998
10. Kinsella JP, Abman SH (1995) Recent developments in the pathophysiology and treatment of persistent pulmonary hypertension of the newborn. J Pediatr 126:853864
11. Chang HK (1984) Mechanisms of gas transport during ventilation by high-frequency oscillation. J Appl Physiol 56:553–563
12. Pokora T, Bing D, Mammel MC, Boros S (1983) Neonatal highfrequency jet ventilation. Pediatrics 72:27–32
13. Boros SJ, Mammel MC, Coleman JM, Lewallen PK, Gordon MJ, Bing DR, Ophoven JP (1985) Neonatal high-frequency jet ventilation: four years' experience. Pediatrics 75:657–663
14. Boros SJ, Mammel MC, Lewallen PK, Coleman JM, Gordon MJ, Ophoven J (1986) Necrotizing tracheobronchitis a complication of high-frequency ventilation. J Pediatr 109:95–100
15. Clark RH, Wiswell TE, Null DM, deLemos RA, Coalson JJ (1987) Tracheal and bronchial injury in high-frequency oscillatory ventilation compared with conventional positive pressure ventilation. J Pediatr 111:114–118
16. Nicklaus PJ (1995) Airway complications of jet ventilation in neonates. Ann Otol Rhinol Laryngol 104:24–30
17. Carlo WA, Chatburn RL, Martin RJ (1987) Randomized trial of high-frequency jet ventilation versus conventional ventilation in respiratory distress syndrome. J Pediatr 110:275–282
18. Carlo WA, Siner B, Chatburn RL, Robertson S, Martin RJ (1990) Early randomized intervention with high-frequency jet ventilation in respiratory distress syndrome. J Pediatr 117:765–770
19. Keszler M, Donn S, Bucciarelli RL, Alverson DC, Hart M, Lunyong V, Mondanlou HD, Noguchi A, Pearlman SA, Puri A, Smith D, Stavis R, Watkins MN, Harris TR (1991) Multicenter controlled trial comparing high-frequency jet ventilation and conventional me-

chanical ventilation in newborn infants with pulmonary interstitial emphysema. J Pediatr 119:85–93
20. Robotham JL, Coalson JJ, de Lemos RA (1987) Dangers of high-frequency ventilation in hyaline membrane disease. Intensive Care Med 13:85–86
21. Bancalari A, Gerhardt T, Bancalari E, Suguihara C, Hehre D, Reifenberg L, Goldberg RN (1987) Gas trapping with highfrequency ventilation:jet versus oscillatory ventilation. J Pediatr 110:617–622
22. Gerstmann DR, Fouke JM, Winter DC, Taylor AF, deLemos RA (1990) Proximal, tracheal, and alveolar pressures during HighFrequency Oscillatory Ventilation in a normal rabbit model. Pediatr Res 28:367–373
23. Marchak BE, Thompson WK, Duffty P, Miyaki T, Bryan MH, Bryan AC, Froese AB (1981) Treatment of RDS by high-frequency oscillatory ventilation: a preliminary report. J Pediatr 99:287–292
24. The HIFI Study Group (1989) High-frequency oscillatory ventilation compared with conventional mechanical ventilation in the treatment of respiratory failure in preterm infants. N Engl J Med 320:88–93
25. Bryan AC (1991) Reflections on the HIFI trial. Pediatrics 87:565–567
26. Clark RH, Gerstmann DR, Null DM, deLemos RA (1992) Prospective randomized comparison of high-frequency oscillatory and conventional ventilation in respiratory distress syndrome. Pediatrics 89:5–12
27. HiFO Study Group (1993) Randomized study of high-frequency oscillatory ventilation in infants with severe respiratory distress syndrome. J Pediatr 122:609–619
28. Gerstmann D, Minton SD (1995) Results of the Provo multicenter surfactant high-frequency oscillatory ventilator controlled trial (abstract). Pediatr Res 37(II):333A
29. Kinsella JP, Clark RH (1993) High-frequency oscillatory ventilation in pediatric critical care. Crit Care Med 21:174–175
30. Arnold JH, Truog RD, Thompson JE, Fackler JC (1993) Highfrequency oscillatory ventilation in pediatric respiratory failure. Crit Care Med 21:272–278
31. Arnold JH, Hanson JH, Toro-Figuero LO, Gutierrez J, Berrens RJ, Anglin DL (1994) Prospective, randomized comparison of high-frequency oscillatory ventilation and conventional mechanical ventilation in pediatric respiratory failure. Crit Care Med 22:1530–1539
32. Mammel MC, Ophoven JP, Lewallen PK, Gordon MJ, Boros SJ (1991) Acute airway injury during high-frequency jet ventilation and high-frequency oscillatory ventilation. Crit Care Med 19:394–398
33. Bell RE, Kuehl TJ, Coalson JM, Ackerman NB, Null DM, Escobedo MB, Yoder BA, Cornish JD, Nalle L, Skarin RM, Cipriani CA, Montos M, Robotham JL, deLemos RA (1984) High-frequency ventilation compared to conventional positive-pressure ventilation in the treatment of hyaline membrane disease in primates. Crit Care Med 12:764–768
34. Traverse JH, Korvenranta H, Adams EM, Goldthwait DA, Carlo WA (1989) Cardiovascular effects of high-frequency oscillatory and jet ventilation. Chest 96:1400–1404
35. Boros SJ, Mammel MC, Coleman JM, Horcher P, Gordon MJ, Bing DR (1989) Comparison of high-frequency oscillatory and highfrequency jet ventilation in cats with normal lungs. Pediatr Pulmonol 7:35–41
36. Zobel G, Dacar D, Rodl S (1994) Proximal and tracheal airway pressures during different modes of mechanical ventilation: an animal model study. Pediatr Pulmonol 18:239–243

The Changing Pattern of Neonatal ECMO: Do we Really Need it?

J. D. Cornish

Introduction

Extracorporeal membrane oxygenation (ECMO) is a modification of classic cardiopulmonary bypass (CPB) intended for the long term support of patients with life threatening cardiac and/or respiratory failure. In terms both of the numbers of patients treated and the success of those treatments, its most important application has been to neonatal patients with acute respiratory failure. Since the first successful neonatal ECMO case was reported in 1976 by Bartlett and colleagues [1], more than 13,000 patients have been supported with this technology, of whom more than 10,000 have been newborns (Table 1).

The most comprehensive summary of neonatal ECMO was recently published by Shanley and colleagues [2] representing Bartlett's life time experience.The number of neonatal patients supported with ECMO was quite small during the early years but increased to about 1,000 per year by 1988 (Figure 1).

Interestingly, there seems to have been a gradual decline in annual number of patients treated since 1992. Although the use of ECMO was quite controversial into the late 1980's, the number of centers offering this treatment has increased each year since 1982 with 20 new centers coming on-line in 1987 (Figure 2).

At present, there are 118 centers registered with the Extracorporeal Life Support Organization (ELSO) worldwide, 96 of which are in the United States. Of these 118 centers, only 110 are currently active. Again, one might question

Table 1. Cumulative ECMO Patient Experience. (International Summary, ECMO Registry Report of the Extracorporeal Life Support Organization, July 1995)

Group	Total Reported	No. Survived	% Survived
Neonatal Respiratory	10391	8352	80
Pediatric Respiratory	982	516	53
Cardiac Support	1491	643	43
Adult	197	80	41
Total	13061	9591	73

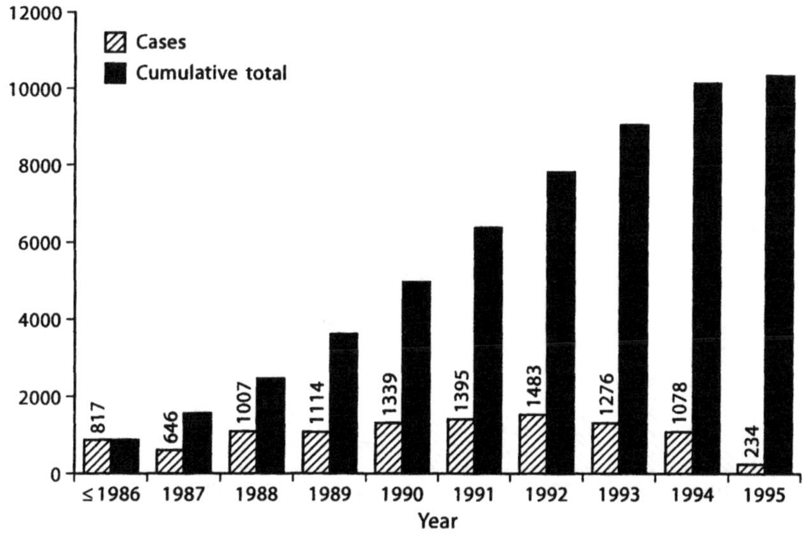

Fig. 1. Neonatal ECMO Cases by Year (Annual and Cumulative). (Data obtained from International ECMO Registry of the Extracorporeal Life Support Organization, January 1995)

whether there is declining interest in this technique as only 2 centers were added to ELSO in each of the years 1994 and 1995. These observations raise the useful questions as to the risks, benefits, and utility of ECMO compared to other available or developing therapies. Investigation of these questions is the focus of this chapter.

Extracorporeal Membrane Oxygenation: An Overview

A brief overview of ECMO may assist those not familiar with this technique before comparing it to the alternatives. ECMO differs from the heart-lung bypass used in the operating room in several meaningful ways. First, a thoracotomy is not necessary. In newborns, a small right cervical incision is generally all that is required to perform ECMO through a catheter inserted into the internal jugular vein, with or without an additional catheter in the common carotid artery. Second, ECMO is considerably simpler than CPB. It does not require multiple pumps, reperfusion systems, or complicated monitors. Although it does necessitate continuous systemic anticoagulation, it can generally be managed by a trained specialist and a nurse without requirement for a perfusionist or anesthesiologist. Third, ECMO does not require a sterile environment but is commonly performed in an intensive care unit under the direction of a neonatal or pediatric intensivist or surgeon. Most significantly, ECMO can be conducted with reasonable safety for periods of days or weeks, meaning that sufficient time can be provided to allow for the intrinsic recovery of injured organs (especially the lungs).

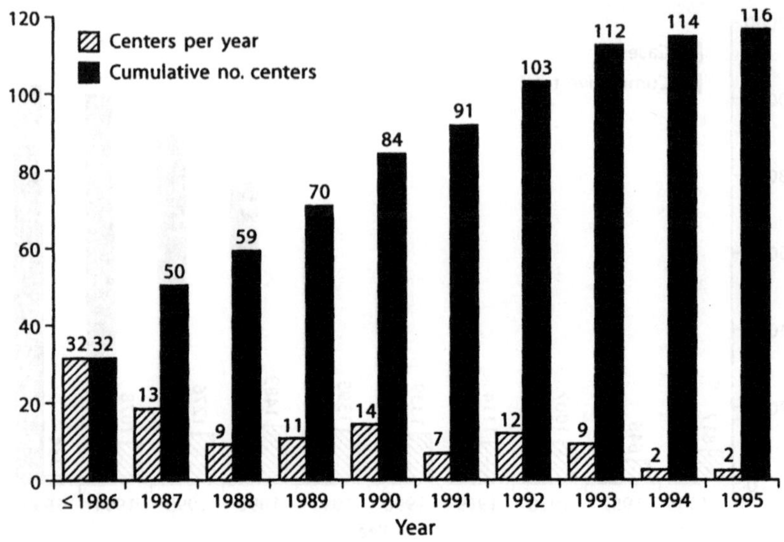

Fig. 2. ECMO Centers Registered (Annual and Cumulative). (Data obtained from International ECMO Registry of the Extracorporeal Life Support Organization, January 1995)

The ECMO system consists essentially of a blood pump, an oxygenator, a countercurrent heat exchanger to rewarm the blood, and a control module that balances the rates of blood drainage and of blood return to the patient. The blood pump is usually a simple roller pump, though some centers employ less traditional devices, the most common of which is a "constrained vortex" type of centrifugal pump. The oxygenator may be the original spiral coil sheet design or one of the newer hollow fiber devices; it exchanges both oxygen and carbon dioxide with the blood. The heat exchanger rewarms the blood by exposing it, across metal tubing, to warm water, which circulates in a direction opposite to that of the blood. A broad variety of control modules are currently in use, but all function by servo regulating pump speed so that the rate of reinfusion cannot exceed the rate of blood drainage from the patient.

Other devices may be added to the basic ECMO system. Pressure monitors are often placed before and after the membrane to monitor the pressure of the circulating blood and to identify increasing resistance in the oxygenator (i.e., increasing transmembrane pressure). Several different types of sensors have been applied to the blood path of ECMO circuits to measure the pO_2, hemoglobin saturation, pCO, Ph, and/or other "blood gas" parameters in the circulating blood. In-line bubble detectors can identify microscopic air bubbles in the arterialized blood and automatically turn off the pump to prevent air embolization. Computerized modules are available from several manufacturers of perfusion equipment which combine pressure monitoring, drainage and return coupling, and bubble detection in a single pump controller system. In addition, other "gadgets" are being introduced to make the system safer, easier to use, and even adaptable to patient transport.

The ECMO procedure is conceptually quite simple. The ECMO system is primed with the freshest available banked blood (which may be leukodepleted and/or irradiated to reduce the risk of graft-versus-host disease). The temperature, acid-base balance, and blood gases in the prime are adjusted to be similar to those of the patient (except for the pO_2, of course). The patient is sedated, and the cervical vessels are isolated and cannulated. In a growing number of neonatal cases, this is accomplished with a single catheter in the internal jugular vein. This catheter has two lumens, allowing blood to both drain and reinfuse through the same cannula. This approach is referred to as venovenous (as opposed to venoarterial) ECMO. In either case, the drainage and return lines of the ECMO system are connected to the catheter(s), and pump flow is begun. Blood flows by gravity from the patient to the control module that regulates pump speed, then onto the pump, the oxygenator, the heat exchanger, and finally back to the patient.

A variety of patient parameters must be carefully monitored during the procedure. These include the patient's vital signs, sedation and analgesia, nutritional and fluid status, acid–base and blood gas data, several coagulation studies (especially the activated coagulation time, prothrombin time, fibrinogen concentration, and platelet concentration), and other clinical and laboratory measurements. Perfusion support is terminated when any of the following conditions is reached: the patient's pulmonary (and/or cardiac) function improves sufficiently to allow survival using more conventional treatments; a contravening complication arises; or it can be reasonably demonstrated that recovery is unobtainable. Although the mechanics of this procedure are relatively straightforward, the risks associated with ECMO are considerable. Exquisitely ill patients who may not only be hypoxic but also infected are at heightened risk of bleeding complications when chronically heparinized. Indeed, hemorrhage into almost every imaginable anatomic site has been documented. Based on their review of the ELSO Registry, Zwischenberger and colleagues [3] reported that 35% of all newborns managed on ECMO suffered some form of hemorrhagic complication. Other patient complications and their reported incidences included cardiopulmonary (43%), neurologic (35%), metabolic (32%), renal (25%), and infectious (9%). Overall, patient complications occurred at a rate of 1.80 ± 2.12 per case. The most common mechanical complications included clots in the circuit (19%), cannula placement problems (9%), and oxygenator failure (4%). The rate of mechanical complications was 0.56 ± 0.84 per case. Notwithstanding these concerning statistics, the overall survival in this group of 7,667 critically ill newborns was 81%. Although outcome studies document a significant incidence of morbidity at 5 years of age when compared to normal controls, 83% of the cohort (103 five-year-olds) studied by Glass and colleagues did not have major neurologic disabilities [4]. Indeed, these ECMO survivors compared quite favorably in a wide array of neuropsychological and behavioral assessments when compared to similarly ill neonates who survived without recourse to ECMO [5]. Also, the incidence and severity of neurodevelopmental impairment seems to correlate with the primary diagnosis and may also correlate with the degree of disease severity prior to ECMO.

The Need for ECMO

Having said that ECMO is conceptually a fairly straightforward procedure but that it is associated with quite significant risks, one must ask whether there is now, or ever has been, a need for it. The anecdotal evidence suggests that a compelling need for ECMO has at least been perceived. After all, on more than 13,000 occasions presumably responsible physicians have made the decision to use it. Any physician who has managed patients on ECMO will confirm that the doing of it is so daunting that ulterior motives would not likely suffice in the absence of anticipated patient benefit. The entry criteria for neonatal ECMO, though applied with varying rigor from institution to institution, are widely published and generally accepted. According to Schwartz and colleagues from the National Perinatal Information Center, as presented in the *Report of the Workshop on Diffusion of ECMO Technology* commissioned by the National Institute of Child Health and Human Development [6], it may be predicted, using these entry criteria, that one in every 1,309 live births in the United States would receive ECMO. Given the 3,979,000 births [7] estimated in 1994, this would amount to a potential treatment group of 3,040 neonates per year in the U.S. If we accept from the foregoing the premise that sizable numbers of neonates could qualify for ECMO each year in the U.S., we must next query whether there is evidence of patient benefit to augment the perception of utility on the part of the prescribing physicians. As it happens, the relevant evidence is somewhat sparse and mostly anecdotal. There have been three prospective controlled clinical trials of ECMO therapy for neonatal respiratory failure. The first of these, conducted by Bartlett and colleagues [8], showed statistically unassailable benefit of ECMO in improving survival ($p=0.00000001$); of the 12 patients treated, only the one randomized to the control group died. Unfortunately, the "play the winner" statistical methodology that resulted in there being only one patient in the control group rendered this study less persuasive than might have been desired. Among the chief critics of Bartlett's study were the intensive care physicians at Boston Children's Hospital. They responded by designing their own study [9]. For ethical reasons, it was divided into two phases. In Phase I, babies were randomly assigned to either conventional treatment or ECMO until the stopping rule (4 deaths in either group) was reached. By this time there had been 10 babies entered into the conventional group and 9 into the ECMO group; all of the ECMO patients had survived. In Phase II, all babies were treated with the more successful therapy (ECMO) until the second stopping rule ($p<.05$) was reached. By this point, 20 additional patients had been treated, of whom 19 had survived. The patients in all groups were comparable in their disease severity. Overall survival for the ECMO group was 28 of 29 (97%) while that for the control group was 6 of 10 (60%). As noted, $p<.05$. Unfortunately, this study has also been criticized for its atypical statistical design. Fortunately, a third and more expansive prospective controlled clinical trial of ECMO has recently been concluded. The United Kingdom Collaborative ECMO Trial began in June of 1993 and was stopped by the data monitoring committee in November of 1995. By that time, 185 infants had been enrolled of whom 93 were selected to receive ECMO and 92 conventional management. The design of this study was unique in that it imposed a transport bias on the ECMO group. Patients were identified as candidates, consent was obtained, and randomization was accomplished after infants were evaluated in a tertiary center. Infants in the control group remained in their respective tertiary centers where aggressive "conventional" treatment was provided. Interestingly, this included high frequency ventilation and use of inhaled nitric oxide in some cases. Those randomized to receive ECMO were transported to one of 5 ECMO centers in the U.K. All data were analyzed on the basis of intention to treat. Study end points included cost-effectiveness, death, survival without disability at 1 year of age, and the presence of severe disabilities.In the ECMO group, 4 patients died prior to receiving ECMO and 4 had spontaneous improvement without receiving ECMO. In the ECMO group 27 (29%) patients died before hospital discharge; in the control group 54 (59%) died before discharge, making the difference between the two groups greater than 3 standard deviations ($p=0.0002$). Interestingly, there were 34 patients with congenital diaphragmatic hernia; 11/17 treated with ECMO survived while none of the 17 conventionally treated babies survived. The incidence of disability and impairment among the infants 1 year of age or older was not different between the two groups. In light of these additional findings, it seems justifiable at long last to conclude that ECMO does indeed improve survival among candidate neonates with life threatening respiratory failure and that it does so without increasing morbidity. With regard to complications, multiple comparisons of neurological and neurodevelopmental outcomes among newborns with severe persistent pulmonary hypertension treated with or without ECMO have been made. Although none of these was conducted as a part of a prospective controlled trial, a summary of these studies suggests that the outcomes for ECMO treated survivors are at least as good as those for non-ECMO treated survivors [10]. Thus, it may be credibly argued that candidate newborns with life threatening respiratory failure who are treated with ECMO are significantly more likely to survive than if ECMO is not offered and should have no greater risk of morbidity.

Appeal of the Alternatives

Any conclusions about the desirability of ECMO today must necessarily take into account the risks and benefits of available alternatives. Among these, the major candidates are conservative ventilation [11], artificial surfactant administration, high frequency ventilation, inhaled nitric oxide, and liquid ventilation. Of course, these are not the only alternatives. An array of lesser-known respiratory support techniques may come to have clinical importance in the future. These include inverse ratio ventilation, airway pressure release ventilation, negative pressure ventilation, and intratracheal pulmonary ventilation among many others. At present, though, the role of each of these in the treatment of neonatal disease is unclear, so no further mention will be made of them in this review.

Surfactant. Exogenous surfactant replacement is not only intuitively appealing for patients with the respiratory distress syndrome (RDS) who have intrinsic surfactant deficiency, but it is also efficacious and cost effective [12]. This brings us back to the observations made from Figure 1 and Figure 2. Given the estimate of 3,000 neonates requiring ECMO in the U.S. each year, a progressive increase in cases would have been predicted as more centers offered the procedure. Instead, the number of cases worldwide seems to have peaked at 1,483 in 1992 and to be stabilizing around 1,000 more recently. Most ECMO practitioners believe that a portion of this downturn may be attributed to the commercial availability of artificial surfactants. A review of data from the ELSO Registry supports this view. As shown in Figure 3, the number of cases treated per year has been relatively stable since about 1990 (discounting the data for 1995 which are yet incomplete) for four diagnostic categories: air leak syndrome (ALS), congenital diaphragmatic hernia (CDH), persistent pulmonary hypertension of the newborn (PPHN), and other. The apparent downturn in numbers of ECMO-treated neonates with sepsis is not easily explained. It is interesting, though, that the number treated for RDS has declined steadily since 1990 as has the number treated for meconium aspiration syndrome (MAS) since 1992. From Figure 4 it appears that there has been a decline in the relative proportion of all ECMO patients treated for RDS over about the same time period. Artificial surfactant became generally available for clinical use in 1990, the year in which the United States witnessed the largest drop in infant mortality in 20 years [12]. Bui and colleagues [13] reported in 1992 that phospholipid and surfactant protein A concentrations were decreased generally in tracheal aspirates from 22 infants requiring ECMO (a finding later validated in a similar population by Lotze and others [14]). They further demonstrated that the 14 infants who increased their phospholipid values more than 200% during the course of ECMO needed shorter periods both of ECMO support and of post-ECMO ventilator support than did the 8 infants with little or more moderate increases in tracheal aspirate phospholipid concentrations. Also of interest is the fact that none of the 22 infants studied bore the diagnosis of RDS (18 with MAS, 4 with pneumonia). There is abundant evidence that meconium inactivates surfactant, making replacement therapy for babies with MAS quite rational. This rationale has been supported by the recent publication of a randomized, controlled trial of Survanta[R] administration in term infants receiving mechanical ventilation for severe MAS [15]. Findlay and colleagues randomly assigned 20 infants to receive up to 4 doses of surfactant and 20 to receive 4 doses of air placebo. None of the treated infants required the fourth dose of surfactant; none developed air leaks; and only 1 required ECMO. By contrast, 5 of the infants in the control group developed air leaks, and 6 required ECMO. The duration of mechanical ventilation, oxygen therapy, and hospital admission were all significantly shorter in the treatment group.In 1993, Lotze et al reported the results from their center of a blinded, randomized, controlled trial of the effect of modified bovine lung surfactant in term infants requiring ECMO [16]. This study not only demonstrated that the duration of ECMO support was approximately 32 hours shorter in the treatment group, but also showed the incidence of post-ECMO complications to be lower with surfactant replacement. In a separate blinded, randomized, controlled trial of surfactant administration in patients treated with ECMO for CDH [17], Lotze and colleagues were not able to demonstrate clinical benefit of surfactant. Finally, Lotze and coworkers recently reported the findings of a 3 year multicenter study of the effects of Survanta[R] in the treatment of term infants with severe respiratory failure [18]. This study varied from the previous controlled trial by Lotze and coworkers in that the surfactant was administered before the infants qualified for ECMO. Of the 154 infants who received surfactant, 45 (29.2%) required ECMO as compared to 60/144 (41.7%) who received placebo ($p = 0.029$). There was no difference in the incidence of severe complications or in mortality between the two groups. Patients were stratified on study entry by disease category and by oxygenation index. The greatest impact of surfactant on the need for ECMO was seen among those neonates who received it earliest in the course of their disease (i.e., in the lowest oxygenation index category). From Figure 3 it may be seen that the number of newborns supported with ECMO declined by about 300 between 1990 and 1994, precisely the time frame when artificial surfactant became clinically available and when it was being shown to be beneficial in ECMO candidates (and more particularly among those with RDS or MAS).

From Figure 4 we see that the combined decline in number of newborns treated with ECMO for RDS and MAS over this time period was about 200 patients. Thus, much of the decrease in utilization of ECMO that we have noted might be the result of the increasing use of artificial surfactant in candidate patients. If appropriate surfactant preparations were more widely applied in

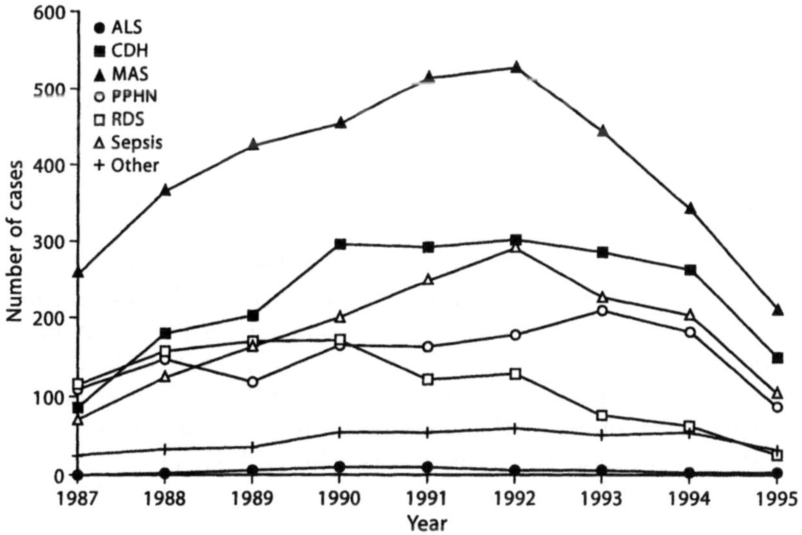

Fig. 3. Number of Neonatal ECMO Cases per Year by Diagnostic Category. (Data obtained from International ECMO Registry of the Extracorporeal Life Support Organization, Januar 1995. Note: Data incomplete for 1995)

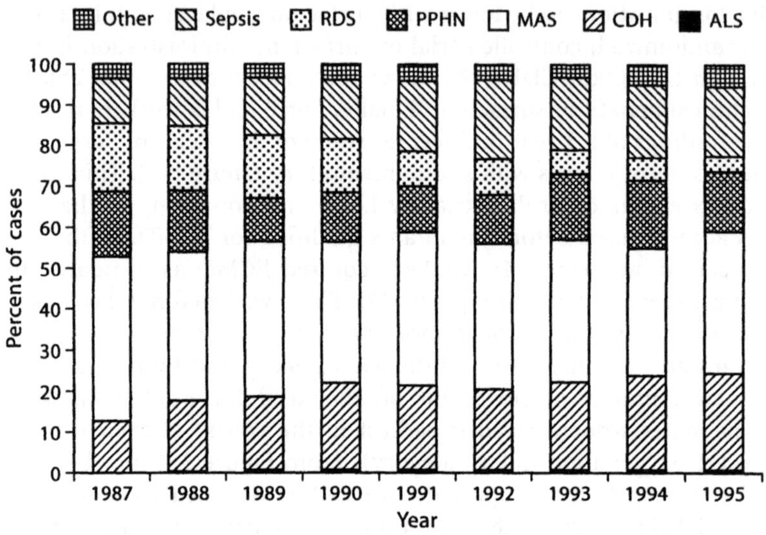

Fig. 4. Proportion of Neonatal ECMO Cases per Year by Diagnostic Category. (Data obtained from International ECMO Registry of the Extracorporeal Life Support Organization, January 1995)

this setting, the decrease in neonatal ECMO cases might be more dramatic still. Without doubt, surfactant is far less expensive and less risky than ECMO, and it should be given clear preference in any setting where there is even a slight chance of benefit. Unfortunately, a large number of infants will probably continue to require ECMO even so. Consequently, we must consider other alternative therapies.

High Frequency Ventilation (HFV). Soon after the introduction of high frequency ventilators, deLemos and colleagues [19] demonstrated the ability of a high frequency oscillatory ventilator (HFOV) to achieve equivalent oxygenation at lower inspired oxygen concentrations than with a conventional mechanical ventilator (CMV) in premature baboons. Several authors have subsequently shown that high frequency ventilators can achieve optimal lung inflation with minimal lung injury in animal models. It has been more difficult in a clinical setting to demonstrate the relative risks and benefits of HFV as compared to CMV. The conclusions, for example, from the original High-Frequency Intervention (HIFI) trial in premature babies [20] were that HFOV did not decrease the risk of bronchopulmonary dysplasia (BPD) but was associated with a higher incidence of grade III and grade IV intraventricular hemorrhage (IVH). One subsequent study supported this conclusion [21], and two did not [22, 23]. In fact, the trial by Ogawa and colleagues [22] failed to show any difference in either favorable or unfavorable outcomes between CMV and HFOV. A review of all of the clinical trials of HFV, supports the conclusion that the risks associated with HFV are quite similar to those seen with conventional ventilation when used with comparable degrees of skill and experience. More recent evidence supports the contention that HFOV may even be less injurious than conventional mechanical ventilation [24].

High frequency ventilators have also been used in term infants with severe respiratory failure who might qualify for ECMO. Cornish and others reported in 1987 that approximately half of term infants referred for possible ECMO could be successfully supported with HFOV without subsequent recourse to ECMO [25]. The efficacy of HFV in supporting term infants with severe respiratory failure was subsequently documented by Carlo [26], Kohelet [27], Tamura [28], Carter [29], deLemos [30], Varnholt [31], and Miguet [32, 33] and their associates. Paranka and others were able to identify predictors of failure of HFOV in term infants in their retrospective review of 190 infants. Of these patients, 111 (58%) responded to HFOV and 79 (42%) required ECMO. Non-responders tended to have congenital diaphragmatic hernia/lung hypoplasia (CDH/LH) or to have arterial/alveolar oxygen ratio (a/A ratio) at initiation of HFOV of 0.05 or lower (sensitivity 74%, specificity 77%). Excluding the CDH/LH group from consideration, the best predictor of HFOV failure was an a/A ratio of 0.08 or less after 6 hours of HFOV (sensitivity 77%, specificity 92%).

It is of note in this series of anecdotal reports that, where HFV was offered at the outset to all candidates, the investigators consistently reported that 50% or so of the patients did not require ECMO support (Cornish–47%, Carter–46%, deLemos–53%, Varnholt–50%, Paranka–58%). This trend makes definitive statements about the relative efficacy of HFV as an alternative to conventional ventilation difficult since most ECMO centers report that around 50% of patients referred to them for ECMO are able to be supported using a broad variety of other therapies. The question of relative efficacy must obviously be addressed in a prospective controlled trial.

The only prospective, randomized comparison of HFV to CMV in newborns who qualified for ECMO was reported by Clark et al [34] in 1994. This study showed HFOV to be a more effective rescue tool than CMV: 63% of patients who did not respond to CMV improved with HFOV while only 23% of those who failed HFOV responded subsequently to CMV. The response to initial assigned therapy was not different between the two groups: 60% in the CMV and 44% in the HFOV group met treatment failure criteria. Once again, 46% of those who met ECMO criteria required ECMO.

Without doubt, the efficacy of HFOV is largely dependent on the strategy used. An approach that optimizes recruitment, avoiding both atelectasis and overdistension, is clearly better [35]. HFV may offer additional benefit over CMV if used early in the course of the disease with a strategy designed to optimize lung volume, even if this results in higher recorded mean airway pressures. Interestingly, this was the conclusion of Arnold and colleagues from their prospective, randomized study of HFOV in pediatric respiratory failure patients [36]. It may be argued that HFV is an effective therapy in many newborns who are considered for ECMO, but it does not appear to prevent the need for ECMO among the most severe of these patients. It is clearly preferable to ECMO among responders, but it is not likely to supplant ECMO overall.

Nitric Oxide. The demonstration that nitric oxide (NO) is a major mediator of vascular relaxation has led to investigations of its potential therapeutic role. Nitric oxide is clearly a selective and effective pulmonary vasodilator. Kinsella and colleagues [37] demonstrated that pulmonary blood flow increases in a dose-dependent fashion when near-term fetal lambs are exposed to 5–20 ppm NO. Roberts showed that inhaled NO at doses of 20–80 ppm reversed the vasoconstrictive effects of both hypoxia and respiratory acidosis in a near-term lamb model [38]. Numerous animal studies verifying these and related points were followed by several anecdotal clinical experiences. Roberts used NO at 80 ppm to treat 6 infants with PPHN [39]. Kinsella and colleagues reported their experience treating 9 neonates with PPHN using doses of 10–20 ppm [40]. Reports have continued to be published from small patient series in multiple centers, but most notably by Kinsella, Abman, and other members of their group in Denver [41–45], by Roberts, Zapol and their coworkers in Boston [46, 47], by Steinhorn, Karamanoukian, and others in Buffalo [48, 49], and by Rossaint, Gerlach and Falke in Berlin [50]. Finer and colleagues in Edmonton have demonstrated that there is no definable dose response at concentrations between 5 and 80 ppm [51] and that NO results in improved oxygenation in prematures with a history of prolonged rupture of the membranes [52]. Gerlach, by showing efficacy of inhaled NO concentrations of 60, 100, and 230 parts per billion has very serviceably demonstrated that the doses currently being used clinically are probably much above that required for therapeutic effect [53, 54].

Many investigators report that the bulk of treated newborns experience a rapid improvement in oxygenation that lasts for hours or days after treatment with NO. Unfortunately, tachyphylaxis occurs in many patients with diminishing clinical response to ever increasing doses. Ultimately, a substantial portion of patients go on to require extracorporeal membrane oxygenation (ECMO) as they are unacceptably compromised and become unstable with discontinuation of NO, perhaps as a result of rebound vasospasm. Finer and colleagues [51], for example, reported that among 23 infants referred for ECMO, 14 responded to NO including 11/13 infants with evidence of PPHN but only 3/11 without PPHN. Unfortunately, 11 of the 23 ultimately required ECMO including 6 of those who had initially improved with NO. This is consistent with our experience as well.

There can be no question that inhaled NO produces virtually immediate improvement in oxygenation and a decrease in pulmonary vascular resistance in animal models and in patients with hypoxia and pulmonary hypertension. The pressing question is whether this initial effect will ultimately alter clinical outcome. Unfortunately, no prospective, controlled clinical trial has yet been published. There are at least 6 prospective clinical trials in progress evaluating the use of inhaled NO to treat persistent pulmonary hypertension of the newborn [55]. It is hoped that light can be shed by these studies not only on the question of short term efficacy but also on the matter of long range clinical impact. Likely the essential consideration here is the one emphasized by Abman and Kinsella [56], namely, that NO is a potent and (when inhaled) selective vasodilator, but it does not treat any associated pulmonary or cardiac diseases. The success of this intervention will probably have more to do with our ability to sort out the multiplicity of underlying pathophysiologic mechanisms (of which pulmonary vasoconstriction is often only a minor one) than with the vasodilatory capacity of NO per se.

It is conceivable that the use of inhaled NO to treat PPHN in neonatal ECMO candidates may not change the frequency with which this "last resort" therapy is employed but may only delay the institution of ECMO. If prospective controlled trials show this to be the case, then NO in this setting may do more harm than good since there is a clear correlation between age at initiation of ECMO and incidence of subsequent chronic lung disease [57].

Liquid Ventilation. Perhaps the most exciting of the new therapies for neonatal respiratory failure is liquid ventilation. A number of perfluorochemicals have been employed as intravascular and intrapulmonary gas exchange media, but the medical grade product being most widely studied today is perfluorooctylbromide, a chemical whose generic name is perflubron and whose trade name is LiquiVent (Alliance Pharmaceutical Corp., San Diego, CA). Structurally, it consists of a single bromide atom at the end of a perfluorinated eight carbon chain. Physically, it is a dense (specific gravity 1.918 g/cm^3), colorless, odorless liquid with remarkable oxygen (53 ml/dl) and carbon dioxide (210 ml/dl) carrying capacity. It is less viscous than water, is an effective surfactant with a surface tension of 18.1 dynes/cm (i.e., about 25% that of normal saline), is radiopaque, and, so far as is known, is biologically inert. The potential benefits that might be realized by the inhalation of such an agent include more complete recruitment of alveoli at lower distending pressures, improvement of ventilation/perfusion balance, maintenance of functional residual capacity, mobilization of debris and inflammatory substances from airways, and decreased tendency for subsequent atelectasis after cessation of liquid ventilation.

Shaffer and colleagues have demonstrated the feasibility of liquid ventilation as a therapy in several animal models. Other investigators have also contributed to the surprisingly large body of laboratory data regarding the effects of inhaled perfluorochemicals in animal models of pulmonary disease states. One of the most instructive recent studies was reported by Leach and colleagues [58]. In a prospective, randomized, controlled study of 11 premature lambs with the respiratory distress syndrome, they demonstrated that liquid ventilation was associated with rapid and significant improvements (over 5–15 minutes) in oxygenation (by four fold), ventilation, and compliance (three fold) in the treated animals as compared to controls.

The first human trial of liquid ventilation was reported in 1989 by Greenspan and colleagues [59] who briefly treated 3 premature infants with severe RDS refractory to CMV and surfactant administration. This trial used the more cumbersome approach called total liquid ventilation (TLV) in which the lungs are filled with the equivalent of their functional residual capacity (about 30 ml/kg) with perfluorocarbon that has been saturated with oxygen. This liquid is then drained from the lungs, and fresh fluid is reinfused. This cycle is repeated at a rate of about 3–5 times per minute. For respiratory support periods of more than a few minutes, it becomes necessary to filter and rewarm the exhaled liquid as well as to circulate it through a gas exchanger to remove carbon dioxide and replace the oxygen.

In the study referenced from Leach and colleagues [58] as well as in essentially all of the ongoing clinical trials [60], a simpler and more appealing approach is used. Known as partial liquid ventilation (PLV) or perfluorocarbon-associated gas exchange (PAGE), this system entails inflation of the lungs with 30 ml/kg of perfluorocarbon followed by 3–4 minutes of tidal liquid ventilation. Then, at end expiration with approximately 30 ml/kg of perfluorocarbon remaining in the lungs, conventional mechanical ventilation is resumed. This approach has been shown to be less injurious than gas ventilation [61] and effective in animal models [62, 63] and in early reports from ongoing human trials. It seems probable that this relatively simple therapy will have an important place in our future treatment strategies for respiratory failure.

Of course, the liquid ventilation story has only begun. There are many unresolved questions. For example, it is known that perfluorochemicals are eliminated for practical purposes only in their evaporated form in the expiratory gases. Small amounts are absorbed in the lungs where they may be engulfed by macrophages but may remain for days or months. Minute quantities may also be found in the fat or in other tissues for much longer. Also, there is evidence that liquid ventilation increases airways resistance and work of breathing and decreases cardiac output [64], all of which may be attributed to the density of the liquids employed. On the other hand, perfluorocarbons may have an anti-inflammatory effect [65], may decrease the requirement for ECMO [66], and are compatible with (but may be better than) surfactant [67]. Obviously, carefully designed and conducted controlled clinical investigations are needed before more general use of this intervention is undertaken.

Hirschl and colleagues [68] have recently reported on their preliminary experience using partial liquid ventilation in 19 adults, children, and neonates with severe respiratory failure who were on extracorporeal life support. These treatments were associated with a decrease in alveolar-arterial oxygen gradient and an increase in static lung compliance, but only 11 (58%) survived. It is thus too early to comment on whether or not liquid ventilation will improve clinical outcomes, much less on whether it will decrease the need for ECMO.

Summary

The number of newborns being supported with ECMO seems to be decreasing even as the efficacy and relative safety of the procedure are being better established. Because ECMO is both invasive and risky, alternative therapies must be sought. The list of options for the management of life threatening neonatal respiratory failure as presented here is by no means complete. Likely, most would agree that the therapies reviewed offer the greatest prospect at present for supplanting ECMO. The evidence certainly suggests that surfactant use in candidate neonates is decreasing the requirement for ECMO. Similarly, early and optimized use of high frequency ventilation may diminish the number of neonates requiring perfusion support. Clinical results do not yet permit speculation as to whether inhaled nitric oxide or liquid ventilation will change clinical outcomes in this population, though the possibilities are exciting. Without question, a key factor impacting the success of any one of these therapies will be the precision with which the true underlying pathogenic mechanisms are identified. Each of these therapies has demonstrable clinical benefit, but they treat distinctly different pathologies. Thus, surfactant normalizes alveolar surface tension, high frequency ventilation achieves quite homogeneous recruitment of airways, nitric oxide dilates pulmonary blood vessels, and liquid ventilation recruits airways, acts as a surfactant, and exchanges respiratory gases. It is most unlikely that inhaled nitric oxide will notably change outcomes in patients with severe underlying lung disease [69]. Similarly, liquid ventilation will probably not significantly alter the outcomes in patients whose respiratory failure is complicated by multi-organ system failure.Recognizing the major physiologic actions of each of these therapies may enable us to use them in potent combinations for specific subpopulations. For example, Karamanoukian and coworkers have demonstrated that inhaled NO is more effective in a lamb model of congenital diaphragmatic hernia if given in conjunction with surfactant [49], and Kinsella and colleagues have shown that inhaled NO in combination with HFOV may be more effective than either therapy alone [56].

Conclusion

For the present, ECMO seems to be the most potent and the most widely applicable of the newer therapies. It seems likely, therefore, that ECMO will retain its position as the treatment of last resort for neonatal respiratory failure, at least until the roles and interactions of alternative therapies are refined.

References

1. Bartlett RH, Gazzaniga AB, Jefferies MR, Huxtable RF, Haiduc NJ, Fong SW. (1976) Extracorporeal membrane oxygenation (ECMO) cardiopulmonary support in infancy. Trans. Am. Soc. Artif. Intern. Organs, 22:80–93.
2. Shanley CJ, Hirschl RB, Schumacher RE, et al. (1994) Extracorporeal life support for neonatal respiratory failure. A 20-year experience. Annals of Surgery, 220:269–80: discussion 281–2.
3. Zwischenberger JB, Nguyen TT, Upp JR, Jr., et al. (1994) Complications of neonatal extracorporeal membrane oxygenation. Collective experience from the Extracorporeal Life Support Organization. J Thorac Cardiovasc Surg, 107:838–48: discussion 848–9.
4. Glass P, Wagner AE, Papero PH, et al. (1995) Neurodevelopmental status at age five years of neonates treated with extracorporeal membrane oxygenation. Journal of Pediatrics, 127:447–457.
5. Rais-Bahrami K, Coffman C, Wagner A, Bulas D, Glass P, Short B. (1995) Outcome of ECMO vs. near miss ECMO patients at five years of age. 11th Annual CNMC Symmposium on ECMO and Advanced Therapies for Respiratory Failure. Keystone, CO, March 1995.

6. Anonymous(1993) Report of the Workshop on Diffusion of ECMO Technology. Extracorporeal Membrane Oxygenation. NIH Publication No. 93-3399, Rockville, MD.
7. Guyer B, Strobino DM, Ventura SJ, Singh GK. (1995) Annual summary of vital statistics-1994. Pediatrics, 96:1029–1039.(Abstract)
8. Bartlett RH, Roloff DW, Cornell RG, Andrews AF, Dillon PW, Zwischenberger JB. (1985) Extracorporeal circulation in neonatal respiratory failure: A prospective randomized study. Pediatrics, 76:479–487.
9. O'Rourke PP, Crone RK, Vacanti JP, et al. (1989) Extracorporeal membrane oxygenation and conventional medical therapy in neonates with persistent pulmonary hypertension of the newborn: a prospective randomized study. Pediatrics, 84:957–963.
10. Schumacher RE. (1993) Extracorporeal membrane oxygenation. Will this therapy continue to be as efficacious in the future?. [Review]. Pediatr Clin North Am, 40:1005–1022.
11. Wung J, James LS, Kilchevsky E, James E. (1985) Management of infants with severe respiratory failure and persistence of the fetal circulation, without hyperventilation. Pediatrics, 76:488–494.
12. Long W, Zucker J, Kraybill E. (1995) Symposium on synthetic surfactant II: perspective and commentary. J Pediatr, 126:S1-S4.(Abstract)
13. Bui KC, Walther FJ, David Cu R, Garg M, Warburton D. (1992) Phospholipid and surfactant protein A concentrations in tracheal aspirates from infants requiring extracorporeal membrane oxygenation. Journal of Pediatrics, 121:271–274.
14. Lotze A, Stroud CY, Soldin SJ. (1995) Serial lecithin/sphingomyelin ratios and surfactant/albumin ratios in tracheal aspirates from term infants with respiratory failure receiving extracorporeal membrane oxygenation. Clinical Chemistry, 41:1182–1188.
15. Findlay RD, Taeusch HW, Walther FJ. (1996) Surfactant replacement therapy for meconium aspiration syndrome. Pediatrics, 97:48–52.(Abstract)
16. Lotze A, Knight GR, Martin GR, et al. (1993) Improved pulmonary outcome after exogenous surfactant therapy for respiratory failure in term infants requiring extracorporeal membrane oxygenation. J Pediatr, 122:261–268.
17. Lotze A, Knight GR, Anderson KD, et al. (1994) Surfactant (beractant) therapy for infants with congenital diaphragmatic hernia on ECMO: evidence of persistent surfactant deficiency. J Pediatr Surg, 29:407–412.
18. Lotze A, The Survanta in Term Infants Study Group. (1996) Survanta pre-ECMO trial: multicenter evaluation of Survanta in treatment of term infants with severe respiratory failure. 12th Annual CNMC Symmposium on ECMO and Advanced Therapies for Respiratory Failure. Keystone, CO, February 1996.
19. Bell RE, Kuehl TJ, Coalson JJ, et al. (1984) High frequency ventilation compared to conventional positive-pressure ventilation in the treatment of hyaline membrane disease in primates. Crit. Care Med. 12:764–767.
20. The HIFI Study Group. (1989) High-frequency oscillatory ventilation compared with conventional mechanical ventilation in the treatment of respiratory failure in preterm infants. New England Journal of Medicine, 320:88–93.
21. HiFO Study Group.(1993) Randomized study of high-frequency oscillatory ventilation in infants with severe respiratory distress syndrome. Journal of Pediatrics, 122:609–619.
22. Ogawa Y, Miyasaka K, Kawano T, et al. (1993) A multicenter randomized trial of high frequency oscillatory ventilation as compared with conventional mechanical ventilation in preterm infants with respiratory failure. Early Human Development, 32:1–10.
23. Clark RH, Gerstmann DR, Null DM, Jr, deLemos RA. (1992) Prospective randomized comparison of high-frequency oscillatory and conventional ventilation in respiratory distress syndrome. Pediatrics, 89, 5–12.
24. Imai Y, Kawano T, Miyasaka K, Takata M, Imai T, Okuyama K. (1994) Inflammatory chemical mediators during conventional ventilation and during high frequency oscillatory ventilation. American Journal of Respiratory & Critical Care Medicine, 150:1550–1554.
25. Cornish JD, Gerstmann DR, Clark RH, Carter JM, Null DM, Jr, deLemos RA. (1987) Extracorporeal membrane oxygenation and high-frequency oscillatory ventilation: potential therapeutic relationships. Crit. Care Med. 15:831–834.

26. Carlo WA, Beoglos A, Chatburn RL, Walsh MC, Martin RJ. (1989) High-frequency jet ventilation in neonatal pulmonary hypertension. Am. J. Dis. Child, 143:233–238.
27. Kohelet D, Perlman M, Kirpalani H, Hanna G, Koren G. (1988) High-frequency oscillation in the rescue of infants with persistent pulmonary hypertension. Crit. Care Med. 16:510–516.
28. Tamura M, Tsuchida Y, Kawano T, et al. (1988) Piston-pump-type high frequency oscillatory ventilation for neonates with congenital diaphragmatic hernia: a new protocol. J Pediatr. Surg. 23:478–482.
29. Carter JM, Gerstmann DR, Clark RH, et al. (1990) High-frequency oscillatory ventilation and extracorporeal membrane oxygenation for the treatment of acute neonatal respiratory failure. Pediatrics, 85:159–164.
30. Delemos R, Yoder B, McCurnin D, Kinsella J, Clark R, Null D. (1992) The use of high-frequency oscillatory ventilation (HFOV) and extracorporeal membrane oxygenation (ECMO) in the management of the term/near term infant with respiratory failure. Early Human Development, 29:299–303.
31. Varnholt V, Lasch P, Suske G, Kachel W, Brands W. (1992) High frequency oscillatory ventilation and extracorporeal membrane oxygenation in severe persistent pulmonary hypertension of the newborn. Eur. J Pediatr, 151:769–774.
32. Miguet D, Cagnin S, Claris O, Lapillonne A, Salle BL. (1994) [Persistence of fetal circulation and high frequency oscillation]. [French]. Cahiers d Anesthesiologie, 42:319–324.
33. Miguet D, Claris O, Lapillonne A, Bakr A, Chappuis JP, Salle BL. (1994) Preoperative stabilization using high-frequency oscillatory ventilation in the management of congenital diaphragmatic hernia. Critical Care Medicine, 22:S77–82.
34. Clark RH, Yoder BA, Sell MS. (1994) Prospective, randomized comparison of high-frequency oscillation and conventional ventilation in candidates for extracorporeal membrane oxygenation. J Pediatr, 124:447–454.
35. Bond DM, Froese AB. (1993) Volume recruitment maneuvers are less deleterious than persistent low lung volumes in the atelectasis-prone rabbit lung during high-frequency oscillation. Crit. Care Med. 21:402–412.
36. Arnold JH, Hanson JH, Toro-Figuero LO, Gutierrez J, Berens RJ, Anglin DL. (1994) Prospective, randomized comparison of high-frequency oscillatory ventilation and conventional mechanical ventilation in pediatric respiratory failure. Critical Care Medicine, 22:1530–1539.
37. Kinsella JP, McQueston JA, Rosenberg AA, et al. (1992) Hemodynamic effects of exogenous nitric oxide in ovine transitional pulmonary circulation. American Journal of Physiology, 263:H875-H880.
38. Roberts JD, Jr., Chen TY, Kawai N, et al. (1993) Inhaled nitric oxide reverses pulmonary vasoconstriction in the hypoxic and acidotic newborn lamb. Circulation Research, 72:246–254.
39. Roberts JD, Polaner DM, Lang P, Zapol WM. (1992) Inhaled nitric oxide in persistent pulmonary hypertension of the newborn. Lancet, 340:818–819.
40. Kinsella JP, Neish SR, Shaffer E, Abman SH. (1992) Low-dose inhalation nitric oxide in persistent pulmonary hypertension of the newborn. Lancet, 340:819–820.
41. Abman SH, Kinsella JP, Schaffer MS, Wilkening RB. (1993) Inhaled nitric oxide in the management of a premature newborn with severe respiratory distress and pulmonary hypertension. Pediatrics, 92, 606–609.
42. Kinsella JP, Toews WH, Henry D, Abman SH. (1993) Selective and sustained pulmonary vasodilation with inhalational nitric oxide therapy in a child with idiopathic pulmonary hypertension. Journal of Pediatrics, 122:803–806.
43. Kinsella JP, Neish SR, Ivy DD, Shaffer E, Abman SH. (1993) Clinical responses to prolonged treatment of persistent pulmonary hypertension of the newborn with low doses of inhaled nitric oxide [see comments]. Journal of Pediatrics, 123:103–108.
44. Kinsella JP, Abman SH. (1993) Inhalational nitric oxide therapy for persistent pulmonary hypertension of the newborn. Pediatrics, 91:997–998.
45. Abman SH. (1994) Pathogenesis and treatment of neonatal and postnatal pulmonary hypertension. [Review]. Current Opinion in Pediatrics, 6:239–247.

46. Roberts JD, Jr. (1993) Inhaled nitric oxide for treatment of pulmonary artery hypertension in the newborn and infant. [Review]. Critical Care Medicine, 21:S374–6.
47. Roberts JD, Jr., Lang P, Bigatello LM, Vlahakes GJ, Zapol WM. (1993) Inhaled nitric oxide in congenital heart disease. Circulation, 87:447–453.
48. Karamanoukian HL, Glick PL, Zayek M, et al. (1994) Inhaled nitric oxide in congenital hypoplasia of the lungs due to diaphragmatic hernia or oligohydramnios. Pediatrics, 94:715–718.
49. Karamanoukian HL, Glick PL, Wilcox DT, Rossman JE, Holm BA, Morin FC. (1995) Pathophysiology of congenital diaphragmatic hernia. VIII: Inhaled nitric oxide requires exogenous surfactant therapy in the lamb model of congenital diaphragmatic hernia. Journal of Pediatric Surgery, 30:1–4.
50. Rossaint R, Gerlach H, Falke KJ. (1994) Inhalation of nitric oxide–a new approach in severe ARDS. [Review]. European Journal of Anaesthesiology, 11:43–51.
51. Finer NN, Etches PC, Kamstra B, Tierney AJ, Peliowski A, Ryan CA. (1994) Inhaled nitric oxide in infants referred for extracorporeal membrane oxygenation: dose response. J Pediatr, 124:302–308.
52. Peliowski A, Finer NN, Etches PC, Tierney AJ, Ryan CA. (1995) Inhaled nitric oxide for premature infants after prolonged rupture of the membranes. Journal of Pediatrics, 126:450–453.
53. Gerlach H, Pappert D, Lewandowski K, Rossaint R, Falke KJ. (1993) Long-term inhalation with evaluated low doses of nitric oxide for selective improvement of oxygenation in patients with adult respiratory distress syndrome. Intensive Care Med 19:443–449.
54. Gerlach H, Rossaint R, Pappert D, Falke KJ. (1993) Time-course and dose-response of nitric oxide inhalation for systemic oxygenation and pulmonary hypertension in patients with adult respiratory distress syndrome. European Journal of Clinical Investigation, 23:499–502.
55. Stark AR, Davidson D. (1995) Inhaled nitric oxide for persistent pulmonary hypertension of the newborn: implications and strategy for future „high-tech" neonatal clinical trials. [Review]. Pediatrics, 96:1147–1151.
56. Abman SH, Kinsella JP. (1995) Inhaled nitric oxide for persistent pulmonary hypertension of the newborn: the physiology matters: [comment]. [Review]. Pediatrics, 96:1153–1155.
57. Kornhauser MS, Cullen JA, Baumgart S, McKee LJ, Gross GW, Spitzer AR. (1994) Risk factors for bronchopulmonary dysplasia after extracorporeal membrane oxygenation. Archives of Pediatrics & Adolescent Medicine, 148:820–825.
58. Leach CL, Fuhrman BP, Morin FC, 3d, Rath MG. (1993) Perfluorocarbon-associated gas exchange (partial liquid ventilation) in respiratory distress syndrome: a prospective, randomized, controlled study. Critical Care Medicine, 21:1270–1278.
59. Fuhrman BP. (1990) Perfluorocarbon liquid ventilation: the first human trial. Journal of Pediatrics, 117:73–74.
60. Gross GW, Greenspan JS, Fox WW, Rubenstein SD, Wolfson MR, ShafferTH. (1995) Use of liquid ventilation with perflubron during extracorporeal membrane oxygenation: chest radiographic appearances. Radiology, 194:717–720.
61. Hirschl RB, Tooley R, Parent AC, Johnson K, Bartlett RH. (1995) Improvement of gas exchange, pulmonary function, and lung injury with partial liquid ventilation. A study model in a setting of severe respiratory failure. Chest, 108:500–508.
62. Tutuncu AS, Akpir K, Mulder P, Erdmann W, Lachmann B. (1993) Intratracheal perfluorocarbon administration as an aid in the ventilatory management of respiratory distress syndrome. Anesthesiology, 79:1083–1093.
63. Tutuncu AS, Faithfull NS, Lachmann B. (1993) Comparison of ventilatory support with intratracheal perfluorocarbon administration and conventional mechanical ventilation in animals with acute respiratory failure. American Review of Respiratory Disease, 148:785–792.
64. Lowe CA, Shaffer TH. (1986) Pulmonary vascular resistance in the fluorocarbon-filled lung. J Appl Physiol, 60:154–159.

65. Lane T, Smith D, Wancewicz E, Funk R. (1992) Inhibition of endotoxin-mediated activation of endothelial cells by a perfluorocarbon emulsion. Biomater. Artif Cells Immobilization. Biotechnol. 20:1051–1057.
66. Hirschl RB, Parent A, Tooley R, Shaffer T, Wolfson M, Bartlett RH. (1994) Lung management with perfluorocarbon liquid ventilation improves pulmonary function and gas exchange during extracorporeal membrane oxygenation (ECMO). Artificial Cells, Blood Substitutes, & Immobilization Biotechnology, 22:1389–1396.
67. Leach CL, Holm B, Morin FC, 3rd, et al. (1995) Partial liquid ventilation in premature lambs with respiratory distress syndrome: efficacy and compatibility with exogenous surfactant. Journal of Pediatrics, 126:412–420.
68. Hirschl RB, Pranikoff T, Gauger P, et al. (1995) Liquid ventilation in adults, children, and full-term neonates. Lancet, 346, 1201–1202.
69. Kinsella JP, Abman SH. (1995) Recent developments in the pathophysiology and treatment of persistent pulmonary hypertension of the newborn. [Review]. Journal of Pediatrics, 126:853–864.

Pediatric ECMO: Is there a Problem?

P. P. O'Rourke

Introduction

Case Report: A three year old boy is transferred from another hospital with presumed viral pneumonia (all cultures are negative). He was previously well with no medical problems. Three weeks ago he developed fever and cough which progressed to respiratory failure. He was admitted to an intensive care unit at another hospital and has been mechanically ventilated for 15 days. He has been on 100% oxygen with peak inspiratory pressures (PIP) > 55 cm H_2O and positive end expiratory pressure (PEEP) > 15 cm H_2O for eight days. He has four chest tubes which show ongoing air leak. Representative arterial blood gases are: PaO_2 35 torr, $PaCO_2$ 78 torr and pH 7.29. The referring hospital does not have access to high frequency ventilation, nitric oxide or ECMO. The child is sent to you.

What is your plan? Should there be a trial of high frequency ventilation? Nitric oxide? Should the child be placed on ECMO? Anecdotal experience claims that each of these options improve survival in children with acute respiratory failure (ARF). But absolute proof is scant and universal acceptance lacking. The decisions of how to responsibly and humanely treat a child with severe ARF can actually be more difficult with the availability of these promising therapies. I will explore this difficulty and focus on the role of ECMO in this dilemma.

Is the use of ECMO for pediatric respiratory failure rescue therapy only? Or is it standard of care? Unfortunately it occupies a rather uncomfortable position somewhere between the two. ECMO for the non-neonate with ARF first caught the fascination of the clinician with Hill's case report of a 24 year old trauma victim with ARDS who was successfully supported with ECMO [1]. But early enthusiasm from this and other case reports was tempered by the results of the National Institute of Health (NIH) adult ARF study which comparing ECMO with conventional management showed a 9.5% and an 8.3% survival respectively [2]. But rather than disgarding the technique, ECMO advocates focused on a different target population, the term neonate with respiratory failure. Dramatic success in this group not only made ECMO standard of care for the term neonate but it also increased interest and research in extracorporeal support [3, 4]. Armed with "new" and hopefully improved ECMO and success in the neonate, the older child and adult again became potential patients.

Table 1. ECMO registry report of ELSO. International Summary, July, 1995

Group	Total	Survival [%]
Neonatal respiratory	10391	80
Pediatric respiratory	982	53
Cardiac support	1491	43
Adult	197	41

The Extracorporeal Life Support Organization (ELSO) maintains a registry of the clinical ECMO experience. Virtually all of the neonatal experience is captured in this registry: pediatric and adult patient reporting is thought to be less reliable. The most recent ELSO Registry Report is provided in the following Table 1 [5].

While nearly 1000 pediatric patients have been reported, this experience pales in comparison to the neonatal experience. Before discussing these specific pediatric patients, it is important to understand the diagnosis of ARF and its non-ECMO treatment and support.

Important Characteristics of Pediatric ARF

There are important differences in the incidence, etiology and natural progression of neonatal versus pediatric ARF. Respiratory failure in neonates is usually primarily caused by or secondarily complicated by persistent pulmonary hypertension of the newborn (PPHN) [4]. This is a pulmonary vascular hyperreactivity which can dramatically and rapidly reverse. In fact, many credit the success of ECMO in the neonatal population with the presence of PPHN as a significant part of the disease process. The non-neonatal patient does not have PPHN. These patients have severe alveolar, interstitial or bronchiolar disease caused by a spectrum of insults including infection, aspiration, metabolic or toxic causes [6, 7,8]. While secondary pulmonary hypertension can occur in the pediatric patient, it is not the twitchy, rapidly reversible hypertension of PPHN. Hence the older patients' survival is dependent on reversal of the parenchymal component rather than relaxation of the pulmonary hypertension. It is important to understand that pediatric ARF is not one disease. While there are a number of causes and histopathologic changes, the pediatric population presents a spectrum of patient ages which presents a range of lung development and maturation. In the first six to eight years of life, the child's lung undergoes dramatic developmental changes [9]. Because of these differences, can the lung of a two month old be compared to the lung of a twelve year old with the identical inciting injury? Do similar physiologic insults encountered at different times in lung development result in the same degree of damage? The same potential for recovery? This is not known.

A very important question is whether or not the alveolar, interstitial or bronchiolar injuries of ARF are reversible. How long does recovery take? Is there a point after which repair is no longer possible?

We have long been taught that fatal ARF is characterized by the presence of pulmonary fibrosis which is an irreversible lesion. This belief was fostered by the routine autopsy findings of pulmonary fibrosis in patients who were ventilated for ARF. The pulmonary fibrosis was seen as terminal scar tissue [6, 7,8]. In fact, some clinicians routinely used the presence of pulmonary fibrosis on lung biopsy to determine whether or not a patient had survivable disease. But now, this is being questioned. We have all cared for the exceptional patient who after surviving severe ARF has taken months to successfully wean from mechanical ventilation. These patients have suggested that given enough time, even severe pulmonary injuries can recover. As will be discussed, the experience with ECMO support may well force us to redefine what is reversible versus irreversible damage. The ability to sustain ARF patients for weeks on ECMO has allowed injured lungs to progress to stages that before were simply impossible. This raises new hope that given enough time, fibrosis may be a reversible lesion. But the uncertainty is concerning. There are necrotizing pneumonitities which completely destroy lung architecture: these will likely only be cured with a lung transplant. But in the absence of overwhelming necrosis, the whole concept of irreversibility is open to speculation.

In addition to lung injury, ARF is often complicated by other organ dysfunction: renal failure, cardiac failure, coagulopathy, coma, seizures and hepatic failure. This is called multi-organ system failure (MOSF). What is the role of MOSF in ARF? Is it a manifestation of global endothelial injury directly caused by the inciting event, or is the result of inadequate gas exchange and the trauma of mechanical ventilation? Regardless of the etiology, the presence of MOSF has a direct impact on the prognosis of the patient: mortality is directly related to the number of organ systems involved [8]. As we evaluate new modes of lung support we must ask if normalization of the blood gases will improve the function of all organ systems, or is supporting gas exchange futile in the presence of severe MOSF?

Specific consideration must be given to abnormalities of the central nervous system (CNS). If there is evidence of significant irreversible CNS damage, than any aggressive support may be inappropriate.

How frequent is pediatric ARF? The numbers are actually quite small. It has been estimated that less than 3% of Pediatric Intensive Care Unit (PICU) admissions have the diagnosis of severe ARF [10, 11, 12]. This means that in one year any specific PICU has relatively few patients with severe ARF. It is instructive to note that both children and adults with ARF rarely die from inadequate gas exchange. The more common causes of death are related to the precipitating event, sepsis or other organ dysfunction (MOSF) [13, 14]. Of note in some pediatric series, CNS injury was the first or second most common cause of death [15, 16]. In the pediatric age group, many victims of ARF have underlying diseases: primary or secondary immune suppression, chronic lung disease or chronic CNS dysfunction. Few patients with no underlying disease develop severe ARF.

The Goals of Therapy

The goals of treatment for a patient with respiratory failure include reversal of the precipitating event, support of gas exchange and support of all other organ systems while hopefully the process reverses and healing occurs. While we had became quite effective supporting gas exchange, we were slow in appreciating the secondary damage being inflicted on already damaged lungs. Lungs were routinely exposed to extreme levels of oxygen, pressures and inflating volumes used in an effort to normalize arterial blood gases. In fact, not so many years age, the overwhelming concern of oxygen toxicity supported our use of even more aggressive levels of pressures and inflating volumes in an effort to minimize the FIO2. We have learned a lot but we have legions more to learn.

While oxygen toxicity and barotrauma are real, the present emphasis is on volutrauma. A number of superb studies demonstrate that absolute volume distension is more injurious than absolute pressures [17]. This has fostered serious caution regarding the manner in which we mechanically ventilate the lung. We now ascribe to the goal of avoiding large inflating volumes.

Permissive hypercarbia is one way of minimizing inflating volumes. Elevated $PaCO_2$ levels are tolerated using an arbitrary lower level of acceptable pH; ie, 7.00 to 7.10. High frequency ventilation and tracheal insufflation are other modes of supporting gas exchange while minimizing tidal volumes [18, 19]. ECMO is obviously very attractive when the goal is maintenance of gas exchange without inflating the lung.

But a word of caution. Providing safer technologies for supporting gas exchange only minimizes secondary lung injury while keeping the patient alive long enough for the disease process to reverse and the lungs to heal. These modes of support are not a cure. Therefore it is imperative that we better understand the histopathologic progression of ARF.

ECMO

ECMO is a technology which supports gas exchange by circulating blood through an externalized artificial lung. While the technology borrows significantly from cardiopulmonary bypass, ECMO is only partial bypass, hence the efficiency of gas exchange is limited. I will not go into the details of veno-arterial (V-A) versus veno-venous (V-V) ECMO other than to note a few differences. In V-V ECMO there is partial recirculation of oxygenated blood. V-A ECMO has no recirculation and hence provides more efficient gas exchange. But V-A ECMO has the main drawback of requiring cannulation of a central artery.

How are ECMO Candidates Selected?

Selection criteria for pediatric ARF patients are relatively arbitrary and institution specific, but there are some generally accepted guidelines. Exclusion criteria are discussed first. One is the presence of any non-pulmonary incurable disease: particular attention should be given to the child with CNS injury. One example is the child after a near-drowning event: while ECMO may support the child through the pulmonary injury, the CNS outcome may be one of devastation. Major burns and active uncontrolled bleeding are contraindications because of the requirement for anticoagulation. Immunosuppressed patients are usually excluded because of their questionable ability to overcome the lung disease. Increased intracranial pressure and intracranial hemorrhage are relative contraindications: cannulation of the internal jugular vein will increase venous stasis in the cerebral system and anticoagulation could likely extend a bleed. While any child with irreversible lung disease should be excluded, as discussed previously, the ability to identify irreversible disease is poor. One clinical attempt has been to disqualify those who have received aggressive mechanical ventilation for prolonged periods of time. Some centers will not consider a patient who has been ventilated in excess of 10 to 14 days [20].

In an attempt to select patients with severe ARF who have little chance of surviving, a number of formulas using ventilator settings and arterial blood gases have been used to try to predict mortality. All of these predictors suffer from the constantly changing concept of "conventional therapy". I will not describe specific predictors because at present there are no validated predictors of mortality. In practice, most clinicians select their ECMO patients as those with severe lung disease with inadequate and worsening pulmonary gas exchange despite escalating aggressive standard therapy. These patients are often described as "failing to respond" to maximum therapy or "treatment failures." In reality, patients are often selected after a consensus is reached by a panel of physicians, respiratory therapists and nurses and not by any specific formula [20].

Another factor which has influenced the selection of potential ECMO patients is the size of the child. Most pediatric ECMO programs started as extensions of neonatal programs. As a result, many of the earlier patients were less than 10 kilograms, because these patients could be supported with the neonatal circuit. As experience with ECMO for larger children and adults has increased, more older/larger children are now being offered this support. But the early registry certainly over-represents the younger child weighing in less than 10 kilograms[20].

Pediatric ECMO Experience

The total numbers of ECMO patients were given in Table 1. Table 2 illustrates the growth of this group pediatric (2 weeks to 18 years) ECMO since 198c [5].

The number of pediatric ARF patients on ECMO has leveled off at slightly less than 200 cases per year. While this number has increased it is nowhere near the frequency of 1000 to 1400 neonates per year [5]. The pediatric num-

Table 2

Year on ECMO	Total	Cum. total	Survival [%]
before 1987	28	28	29
1987	14	42	50
1988	39	81	33
1989	51	132	51
1990	120	252	47
1991	138	390	55
1992	152	542	50
1993	194	736	54
1994	179	915	62
1995 (July)	67	982	57

bers given here may be conservative, many believe that more cases are being done, than are reported.

The primary diagnoses of these patients are listed in Table 3 [5]. Although viral pneumonia is the largest single diagnosis, it is a presumptive diagnosis and not culture proven.

The clinical reasons for starting ECMO support are given in Table 4.

Each of these criteria is defined separately in each institution. The majority are very broad categories and open to much interpretation. The largest single category is "failure to respond", which as previously described is the situation in which the patient is failing to improve despite all other known therapy. It is virtually impossible to compare patient care between institutions. Each institution uses conventional pressure limited and volume limited ventilation differently and each institution has different access to oscillators, nitric oxide, surfactant. Therefore, "failure to respond" is very institution-specific.

While identifying entry criteria for ECMO was also a huge problem for neonatal ECMO, the problem is magnified by the heterogeneity of diseases and therapies in the older child.

Eighty percent of the patients in this registry received some amount of V-A ECMO and 20% only V-V ECMO [5]. Most of the patients could not be put on the routine neonatal level of total lung rest with room air and negligible lung

Table 3

Primary diagnosis	Total	Survival [%]
Bacterial pneumonia	88	45
Viral pneumonia	304	56
Intrapulmonary hemorrhage	13	62
Aspiration	88	65
Pneumocystis	13	38
ARDS	61	51
Other	415	49

Table 4

Criteria	Total	Survival [8%]
$AaDO_2$	38	42
Oxygenation Index Score	96	52
Acute deterioration	88	48
Barotrauma	139	60
Failure to respond	548	52
Cardiac arrest	22	45
Transpulmonary shunt >30%	5	80
Others	46	52

inflation. In this Registry review, routine ventilator settings while on ECMO were: 15 breaths per minute with an FIO_2 of 0.38, PIP of 29 cm H_2O and PEEP of 8 cm H_2O. This compared to pre-ECMO ventilator settings of: 62 breaths per minute at FIO_2 of 1.00, PIP 48 cm H_2O and PEEP of 11 cm H_2O [20].

The duration of ECMO was 2 to 1256 hours (52 days) with a mean of 254 ± 185 hours (10+ days). The incidence of complications was directly related to the amount of time on ECMO. This is also true for the neonatal population. Complications are subcategorized into mechanical and patient. Mechanical complications are defined as problems with the ECMO circuit: mechanical problems may or may not have a direct effect on the patient. Patient complications describe clinical patient events. In a review of the first 238 pediatric ECMO cases, 79% of the patients had a patient complication at a rate of 2.4 ± 2.1 complications per patient. Survivors had fewer complications than nonsurvivors (1.6 ± 1.6 vs 3.2 ± 2.2 per patient, $p < 0.001$). Mechanical complications occurred in 50% of the patients. Survivors had fewer mechanical complications than nonsurvivors (0.5 ± 0.84 vs 0.84 ± 0.91 per patient, $p < 0.001$). Hence complications are more than merely problematic. While there is no proof that they cause death, they certainly are associated with diminished survival.

The longer duration of ECMO for the pediatric patient versus the neonate reflects the differences in disease pathophysiology. The range of ECMO was as long as 52 days. Is this reasonable? Should there be a time limit for ECMO? What is the possibility of improvement after two weeks, three weeks, four weeks? At what point is ECMO merely prolonging death? These questions and the possibility of providing futile support gnaw at every ECMO clinician. Some ECMO programs have a defined time limit for ECMO support: 7 days, 14 days, 21 days or 28 days. Others continue ECMO until there is a complication that mandates removal. The fact that a European center [25] reported a good survivor after 76 days of ECMO [21] is marvelous for that survivor, but is it the rule or the exception?

Green et al [22] looked at this issue through a retrospective review of the ELSO Registry to determine the survival rate of pediatric ARF patients who were ECMO supported in excess of 14 days. Survival after 14 days and in fact after 21 days was as good as survival in those supported with ECMO less than

14 days. This report raises doubts about the use of arbitrary time limits. What then is the answer? Should all patients be treated indefinitely pending an ECMO complication? Even without a complication is there some time limit that most would agree is consistent with futility? Would that be one month, two months, three months? ECMO has forced us into uncharted territory that is filled with new questions.

Autopsy findings of patients supported with ECMO for three to four weeks often demonstrate fibrosis and destruction of the lung architecture. Many still interpret this as irreversible disease and see it as an excellent reason why we should limit the duration of ECMO support. In contrast, others say that if these patients had been supported for a longer period of time, some if not all of these lesions would have proven to be reversible. Clearly the answer is not known.

Prolonged ECMO courses focus the problem of allocation of relatively scarce ECMO technology. Most centers can provide ECMO for one or two patients at one time. If a single patient is on ECMO for 50 or 70 days will other patients be turned away or sent to other ECMO facilities?

Did ECMO Improve the Survival of These Pediatric ARF Patients?

While selection of patients is so difficult, how do we know whether or not ECMO in fact improved survival? Without a prospective randomized study with a control group, absolute proof is lacking. I will not address the question as to whether or not a pediatric ECMO trial can be or should be done; but rather, with the limited data we have, is there any evidence that ECMO improves survival? The anecdotal response is: YES. Many clinicians are certain that patients who were dying with "routine" therapy were only able to survive because of ECMO support. I refer the reader to an excellent study by Green et al, in which he compared cohorts of ECMO and non-ECMO patients with similar etiology and severity of disease. He looked for features that correlated with survival. Of interest, high frequency ventilation had no correlation, ECMO was correlated with an improved survival, especially in the group that met criteria for 25–50% mortality.

Data which does not support an improvement with ECMO include the NIH study [2] and a randomized study by Morris et al. The NIH study was completed in the 1970's at a time when ECMO was in its early development. At that time, ECMO technology was quite primitive compared to today. In addition, the NIH study limited ECMO support to five days: present experience with pediatric ECMO suggests that this is much too short a period of time to see any effect. As a result, the results of the NIH study have enjoyed less and less acceptance over time. The study by Morris et al, randomized adult ARF patients into a computer-driven standard therapy protocol versus Extracorporeal CO_2 Removal ($ECCO_2R$) which is a form of V-V ECMO. There was no difference in survival between the groups. The study was criticized for the fact that the first $ECCO_2R$ patients were study patients and hence exposed to the risks of a steep learning curve. In fact, these patients had an extraordinary amount of bleeding complications. Despite the fact that both of these studies deserve critical review, it is interesting that the only randomized studies performed revealed no difference with conservative therapy.

I return to the patient presented at the beginning. What is the appropriate therapeutic approach? What do you do? Do you offer ECMO? Do you offer it immediately?

Does this child have reversible disease? The primary diagnosis of viral pneumonia is a presumptive one because cultures have been negative. But if that diagnosis is correct, then the disease may well be reversible. This child has had 15 days of mechanical ventilation with elevated oxygen, inflating pressures and inflating volumes: how much secondary injury have the lungs sustained? I think that at this time, decisions to offer or not offer ECMO can both be defended. ECMO should only be offered if your clinical assessment is that the lung disease is reversible; otherwise, ECMO would do nothing more than prolong the death of the child.

Should ECMO be offered immediately? Or should other less aggressive therapies be offered first. I would argue that this child's lungs have already been exposed to near maximal iatrogenic injury. If the child has any chance of reversing his lung disease, then further trauma to the lungs must be avoided. In contrast if this child had only been ventilated for two days, a decision to try high frequency ventilation, nitric oxide or other therapies would be more defensible.

What do you tell the parents regarding the child's prognosis and how long ECMO will be offered? Do you give them a time limit or do you tell them ECMO will be continued until the child's lungs are improved or until there is a complication that precludes a continuation of ECMO?

I fear that none of the questions posed by the case report have absolute answers. This is the present dilemma of ECMO support.

Why ECMO is Problematic

ECMO technology has seen great advances in the past ten years. The steadily increasing clinical experience with ECMO has allowed us to better anticipate and prevent many of the associated morbidities. But while it is decidedly safer procedure than it was ten years age, it still carries significant costs to the institution and serious risks to the patient.

But I do not see ECMO itself as the main problem. The problem is our poor understanding of the diseases we are trying to treat. While we may be able to offer reasonably safe ECMO, if the patient has irreversible lung disease, then any form of ECMO is inhumane prolongation of death.

It is imperative that while ECMO continues to be offered we meticulously collect patient data so that we can learn from our best efforts. No one should be offering ECMO in a vacuum: we have to share our experiences, learn from each other's experience and be willing to change our practice as suggested by new information.

References

1. Hill JD, O'Brien TG, Morray JJ, et al. (1972) Prolonged extracorporeal membrane oxygenation for acute post-traumatic respiratory failure (shock-ling syndrome). N. Eng. J.Med. 286:629–634.
2. Zapol MW, Snider MT, Hill JD et al (1979) Extracorporeal membrane oxygenation in severe acute respiratory failure. A randomized prospective study. JAMA 242:2193-2196.
3. Stolar CJ, Snedecor SS, Bartlett RH (1991) Extracorporeal membrane oxygenation and neonatal respiratory failure: Experience from the extracorporeal life support organization. J.Pediatr.Surg. 26:563–571.
4. O'Rourke PP, Crone RK, Vacanti JP et al (1989) A prospective randomized study of extracorporeal membrane oxygenation (ECMO) and conventional medical therapy in neonates with persistent pulmonary hypertension of the newborn. Pediatrics 84:957-963.
5. Registry Report of the Extracorporeal Life Support Organization (ELSO). Ann Arbor, Michigan, July 1995
6. Royall JA, Levin DL (1988) Adult respiratory distress syndrome in pediatric patients. I. Clinical aspects, pathophysiology, pathology and mechanisms of lung injury. J.Pediatr 112:169–180.
7. Royall JA, Levin DL (1988) Adult respiratory distress syndrome in pediatric patients. II. Management. J.Pediatr 345:335–345.
8. Davis SL, Furman DP, Costarino AT Jr (1993) Adult respiratory distress syndrome in children: associated disease, clinical course, and predictors of death. J.Pediatr 123:35-45.
9. O'Rourke PP, Crone RK (1989) The Respiratory System. In: Gregory GA (ed): Pediatric Anesthesia (ed 2), New York, NY. Churchill Livingston, p.63
10. Rivera RA, Butt W, Shann F (1990) Predictors of mortality in children with respiratory failure. Possible indications for ECMO. Anaesth Intensive Care 18:385-389.
11. Tamburro RF, Bugnitz MC, Stidham GL (1991) Alveolar-arterial oxygen gradient as a predictor of outcome in patients with non-neonatal pediatric respiratory failure. J Pediatr 119:935–938.
12. Timmons OD, Dean JM, Vernon DD (1991) Mortality rates and prognostic variables in children with adult respiratory distress syndrome. J. Pediatr 119:896–899.
13. Fowler AA, Hamman RF, Zerbe GO, et al (1985) Adult respiratory distress syndrome. Prognosis after onset. Am.Rev.Respir.Dis. 132:472–478.
14. Montgomery AB, Stager MA, Carrico CJ, et al (1985) Causes of mortality in patients with adult respiratory distress syndrome. Am.Rev.Respir.Dis. 132:485–489.
15. Katz R (1987) Adult respiratory distress syndrome in children. Clin .Chest.Med. 8:635–639.
16. Pfenninger J, Gerber A, Tschappleler H, et al (1982) Adult respiratory distress syndrome in children. J.Pediatr 101:352–357.
17. Parker JC, Hernandez LA, Peevy KJ. (1993) Mechanisms of ventilator-induced lung injury. Crit.Care Med. 21:131–143.
18. Clark RH, Gerstmann DR, Null DM, deLemos RA. (1992) Prospective randomized comparison of high-frequency oscillatory and conventional ventilation in respiratory distress syndrome. Pediatr 89:5–12.
19. Arnold JH, Hanson JH, Toro-Figuero LO, et al (1994) Prospective randomized comparison of high-frequency oscillatory ventilation and conventional mechanical ventilation in pediatric respiratory failure. Crit.Care Med. 22:1530–1539.
20. O'Rourke PP, Stolar CJH, Zwischenberger JB et al (1993) Extracorporeal Membrane Oxygenation: Support for overwhelming pulmonary failure in the pediatric population. Collective experience from the Extracorporeal Life Support Organization. J.Pediatr.Surg. 28:523–529.
21. personnal communication
22. Green TP, Moler FW, Goodman DM (1995) Probability of survival after prolonged extracorporeal membrane oxygenation in pedieatric patients with acute respiratory failure. Crit.Care Med. 23:1132–1139.

Inhaled Nitric Oxide Therapy in Neonatal and Pediatric Cardiorespiratory Disease

S. H. Abman

Introduction

Abnormalities of pulmonary vascular function and structure contribute significantly to morbidity and mortality in many pediatric cardiopulmonary diseases, including persistent pulmonary hypertension of the newborn (PPHN), respiratory distress syndrome (RDS) in premature neonates, acute hypoxemic respiratory failure, postoperative heart disease, primary pulmonary hypertension (PPH) and others. Clinical approaches of these diseases have long been hampered by the lack of agents which could effectively lower pulmonary vascular resistance (PVR) without adversely affecting systemic hemodynamics or impairing oxygenation. Although many pharmacologic agents cause potent vasodilation, their clinical utility is often limited by systemic hypotension or worsened gas exchange, especially in the setting of advanced lung disease.

Since the discovery of endothelium-derived relaxing factor (EDRF) and its subsequent identification as nitric oxide (NO) or an NO-containing substance, there has been an explosion of information regarding fundamental physiologic roles for NO in diverse biologic systems. In addition to modulating vascular tone as originally described, NO has been shown to also play critical roles in host defense, inflammation, central and peripheral neurologic function, myocardial function, systemic hypotension in shock, penile erection and others. Recognition of its potent vasodilator properties and its unique ability to be delivered as a gas to the lung led to the use of inhaled NO (iNO) as a new treatment for several disorders characterized by pulmonary hypertension and altered pulmonary vasoregulation. The purpose of this review is to briefly summarize our current understanding of iNO in the lung circulation and its potential therapeutic applications.

Endogenous NO and the Pulmonary Circulation

As first discovered by Furchgott, the vascular endothelium produces a short-lived dilator substance which has been identified as NO or an NO- containing substance [1–3]. In the vessel wall, NO is synthesized from the amino acid, L-arginine, by an endothelium- specific isoform of *NO synthase* (eNOS; or Type III NOS). NOS is a large and complex enzyme, consisting of a dimeric, calmodulin -dependent cytochrome P450-like hemoprotein, and requires several cofactors for the five electron oxidation of the L-arginine guanidine group to produce NO. Molecular O_2 is incorporated into both NO and citrulline during the 2 step reaction with arginine and NADPH. NOS activity is dependent upon availability of such substrates as L-arginine, NADPH, FAD, FMN, and tetrahydrobiopterin. Once produced, NO is released from the endothelial cell, and stimulates soluble guanylate cyclase in vascular smooth muscle, increasing cGMP levels and lowering intracellular calcium. The exact signal transduction mechanisms by which cGMP mediates vasodilation remain uncertain, but appear to involve *GMP kinase* mediated activation of *calcium-gated K^+-channels* [4]. NO may also have non-GMP mechanisms of vasodilation via direct hyperpolarization of smooth muscle cells, which causes vasodilation by closure of voltage-dependent calcium channels [5].

NO-induced vasodilator activity is also dependent upon *cGMP-specific (type V) phosphodiesterase (PDE5)* activity, which inactivates cGMP by hydrolysis to 5'-GMP [6]. Recent studies suggest that PDE5 activity may contribute to high PVR in the normal fetus and in animal models of pulmonary hypertension [7–9]. Inhibition of PDE5 with selective antagonists (including zaprinast, dipyridamole, and E4021) may augment the vasodilator response to endogenous or exogenous NO (see below).

In addition to its vasodilator properties, NO modulates *vascular growth and structure*. NO also has other important properties, such as decreasing *platelet* aggregation, *neutrophil* adherence, and *vascular permeability*. These findings raise exciting speculations regarding its potential role in modulating lung inflammation, such as with acute respiratory distress syndrome (ARDS), pneumonia, and various interstitial lung diseases. NO also affects non-vascular aspects of lung function, including as bronchomotor tone and respiratory epithelial function (such as sodium transport and fluid flux). Its role in airway function is under active investigation, but most early studies suggest that iNO has weak bronchodilator activity in animal and that endogenous NO has a minimal role in regulating airway caliber.

Multiple mechanisms contribute to regulation of eNOS activity, such as shear stress, exercise, acute hypoxia, and certain growth factors. Although under most circumstances, availability of L-arginine is not rate-limiting, L-arginine supplementation increases NO activity in some experimental settings. End-product inhibition of NOS by NO may inhibit its activity through formation of heme-NO complex formation [10]. The physiologic roles of feedback inhibition are unclear, but it may be especially important in the "rebound" effect on pulmonary artery pressure or oxygenation after the rapid withdrawal of inhaled NO during clinical use.

Physiologic stimuli, including increased PO_2 and hemodynamic forces, such as pulsatile flow or shear stress, activate eNOS activity, and over hours, can upregulate eNOS gene expression. NO contributes to basal tone in many vascular beds, as demonstrated by vasoconstriction induced by infusions of arginine analogues, such as nitro-L-arginine (L-NA). Acute hypoxia decreases basal and stimulated NO release from cultured bovine pulmonary artery endothelial cells, which is associated with decreased GMP generation in pulmonary artery rings. A recent study demonstrated a 40–60% reduction in eNOS mRNA levels in human umbilical vein endothelial cells during exposure to hypoxia for 48 hours due to decreased gene transcription and decreased RNA stability. However, several studies suggest that NO release is stimulated by acute hypoxia and attenuates the severity of vasoconstriction. Hypoxic suppression of EDRF/NO activity may contribute to hypoxic vasoconstriction. Some reports suggest augmented hypoxic vasoconstriction in human conduit pulmonary arteries under the same conditions, and that suppression of basal NO release is unlikely to contribute to hypoxic constriction. In whole animals, chronic hypoxia has been shown to impair or augment. EDRF/NO activity. In addition to hypoxia, shear stress (stress exerted along the endothelial surface in the same plane as the blood flow through the vessel lumen) induces NO release, causing additional vasodilation.

Physiologic Role of NO in the Pulmonary Circulation

Endogenous NO plays a central role in pulmonary vascular function, especially during the *perinatal period*. The presence of eNOS in the developing lung has been reported at least as early as 0.3 term in the sheep fetus, and appears to peak in the immediate postnatal period before decreasing with age. Despite high fetal PVR, basal NO activity modulates vascular tone throughout late-gestation. NOS activity may be partly limited by high PDE5 activity, which limits its vasodilator effects. At birth, high fetal PVR must decrease to allow the 8–10 fold increase in pulmonary blood flow which is essential for postnatal adaptation. Mechanisms contributing to this decline in PVR include the release of endogenous NO, as NOS inhibition in experimental models leads to sustained PVR. Shear stress, ventilation and increased oxygen tension each contribute to NOS activity. Endogenous NO contributes to drop in PVR in immature animals as well.

During *postnatal* life, endogenous NOS activity contributes to low basal PVR in most species, modulates the response to vasoconstrictor activity (such as hypoxia), and appears to augment the decline in PVR during exercise. These findings have not been consistent between studies, however, and the role of eNOS remains somewhat controversial. Although eNOS activity is low and mRNA gene expression falls during postnatal life in normal rat lungs, exposure to chronic hypoxia upregulates eNOS content. In contrast, *clinical studies* tend to suggest that eNOS activity is present in the lung circulation in normal children and adults but decreases in the setting of chronic pulmonary hypertension. First, several clinical studies have shown that NOS antagonists increase PVR in normal subjects, suggesting that basal NO modulates low PVR in the normal setting [11, 12]. Second, patients with pulmonary hypertension respond poorly to endothelium-dependent vasodilators (especially acetylcholine) in comparison with inhaled NO or NO donors [13]. Third, *in vitro* studies of pulmonary arteries harvested from the lungs of patients with chronic pulmonary hypertension (including cystic fibrosis, Eisenmenger's complex, and primary pulmonary hypertension) have impaired endogenous NO activity [14]. Finally, recent studies of lung biopsy or autopsy samples from patients with pulmonary hypertension demonstrate decreased endogenous eNOS [15]. Thus, most clinical studies support the hypothesis that endogenous NOS activity modulates PVR in the normal lung and is impaired in chronic pulmonary hypertension.

Mechanisms Underlying Clinical Uses of Inhaled NO Therapy

Two early clinical observations provided insight into physiologic responses to iNO which led to the explosion of interest in its therapeutic applications. iNO was first shown to cause potent and selective pulmonary vasodilation in the clinical setting in adults with primary pulmonary hypertension by Dr. Higenbottam's group [16]. Although high doses of intravenous prostacyclin (PgI_2) decreased PVR as effectively as iNO, PgI_2 also lowered systemic vascular resistance (SVR). In contrast, iNO (at 40 ppm) decreased PVR as effectively as PgI_2, but did not affect systemic hemodynamics. Later studies demonstrated that iNO does not effect basal pulmonary vascular tone [17], emphasizing that the normal pulmonary circulation is maximally dilated under normal conditions. Experimental studies confirmed and expanded the observations of iNO's for the lung circulation in the setting high PVR [18–20]. INO reversed pulmonary hypertension without reducing systemic blood pressure in awake spontaneously breathing lambs with high PVR due to hypoxia or pharmacologic vasoconstrictor (thromboxane analogue, U46619) [18]. Marked responsiveness to iNO of the developing lung circulation was also demonstrated [19, 20]. One study emphasized the responsiveness of the immature pulmonary circulation to low doses (< 20 ppm), lack of tachyphylaxis over 2 hours, and the sensitivity of fetal lung circulation [20]. These strategies were later successfully applied in early clinical trials (see below).

INO's selective effects on the lung circulation are due to its direct administration within the lung, allowing NO to diffuse directly to vascular smooth muscle cells, stimulating soluble guanylate cyclase, increasing cGMP production, and causing vasodilation. Excess NO enters the bloodstream, avidly binds hemoglobin, and is rapidly metabolized to nitrites and nitrates, thereby limiting its action to the pulmonary vascular bed. Likely sites of vasodilator activity include resistance vessels on the pulmonary arterial side of the lung circulation and but may also lower tone in small pulmonary veins.

The *second critical clinical observation* was that iNO also selectively lowered PVR in adults with severe ARDS, but unlike systemic vasodilators, iNO improves oxygenation [21]. ARDS is characterized by ventilation-perfusion (v-q) mismatch due to continued perfusion of poorly aerated lung regions. As a gas, iNO is delivered to better aerated distal lung regions, causing greater vasodilation and hence better perfusion, to the better ventilated lung units. Thus, this redistribution of pulmonary blood flow lowers intrapulmonary shunt and improves gas exchange, an effect which may be lost with high doses of iNO (see below). Based on these physiologic effects, iNO has been studied in diverse clinical settings, some of which are discussed below.

Persistent Pulmonary Hypertension of the Newborn (PPHN)

At birth, survival is dependent upon the marked fall in PVR at birth, which enables the lung to assume its postnatal role in gas exchange. PPHN is a *clinical syndrome* which is characterized by the inability to achieve this decline in PVR during the immediate postnatal period, leading to severe hypoxemia due to marked right-to-left shunting of blood across the patent ductus arteriosus or foramen ovale [22]. PPHN is associated with a variety of diseases, including asphyxia, sepsis, meconium aspiration syndrome, congenital diaphragmatic hernia (CDH), respiratory distress syndrome (RDS), lung hypoplasia, and others. Each of these disorders is associated with high PVR, abnormal pulmonary vasoreactivity, and at least in fatal cases, hypertensive structural disease. Despite aggressive therapy with hyperoxia, hyperventilation, metabolic alkalosis, and cardiotonic drugs, morbidity and mortality remain high. Therapeutic interventions often include attempts to lower PVR with vasodilator drugs, such as tolazoline, sodium nitroprusside, PgI_2 and others. Vasodilator therapy is often ineffective, however, due to concomitant systemic hypotension (due to the lack of selectivity for the pulmonary circulation), an inability to acutely lower PVR, the inability to sustain vasodilation (tachyphylaxis), or adverse side effects. Patients who fail conventional therapy often require treatment with extracorporeal membrane oxygenation (ECMO). Despite ECMO, PPHN remains a significant cause of neonatal mortality (20%) and morbidity, including chronic lung disease (up to 30%), intracranial hemorrhage, cerebral infarction, hearing loss, and related neurodevelopmental sequelae.

As observed in previous studies of older animals, iNO caused potent and selective pulmonary vasodilation in the developing lung circulation [19, 20], achieving maximal effects at 20 ppm in the normal late-gestation fetus [20]. These animal studies set the stage for the first clinical studies examining the acute effects of iNO therapy in newborns with severe PPHN. Roberts et al. reported increased oxygen saturation in a small group of neonates with severe PPHN during brief iNO treatment at doses of up to 80 ppm [23]. In a concomitant report, Kinsella et al. demonstrated that lower doses of iNO (less than 20 ppm) acutely improved PaO_2 and decreased PVR, as assessed by echocardiography [24]. This same study also reported sustained improvement and recovery without the need for ECMO therapy in 6 patients during prolonged iNO therapy by utilizing a low dose strategy (20 ppm for 4 hours, then 6 ppm) [24]. Treatment for 24 hours of low dose iNO did not cause any apparent adverse effects, such as methemoglobinemia, systemic hypotension, or signs of lung toxicity. A subsequent report of 9 consecutive patients with severe PPHN meeting ECMO criteria further demonstrated the efficacy of this approach [24, 25]. Overall, 13 of the initial 15 patients treated with prolonged iNO were recovered from severe PPHN without the need for ECMO therapy. Two patients transiently improved oxygenation with iNO, but subsequently required ECMO therapy because of concomitant cardiac insufficiency and multiorgan failure associated with "sepsis syndrome."

PaO_2 did not fall after dropping from 20 to 6 ppm in these patients; however, withdrawal of iNO was associated decreased oxygenation and a rise in pulmonary artery pressure in most patients [25]. This was also observed in adults with ARDS [21]. The mechanisms of this so-called "rebound" effect with rapid iNO withdrawal is uncertain, but can occur in any patient treated with iNO, and can lead to life-threatening elevations of PVR. Although this may be due suppression of endogenous NO, similar responses also occur after rapid withdrawal of other vasodilators such as PgI_2 in PPH.

Early clinical experience led to the recognition of important clinical issues regarding the application of iNO to term neonates with PPHN. Clinical improvement during iNO therapy occurs with many disease-specific entities associated with PPHN, including congenital diaphragmatic hernia, meconium aspiration syndrome, severe sepsis, idiopathic, and others. In many cases, however, greater clinical improvement is achieved with inhaled NO *in combination with* HFOV than with either treatment alone. As observed by Finer and coworkers, neonates with hypoxemic respiratory failure in the absence of echocardiographic confirmation of PPHN tend to not respond as well to inhaled NO therapy as neonates with PPHN [26]. We speculate that improved lung inflation and the use of low doses of NO will lead to more successful outcome in this setting.

Subsequent clinical experience demonstrated that although iNO often causes acute improvement in PaO_2, the response to iNO can be transient, poor or incomplete. Studies of mechanisms underlying poor responsiveness to iNO in severe PPHN have provided insight into the underlying cardiopulmonary interactions of PPHN and highlight the need for an individualized and integrative therapeutic approach in the management of severe PPHN.

Several mechanisms may explain clinical variability in responsiveness to iNO therapy (Table 1).

First, the inability to effectively deliver NO to the pulmonary circulation due to *poor lung inflation* or distribution of gas within the lung may be the major cause of poor responsiveness. In some settings, administration of iNO with HFOV has improved oxygenation more effectively than during conventional ventilation in the same patient. Recruitment of lung volume provides better exposure of the pulmonary circulation to iNO, and decreases adverse effects of low lung volumes on PVR (low lung volumes increase PVR due to lack of vessel distension and regional hypoxia). Clinical improvement during iNO therapy occurs with many disorders associated with PPHN, such as congenital diaphragmatic hernia (CDH), meconium aspiration syndrome, severe sepsis, idiopathic, and others. Some diseases appear less responsive than others, and sustained improvement in oxygenation may vary between disorders. For example, a recent report suggested no improvement in lung hypoplasia with or without CDH [27]. These authors speculated that surfactant deficiency may be related to poor NO responsiveness in CDH; however, several patients had received surfactant prior to NO therapy. Several centers have successfully managed severe

Table 1. Potential mechanisms contributing to variable clinical responses to inhaled NO therapy in severe PPHN

1. *NO Delivery:*
   a. *Poor lung inflation, alveolar recruitment,* causing decreased NO delivery to the distal lung and small pulmonary arteries;
   b. *Low dose of NO,* leading to inability to maximally dilate the pulmonary vascular bed;
   c. *High-doses of NO,* paradoxical worsening of ventilation-perfusion mismatch in the presence of parenchymal lung disease, or NO-related toxicity, altering vascular reactivity or potentiating lung injury (e.g., peroxynitrite injury).
2. *Abnormal Pulmonary Vascular Structure:*
   a. *Hypertensive structural lesions,* such as smooth muscle hypertrophy and thickened adventitia, due to poor NO diffusion and mechanical restriction of vasodilation;
   b. *Congenital lung lesions,* such as alveolar capillary dysplasia, lung hypoplasia or pulmonary veno-occlusive disease;
3. *Missed or Unsuspected Congenital Heart Disease,* such as coarctation of the aorta, total anomalous pulmonary venous return, others;
4. *Myocardial Dysfunction,* due to asphyxia, sepsis;
5. *Systemic Hypotension* due to sepsis, hypovolemia, other causes;
6. *Altered Smooth Muscle Cell Responsiveness,* with multiple possibilities, such as:
   - high superoxide production, decreased SOD activity;
   - decreased guanylate cyclase activity,
   - increased cGMP-specific (Type V) phosphodiesterase activity,
   - changes in myosin isoforms, ion channels, other mechanisms.

CDH with inhaled NO and lung hypoplasia, including cases with severe renal agenesis. In some cases, greater clinical improvement was achieved with *iNO in combination with HFOV* than with either treatment alone, suggesting that variability in successful management of PPHN with inhaled NO is likely to reflect different strategies in clinical management.

In some cases, iNO reverses right-to-left shunting by lowering PVR (by echocardiogram), but hypoxia persists because of intrapulmonary shunt, suggesting undertreatment of associated lung disease. In this setting, improving lung inflation with changes in ventilator management or HFOV can further improve PaO_2. Management strategies which optimize lung recruitment (surfactant, perfluorocarbons, ventilator strategies) are likely to enhance responsiveness to iNO in patients with persistent pulmonary hypertension despite these interventions.

High doses of iNO can paradoxically worsen oxygenation in acute respiratory distress syndrome (ARDS) due to the loss of selective pulmonary vasodilation within the lung due to increased ventilation-perfusion mismatch. Similar effects are possible in hypoxic neonates with pulmonary hypertension and parenchymal lung disease. As reported by Finer, high doses (up to 80 ppm) of inhaled NO in hypoxemic neonates often do not provide further improvement in oxygenation [26]. Another potential cause of poor responsiveness may be due to the use of NO at *doses which are too low* to achieve maximal lowering of PVR. Our experience at the University of Colorado suggests that neonates with severe PPHN who do not respond well to 20 ppm do not improve with 40 ppm. In contrast, we and others have observed greater clinical effects at higher doses in selected congenital heart disease patients with pulmonary hypertension. In light of persistent concerns persist regarding possible *NO toxicity,* the lack of enhanced responsiveness at high doses (especially above 40 ppm) suggests that the use of iNO at these levels is unwarranted. Although chronic treatment with low dose iNO does not cause significant methemoglobinemia, potential toxicities such as surfactant inactivation, lung injury and inflammation remain. Such toxicities have not been noted with the clinical use of low dose NO therapy; most patients do not develop decreased lung compliance, new lung infiltrates, and increasing ventilator requirements during therapy. In fact, recent experimental data suggest that iNO may protect against oxidant injury and inflammation, as reflected by decreased vascular permeability and pulmonary edema. In some cases, however, it would be difficult to distinguish clinical worsening due to iNO-related toxicity from progression of the underlying disease itself. Some patients who become "unresponsive" to iNO during therapy despite an early response are likely to have alternate reasons for "losing" this effect (for example, progressive lung disease with loss of lung volume and intrapulmonary shunting).

Failure to respond to iNO may be due to *abnormal pulmonary vascular structure* or *altered smooth muscle cell responsiveness.* In addition to vascular wall thickening, hypertensive structural lesions often include a thickened adventitia, which can decrease vessel wall compliance and mechanically restrict the vessel's ability to dilate. In addition, vascular remodeling may produce a barrier to NO diffusion to vascular smooth muscle. Hypertension may also alter smooth muscle cell responsiveness to iNO by several potential mechanisms. Since response to iNO is dependent on sustaining intracellular elevations of cGMP, decreased *soluble guanylate cyclase* or increased *cGMP-specific (Type V) phosphodiesterase* (PDE5) activities could potentially limit the vasodilator response to NO. Preliminary data suggest that inhibition of PDE5 activity with dipyridamole or zaprinast augments the pulmonary vasodilator response to iNO in several experimental settings, including the normal fetus, acute pulmonary hypertension in the normal newborn, PPHN and ARDS. Preliminary clinical data suggests that *dipyridamole* enhances the iNO response in some patients with pulmonary hypertension, but is still under active investigation. (Note that systemic hypotension and bronchospasm can occur with intravenous dipyridamole).

Another category of poor responders includes patients with unsuspected or missed anatomic cardiovascular lesions (such as total anomalous pulmonary venous return, coarctation of the aorta, and others). In addition, poor iNO responsiveness may be related to myocardial dysfunction or systemic hypotension . Since the degree of right-to-left shunting is dependent upon the ratio of pulmonary and systemic arterial pressures, low systemic blood pressure will limit clinical improvement despite lowering of PVR during iNO therapy. Although commonly observed with sepsis, aggressive management of systemic pressure is required to sustain clinical improvement in many disorders associated with PPHN. Rapid availability of ECMO is needed in hemodynamically unstable neonates. In addition to hypotension, severe left ventricular dysfunction contributes to pulmonary hypertension by elevating left ventricular end diastolic, left atrial and pulmonary venous pressures. Although these patients may demonstrate a partial response to iNO, clinical improvement may be more dependent on systemic afterload reduction.

Inhaled NO Therapy of Severe Respiratory Failure in Premature Neonates

INO therapy has also been suggested for the premature neonate with severe respiratory distress syndrome (RDS) with marked hypoxemia which persists despite surfactant therapy [28]. The predominant mechanism underlying respiratory failure in the premature newborn is surfactant deficiency or dysfunction due to interactive effects of lung immaturity, lung injury and pulmonary edema, which cause decreased lung compliance, diffuse atelectasis and abnormal gas exchange. Surfactant therapy with mechanical ventilation improves lung compliance and gas exchange in most cases of RDS, improving their clinical course and outcome. Despite the success of surfactant therapy, some premature neonates with severe RDS fail to have sustained clinical improvement after surfactant treatment. Persistent hypoxemia despite multiple doses of surfactant has been estimated at between 5–50%, depending upon criteria. Some premature neonates with severe RDS have evidence of high PVR, which can exacerbate hypoxemia due to right-to-left shunting across the ductus arteriosus or foramen ovale. Pulmonary hypertension may be due in part to the mechanical effects of low lung volumes or low alveolar PO2 on PVR. This is supported by studies of Kaapa and coworkers, who recently demonstrated that surfactant treatment acutely lowers pulmonary artery pressure, perhaps by improving lung volume, increasing perfusion of distal lung units and aiding capillary recruitment [29].

In some cases, however, pulmonary vasoconstriction contributes to high PVR, as suggested by echocardiographic evidence of reversal of right-to-left shunting and improved oxygenation with vasodilator therapy. Although pharmacologic agents, such as tolazoline and sodium nitroprusside, can improve oxygenation in selected premature neonates with RDS, these agents can have adverse side effects, including systemic hypotension, gastrointestinal bleeding, and others, leading to marked clinical complications. In addition, despite lowering PVR, vasodilator drugs may worsen hypoxemia due to deterioration of ventilation-perfusion mismatch by increasing perfusion of poorly aerated lung regions in the presence of severe parenchymal lung disease.

As hypoxemic premature neonates are not ECMO candidates due to size limitations and risks associated with heparinization, including severe intracranial hemorrhage, novel approaches to treating pulmonary hypertension and improving gas exchange may enhance outcome. Low dose iNO has been reported to improve oxygenation in a premature neonate with severe RDS [28]. As illustrated in this case, iNO caused rapid improvement in oxygenation by abrupt reversal of right-to-left ductal shunting. A few days later, oxygenation worsened off therapy. At this time, reinitiation of therapy improved gas exchange in the absence of extrapulmonary shunting, suggesting that the clinical response was due to enhanced matching of ventilation with perfusion. Subsequent clinical experience with inhaled NO in hypoxemic premature neonates without echocardiographic evidence of pulmonary hypertension supports this mechanism. In these cases, the rate of improvement in oxygenation is slower than in cases with rapid reversal of ductal shunting. Recent reports have confirmed the responsiveness of prematures to iNO therapy [30]. Concerns persist regarding iNO therapy, however, regarding several potential adverse effects. These include possible extension of ICH due to prolonged bleeding time, pulmonary hemorrhage, or increased risk for chronic lung disease. Data from clinical trials with long term follow-up is necessary before iNO treatment of premature neonates can be recommended.

Adult Respiratory Distress Syndrome

ARDS remains a major cause of morbidity and mortality in intensive care units, with mortality ranging between 50–70%. ARDS is physiologically characterized by non-cardiogenic pulmonary edema, inflammation, surfactant dysfunction, pulmonary hypertension, decreased lung compliance, and progressive hypoxemia due to severe intrapulmonary shunt. Although death is often due to non-respiratory causes, improved management of respiratory failure is likely to enhance outcome. Pulmonary hypertension and altered vasoreactivity due to progressive lung injury contribute to marked intrapulmonary shunt with profound hypoxemia impaired cardiac performance [31–33]. Based on the original observation that iNO lowers PVR and improves oxygenation in ARDS, it has been hoped that iNO therapy may enhance outcome in patients with ARDS [21]. This has yet to be proven, but serves as the hypothesis of several ongoing multicenter trials.

The rationale for improved outcome with iNO therapy is primarily based on *decreased PVR*. Pulmonary hypertension in ARDS increases right ventricular afterload, which may depress RV contractility and ejection fraction [33–35]. In contrast with dying patients, survivors demonstrate a fall in PVR during their clinical course. In selected patients, including children, iNO therapy improved RV function and cardiac output [36, 37]. Although pulmonary hypertension can adversely affect right ventricular function, most ARDS patients do not have impaired cardiac function. However, high pulmonary artery pressure also increases microvascular pressure and worsens pulmonary edema. Reduction of lung microvascular pressure may attenuate fluid filtration and improve outcome. These physiologic effects have been recently demonstrated in animal and clinical studies [38, 39].

Another rationale for iNO therapy of ARDS is related to its "microselective" effects within lung; that iNO improves PaO_2 by improving *v-q mismatch* was convincingly demonstrated by Rossaint et al. using the multiple inert gas technique [21]. Improved oxygenation tends to be modest (roughly 50% increase in PaO_2/FiO_2 in most studies); however, clinical responsiveness is variable, and in some cases, this improvement allows for greater clinical stability and strategies which allow greater lowering of FiO_2 or ventilator settings. Whether responses to iNO represent a "cosmetic" effect on blood gases or real improvement, as demonstrated by improved clinical outcome, remains to be proven.

INO doses as low as 0.01 ppm improved PaO_2 in ARDS patients; oxygenation continued to improve up to 10 ppm, but fell at 100 ppm (40–100 ppm) [40]. Although data from that study was limited by the lack of study points between 10 and 100 ppm, subsequent workers have shown that an optimal dose is generally <20 ppm [36, 37]. Studies which compare such endpoints as outcome, instead of acute responsiveness, are needed to determine optimal dosing strategies. As discussed above (under PPHN), multiple mechanisms are likely to contribute to the marked variability in responsiveness to iNO in ARDS. Clinical strategies to improve responsiveness to iNO may include almitrine or the use of PDE5 antagonists. Although in some patients, almitrine improves oxygenation during iNO therapy, it also elevates pulmonary artery pressure, which may potentially aggravate pulmonary edema formation and worsen outcome [41].

New excitement has been generated by observations that iNO therapy may limit lung inflammation by decreasing neutrophil and monocyte adherence to vascular endothelium, decreasing thrombosis in situ, augmenting antioxidant defenses, and directly improving vascular permeability [39]. These potential effects may be of marked benefit in the clinical course of ARDS patients *independent* of the hemodynamic effects described above.

Acute Hypoxemic Respiratory Failure (non-ARDS)

In addition to ARDS, an important cause of acute hypoxemic respiratory failure are children with chronic lung disease or bronchopulmonary dysplasia (BPD) with respiratory viral infection [37]. RSV and influenza remain major causes of late morbidity and mortality in chronic lung disease. In many centers, these patients often require ECMO therapy for survival. In some BPD infants without an acute exacerbation, we have observed modest improvement in ventilation (decreased $PaCO_2$) with small changes in oxygenation (unpublished observations). Further studies in these infants are needed before recommendations for expanded iNO use can be made.

Pulmonary Hypertension Associated with Heart Disease

INO has been shown to provide a safe and effective approach toward assessing pulmonary vasoreactivity during cardiac catheterization [42], as well as utility in the treatment of pulmonary hypertension in adults and children after cardiac surgery [13,43,44]. Assessments of pulmonary vasoreactivity are often necessary to determine operability in candidates for heart or heart-lung transplantation, as well as congenital heart disease. Past use of pharmacologic vasodilators can lead to dangerous systemic hypotension, worsening of right-to-left shunting, cardiac dysrhythmias, or complex effects on myocardial function. Due to its rapid onset and lack of adverse effects on systemic hemodynamics, iNO appears to be the safest agent to assess responsiveness of such patients with pulmonary hypertension. Although iNO responsiveness is variable, several studies have consistently demonstrated that the fall in PVR is directly proportional to resting PVR.

INO appears to have no direct effects on myocardial function; however, pulmonary capillary wedge pressure often increases during iNO treatment in patients with left ventricular dysfunction [45]. This rise in pressure is most likely related to increased LV end-diastolic volume to a poorly compliant left ventricle, but has not been proven. In the setting of LV dysfunction, systemic afterload reduction may provide additional benefit in the hemodynamic response to iNO therapy.

INO therapy effectively relieves right heart failure in postoperative cardiac patients, but its most dramatic application is during treatment of *acute pulmonary hypertensive crises.* For patients who are undergoing iNO therapy, rapid withdrawal of iNO can precipitate sudden, life-threatening rises in PVR. Problems can occur during routine bedside procedures, especially during hand-bagging or endotracheal suctioning, but also during patient transport to the radiology suite or operating room. Precautions must be taken to anticipate such risks. We also maintain a tank of NO as part of the resuscitation cart to provide for rapid use in patients who may undergo sudden pulmonary hypertensive crisis but are not currently on iNO therapy.

Potential Toxicities and Safety Issues with iNO Therapy

As stated above, one of the major safety issues with iNO therapy is to avoid inadvertent withdrawal of iNO, leading to a pulmonary hypertensive crisis and severe hypoxemia. Staff must anticipate such risks by providing bedside availability of an NO tank set-up for *hand bagging* during endotracheal tube suctioning, bag mask ventilation after extubation or tube changes. Similarly, moving patients from the ICU to other areas of the hospital require the availability of a portable iNO delivery system, managed by experienced personnel, to avoid accidental administration of toxic NO doses.

In addition to methemoglobinemia and NO_2-related toxicity, potential toxicities from inhaled NO therapy include the formation of peroxynitrite from the reaction of NO reacting with superoxide anion. Peroxynitrite can damage surfactant protein and is cytotoxic *in vitro* . More recent observations, however, suggest that iNO may inactivate reactive oxygen species, thereby serving as an antioxidant. NO protection against cellular damage from reactive oxygen species generated from hypoxanthine and xanthine oxidase has been demonstrated in the isolated perfused lung [46].

Conclusions

The Future of Inhaled NO Therapy

Clearly, few developments in vascular biology have had the dramatic clinical impact which followed the "simple" observation that vascular endothelium produces a potent dilator substance, EDRF [1]. Multiple demonstrations of its remarkable ability to acutely lower PVR and improve oxygenation in diverse clinical settings suggest that iNO therapy provides a unique tool to expand our current armamentarium in treating severe cardiopulmonary disease. Current multicenter and single center studies will help to better define which patients are the best candidates for therapy, how NO fits with other therapies, and optimal delivery approaches to optimize efficacy and safety. Unfortunately, iNO therapy has been mislabelled as a "magic bullet." As iNO therapy is commonly used in diverse and complex clinical settings, it is unrealistic to expect that improvement in PVR or PaO_2 alone will be sufficient in reversing conditions associated with multiorgan failure. Randomized, large scale clinical studies are necessary to improve our understanding of its clinical applications; however, these studies must include realistic clinical endpoints, and allow approaches which include iNO therapy with appropriate management strategies.

References

1. Furchgott RF, Zawadzki JV (1980) The obligatory role of endothelial cells in the relaxation of arterial smooth muscle by acetylcholine. Nature 288:373–6.
2. Ignarro LJ, Buga GM, Wood KS, Byrns RE, Chaudhuri G. (1987) EDRF produced and released from artery and vein is NO. Proc Natl Acad Sci USA 84:9265–9.
3. Palmer RM, Ferrige AG, Moncada S. (1987) NO release accounts for the biological activity of EDRF. Nature 327:524–6.
4. Archer SL, Huang JC, Hampl V et al. (1994) NO and cGMP cause vasorelaxation by activation of a charybdotoxin-sensitive K channel by cGMP-dependent protein kinase. Proc Natl Acad Sci 91:7583–7.
5. Kuriyama H, Kitamura K, Nabata H. (1995) Pharmacological and physiological significance of ion channels and factors that modulate them in vascular tissues. Pharmacol Reviews 47:387–530.
6. Beavo JA. (1995) Cyclic nucleotide phosphodiesterases: functional implications of multiple isoforms. Physiol Rev 75:725–48.
7. Ziegler JW, Ivy DD, Kinsella JP, Clarke WR, SH Abman. (1995) Dipyridamole, a cGMP phosphodiesterase inhibitor augments inhaled NO-induced pulmonary vasodilation in the ovine transitional circulation. Am J Physiol. 269:473–9.
8. Braner D, Fineman J, Change R et al. (1993) M & B 22948, a cGMP phosphodiesterase inhibitor, is a pulmonary vasodilator in lambs. Am J Phsyiol. 264:H252–58.
9. Clarke WR, Uezono S, Chambers A, Doepfner P. (1994) The type III phosphodiesterase inhibitor milrinone and type V PDE inhibitor dipyridamole individually and synergistically reduce elevated PVR. Pulm Pharmacol. 7:81–9.
10. Assreuy J, Cunha FQ, Liew FY, Moncada S. (1993) Feedback inhibition of NOS activity by NO. Br J Pharmacol 108:833–7.
11. Celermajer DS, Cullen S, Deanfield JE. (1993) Impairment of endothelium-dept pulmonary artery relaxation in children with congenital heart disease and abnormal pulmonary hemodynamics. Circulation 87:440–6.

12. Stamler JS, Loh E, Roddy MA et al. (1994) NO regulates basal systemic and pulmonary vascular resistance in healthy humans. Circulation 89:2035–40.
13. Wessel DL, Adatia I, Giglia TM et al. (1993) Use of iNO and acetylcholine in the evaluation of pulmonary hypertension and endothelial function after cardiopulmonary bypass. Circulation 88:2128–38.
14. Dinh-Xuan AT, Higenbottam TW, Clelland CA et al. (1991) Impairment of endothelium-dependent pulmonary artery relaxation in COLD. N Engl J Med. 324:1539–47.
15. Giaid A, Saleh D. (1995) Reduced endothelial NO synthase expression in the lungs of patients with pulmonary hypertension. N Engl J Med. 333:214–220.
16. Pepke-Zaba J, Higenbottam T, Dinh-Xuan AT, Stone D, Wallwork J. (1991) Inhaled NO as a cause of selective pulmonary vasodilatation in pulmonary hypertension. Lancet 338:1173–4.
17. Frostell CG, Blomquist H, Hedenstierna G et al. (1993) INO selectively reverses human hypoxic pulmonary vasoconstriction without causing systemic vasodilation. Anesthesiology 78:427–35.
18. Frostell C, Fratacci MD, Wain JC, Jones R, Zapol WM. (1991) Inhaled iNO. a selective pulmonary vasodilator reversing hypoxic pulmonary vasoconstriction. Circulation 83:2038–47.
19. Roberts JD, Chen TY, Kawai et al. (1993) Inhaled NO reverses pulmonary vasoconstriction in the hypoxic and acidotic newborn lamb. Circ Res 72:246–54.
20. Kinsella JP, JA McQueston, AA Rosenberg, and SH Abman (1992) Hemodynamic effects of exogenous nitric oxide in ovine transitional pulmonary circulation. Am J Physiol. 263:H875–880.
21. Rossaint R, Falke KJ, Lopez F, Slama K, Pison U, Zapol WM. (1993) Inhaled NO in ARDS. N Engl J Med. 328:399–405.
22. Kinsella JP, Abman SH. (1995) Recent developments in the pathophysiology and treatment of PPHN. J Pediatr 126:583–64.
23. Roberts JD, Polander DM, Lang P, Zapol WM. (1992) Inhaled NO in PPHN. Lancet. 340:818–9.
24. Kinsella JP, Neish SR, Shaffer EM, Abman SH (1992) Low-dose inhalational NO in PPHN. Lancet 340:819–820.
25. Kinsella JP, Neish SR, Ivy DD, Shaffer E, Abman SH. (1993) Clinical responses to prolonged treatment of PPHN with low doses of iNO. J Pediatr 123:103–8.
26. Finer NN, Etches PC, Kamstra B, Tierney AJ, Peliowski A and CA Ryan. (1994) Inhaled NO in infants referred for ECMO: dose response. J Pediatr 124:302–8.
27. Karamanoukian H, Glick P, Zayek M, Steinhorn RH, Zwass MS, Fineman JR, Morin FC. (1994) Inhaled NO in congenital hypoplasia of the lung due to diaphragmatic hernia or oligohydramnios. Pediatrics 94:715–8.
28. Abman SH, JP Kinsella, MS Schaffer, and RB Wilkening. (1993) Inhaled nitric oxide therapy in a premature newborn with severe respiratory distress and pulmonary hypertension. Pediatrics 92:606–9.
29. Kaapa P, Seppanen M, Kero P, and MM Saraste. (1993) Pulmonary hemodynamics after synthetic surfactant replacement in neonatal RDS. J Pediatr 123:115–9.
30. Peliowski A, Finer NN, Etches PC et al. (1995) INO for premature infants after prolonged rupture of membranes. J Pediatr 126:450–3.
31. Zapol WM, Snider MT. (1977) Pulmonary hypertension in severe acute respiratory failure. N Engl J Med. 296:476–80.
32. Zapol WM, Snider MT, Rie MA, Frikker M, Quimm DA. (1985) Pulmonary circulation during ARDS. In: Zapol WM, Falke KJ (eds). Acute Respiratory Failure. NY: Marcel Dekker, p 241–273.
33. Radermacher P, Santak B, Becker H, Falke KJ. (1989) Prostaglandin E1 and nitroglycerin reduce pulmonary capillary pressure but worsen ventilation-perfusion distributions in patients with ARDS. Anesthesiology 70:601–6.
34. Sibbald WJ, Driedger AA, Myers ML, Short AI, Wells GA. (1983) Biventricular function in the ARDS. Chest 84:126–34

35. Dhainaut JF, Brunet F. (1990) Right ventricular performance in ARDS. Eur Respir J 3 (supp 11):490–5.
36. Wysocki M, Vignon P, Roupie E, Humbert M, Adnot S, Lemaire F, Brochard L. (1993) Improvement in RV function with iNO in patients with the ARDS and permissive hypercapnia. Am Rev Resp Dis 147:A350.
37. Abman SH, Greibel J, Parker D et al. (1994) Acute effects of iNO in children with severe acute hypoxemic respiratory failure. J Pediatr 124:881–8.
38. Benzing A, Gieger K. (1994) Inhaled NO lowers pulmonary capillary pressure and changes longitudinal distribution of pulmonary vascular resistance in patients with acute lung injury. Acta Anaesthesiol Scand. 38:640–5.
39. Benzing A, Brautigam P, Gieger K et al. (1995) Inhaled NO reduces pulmonary transvascular albumin flux in patients with acute lung injury. Anesthesiology 83:1153–61.
40. Gerlach H, Rossaint R, Pappert D, Falke KJ. (1993) Time-course and dose-response of NO inhalation for systemic oxygenation and pulmonary hypertension in patients with ARDS. Eur J Clin Invest 23:499–502.
41. Lu Q, Mourgeon E, Law-Koune JD et al. (1995) Dose-response curves of iNO with and without intravenous almitrine in NO-responding patients with acute respiratory distress syndrome. Anesthesiology 83:929–43.
42. Roberts JD, Lang P, Bigatello LM et al. (1993) INO in congenital heart disease. Circulation 87:447–53.
43. Journois D, Pouard P, Mauriat P et al.(1994) INO as a therapy for pulmonary hypertension after operations for congenital heart defects. J Thorac Cardiovasc Surg 107:1129–35.
44. Rich GF, Murphy GD, Roos CM et al. (1993) INO: selective pulmonary vasodilation in cardiac surgical patients. Anesthesiology 78:1028–35.
45. Semigran MJ, Cockrill BA, Kacmarek R et al. (1994) Hemodynamic effects of iNO in heart failure. JACC 24:882–8.
46. Kavanaugh BP, A Mouchawar, J Goldsmith and RG Pearl (1994) Effects of inhaled NO and inhibition of endogenous NO synthesis in oxidant-induced lung injury. J Appl Physiol. 76:1324–9.

Airflow Obstruction in Asthma: There is More than Smooth Muscle

H. A. W. M. Tiddens and J. C. de Jongste

Introduction

Airways can obstruct in many different ways. Basically, airflow obstruction can be the result of increased smooth muscle force generation, airway wall thickening, loss of lung elastic recoil, increased compliance of the airway wall, and secretions in the airway. In severe asthma most of these factors can be responsible for the airflow obstruction. Knowledge of these factors is required to optimize treatment for these patients.

Structural Changes in Asthma

Smooth muscle area. The amount of smooth muscle has been found to be increased in airways of patients who died from asthma or who died of non-respiratory diseases but with a history of asthma [1–3]. However, Bramley and coworkers did not find a difference in the smooth muscle area between a single asthmatic patient in comparison to 6 non-asthmatic patients when the extracellular matrix was subtracted from the muscle bundle area. They hypothesized that the extracellular matrix is increased in asthmatics but not the amount of smooth muscle [4].

Airway Wall Thickening

Thickening of the airway wall was found in patients who died from asthma or who died of non-respiratory diseases but with a history of asthma [1–3]. This thickening is related to airway inflammation [5], and is caused in part by deposition of fibrous tissue due to this chronic inflammation [6, 7]. Highly hydrated proteoglycans are deposited in the submucosa and contribute to this wall thickening [8]. In addition, a thickened layer of matrix composed of collagen type III and V and fibronectin has been found below the basement membrane [9]. These abnormal features of the basement membrane are likely to represent the results of repeated bronchial injury and are found early in the course of asthma. In acute asthma plasma exudation and cellular infiltration has been described [10].

Airway Cartilage

Cartilage is important to maintain airway patency especially during forced expiration. Inflammatory destruction of bronchial cartilage is thought to increase airway collapsibility and could contribute to airflow obstruction. Decreased cartilage volume in relation to chronic bronchitis was found by several authors [11–14], but not by others [15–17]. Whether the mechanical properties of airway cartilage in chronically inflamed airways such as asthma are normal is not known. Even morphologically normal airway cartilage does not guarantee normal mechanical properties. In rabbits it was shown that papain reduced cartilage stiffness and decreased its ability to withstand compression. However, its morphology remained unchanged in comparison to control rabbits [18].

Epithelium

The airway epithelium acts as a barrier against leakage of water and solutes into the airways, and prevents penetration of inhaled material into the interstitium [19, 20]. In addition human epithelial cells are a source of biologically active compounds which modulates the function of neighboring cells and tissues and can inactivate inflammatory mediators. Damage of the epithelium could therefore lead to changes in bronchial responsiveness. In asthma extensive epithelial damage was in fact found in bronchial biopsies [21]. Furthermore, the loss of epithelium was found related to bronchial hyperresponsiveness [21–23].

Vascular Plexus

The airway mucosa contains a dense subepithelial vascular plexus that is densely innervated [24, 25]. The vascular plexus has been shown to be responsive to inflammatory mediators. These mediators can increase its permeability due to the opening of gaps in the endothelium [26]. Changes in vascular permeability can occur within seconds after exposure to irritants. Massive changes in its permeability could therefore lead to sudden and severe changes in airflow obstruction. There are several reports describing sudden death from asthma in relatively stable patients. In a patient described by Saetta edematous thickening of the bronchial walls associated with dilatation of the bronchial vessels was found [10]. It was suggested that the mechanism of airway inflammation as well as airway narrowing in sudden onset fatal asthma may be quite distinct from slow onset fatal asthma [27, 28].

Inflammatory Exudate

Plasma extravasation from the subepithelial vascular plexus into the interstitium of the airway wall might worsen or even cause airflow obstruction in asthma. Mucus, epithelial debris, leukocytes and exudate are all found in the airway lumen of postmortem specimen. This sputum can contribute to airflow obstruction in the following ways. Firstly, it can fill all interstices in between the folds of the bronchial mucosa, reducing the airway lumen. It was estimated that only 6 ml of fluid is sufficient to fill these interstices [29]. Secondly, the appearance of an exudate on the surface of the smaller airways increases their tendency to close because the replacement or inactivation of airway surfactant by plasma greatly increases the airways surface tension [30]. Thirdly, mucous plugs can obstruct large bronchi.

Functional Implications of Structural Changes

Smooth Muscle Contraction and Airway Wall Thickening

The combination of airway wall thickening and smooth muscle shortening is thought to substantially increase airway resistance. When the smooth muscle contracts, the tissue located inside the smooth muscle layer (inner wall area) will fold and encroach upon the lumen (Figure 1).

In a computational model it was estimated that moderate airway wall thickening has little effect on baseline resistance but can profoundly affect airflow obstruction in combination with smooth muscle shortening especially in the peripheral airways [31]. In patients suffering from chronic bronchitis with se-

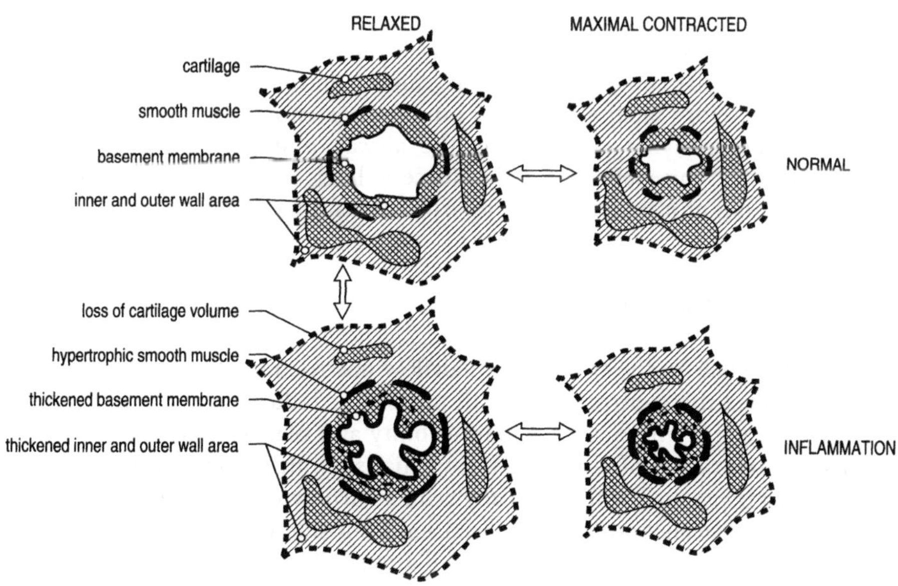

Fig. 1. Schematic drawing of a normal airway and of an inflamed airway in the relaxed and contracted state. In the relaxed state thickening of the inner wall area has relatively little effect on airway resistance. In the maximal contracted state thickening profoundly increases airway resistance.

vere airflow obstruction the inner wall area in the smaller cartilaginous airways was increased by 64% in comparison to non obstructed patients. Airway dimensions of these patients were fed into a computational model. It was estimated that without smooth muscle shortening airway resistance was only 8% higher for the obstructed patients in comparison to the non-obstructed patients. In case of a maximal smooth muscle shortening resistance was 48% higher for the obstructed patients in comparison to the non-obstructed patients [5].

To what extent the smooth muscle can shorten will depend on the balance between the force that the smooth muscle can generate and the load against which it has to contract [32]. The force which smooth muscle of asthmatic patients can generate was found to be increased [2, 4, 33]. It is not clear whether the load on the smooth muscle is increased or decreased. The load on the smooth muscle is provided by the extracellular matrix surrounding the smooth muscle, the inner and outer airway wall area, and by the surrounding lung parenchyma. There is some evidence that the extracellular matrix surrounding the smooth muscle cells is degraded in asthma [34]. This would reduce the load upon the contracting smooth muscle allowing it to shorten further for a given smooth muscle tone. In fact the elastance of airways from a single asthmatic patient was found to be reduced in comparison to controls [4].

The inner wall area has to be deformed into folds when the smooth muscle contracts. One would expect the thickened and fibrotic inner airway wall of asthmatic patients to be stiffer. In fact airway wall distensibility was shown to be decreased in asthmatics [35]. This would increase the load for the contracting smooth muscle and therefore limit airway narrowing for a given smooth muscle tone. Thickening of the airway wall outside the smooth muscle layer (outer airway wall) could uncouple the smooth muscle from its surrounding tissue and therefore facilitate smooth muscle shortening [31, 36].

The lungparenchyma surrounding the airway opposes shortening of the smooth muscle. This outward pulling force is likely to be maximal in the hyperinflated lung of a patient suffering from an asthma attack.

Therapeutical Implications

The possible goals in the treatment of airflow obstruction in acute severe asthma are to relax the contracted smooth muscle, to reduce airway wall thickening, and to reduce microvascular permeability and plasma exudation.

Effective relaxation of contracted bronchial smooth muscle around a thickened inner airway wall will drastically reduce airflow obstruction. Continuous nebulization of bronchodilators in children is considered to be the most effective and safe method to obtain bronchodilation [37, 38]. Continuous nebulization of β_2- agonists was even more efficacious and less toxic than intravenously administered β_2-agonists in adults admitted to hospital for severe acute asthma. However, it remains puzzling why in some patients nebulization of even high doses of bronchodilators does not result in a reduction of airflow obstruction. The effectiveness of nebulization might be reduced due to an irregular distribution pattern of the aerosol [39]. This can be caused by the narrowed airways in combination with sputum covering the epithelial layer or obstructing the airways. For some severely obstructed patients bronchodilators administered intravenously might be more homogeneously distributed throughout the lung and therefore more effective to obtain bronchodilation. Bronchoscopy with the use of a mucolytic agent may provide effective therapy for selected patients who require mechanical ventilation and who have mucous plugs [40].

Corticosteroids are essential in the management of acute severe asthma. They are known to decrease inflammatory cell recruitment and activation, to upregulate β_2-receptors, to decrease microvascular permeability, and the may decrease mucus production [41]. Corticosteroids will reduce inflammatory airway wall thickening and as a result airway resistance will drop drastically even in the presence of smooth muscle contraction [1].

Oedema of the airway walls can be a prominent feature in some cases of sudden onset severe asthma. Although β_2-agonists are the first choice potent bronchodilators they do not affect vascular permeability effectively. Epinephrine, an agent with vasoconstrictor effects, should be used in particularly severe attacks of asthma not reversed by the usual therapy [10].

Conclusion

The relation between structural changes in airways on airflow obstruction in acute severe asthma is complex. For each individual patient suffering from a severe asthma attack a different combination of factors like smooth muscle contraction, oedema of the airway walls, dilatation of bronchial vessels, and mucosal plugs can have lead to the severe airflow obstruction. Causal therapy should be directed against as many factors as possible. It also explains why some patients will not react on maximal bronchodilator therapy since other mechanisms than increased smooth muscle tone might be involved. The additional value of vasoconstrictor agents like epinephrine in the treatment of sudden onset severe asthma should be further investigated.

References

1. James AL, Paré PD, Hogg JC (1989) The mechanics of airway narrowing in asthma. Am Rev Respir Dis 139(1):242–246.
2. Bai TR (1990) Abnormalities in airway smooth muscle in fatal asthma. Am Rev Respir Dis 141:552–557.
3. Carroll N, Elliot J, Morton A, James A (1993) The structure of large and small airways in nonfatal and fatal asthma. Am Rev Respir Dis 147:405–410.
4. Bramley AM, Thomson RJ, Roberts CR, Schellenberg RR (1994) Hypothesis: excessive bronchoconstriction in asthma is due to decreased airway elastance. Eur Respir J 7(2):337–341.

5. Tiddens HAWM, Paré PD, Hogg JC, et al (1995) Cartilaginous airway dimensions and airflow obstruction in human lungs. Am J Respir Crit Care Med 152:260–266.
6. Brewster CE, Howarth PH, Djukanovic R, et al (1990) Myofibroblasts and subepithelial fibrosis in bronchial asthma. Am J Respir Cell Mol Biol 3(5):507–511.
7. Wilson JM, Li X (1994) The measurement of airway collagen in asthmatic airways. Am J Respir Crit Care Med 149(4):A959.
8. Roberts CR (1995) Is asthma a fibrotic disease. Chest 107(suppl):111s–117s.
9. Roche WR, Beasley R, Williams JH, Holgate ST (1989) Subepithelial fibrosis in the bronchi of asthmatics. Lancet 1(8637):520–524.
10. Saetta M, Thiene G, Crescioli S, Fabbri LM (1989) Fatal asthma in a young patient with severe bronchial hyperresponsiveness but stable peak flow records. Eur Respir J 2:1008–1012.
11. Tandon MK, Cambell AH (1969) Bronchial cartilage in chronic bronchitis. Thorax 24:607–612.
12. Thurlbeck WM, Pun R, Toth J, Frazer RG (1974) Bronchial cartilage in chronic obstructive lung disease. Am Rev Respir Dis 109:73–80.
13. Nagai A, West WW, Paul JL, Thurlbeck WM (1985) The national institutes of health intermittent positive pressure breathing trial: pathology studies. Am Rev Resp Dis 132:937–945.
14. Nagai A, Thurlbeck WM, Konno K (1995) Responsiveness and variability of airflow obstruction in chronic obstructive pulmonary disease. Am J Respir Crit Care Med 151:635–639.
15. Dunhill MS, Massarella GR, Anderson JA (1969) A comparison of the quantitative anatomy of the bronchi in normal subjects, in status asthmaticus, in chronic bronchitis, and in emphysema. Thorax 24:176–179.
16. Mullen JB, Wright JL, Wiggs BR, Paré PD, Hogg JC (1985) Reassessment of inflammation of airways in chronic bronchitis. Br Med J (Clin Res Ed) 291 (6504):1235–1239.
17. Tiddens HAWM, Boogaard JM, Jongste JC, et al (1996) Physiologic and morphologic determinants of maximal expiratory flow in chronic obstructive lung disease. Submitted.
18. Moreno RH, McCormack GS, Brendan J, et al (1986) Effect of intravenous papain on tracheal pressure-volume curves in rabbits. J Appl Physiol 60(1):247–52.
19. Munakata M, Huang I, Mitzner W, Menkes H. (1989) Protective role of epithelium in the guinea pig airway. J Appl Physiol 66(4):1547–1552.
20. Hulsmann AR, Raatgeep HR, Den Hollander JC, Bakker WH, Saxena PR (1996) Permeability of human isolated airways increases after hydogen peroxide and poly-L-arginine. Am J Respir Crit Care Med: in press
21. Jeffery PK, Wardlaw AJ, Nelson FC, Collins JV, Kay AB (1989) Bronchial biopsies in asthma. An ultrastructural, quantitative study and correlation with hyperreactivity. Am Rev Respir Dis 140(6):1745–1753.
22. Laitinen LA, Heino M, Laitinen A, Kava T, Haahtela T (1985) Damage of the airway epithelium and bronchial reactivity in patients with asthma. Am Rev Respir Dis 131:505–606.
23. Hulsmann AR, Raatgeep HR, Den Hollander JC, et al (1994) Oxidative epithelial damage produces hyperresponsiveness of human peripheral airways. Am J Respir Crit Care Med 149:519–525.
24. Widdicombe J (1993) Why are the airways so vascular. Thorax 48:290–295.
25. Strek P, Nowogrodzka-Zagorska M, Litwin JA, Miodonski AJ (1994) The lung in closeview: A corrosion casting study on the vascular system of human foetal trachea. Eur Respir J 7:1669–1672.
26. Persson CGA (1994) Airway epithelium and microcirculation. Eur Respir Rev 4(23):352–362.
27. Wasserfallen J-B, Schaller M-D, Feihl F, Perret CH (1990) Sudden aspyxic asthma: a distinct entity. Am Rev Respir Dis 142:108–111.
28. Sur S, Crotty TB, Kephart GM, et al (1993) A distinct entity with few eosinophils and relatively more neutrophils in the airway mucosa? Am Rev Respir Dis 148:713-719.

29. Yager D, Butler JP, Bastacky J, et al (1989) Amplification of airway constriction due to liquid filling of airway interstices. J Appl Physiol 66(6):2873–2884.
30. Macklem PT, Proctor DF, Hogg JC (1970) The stability of peripheral airways. Respir Physiol 8:191–203.
31. Wiggs BR, Bosken C, Paré PD, James A, Hogg JC (1992) A model of airway narrowing in asthma and in chronic obstructive pulmonary disease. Am Rev Respir Dis 145:1251–1258.
32. Moreno R, Taylor R, Muller N, et al (1986) In vivo human tracheal pressure-area curves using computerized tomographic scans. Correlation with maximal expiratory flow rates. Am Rev Respir Dis 134(3):585–589.
33. De Jongste JC, Mons H, Bonta IL, Kerrebijn KF (1987) Human asthmatic airways responses in vitro. Eur J Respir Dis 71:23–29.
34. Bousquet J, Chanez P, Lacoste JY, et al (1992) Asthma: a disease remodeling the airways. Allergy 47:3–11.
35. Wilson JW, Li X, Pain MCF (1994) Airway collagen and airway distensibility in asthmatic airways. Am J Respir Crit Care Med 149(4):A959.
36. Ishida K, Paré PD, Hards J, Schellenberg RB (1992) Mechanical properties of human bronchial smooth muscle in vitro. J Appl Physiol 73:1481–1485.
37. Papo MC, Frank J, Thompson AE (1993) A prospective, randomized study of continuous versus intermittent nebulized albutarol for severe status asthmaticus in children. Critical Care Medicine 21:1479–1486.
38. Schuh S, Johnson DW, Callahan S, Canny G, Levison H (1995) Efficacy of frequent nebulized ipratropium bromide added to frequent high-dose albuterol therapy in severe childhood asthma. J Pediatrics 126:639–645.
39. O'Riordan TG, Walser L, Smaldone GC (1993) Changing patterns of aerosol deposition during metacholine bronchoprovocation. Chest 103:1385–1389.
40. Henke CA, Hertz M, Gustafson P (1994) Combined bronchoscopy and mucolytic therapy for patients with severe refractory status asthmaticus on mechanical ventilation: A Case report and review of the literature. Crit Care Med 22(11):1880–1883.
41. Barnes NC (1992) Effects of corticosteroids in acute severe asthma. Thorax 47:582–583.

Treatment of Severe Acute Asthma in the Child

J. P. Piva, S. Amantéa and P. C. R. Ramos Garcia

Introduction

The admission of children with respiratory insufficiency, mainly by compromise of the lower airways is a common finding in our ICUs [1, 2,3]. The obstruction of the lower airways may be a consequence of many processes: congenital (cystic fibrosis), viral infectious disease (bronchopneumonia, bronchiolitis), microaspirations (pneumopathy by gastroesophageal reflux and/or sinusitis), pulmonary sequelae (bronchopulmonary dysplasia, post viral disease bronchiolopathy), chronic inflammation (asthma), and others [3].

The severe obstruction of the airways may occur as an acute episode of severe asthma, with rapid progression in a patient previously stable, or most frequently, in patients with a chronic obstructive setting (or sequela), which presents a clinical occurrence that contributes to worsen and decompensate this clinical setting. In this last case, one can observe less reversibility, major severity and worse prognosis [4, 5]. In this group, an increasing number of admissions to the ICUs is observed, of patients with chronic pulmonary disorders related to asthma or secondary to other chronic diseases with associated bronchospastic components [3].

The severe crisis of acute asthma may be defined as an acute crisis of bronchospasm accompanied by hypoxemia, important respiratory distress, with exhaustion or alteration of conscience, as consequence of the absent or poor response to the initial therapy with oxygen, bronchodilators and corticosteroids. The rapid identification of this circumstances and the early start with bronchodilator therapy contributes to a minor morbidity/mortality.

There are many aspects in the patient with severe acute asthma (SAA) which are related to the increase of morbidity/mortality, being detached:

- underestimation of the severity of the crisis (undertreatment): The increased mortality due to asthma, as observed in many countries, is related to the inability in early recognizing and treating this circumstances, either by the family or by the medical staff. For this reason, even those mild crisis of asthma should be treated as they could rapidly progress to a more intense and intractable crisis;
- patients with previous admissions in ICUs and emergency rooms, tend to have more severe recurrent crisis. This patients demand special care even when presenting mild crisis;

- children up to 3 years old have a small caliber airway leading to an increased obstruction and resistance, producing turbulent air flow, and, as a consequence, more intractable crisis with poor response to the treatment with nebulized bronchodilators when compared with older children;
- patients with low socio-economic and cultural level use to present with severe crisis, the same as with patients with psychiatric disease;
- patients with chronic pulmonary disease, bronchopulmonary sequelae (bronchopulmonary dysplasia, emphysema) frequently present with a bronchial hyperactivity associated to their basic setting, which is very similar to what is found in the asthma. In the majority of these patients, the associated bronchospasm will cause the decompensation of the clinical setting, simulating an acute crisis of asthma being almost indistinguishable;
- previous treatment not adopted (circumstance frequently found among teenagers)
- common use or recent interruption in corticotherapy.

Pathophysiology

Up to 5 years of age, the resistance of the airways is almost exclusively related to the small diameter of the little lower airways. Thus, in the crisis of asthma, when bronchospasm, edema of the mucosa and hypersecretion are present, will occur an accentuated increase in this resistance to the air flow. For the tidal volume to be maintained, it is necessary that the child produces a greater negative intrathoracic pressure increasing the use of accessory respiratory muscles. While the obstruction progresses, the tidal volume progressively diminishes. Frequently, despite the attempt of the child to produce increased negative inspiratory pressures and to compensate the respiratory insufficiency, this mechanism fails due to the increased thoracic compliance, the muscular fatigue or the turbulent airflow in the airways. As consequence, with the progression of the crisis of asthma, one can observe a progressive diminishing in the tidal volume. In this attempt to compensate, and trying to maintain the same volume/minute, these children with severe crisis of acute asthma also increase the respiratory frequency, hyperventilating not obstructed areas.

The pulmonary compromise in children with severe crisis of acute asthma does not occur homogeneously (Figure 1). There are partially obstructed areas which are partially ventilated ones. In this areas, during inspiration, by retraction of the thoracic wall, an increase in the airway diameter occurs permitting to ingress a small amount of air. However, during expiration, when the retraction of the thoracic wall is over, there is a narrowing of the airway making difficult the egress of air from the alveolus producing an increase in the residual functional capacity and emphysema (areas of hypoventilation). There are still areas with complete obstruction (atelectasis) which are not ventilated and present shunt effect. In the other hand, there are some areas not yet compromised which are hyperventilated in order to compensate the hypoxemia and maintain the volume/minute. The final goal of this disorder in the relation

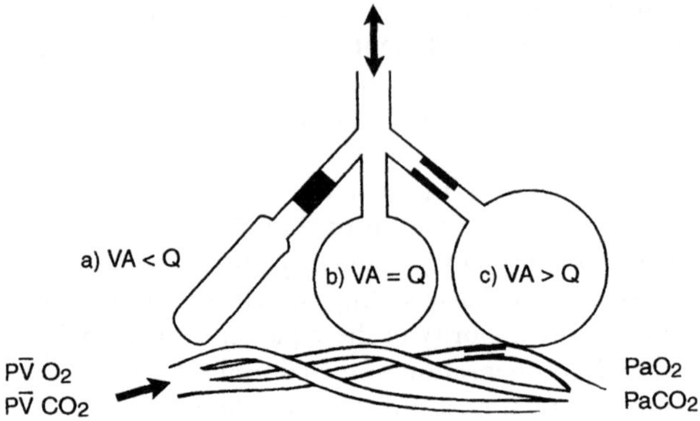

Fig. 1. Ventilation/Perfusion (V/Q) Abnormalities in Asthma. **a** "Shunt Unit" (Perfused but not ventilated); **b** Normal Unit (Ventilated and perfused); **c** "Dead Space" Unit (Ventilated but not perfused)

ventilation/perfusion is manifested by hypoxemia accompanied by variable levels of pCO_2, depending on the predominance of hypoventilated areas or atelectasis.

As the obstruction progresses and the hypoxemia worsens, there is an increase in the muscular activity. This may lead to a metabolic acidosis which may be associated to a CO_2 retention and result in a mixed acidosis having a worse prognosis and requiring more aggressive measures.

The progression in the hypoxemia (associated or not to hypercapnia) may lead to alterations of conscience (agitation/prostration), cardiovascular response with tachycardia and posterior brachycardia and hypotension resulting in shock and cardiorespiratory arrest.

Clinical and Laboratory Evaluation

The continuous evaluation and determining the severity of the crisis are essential to follow-up and to decide for more aggressive maneuvers. There is not only one criteria or score with predictive power that could be secure and suitable to all patients. So, it is advisable to use data (Table 1) and, based on the findings, classify the crisis as mild, moderate or acute [6]. There are some findings in the physical examination which present a good correlation with the severity of the situation: the use of the accessory respiratory muscles is well correlated with the degree of the airway obstruction (PEFR and VEF1 around 50% of the expected vale to that age). The state of conscience is directly related to the degree of fatigue and hypoxemia, where mental confusion and disturbance are data of late evaluation and associated to extremely severe settings. The use of the accessory respiratory muscles is the isolated item which is better correlated with the severity of the crisis, while the hemoglobin saturation obtained by pulse oxymetry is the most objective measure [6, 7, 8].

The paradoxical pulse should be measured whenever possible. Values above 20 mmHg are associated to very severe crisis.

Subjective dyspnea, subjective wheezing, prolonged expiration, auscultatory rhonchi have no discriminated value in differentiating patients with severe from those with minimal measured function impairment.

The laboratory evaluation can be performed using tests of function to determine the degree of obstruction (FEV1 and PEFR), or measuring the degree of hypoxemia and/or ventilation obtained determining the hemoglobin saturation and/or arterial gasometry [Rubin].

Ideally, all places dealing with asthmaticus in acute crisis should have spirometry available. Meanwhile, not all the patients are used or trained to perform such maneuver, becoming difficult, in a practical viewpoint, to adopt this measure during and acute crisis. In children, the measurement of the hemoglobin saturation (pulse oxymetry) has proved to be useful and secure in the evaluation and follow-up of the severity of the crisis. Hemoglobin saturation in atmospheric air up to 91–93% suggests a severe crisis requiring a careful follow-up and an aggressive treatment [8]. In cases of an intense respiratory distress associated or not to hypoxemia, it is imperative the evaluation using ar-

Table 1. Classification according to the intensity of the asthma crisis*

	Mild	Moderate	Severe
Dyspnea	Absent or mild; talk complete sentences	Moderate, incomplete sentences/partial; short cry, feeding difficulties	Severe; talk short sentences/monosyllable; half-seated position, >feeding difficulties
Conscience	Normal	Normal or excited	Excited or depressed
Respiratory Frequency**	From normal to >1 DP/age	Increased to 2 DP/age	Increased and >2 DP
Use of accessory respiratory muscles	Mild or absent Intercostal retractions	Moderate subcostal retractions and Sternocleidomas	Intense retractions and Beating of the Nasal Wings-BNW
Auscult	Wheezing at the end of inspiration	Inspiratory and expiratory wheezing	Unheard murmur Poor airflow
Paradoxical pulse	<10 mmHg	10–20 mmHg	20–40 mmHg
PEF	70–90%	50–70%	<50%
O_2 saturation in atmospheric air	>95%	91–95%	<90%
pO_2 (atmospheric air)	Normal	~60 mmHg	<60 mmHg
pCO_2	≤50 mmHg	≤40 mmHg	>45 mmHg

* The presence of several parameters, not necessarily all of them, indicates the general classification of the acute crisis.

** Table of Respiratory Frequency in normal children.

terial gasometry (pH, pCO_2, pO_2 and bicarbonate). The evaluation of the oxygenation is better accomplished through the relation paO_2/FiO_2 (when up to 250, reveals a severe compromise in the relation ventilation: perfusion). In the severe acute asthma, no other test of evaluation is equal or better than the arterial gasometry, ånd should be performed in all patients.

In critical patients with severe acute asthma, it is also suggested to measure the electrolytes serum concentration (especially potassium due to the possible utilization of high doses of beta-adrenergics) and the rate of hemoglobin (which should be above 10g% in these critical patients with insufficient ventilation). The leukogram has a poor value in this situation due to the stress and the use of adrenergics and corticoids, thus being the leukocytosis a common finding [9].

The chest X-ray has a poor value in the acute crisis being performed to exclude a different diagnosis (foreign body, etc.) or to evaluate the presence of pneumothorax (uncommon in children) or bacterial complications such as pneumonia (uncommon finding in the crisis of acute asthma in childhood).

Treatment in the ICU

In the last decade, not any newer medication appeared proving to be efficient and secure in the treatment of the severe acute asthma. Even so, there were many therapeutic advances improving the use of some drugs, giving priority to others, and adopting more aggressive therapeutic maneuvers earlier. In this viewpoint, even mild crisis of asthma have been treated as if they could rapidly progress to a more intense and intractable crisis.

The environment must be calm, secure and organized, no matter the severity of the setting. This situation does not permit improvisations or the patients being submitted to the subjective evaluation of each physician on call.

Considering this assertion, we suggest that each service develop its own protocol, based in their conditions, difficulties and experience.

The protocol adopted by us is as follows:

Oxygen: By the reason it is an hypoxemic disease, oxygen should be always administered using the most comfortable method (mask, catheter, tent) with the purpose of maintaining the hemoglobin saturation above 95%, remembering that systems of low flux may be inadequate to tachypneic patients.

Hydration: Some patients when admitted in the ICUs present with dehydration due to the vomiting, fever, feeding abnormalities and tachypnea. In this case, it is administered as glucose and a normal saline solution in the proportion 1:1, speed of 10–20 ml/kg/h, during a period of 1 hour and 15 minutes. After hydration has been controlled, we prescribe the hydroelectrolytic maintenance with clinical monitoring of diuresis and electrolytes avoiding hyperhydration as much as dehydration. Special attention should be paid to the administration of potassium, mainly in the case of being necessary to use high doses of beta-adrenergics.

Medication: Among the therapeutic options there are many drugs: beta-adrenergics, xanthines, ipratropium bromide, corticoids, furosemide, magnesium sulfate, halothane, ketamine, and others. In spite of have being used during many years, the true effectiveness of many of these drugs is still discussed today. In the last years, a different priority in the use of these drugs is being adopted. The sequence of medications used in our Service in this situation is as follows:

Nebulizations with beta-2 agonist: Many studies in the recent decades demonstrate the benefits (lasting and earliest bronchodilation) using greater and more frequent doses of nebulized fenoterol and salbutamol in patients with severe acute asthma without a significant increase in the side effects. The frequency of nebulizations is related to the intensity of the crisis and the patients response to the medication used. Thus, the nebulized bronchodilators will be administered in the frequency necessary to obtain a clinical improvement [6, 10, 11].

We start the treatment with salbutamol or fenoterol (0.15 mg/kg/max.dose: 5 mg/dose or 20 dps.), dissolved in 3 ml of SF, with an oxygen flux of 6 to 8 l/min, each 20 minutes, with an average of 3 nebulizations each hour. In the majority of the patients, after 1 or 2 hours, 3 to 6 nebulizations) stabilization is achieved with improvement in the tidal volume, decrease in the respiratory effort, and the interval between each nebulization is then prolonged (one each 30 minutes, 1 hour, and so progressively). In case there is no improvement, and the patient does not present with a clinical impairment, we maintain the nebulizations each 20 minutes during 3 or 4 hours. If, after this period, the patient does not present with better results, more likely this will not occur with this kind of treatment due to the small tidal volume of the patient which avoids an adequate deposition of the bronchodilators in the lower airways.

Infants, in consequence of the small caliber of the airways, present with a turbulent airflow making difficult the distribution of nebulized bronchodilators in severe crisis of acute asthma. In our Service, according to some reports of the literature, we have used a mixture of 40% of oxygen and 60% of helium with a flux of 6–8 l/min. This mixture, which presents a coefficient of resistance lesser than the oxygen coefficient, allows a better distribution of these medications in the lower airways of these patients [12]. Our results are still in phase of data collection, but, as seen in the preliminary results, they permit to foresee a reasonable alternative for these cases.

Corticoids: Corticoids present, at least, two benefits, in the severe acute asthma: enhances the bronchodilator effects of beta-adrenergics (in 4 to 6 hours after administration) and has an anti-inflammatory effect (later) [6]. Because of this interval, they should be early administered intravenously – hydrocortisone (5 mg/kg/dose in 6/6 hours) or methyl-prednisolone (1–2 mg/kg/dose in 6/6 hours). Excepting some anecdotal trials, there are no factual evidences of a significant difference in the outcome when using high doses of corticoids. For the same reason, we avoid to use dexamethasone or betamethasone due to their long-term effects.

Xanthines: The use of aminophylline as a first-line drug in the treatment of the severe asthma is already discussed. Some trials does not report any benefit of its use associated with beta-adrenergics and/or corticoids. Likewise, it should be noted that the majority of this papers exclude for study patients with severe acute asthma and patients above 3 to 5 years [13, 14]. Thus, for this age, and in those cases in which an improvement is not achieved with the use of appropriate doses (frequent) of nebulized beta2 and corticoid, we believe the xanthines should be indicated.

The parenteral administration of aminophylline may be done in bolus each 6 hours (infusion in 20–30 minutes) or continuous. Whenever possible, the patient using intravenous aminophylline should have dosed the serum concentration (which should be, ideally, between 5 and 15 mcg/dl). The initial dose may be used in patients which have not used theophylline previously (7mg/kg/dose) and the maintenance dose used from this moment (5mg/kg/dose each 6 hours or 0.9 mg/kg h). In case of having used xanthine during the last hours, ones may start using the maintenance dose (0.7 to 0.9 mg/kg/hour), until be available the serum concentration levels.

Ipratropium bromide: It is derived from atropine, has the double bronchodilator effect and does not pass through the hematoencephalic barrier. Although the ipratropium bromide is being used in nebulizations for the treatment of asthma since more than one decade, its effectiveness is already discussed nowadays [2, 15]. In our Service, we have use associated therapy with ipratropium bromide when the response to the nebulized beta-adrenergics and intravenous corticoids is not satisfactory. We add ipratropium bromide (0.5ml/dose each 4–6 hours in children above 1 year and 1 ml/dose when older) to the solution for nebulization with beta-adrenergics. Recently, it has been shown advantages with the frequent nebulized ipratropium bromide associated to high doses of albuterol achieving better bronchodilation than when this drugs are used separately or in prolonged intervals.

Intravenous beta-adrenergics: They are indicated in the treatment of the severe acute asthma when: a) there is a progressive retention of pCO_2 (hypoventilation); b) clinical improvement is not observed with the conservative treatment, and there is a poor outcome with the nebulizations due to the small tidal volume; c) signs of eminent respiratory fatigue, which progression will lead to exhaustion and to the necessity of using mechanical ventilation.

There are three types of beta-adrenergic solution for intravenous infusion: isoproterenol (older and with greater beta1 effect), salbutamol and terbutaline. Like in other services, we prefer the use of salbutamol and terbutaline due to their preferential $beta_2$ effect causing less tachycardia and less vasomotor phenomenon. Beta-adrenergics may cause an accentuated decrease in the potassium serum concentration, which should be maintained under overzealous monitoring. After the initial infusion (initial dose), it is expected an increase in the cardiac frequency from 10 to 15% and, posteriorly, even with progressive increases of the medication, the cardiac frequency keeps stable. As the bronchodilation occurs, there is an improvement in the tidal volume, in the volume/minute, in the oxygenation, a decrease in the respiratory effort, and as a consequence, a decreasing in the tachycardia, even that intravenous salbutamol/terbutaline is still being used [9,16,17]. The doses of these drugs, as used in our Service, has been as follow:

a) Salbutamol (amp. 1ml/500mcg): A initial dose of 10mcg/kg in 10 minutes, followed by a maintenance dose of 0.6–0.8 mcg/kg/min, increasing to 0.2mcg/kg/min each 15 to 20 minutes, up to a maximum of 4 to 8 mcg/kg/min.
b) Terbutaline (amp. 1ml/500mcg): A initial dose of 5mcg/kg/min in 10 minutes followed by a maintenance dose of 0.4 to 0.6mcg/kg/min up to a maximum of 4 to 8mcg/kg/min. Either with the salbutamol or the terbutaline, we have started with maintenance doses greater than the ones initially described in the literature, based in previous observation where we verified that the effective dose in many patients is around 0.8 to 1.2mcg/kg/mi [9, 16, 17].

As soon as there is an improvement in the ventilatory function (reversion of the bronchospasm), the intravenous beta2 agonist should be slowly diminished to re-start with the use of nebulized bronchodilators. Exceptionally, this drug is withdrawn in the first 24 hours of use. In case of the patient presents with an enhanced improvement, we reduce the infusion till next to 1.0mcg/kg/min, and maintain like that, associated with nebulizations with beta-adrenergics each hour, during a period of 12 to 24 hours.

Mechanical Ventilation

When the aggravation of the disease can not be controlled with the conventional therapy, the mechanical ventilation should be employed. Clinical findings as exhaustion or hemodynamic compromise are more significant to indicate ventilatory support than controversial gasometric values.

The purpose of the mechanical ventilation is to maintain an adequate oxygenation of the child, until the bronchodilator and anti-inflammatory medications be effective and the bronchodilation occurs.

The main concern is oriented to an adequate oxygenation, even though the patient presents with increased rates of arterial pCO_2. Reaching this purpose assumes the patient be completely under sedation. Among the variety of proposals to sedate the asthmatic patient under ventilation, we have chosen to start with benzodiazepines, with good response in preventing the respiratory asynchrony in some patients. Many times, to obtain a complete sedation, thionembutal is used associated or not to curarizing agents according to individual needs [18]. The use of anesthetics as halothane and ketamine, although having some benefits described in relation to its use for bronchodilation, is not currently adopted in the management of these patients, in our Service.

For mechanical ventilation, we employ regimens with oxygen concentrations sufficient to establish the equilibrium in the V/Q relation, a low respiratory frequency, a high inspiratory flow, a prolonged expiratory time and a minimal final expiratory pressure. Following these principles, employing the pressures necessary to obtain an adequate thorax expendability (generally between 30–35 cmH_2O) or with tidal volume sufficient to proceed the ventilation (generally 10 ml/kg), it is possible to win the resistance of the obstructed airways and prevent the alveolar ventilation. Aiming a better distribution of this volume in the lower airways (different time constants), we use lower respiratory frequencies to maximize the expiratory times and prevent air-trapping.

It is important to highlight that, even with an increased pCO_2, ones should not use exceedingly high pressures or increase the respiratory frequency due to the risk of barotrauma and air-trapping. The pCO_2 will gradually decrease as the bronchodilation occurs.

In the severe acute asthma, the mechanical ventilation is used as a therapeutic support. During all the time these patients are in mechanical ventilation, they are kept under continuous infusion of beta-adrenergics which are withdrawn only after extubation.

References

1. Helfaer MA, Nichols D, Rogers MC et al (1992) Lower airway disease: Bronchiolitis and asthma. In: Rogers MC (ed) Textbook of Pediatric Intensive Care, 2nd edn. Williams & Wilkins, Baltimore, pp 258–295.
2. Downs JB & Pillmer SL (1995) Distal airway disorders in infants and children: Bronchiolitis and asthma. In: Ayres SM, Grenvik A, Holbrook P, Shoemaker WC (eds) Textbook of critical care, 3rd edn. W.B. Saunders Co., Philadelphia, pp 739–749.
3. Lanier B (1981) Who is dying of asthma and why ? J Pediatr 115:38–40.
4. Campbell DA, McLennan G, Coates JR et al (1994) A comparison of asthma deaths and near-fatal asthma in South Australia. Eur resp J 7:490–497.
5. Schuh S, Johnson DW, Callahan S, et al (1995) Efficacy of frequent nebulized ipratropium bromide added to frequent high-dose albuterol therapy in severe childhood asthma. J Pediatr 126:639–645.
6. Kerem E, Canny G, Tibshirani R, et al (1991) Clinical-physiologic correlations in acute asthma of childhood. Pediatrics 87:481–486.
7. Rubin BK, Marcushamer S, Priel I, et al (1990) Emergency management of the child with asthma. Pediatr Pulmonol 8:45–57.
8. Fugisang G, Pedersen S, Borgströn (1989) Dose-response relationship of intravenously administered terbutaline in children with asthma. J Pediatr 114:315–320.
9. Santana JC (1995) Fatores relacionados a asma aguda em pacientes internados em Unidade de Terapia Intensiva Pediatrica. {Dissertacao de Mestrado. Universidade Federal do da UFRGS - Brazil}.
10. Geelhoed GC, Landau L, LeSouër PN (1990) Oxymetry and peak flow in assessment of acute childhood asthma. J Pediatr 117:907–909.
11. Stein RT, Gervini MG, Chaves D (1992) Asma aguda grave. In: Piva JP, Carvalho PA, Garcia PC (eds) Terapia Intesiva em Pediatria (3rd ed) Medsi, Rio de Janeiro, pp 167–183.

12. Bentur L, Canny GJ, Shields MD, et al (1990) Controled trial of nebulized albuterol in children younger than 2 years of age with acute asthma. Pediatrics 89:133–137.
13. Papo MC, Frank T, Thompson AE (1993) A prospective, randomized study of continuous versus intermittent nebulized albuterol for severe status asthmaticus in children. Crit Care Med 21:1479–1486.
14. Wolfson MR, Bhutani VK, Shaffer TH, et al (1984) Mechanics and energetics of breathing helium in infants with bronchopulmonary dysplasia. J Pediatr 104:752–757.
15. Carter E, Cruz M, Chesrow S, et al (1993) Efficacy of intravenously administered theophyline in children hospitalized with severe asthma. J Pediatr 122:470–476.
16. Di Giulio GA, Kerscsmar CM, Krug SE, et al (1993) Hospital treatment of asthma: lack of benefit from theophyline given in addition to nebulized albuterol and intravenously administered corticosteroid. J Pediatr 122:464–469.
17. Piva JP, Giugno K, Maia TR (1990) Asma aguda severa. I Congresso de Emergencias em Pediatria. Porto Alegre (Brazil), Anais, pp 61.
18. Grunberg G, Cohen JD, Keslin J, et.al. (1991) Facilitation in status asthmaticus with continuous intravenous thiopental. Chest 99:1216–1219.

Treatment of Respiratory Syncytial Virus Bronchiolitis: Hope and Despair

J. L. L. Kimpen

Introduction

Respiratory syncytial virus (RSV) is the most important cause of bronchiolitis in infants and young children. The disease is characterized by tachypnea, wheezing, inter-and subcostal retractions and low-grade fever. Oxygen saturation is usually impaired. Children with congenital heart disease and ex-prematures with or without bronchopulmonary dysplasia are at increased risk for severe disease. Every year approximately 1000–1500 children are admitted with bronchiolitis in the Netherlands. Nearly every individual is infected before the age of 3 years. Evidence has accumulated that RSV bronchiolitis is an immune-mediated disease [1]. All cells of the immune system have been suggested as contributing to the inflammation of the airways during RSV bronchiolitis (Table 1).

Table 1. Role of different cell types in immunity and immune injury during RSV bronchiolitis (clinical and animal data)

	Immunity	Immunopathology
Lymphocytes		
NK cells	+	+
B cells		
IgG	+	–
IgM	+	–
IgA	+	–
IgE	–	+
T cells		
CD4	+	+
CD8	+	+
Macrophages	+	+
Granulocytes		
Eosinophils	–	+
Neutrophils	?	?
Basophils	–	+

Most probably an intricate network of immune reactions is activated during infection with RSV, of which T cells, pulmonary macrophages and infected epithelial cells could be the orchestrators.

Almost half a century after discovery of the virus there is no effective treatment or vaccine available.

Possible Treatment Strategies

Two aspects of RSV bronchiolitis are of paramount importance in our thinking about possible therapeutic strategies. First the immunopathogenetic mechanisms involved in the disease process dictate that treatment ideally should not only deal with the viral infection per se, but also modulate the immune response, in order to curtail the damage done to the airways, leading both to acute disease and long term sequelae. Second the epidemiological, clinical and pathological similarities between RSV bronchiolitis and childhood asthma have influenced treatment of bronchiolitis in the past decades. Indeed, Landau has formulated in a recent editorial the question that puzzles many researchers on RSV immunology and asthma: Are the two disease entities related? [2]. Antiviral therapy has been shown to be marginally effective. Treatment of RSV bronchiolitis has mainly focused on therapeutics active in asthma: bronchodilators and corticosteroids (Table 2).

Finally passive and active immunization is still a topic of considerable interest. The present paper will review the most important data on the medical treatment of RSV bronchiolitis and the possible role of passive immunization. Vaccine trials will not be discussed.

Medical Treatment

Antiviral Therapy

Ribavirin, a guanosine analogue, has in vitro activity against many respiratory and non-respiratory viruses including RSV. Since 1982 several trials of ribavirin for RSV bronchiolitis have been published, both in non-ventilated and ventilated pediatric patients (Table 3 and 4).

On the basis of the first three studies [3–5] the American Academy of Pediatrics issued guidelines for the use of ribavirin in a considerable proportion of

Table 2. Therapeutic strategies for asthma and bronchiolitis

	Asthma	Bronchiolitis
Bronchodilators	+	±
Antiviral drugs	–	±
Corticosteroids	+	?

Table 3. Ribavirin (non-ventilated patients)

	n	Study design	Results
Hall (1983)	33	DB, PC (17/16)	↓ severity score ↓ LRT signs ↑ oxygen saturation ↓ viral shedding
Taber (1983)	26	DB, PC (12/14)	↓ severity score ~ viral shedding
Hall (1985)	13 (HR)	DB, PC (6/7)	↓ severity score
Rodriguez (1987)	30	DB, PC (20/10)	↓ severity score ↑ oxygen saturation ~ viral shedding
Conrad (1987)	33 (HR)	open study	↓ severity score
Groothuis (1990)	47 (HR)	DB, PC (20/27)	↓ severity score ↑ oxygen saturation
Janai (1993)	19	DB, PC (10/9)	no clinical effect no effect on lung function
Wheeler (1993)	158	historical cohort/ multicenter (100/52)	no clinical effect

DB = double-blind; PC = placebo-controlled; HR = high risk; LRT = lower respiratory tract

high risk children [6]. Three studies confirmed the data of Hall et al. and Taber et al. after FDA approval of the drug [7–9]. However, not many therapies in infectious diseases have been as controversial as the treatment of RSV bronchiolitis with ribavirin. Small numbers of heterogeneous patients have been included in the studies leading to possible bias. Most important however is the fact that, although the differences between the treatment and placebo groups in the various studies reached statistical significance, it is not clear if these differences are indeed clinically relevant. No difference in important data as duration of hospitalization, days in intensive care, prevention of artificial ventilation, death and complications could be demonstrated. Moreover two recent publications (one double-blind placebo-controlled trial and one multicenter historical cohort study) did not find any clinical or lung function effect of ribavirin in the treatment of bronchiolitis [10, 11].

In 1991 a hallmark study was reported by Smith et al. showing a considerably faster improvement of ribavirin-treated ventilated patients versus controls. Ribavirin was administered via the respirator and water was used as a placebo [12]. Unfortunately the results of this promising trial could not be reproduced by Meert et al. [13].

The reason for this discrepancy is not clear although the use of water as a placebo in the Smith study (versus saline in the Meert study) could have in-

Table 4. Ribavirin (ventilated patients)

	n	Study design	Results
Smith (1991)	28	DB, PC (14/14)	↓ duration mechanical ventilation ↓ supplemental oxygen ↓ duration hospitalization
Meert (1994)	41	DB, PC (22/19)	no clinical effect

DB = double-blind; PC = placebo-controlled

fluenced the results in favor of ribavirin because of the possible irritating effect of water on the airways resulting in bronchoconstriction.

In addition practical and economical considerations as well as the fear for teratogenicity preclude the widespread use of ribavirin in the treatment of RSV bronchiolitis awaiting well-controlled trials with larger numbers of stratified patients.

Bronchodilator Therapy

Several bronchodilator drugs, with have proven effectivity in the treatment of asthma, have been tested in the treatment of RSV bronchiolitis. Therapeutic trials with theophylline, aerosolized epinephrine and ipratropium bromide have been reported. However the drug tested most extensively is albuterol. When clinical parameters, as well as lung function tests and changes in oxygen saturation are compared between treated patients and controls, controversial results have been obtained (Table 5).

Stokes et al. and Hughes et al. demonstrated a negative effect of albuterol in the treatment of RSV bronchiolitis when different lung function parameters

Table 5. Bronchodilator therapy (albuterol)

	n	Study design	Parameter	Results
Stokes (1983)	25	DB, PC	Lung function	negative
Soto (1985)	50	Open study	Lung function	no difference
Hughes (1987)	17	Open study	Lung function	negative
Schuh (1990)	40	DB, PC	Clinical score Oxygen saturation	positive positive
Ho (1991)	21	DB, PC	Oxygen saturation	negative
Klassen (1991)	83	DB, PC	Clinical score Oxygen saturation	positive no difference
Gadomski (1994)	128	DB, PC	Clinical score Oxygen saturation	no difference no difference

DB = double-blind; PC = placebo-controlled

were measured [14, 15], while Ho et al. found a disadvantagous effect on oxygen saturation after inhalation of albuterol [16]. Several studies did not show any effect, nor beneficial neither detrimental, on the clinical score, oxygen saturation or lung function when treated patients were compared to controls [17–19]. On the contrary Klassen et al. showed a beneficial effect on the clinical score of the treated patients confirming data of Schuh et al. [18, 20]. Most clinicians feel that bronchodilator treatment should be used on admission on a trial and error basis under close supervision. Therapy is continued when the patient responds well and is stopped if the clinical condition, lung function or oxygen saturation deteriorates or does not improve after inhalation.

Corticosteroids

The next logical step in the treatment of RSV bronchiolitis is the use of systemic or inhalation corticosteroids. Several studies have been reported since the end of the 1960's (Table 6).

Only one study by Tal et al. showed a beneficial effect in a small subgroup of children with RSV bronchiolitis who were treated with corticosteroids and albuterol [21]. All other studies did not show a beneficial effect of corticosteroids on the clinical course of RSV bronchiolitis [22–24]. However, no study verified the presence of RSV before inclusion of the patients, resulting in a probable selection bias. The early studies certainly included patients with diseases other than RSV bronchiolitis e.g. bacterial respiratory infections [22, 23]. A randomized double-blind placebo-controlled trial of oral prednisolone in the treatment of hospitalized patients with proven RSV bronchiolitis was initiated in our center 2 years ago. Preliminary results show a beneficial effect in the subgroup of patients with an initial high severity score. The effect was most marked in the ventilated patients. Prednisolone-treated patients could be discharged earlier and had a faster decrease of the severity score as placebo recipients (van Woensel et al., manuscript submitted).

Table 6. Corticosteroids

	n	Diagnosis	Treatment	Effect
Dabbous (1966)	44	Clinical	Prednisolone Tetracycline Epinephrine	–
Leer (1969)	297	Clinical	Betamethasone	–
Tal (1983)	32	Clinical	Dexamethasone	+
Springer (1990)	50	Clinical	Hydrocortisone Prednisone	–

Immunological Treatment – Immunoglobulin Treatment

The rationale behind treatment of children at risk for severe RSV disease prophylactically or therapeutically with parenteral immunoglobulins lies in the experimental finding that the presence of high-titer neutralizing antibody in the serum of laboratory animals and human infants before infection with RSV is relatively protective for development of RSV-induced disease. Additionally RSV-specific immunoglobulins (IgG, IgM, IgA) do not seem to play a role in immunopathogenesis.

Passive immunotherapy with intravenous immunoglobulins (IVIG) of cotton rats and owl monkeys resulted in an enhanced clearance of virus from the lungs [25]. Hemming et al. treated children hospitalized with RSV bronchiolitis in a double-blind placebo-controlled trial with IVIG and found a faster increase in oxygen saturation after 24 hr, a faster decrease of viral shedding from the nose but no difference in the duration of hospitalization or clinical recovery [26].

The next step was to use IVIG prophylactically in children at high risk for severe disease. Meissner et al. showed a reduction in the severity of disease after natural RSV infection in the group who received IVIG versus placebo. However the number of infections was equal in both groups [27]. They concluded that treatment with IVIG was safe but the neutralizing antibody titer in the IVIG lots was probably too low to induce protection against infection. A technique to obtain high-titer RSV-specific IVIG (RSIVIG) lots from selected high-titer plasma units was developed and in 1993 Groothuis et al. demonstrated in a large multicenter trial that administration of monthly infusions of high-dose-RSIVIG (750 mg/kg) to high-risk patients resulted in less severe disease after natural infection, a shorter duration of hospitalization, less hospital and intensive care days and less ribavirin use as compared to low-dose-RSIVIG (150 mg/kg) or controls [28]. However administration of IVIG on a monthly basis to children with a complex past history, a tendency for fluid retention in addition to logistic and practical problems inherent to intravenous therapy, is cumbersome. Therefor, future trials will concentrate on the administration of less voluminous immunoglobulin suspensions by the intramuscular or subcutaneous route. Much effort will be devoted to engineering immunoglobulin lots with high-titer anti-RSV antibodies in the form of monoclonal antibodies to the most immunogenic determinants of the virus [29]. Trials with these products are in progress.

Conclusions

Treatment of RSV bronchiolitis is still a matter of much debate. New insights in the immunological nature of the disease and its correlation with childhood asthma will determine future treatment strategies. For the time being treatment of bronchiolitis is still discouraging. Ribavirin has not lived up to the high expectations following its discovery. Bronchodilator drugs should be used with caution in view of the possible disadvantageous effects on the lung function, although a clinical trial in the individual patient seems to be warranted. The use of corticosteroids holds promise for severely ill patients but awaits further study. Finally the prophylactic and even less the therapeutic use of RSV-specific immunoglobulins or monoclonal antibodies will only buy time for researchers to come up with an effective vaccine that can be administered immediately after or even before birth to be protective for the most vulnerable of patients, the small infant with underlying cardio-pulmonary disease.

References

1. Kimpen JLL, Heymans HSA (1993) Respiratory syncytial virus: immunity and immune injury. Immunol Infect Dis 3:281–288.
2. Landau LI (1994) Bronchiolitis and asthma: are they related? Thorax 49:293–296.
3. Hall CB, McBride JT, Walsh EE, et al (1983) Aerosolized ribavirin treatment of infants with respiratory syncytial viral infection. A randomized double-blind study. N Engl J Med 308:1443–1447.
4. Taber LH, Knight V, Gilbert BE, et al (1983) Ribavirin aerosol treatment of bronchiolitis associated with respiratory syncytial virus infection in infants. Pediatrics 72:613–618.
5. Hall CBN, McBride JT, Gala CL, Hildreth SW, Schnabel KC (1985) Ribavirin treatment of respiratory syncytial viral infection in infants with underlying cardiopulmonary disease. JAMA 254:3047–3051.
6. Committee on Infectious Diseases (1993) Use of ribavirin in the treatment of respiratory syncytial virus infection. Pediatrics 92:501–504.
7. Rodriguez WJ, Kim HW, Brandt CD, et al (1987) Aerosolized ribavirin in the treatment of patients with respiratory syncytial virus disease. Pediatr Infect Dis J 6:159–163.
8. Conrad DA, Christenson JC, Waner JL, Marks MI (1987) Aerosolized ribavirin treatment of respiratory syncytial virus infection in infants hospitalized during an epidemic. Pediatr Infect Dis J 6:152–158.
9. Groothuis JR, Woodin KA, Katz R, et al (1990) Early ribavirin treatment of respiratory syncytial viral infection in high-risk children. J Pediatr 117:792–798.
10. Janai HK, Stutman HR, Zaleska M, et al (1993) Ribavirin effect on pulmonary function in young infants with respiratory syncytial virus bronchiolitis. Pediatr Infect Dis J 12:214–218.
11. Wheeler JG, Wofford J, Turner RB (1993) Historical cohort evaluation in ribavirin efficacy in respiratory syncytial virus infection. Pediatr Infect Dis J 12:209–213.
12. Smith DW, Frankel LR, Mathers LH, Tang ATS, Ariagno RL, Prober CG (1991) A controlled trial of aerosolized ribavirin in infants receiving mechanical ventilation for severe respiratory syncytial virus infection. N Engl J Med 325:24–29.
13. Meert KL, Sarnaik AP, Gelmini MJ, Lieh-Lai MW (1994) Aerosolized ribavirin in mechanically ventilated children with respiratory syncytial virus lower respiratory tract disease: a prospective, double-blind, randomized trial. Crit Care Med 22:566–572.
14. Stokes GM, Milner AD, Hodges IGC, Henry RL, Elphick MC (1983) Nebulised therapy in acute severe bronchiolitis in infancy. Arch Dis Child 58:279–283.
15. Hughes DM, Le Souef PN, Landau LI (1987) Effect of salbutamol on respiratory mechanics in bronchiolitis. Pediatr Res 22:83–86.
16. Ho L, Collis G, Landau LI, Le Souef PN (1991) Effect of salbutamol on oxygen saturation in bronchiolitis. Arch Dis Child 66:1061–1064.
17. Soto ME, Sly PD, Uren E, Taussig LM, Landau LI (1985) Bronchodilator response during acute viral bronchiolitis in infancy. Pediatr Pulmonol 1:85–90.
18. Klassen TP, Rowe PC, Sutcliffe T, Ropp LJ, McDowell IW, Li MM (1991) Randomized trial of salbutamol in acute bronchiolitis. J Pediatr 118:807–811.

19. Gadomski AM, Lichenstein R, Horton L, King J, Keane V, Permutt T (1994) Efficacy of albuterol in the management of bronchiolitis. Pediatrics 93:907–912.
20. Schuh S, Johnson D, Canny G, et al (1992) Efficacy of adding nebulized ipratropium bromide to nebulized albuterol therapy in acute bronchiolitis. Pediatrics 90:920–923.
21. Tal A, Bavilski C, Yohai D, Bearman JE, Gorodischer R, Moses SW (1983) Dexamethasone and salbutamol in the treatment of acute wheezing in infants. Pediatrics 71:13–18.
22. Dabbous IA, Tkachyk JS, Stamm SJ (1966) A double blind study on the effects of corticosteroids in the treatment of bronchiolitis. Pediatrics 37:477–484.
23. Leer JA Jr, Green JL, Heimlich EM, et al (1969) Corticosteroids treatment in bronchiolitis. A controlled, collaborative study of 297 infants and children. Am J Dis Child 117:495–503.
24. Springer C, Bar-Yishay E, Uwayyed K, Avital A, Vilozni D, Godfrey S (1990) Corticosteroids do not affect the clinical or physiological status of infants with bronchiolitis. Pediatr Pulmonol 9:181–185.
25. Hemming VG, Prince GA, Groothuis JR, Siber GR (1995) Hyperimmune globulins in prevention and treatment of respiratory syncytial virus infections. Clin Microbiol Rev 8:22–33.
26. Hemming VG, Rodriguez W, Kim HW, et al (1987) Intravenous immunoglobulin treatment of respiratory syncytial virus infections in infants and young children. Antimicrob Agents Chemother 31:1882–1886.
27. Meissner HC, Fulton DR, Groothuis JR, et al (1993) Controlled trial to evaluate protection of high-risk infants against respiratory syncytial virus disease by using standard intravenous immune globulin. Antimicrob Agents Chemother 37:1655–1658.
28. Groothuis JR, Simoes EAF, Levin MJ, et al (1993) Prophylactic administration of respiratory syncytial virus immune globulin to high-risk infants and young children. N Engl J Med 329:1524–1530.
29. Wyde PR, Moore DK, Hepburn T, et al (1995) Evaluation of the protective efficacy of reshaped human monoclonal antibody RSHZ19 against respiratory syncy tial virus in cotton rats. Pediatr Res 38:543–550.

Pharmacology

Fetal Pharmacology and Therapy

E. Jacqz Aigrain

Introduction

Major progresses have been made in recent years in investigating fetal disorders. Echography now allows precise diagnosis of congenital malformations (such as digestive, urinary tract or cardiac abnormalities). Diagnosis of abnormal karyotype is possible with chorion biopsy, amniocentesis or fetal blood sampling. Such procedures have their own complications but their frequency is reduced in experienced hands. The therapeutic decision of whether to carry on pregnancy and to treat fetal diseases or to induce abortion is obviously a matter of individual cases and differences in legislation in various countries.

Clinicians may deal with a large variety of situations where the mother and the fetus are exposed to drugs and the evaluation of the risk to benefit ratio of drug administration during pregnancy remains often a challenge.

Obviously, the human teratogenic effects of thalidomide is demonstrated and the use of this drug is banished during pregnancy. In the case of retinoic acid, the drug is teratogenic in animal strains and human effects are established. Warfarin derivates cross the placenta during pregnancy and can induce fetal malformations and fetal hemorrhages by competing with vitamine K. Therefore, the administration of these drugs is contraindicated during pregnancy. Long term consequences of fetal exposure to drugs is unpredictable: the high incidence of vaginal adenocarcinoma developing in young women exposed to stilbestrol during pregnancy is a well-known example of possible delayed side-effects of drugs administered during pregnancy.

Apart from these drastic situations, clinicians are more frequently facing compromises, between either a mandatory maternal treatment and its potential fetal effects or the maternal and fetal side-effects when fetal treatment is required. Hypertension, life-threatening maternal arrhythmias or epilepsy are situations where maternal therapy is required, not only for maternal reasons but also for the possible fetal consequences of the maternal disease. Most practitioners are now aware of potential fetal risks, including teratogenic effects, fetal growth retardation and fetal and neonatal distress. Therefore, such treatments are associated with a close monitoring of the fetus.

Applications of fetal therapy are multiple. Our aims are to present some of the recent progresses in performing fetal diagnosis, in understanding the pharmacokinetics of drugs during pregnancy and in evaluating the risk to benefit ratios of these drugs in different areas of fetal therapy [1].

Pharmacokinetics During Pregnancy

Physiological Changes in the Mother

The physiological changes which occur during pregnancy in the mother can alter the uptake, distribution and metabolism of drugs which may be used to treat maternal, fetal or pregnancy associated diseases.

Absorption is modified by decreased intestinal motility and increased gastric emptying time. This may delay the time to peak concentration in the mother and either decrease or increase drug absorption.

Modifications in body weight and body fat, total body water and plasma proteins can alter the distribution of drugs and the amount of drug needed for therapeutic effectiveness.

Maternal hepatic and extrahepatic metabolism may be affected by hormonal changes and increase in hepatic blood flow.

Elimination of xenobiotics are modified by major changes in renal blood flow and glomerular filtration rate.

Placental Physiology

For ethical and procedural reasons, studies of physiology and metabolism of the placenta, as well as factors determining placental transfer are limited and have been conducted using term human placenta.

The physiology of the placenta changes throughout pregnancy: surface area increases, thickness of tissue layers decreases, the placenta can carry out oxidations in vitro. However, the metabolism of xenobiotics is less important than the biotransformation of endogenous substrates such as steroidal hormones.

Placental drug transfer is dependent on the physicochemical characteristics of drugs: most drugs have a molecular weight from 250 to 500 and cross the placenta easily. The rate of transfer is dependant upon: lipid solubility, degree of ionization measured by the P_K value, protein binding in the maternal and fetal circulation. Only the free and nonionized drug in the maternal circulation is available for transfer [2].

Drug Disposition in the Fetus [3]

Following their transfer across the placenta, drugs enter the umbilical vein. The umbilical venous blood flow is either diverted into the portal vein to perfuse the hepatic tissue or bypass the liver via the ductus venosus. This relative distribution between the two circulations may be of major importance in determining the quantity of drug reaching fetal tissues and in particular the central nervous system.

The human fetal liver is able to oxidize numerous substrates. Among cytochromes P450, CYP3A subfamily is present as early as twenty weeks' gestation. In contrast, CYP2D exhibits a perinatal ontogenesis and CYP1A a postnatal ontogenesis. Other factors affecting drug disposition in the fetus include: excretion by fetal kidney, swallowing of amniotic fluid. Some drugs accumulate in the amniotic fluid compartment after urine excretion and exchanges occur across the fetal skin.

In most cases, drugs exert their effects through interactions with receptor sites. Adrenergic receptor function develops early during fetal life. In addition, receptor interactions exist with digoxin, insulin and glucocorticoids. However, major differences between adults and fetuses have been reported in the number of receptors or in drug affinity for these receptors. Much more information is needed to understand the factors controlling drugs disposition and effects in the fetus.

Pharmacokinetics of Various Drugs during Pregnancy

The pharmacokinetics of many drugs are modified during pregnancy [1]. For ampicillin, the effect of increased rate of elimination and volume of distribution doubles the amount of drug needed to obtain the same plasma concentrations.

Caffeine is characterized by an increased volume of distribution and a decreased rate of elimination. Therefore, it is necessary to decrease the dose of caffeine throughout pregnancy to obtain the plasma concentration time that characterizes non pregnant women.

A pharmacokinetic study of digoxin administered intravenously in pregnant women receiving the drug for fetal supraventricular arrhythmia was performed [4]. Digoxin is mainly excreted unchanged by the kidney. During pregnancy, the systemic clearance of digoxin was increased, probably due to increased renal blood flow and glomerular filtration rate. As a consequence, elimination half-life was shortened. Using these informations the modalities of digoxin administration for the treatment of fetal arrhythmias was modified.

Examples of Medical Fetal Therapy

An historical example of fetal therapy is the maternal administration of penicillin for the treatment of fetal syphilis. But other examples could be given such as the use of maternal administered phenobarbital in late pregnancy for it's inductive effects on metabolizing enzymes, reducing hyperbilirubinemia in neonates. Recently, major improvements in investigational procedures, particularly the routine use of cord taps, increased the diagnostic and management potentials of life threatening fetal disorders becoming accessible to fetal treatment. Administration of intravenous gamma globulins increases the fetal platelet count in fetuses with alloimmune thrombocytopenia and reduces the risk of intracranial hemorrhage. Fetal blood transfusion are performed for the treatment of severe rhesus immunization (erythroblastosis fetalis). The efficiency of antenatal glucocorticoid therapy in reducing both the incidence of hyaline membrane disease and perinatal mortality is demonstrated.

The situations requiring fetal drug therapy are numerous and only some examples, classified in 1) high risk fetal diseases, 2) alterations in hormonal milieu, 3) treatment of maternofetal diseases of pregnancy are presented.

Treatment of High Risk Fetal Diseases

Treatment of Fetal Supraventricular Tachyarrhythmias

Fetal supraventricular tachyarrhythmias with normal cardiac anatomy are estimated to complicate the course of 1/10.000 pregnancies. The diagnosis, the mechanism and tolerance of the arrhythmia can be evaluated by M. Mode and doppler echocardiography. The prognosis is dependent on the cardiac function and risk of cardiac failure, the mechanism of the arrhythmia and the response to treatment.

Antiarrhythmic drugs are usually administered to the mother for fetal treatment. The choice between antiarrhythmic drugs is based on the efficacy of the drug and its pharmacokinetics during pregnancy, the potential maternal and fetal toxic effects [4].

The drug administered as first choice is usually digoxin and the control of the arrhythmia is obtained in 30 to 40% of cases. When return to sinus rhythm is not obtained, various second drugs are prescribed in association. Amiodarone or blockers are frequently used in France [4].

Flecainide is a promising antiarrhythmic drug for this indication. However, data on its use during pregnancy are limited, particularly the evaluation of maternal and fetal toxic effects.

The overall efficacy of treatment is over 80% in the few series available in the literature [4–6]. However, a large discrepancy is noted in terms of drugs and doses administered, due to differences in the prescription habits and in the analysis of benefit/risk ratios in various countries.

Treatment of Fetal Toxoplasmosis

Congenital toxoplasma infection is defined by the transmission of the parasite to the fetus and is dependant on the time of acquisition of maternal infection during pregnancy. The later maternal infection is acquired, the more frequently parasites are transmitted to the fetus, reaching 90% of transmission during the last weeks before delivery [7].

Congenital toxoplasmosis is defined by the clinical manifestations of the disease in the newborn. It is subclinical, mild or severe and depends on the age of the fetus at the time of transmission. The period of higher risk is between 10 and 24 weeks. It is known that most of the infants with congenital toxoplasmosis have major sequelae. In the early fifties at a time when treatment was not undertaken, the major sequelae among 105 children less than five years of age, were mental retardation (96%), convulsions (84%), impaired vision (61%) and deafness (15%).

Epidemiological surveys of the prevalence of specific antibodies in women in the child bearing age were conducted in 1960 and 1985 and demonstrate that the frequency of high-risk negative women varies widely between countries. The observed decrease in prevalence in France (87% in 1960–1970 and 73% in 1985) is probably related to changes in eating habits [7, 8].

Antenatal diagnosis of fetal toxoplasmosis is performed by fetal blood sampling, ultrasonography and amniocentesis. Specific diagnosis tests include demonstration of fetal toxoplasma IgM and presence of Toxoplasma Gondii in fetal blood amniotic fluid or both by inoculation into mice or tissue cultures. P.C.R. reaction tests on amniotic fluid are recent technics used to detect toxoplasmic DNA. They are rapid, highly specific and sensitive but need further evaluation [9].

The treatment of congenital toxoplasma infection is based on the administration of spiramycin and if the fetal infection is confirmed, an additional treatment with pyrimethamine and sulfadiazine is administered in 3 weeks courses alternating with 3 weeks of daily spiramycin [10].

Spiramycin is a macrolide antibiotic active against toxoplasma. This drug is known to concentrate in the placenta. Under the recommended dose of 3 mg daily, plasma concentrations are 1.7, 0.8 and 6.2 mg per microliters in the mother, fetus and placenta with a fetal to maternal ratio of 0.5. The incidence of fetal toxoplasmosis is reduced from 60% to 23% by spiramycin administration. This effect may reflect a limitation of placental infection and transplacental passage to the fetus [11].

Pyrimethamine is a folic acid antagonist and sulfadiazine is a sulfonamide. They act synergistically against toxoplasma as demonstrated by their combined activity which is eight times what would be expected if their effects were additive.

A large survey of 1.270 referred cases of acquired maternal toxoplasma infection during pregnancy [12] demonstrated 89 fetal infections in 86 pregnancies with a overall fetal risk of 7%. The time of fetal infection varied from the periconceptional period to the third trimester of pregnancy. 34 terminations of pregnancy were performed on parent's request according to the French law. Comparison of spiramycin alone versus courses of pyrimethamine-sulfamines alternating with courses of spiramycin demonstrates a lower incidence of positive placenta and IgM in cord blood at birth in the second group of patients. In addition, progresses in fetal diagnosis and treatment improved infant outcome. The outcome of liveborn infants with congenital toxoplasma infection of the first, second or third trimester of pregnancy has been analyzed over two periods: 1972–1981 and 1982–1988 [12]. The severity of the infection is decreased during the second period whatever the time of infection, with predominance of subclinic infection and disappearance of severe forms of infection. This is particularly clear for fetal infection which occurred during the second trimester: severe forms were 18% on 62 cases during the period 1972–1981 and none in 43 cases during the period 1982–1988.

Pyrimethamine and sulfadiazine are both potentially toxic. Sulfonamides may induce hypersensitivity and pyrimethamine exhibits dose related toxicity inducing platelet depression and leukopenia. In addition teratogenic effects are reported in rats, but their frequency seems to be reduced by the co-administration of folinic acid. Very little is known on the pharmacology of the association during pregnancy [10].

Future tools in the fetal treatment of congenital toxoplasmosis include to improve the reliability of prenatal diagnosis, particularly using P.C.R and to conduct large trials of treated patients to analyze maternal and fetal tolerance of treatment.

Alterations in Fetal Hormonal Milieu

Fetal Treatment of Congenital Adrenal Hyperplasia (CAH)

The sexual differentiation occurs very early in male fetuses under the influence of testosterone. In contrast, sexual differentiation occurs later and is not stimulated by any hormones in female fetuses. As early as 7 week's gestation circulating concentrations of testosterone are higher in male than in female fetuses but the peak concentration of testosterone occurs at 17 week's gestation.

The congenital adrenal hyperplasia (CAH) is related in most cases (>90%) to a deficit in steroid 21 hydroxylase, leading to overproduction of D4 epiandrosterone and testosterone. 21 hydroxylase deficiency is transmitted as an autosomal recessive trait. The "classic form" causes ambiguous external genitalia in females with or without salt wasting. But there is also a "wild-late, form" causing symptoms of masculinization at puberty and infertility.

The prenatal treatment of congenital adrenal hyperplasia due to 21 hydroxylase deficiency is instituted with the aim of preventing the in utero virilization of CAH affected female fetuses which is caused by overproduction of adrenal androgens.

Fetal adrenal suppression is based on maternal administrated glucocorticoids that induce suppression of the increased adrenocorticotropin (ACTH) levels by the fetal pituitary-adrenal axis. It must be started early, before 7 week's gestation and therefore, before the possible antenatal diagnosis of CAH in an high risk mother, and either continued until term in case of a CAH female or stopped in the other cases.

Until recently, prenatal diagnosis was made in females after amniocentesis at sixteen to eighteen week's pregnancy. It was based on informations provided by an index case, using HLA typing. Prenatal diagnosis is now made earlier during pregnancy, by direct molecular studies of the 21 hydroxylase genes on chorionic villus biopsies [13].

If the baby is affected, treatment is maintained throughout pregnancy. Concentrations of several steroids including 17 hydroxyprogesterone and adrenal androgens are determined in order to verify fetal adrenal gland suppression [14].

It is now admitted that the first choice drug for the treatment of CAH is dexamethasone. The drug is not inactivated by the placenta, but crosses the placenta with a fetal to maternal ratio near unity. It is not linked with transcortin, had a long half life of 4 to 6 hours.

The administered dose was initially 1 mg/day but was increased to 1.5 mg/day in 2 to 3 divided doses. The minimal effective dose is required. The analysis of failures of antenatal treatment in the literature suggests that they may be related to low doses, sometimes administered once daily, late initiation or interruption of treatment and individual variations in dexamethasone disposition during pregnancy. The maternal side-effects of treatment are very limited and the benefits of treatment clearly outweigh the risks [15].

Treatment of Fetal Dysthyroidism

The development of the fetal thyroid function begins during the tenth week of gestation [16]. Fetal thyroid function during pregnancy can be evaluated by ultrasound examination and measurement of thyroid hormones in cord blood. The treatment of fetal hyperthyroidism is based on maternal administration of antithyroid drugs which easily cross the placenta. Fetal hypothyroidism with goiter was successfully diagnosed in utero by obstetrical ultrasound revealing a goiter. Congenital hypothyroidism occurs with a incidence of 1/4.000 and 1/5.000 and only 10 to 20% may be attributed to dyshormonogenesis. Intra-amniotic administration of levothyroxine sodium (T4) every 2 weeks increased fetal concentrations of T4 and decreased fetal concentrations of TSH. The usefulness of such treatment is to be evaluated. However, it may reduce the central nervous system deficits and the specific defects in hearing and speech associated with late post-natal treatment [17].

Treatment of Maternofetal Diseases. The Use of Non Steroidal Anti-Inflammatory Agents During Pregnancy

Non steroidal anti-inflammatory agents are inhibitors of prostaglandin synthesis. They are administered to pregnant women to treat various diseases. Acetyl salicylic acid is currently administered to prevent idiopathic fetal growth retardation of vascular origin. Indomethacin is prescribed to try to stop premature labor and to reduce polyhydramnios.

The Role of Prostaglandins During Pregnancy – Pharmacology of Non Steroidal Anti-Inflammatory Agents

Various chemical, physical, neuronal and hormonal factors can stimulate the synthesis of prostaglandins. Phospholipase A_2 is activated and this enzyme is regarded as the limiting step in the rate of synthesis. It cleaves from the phospholipids of the cell membranes the precursors for prostaglandin synthesis, e.g., arachidonic acid. In the next step a membrane bound enzyme complex, "prostaglandin synthetase or cyclo-oxygenase", catalyzes the formation of endoperoxides, PGG_2 and PGH_2 from the precursor fatty acids. Endoperoxides are then transformed to prostaglandins by peroxidase or endoperoxide isomerase. The same endoperoxides are also changed to thromboxane A_2 and PGI_2 (called prostacyclin or PGX). PGI_2 is a potent vasodilator and anti-aggregatory agent formed by the endothelial wall, while thromboxane A_2 is formed in platelets and is a vasoconstrictor and aggregatory agent.

During pregnancy, the production of prostacyclin and thromboxane A_2 increases in the mother and in the feto-placental tissues. They play a major role in the regulation of: maternal vascular tone, placental and fetal circulation (placenta, umbilical blood flow, ductus arteriosus), uterine contractility and induction of labor [18].

Aspirin is known to irreversibly acetylating and therefore inactivating cyclo-oxygenase while indomethacin is a competitive inhibitor of the enzyme. Aspirin is extensively protein bound and during pregnancy, crosses the placenta. The fetal to maternal ratio of aspirin was reported to be over 1.5 at birth and is related to the binding characteristics of fetal serum. Indomethacin is highly absorbed and protein-bound. It is metabolized by the liver and excreted by the kidney. Its elimination half-life is longer in neonates than in adults.

Aspirin and Idiopathic Fetal Growth Retardation

Idiopathic fetal growth retardation is associated with reduced uteroplacental perfusion, abnormal platelet behavior and local thrombosis resulting in placental infarction. In vitro platelet cyclo-oxygenase is more sensitive to inhibition by low doses aspirin than is vascular endothelial cyclo-oxygenase. Maternal serum levels of 6 keto $PGF_{1\alpha}$ and thromboxane B_2, which are the inactive metabolites of prostacyclin and thromboxane A_2 were measured after one and two weeks administration of various doses of aspirin. Thromboxane B_2 generated by maternal blood during clotting was decreased while 6 keto $PGF_{1\alpha}$ levels were not affected by aspirin although they tend to decrease during treatment in the groups receiving 60 mg and 80 mg aspirin. Therefore, low-dose aspirin may direct prostacyclin/thromboxane balance to the dominance for prostacyclin [19].

Many studies have been conducted since 1978 to treat pre-eclampsia and other chronic insufficiency syndromes [20, 21]. The inclusion criteria were initially a past history of pregnancy complicated with severe fetal growth retardation, placental infarction, idiopathic fetal growth retardation, fetal or neonatal death, or pregnancy induced hypertension.

Low doses aspirin in most cases 150 mg/day, were administered daily associated with dipyridamole in some cases. In all the published studies, the incidence of intra-uterine growth retardation was reduced, the birth weight was higher and the incidence of fetal death, eclampsia and pre-eclampsia, reduced even if it did not reach statistical significance in some studies. The Epreda trial is an European controlled randomized double blind trial including 319 women with either 1 (220 patients) or 2 (103 patients) of previous fetal growth retardation or hypertension induced complication. This study demonstrated that low doses aspirin has a preventive effect on recurrent fetal growth retardation or fetal death in high-risk mothers [20].

Conclusion

There are many other indications of drug administration during pregnancy for fetal treatment. In most cases, major questions remain to be elucidated and fetal drug therapy will benefit of investigations conducted in the following areas: investigations of normal and pathological fetal development using non invasive procedures, development of pharmacokinetic modelling for fetal drug therapy, evaluation of non invasive versus invasive drug administration, evaluation of the immediate benefit and the immediate and long term risks of treatment by large clinical trials, validation of animal models for toxicity and teratogenicity. In addition, the possible implications of pharmacogenetics in the fetal side-effects of drugs, including teratogenic effects remain to be investigated. The initial study performed by Spielberg in Toronto, using an "in vitro cytotoxic assay" demonstrated that a genetic predisposition was associated with the major birth-defects complicating the treatment with phenytoin during pregnancy [22]. This certainly is an area of future research on fetal pharmacology and therapy.

References

1. Ward RM (1995) Pharmacological treatment of the fetus. Clinical pharmacokinetic considerations. Clin Pharmacokinet 28:343–350.
2. Pacifici GM, Nottoli R (1995) Placental transfer of drugs administered to mothers. Clin Pharmacokinet 28:235–269.
3. Levy G (1981) Pharmacokinetics of fetal and neonatal exposure to drugs. Obstet Gynecol 58:9S–16S.
4. Azancot Benisty A, Jacqz Aigrain E, Guirgis NM, De Crepy A, Oury JF, Blot P (1992) Clinical and pharmacological study of fetal supraventricular tachyarrhythmias. J Pediatr 121:608–613.
5. Maxwell DJ, Crawford DC, Curry PVM, Tynan MJ, Allan LD (1988) Obstetric importance, diagnosis and management of fetal tachycardias. BMJ 297:107–110.

6. VanEngelen AD, Weijtens O, Brenner JI, Kleinman CS, Copel JA, Stoutenbeek P, Meijboom EJ (1994) Management outcome and follow-up of fetal tachycardia. J Am Coll Cardiol 24:1371–1375.
7. Dupouy Camet J, Gavinet MF, Paugam A, Tourte-Schaefer C (1993) Mode de contamination, incidence et prevalence de la toxoplasmose. Med Mal Inf 23:139–147.
8. Wong SY, Remington JS (1994) Toxoplasmosis during pregnancy. Clin Infect Dis 18:853–862.
9. Hohfeld P, Daffos F, Costa JM, Thulliez P, Forestier F, Vidaud M (1994) Prenatal diagnosis of congenital toxoplasmosis with a polymerase chain reaction test on amniotic fluid. N Eng J Med 331:695–699.
10. Wilson CB (1990) Treatment of congenital toxoplasmosis during pregnancy. J Pediatr 116:1003–1004.
11. Couvreur J, Desmonts G, Thulliez P (1988) Prophylaxis of congenital toxoplasmosis: effects of spiramycin on placental infection. J Antimicrob Chemother 22:193–200.
12. Hohfeld P, Daffos F, Thulliez P, Aufrant C, Couvreur J, MacAleese J, Descombey D, Forestier F (1989) Fetal toxoplasmosis: outcome of pregnancy and infant follow-up after in utero treatment. J Pediatr 115:765–769.
13. Morel Y, Miller WL (1991) Clinical and molecular genetics of congenital adrenal hyperplasia due to 21-hydroxylase deficiency. Adv Hum Genet 20:1–68.
14. Forest MG, David M, Morel Y (1993) Prenatal diagnosis and treatment of 21-hydroxylase deficiency. J Steroid Biochem Mol Biol 45:75–82.
15. Forest MG, Dörr HG (1993) Prenatal treatment of congenital adrenal hyperplasia (CAH) due to 21-hydroxylase deficiency: European experience in 223 pregnancies at risk. Pediatr Res 33:S3.
16. Burrow GN, Fisher DA, Larsen PR (1994) Maternal and thyroid function. N Engl J Med 331:1072–1078.
17. Perelman AH, Johnson RL, Clemons RD, Finberg HJ, Clewell WH, Trujillo L (1990) Intrauterine diagnosis and treatment of fetal goitrous hypothyroidism. J Clin Endocrinol Metab 71:618–621.
18. Friedman SA (1988) Pre-eclampsia: a review of the role of prostaglandins. Obstet Gynecol 71:1.
19. Schiff E, Peleg E (1989) The use of aspirin to prevent pregnancy induced hypertension and lower the ratio of thromboxane A_2 to prostacyclin in relatively high risk pregnancies. N Engl J Med 321:351–356.
20. Uzan S, Beaufils M (1989) Idiopathic recurrent fetal growth retardation and aspirin-dipyridamole therapy. Am J Obstet Gynecol 160:763–764.
21. Wallenburgh HCS, Rotmans N (1987) Prevention of recurrent idiopathic fetal growth retardation by low dose aspirin and dipyridamole. Am J Obstet Gynecol 157:1230–1235.
22. Spielberg SP, Strickler SM, Miller MA, Andermann E, Dansky LV, Seni MH (1985) Genetic predisposition to phenytoin-induced birth defects. Lancet pp: 746.

Principles of Neonatal Pharmacology

C. M. A. Rademaker, A. Fleer and J. N. van den Anker

Introduction

The pharmacologic behavior of drugs administered to newborns shows unique characteristics which in general cannot be extrapolated from data derived from older infants and adults. Rapidly changing physiological processes characteristic of the neonatal period may profoundly affect the pharmacokinetics of drugs and result either in subtherapeutic or toxic drug concentrations. Therefore, the pharmacokinetics but also the safety and efficacy of drugs need to be determined by trials specifically designed to include term and preterm infants. Since the 1950s investigators have reported serious side effects associated with the inadvertent use of drugs in newborns. Sulfonamides displaced bilirubin from albumin-binding sites which resulted in an increased incidence of kernicterus in preterm infants. The "grey baby syndrome" was described in three newborns treated with chloramphenicol. The occurrence of cardiovascular collapse and shock in these neonates was due to the accumulation of free drug caused by deficient glucuronidation in the presence of a reduction in glomerular filtration. More recent examples of the consequences of ignorance about the unique transitional metabolic and physiological characteristics of neonates are easily found. These include poisoning of very low birth weight infants by inadvertent exposure to toxic doses of benzyl alcohol contained in bacteriostatic water or saline used to reconstitute medications or to flush intravascular catheters, and the excessive mortality associated with the intravenous administration of vitamin E to low birth weight infants. As a result of these adverse experiences both the pharmaceutical industry and pediatricians have become more careful with the introduction of new compounds in neonates. They have recognized that rational drug therapy for newborns is often confounded by a combination of poorly understood pharmacokinetic and pharmacodynamic interactions [1]. However, new drugs are currently still introduced into neonatal intensive care units, even though most of these have neither been tested in neonatal animals nor studied in human infants. In addition most studies on pharmacokinetics, safety and efficacy of drugs in newborns have only included term infants. Nowadays neonatal intensive care units are increasingly occupied with preterm infants with gestational ages of less than 32 weeks and a birth weight below 1500 g. Even pharmacokinetic data on commonly used drugs such as penicillin G, flucloxacillin, dobutamine and tolazoline are not available in these infants.

Effective and safe drug therapy requires a thorough understanding of human developmental biology and of the dynamic ontogeny of drug absorption, drug disposition, drug metabolism, and drug excretion. It is apparent that maturation of organ system function and changes in body composition during gestation and during the neonatal period exert a significant effect on the disposition of drugs. Hence, specific dosage recommendations are required for newborn infants.

Clinical Pharmacokinetics

Pharmacokinetics is the mathematical description of the biologic rate processes in the body by which drug concentrations are altered. This includes the study of the plasma concentration versus time course of a drug after its administration and the development of mathematical models to predict these concentrations. Knowledge of a drug's physicochemical and pharmacokinetic properties allows the clinician to predict plasma concentrations at any given time after administration and to make fairly reliable estimates of the magnitude and duration of drug response. The application of pharmacokinetic principles provides an invaluable tool that will lead to optimal drug therapy in the individual patient.

Four pharmacokinetic parameters are critical to the characterization of plasma concentrations after drug administration and hence necessary for the determination of appropriate drug dosing regimens: systemic availability, volume of distribution, clearance, and half-life.

Systemic Availability

In order to accurately predict plasma concentrations and clinical response after administration of a drug to a patient, it is necessary to know the exact amount of drug in the body, i.e. the systemic availability. Administration by an intravenous bolus is assumed to provide 100 percent systemic availability. The systemic availability of other routes of administration is commonly calculated from the comparison of plasma concentration following administration of a single dose by intravascular and extravascular routes.

Volume of Distribution

Drugs will not remain exclusively in the blood but may distribute into various tissues and other fluids. The rate at which a particular tissue-plasma concentration equilibrium is achieved depends on the blood perfusion to the organ. The extent to which a drug distributes extravascularly depends on its lipophilicity and its affinity for plasma and tissue proteins. The parameter volume of distribution (V) is used to identify the proportionality factor relating the amount of drug in the body (A) with the blood or plasma concentration (C). This can be expressed with use of the following equation:

$$A = V \cdot C.$$

Volume of distribution does not represent a true physiological volume. The volume of distribution of a drug that is highly bound to plasma proteins with no significant tissue binding is equal to the volume of distribution of albumin. If a drug has a very low affinity for plasma proteins, the minimum volume of distribution would equal the extracellular fluid space. There is no upper limit for volume of distribution, and calculation of the volume of distribution frequently exceeds total body water. This would indicate significant storage of the drug in peripheral tissue sites.

Clearance

Just as volume of distribution relates the amount of drug in the body to the plasma concentration, body clearance refers to the proportionality factor between the rate of elimination of the drug from the body and the plasma or blood concentration. Body clearance is a more precise measurement of the body's ability to eliminate drugs than half-life because it has a physiological basis. It directly reflects physiological processes of elimination. Clearance does not measure the quantity of drug eliminated by the body, but it quantifies the volume of blood or plasma that can be completely cleared of drug per unit time. Clearance is the most important pharmacokinetic parameter for calculation of maintenance doses. The kidney and liver are the major routes of elimination for most drugs. Renal clearance depends on renal blood flow, plasma drug protein binding, and glomerular filtration, tubular secretion and reabsorption. Similarly, hepatic clearance depends on the hepatic blood flow, plasma drug protein binding, and the intrinsic capability of the liver to metabolize a drug.

Half-Life

The half-life ($t_{1/2}$) of a drug is defined as the amount of time necessary to decrease plasma drug concentrations by 50 percent. In order to be eliminated from the body, a drug must be present in the plasma without being bound to proteins. Plasma half-life depends on the physiologically based parameters volume of distribution and total body clearance (CL). This can be expressed with use of the following equation: $t_{1/2} = 0.693.V/CL$. Although half-life is not an independent pharmacokinetic parameter, it is an useful estimation of the time required to eliminate the drug entirely from the body, as well as the time needed to reach steady state during a multiple dosing regimen.

Developmental Physiology and Drug Disposition

Disposition of drugs in preterm infants differs substantially from that in term infants as a result of differences in absorption, distribution, biotransformation, and excretion [1]. The unique characteristics of these processes in the small preterm infant are briefly reviewed below.

Drug Absorption

Absorption refers to the translocation of a drug from its site of administration into the bloodstream. Absorption of drugs from the gastrointestinal tract, skin, or an intramuscular injection site is significantly different in newborns as compared to older children and adults. The gastric and duodenal pH, gastro-intestinal motility, the maturational state of intestinal mucosa, concomitant feedings and fluctuating gastro-intestinal perfusion have been implicated as factors contributing to the variability in the gastrointestinal absorption of enterally administered drugs [2, 3].

Gastric Acid Production

An acidic pH favors absorption of acidic drugs because in such an environment the drug will be largely in an un-ionized, more lipid-soluble form. However, on the other hand an acidic pH also will lead to a rapid degradation of for instance penicillins and erythromycin. A relatively high pH, as in states of achlorhydria, will enhance the absorption of basic drugs. For instance during hypochlorhydria the absorption of penicillin, ampicillin, nafcillin and erythromycin is enhanced, whereas the oral absorption of phenobarbitone, diphenylhydantoin, nalidixic acid, acetaminophen, rifampicin and ketoconazole is reduced.

Gastric Emptying

Gastric emptying rate during the neonatal period is prolonged relative to that of the adult. It is directly affected by gestational and postnatal age, as well as the type of feeding used [4]. Gastric emptying time appears to approach adult values within the first 6–8 months of life. Since most orally administered drugs are absorbed in the small intestine, the rate of gastric emptying is an important determinant of the rate and extent of drug absorption.

If gastric emptying is prolonged, the decreased rate of intestinal drug absorption will lead to lowering of the peak serum drug concentration.

In summary, the relatively high gastric pH, a prolonged gastric emptying, the presence or absence of food, and underlying diseases of the newborn will influence the gastrointestinal absorption of drugs. This variability and the limited data on the bioavailability of enterally administered drugs have restricted oral administration of many compounds in the preterm infant [5, 6].

Transdermal absorption is increased in the preterm infant because of the relatively thin layer of epidermal tissue at birth. In the past this has resulted in intoxications. More recently attention has been given to potential beneficial effects. In a study of Evans et al. [7] therapeutic concentrations of theophylline were obtained after topical application of theophylline gel in preterm infants.

The systemic absorption of many intramuscularly administered drugs in newborns who are hemodynamically stable results in a similar therapeutic efficacy as intravenous administration [8]. However, the clinical condition of the patient must be taken into account since hemodynamically unstable newborns may lack adequate tissue perfusion to effectively absorb drugs given by the intramuscular route. In addition muscle activity may affect the rate of absorption and consequently the peak serum concentration of a drug. Sick, immobile newborns or those receiving a paralyzing agent such as vecuronium may show reduced absorption rates after intramuscular drug administration. Finally, intramuscular administration of drugs in very low birth weight infants is not practical because of their small muscle mass. Therefore intravenous administration remains the main route for drug therapy in this patient population.

Drug Distribution

The movement of drugs and other compounds from the systemic circulation into various body compartments, tissues, and cells is termed distribution. The distribution of most drugs in the body is influenced by several age-dependent factors including protein binding, body compartment size, hemodynamic factors e.g. cardiac output and regional blood flow, and membrane permeability [9].

Protein Binding

The serum protein binding of drugs is dependent on the amount of binding proteins, the affinity constant of the drug for the protein, the number of available binding sites, and the presence of pathophysiological conditions or endogenous compounds which may alter the drug protein binding interaction. Acidic and uncharged compounds are primarily bound by albumin. Basic drugs bind to albumin, alpha-1-acid glycoprotein and lipoprotein [1]. Albumin concentrations are lower in term infants than in older children and adults and are further reduced with increasing prematurity. Plasma concentrations of alpha-1-acid glycoprotein are significantly lower in term infants than in normal adults and are even lower in premature infants. Substantial differences exist between the degree of drug–protein binding for various agents in newborn and adult serum. Increased concentrations of unbound drug have been reported in neonatal or fetal plasma samples of antibiotics such as ampicillin, benzylpenicillin, chloramphenicol and sulfonamides [1].

Consequently the therapeutic and adverse effects of the drug may be accentuated.

Protein binding may also be affected by endogenous competitors for binding sites. There are a number of endogenous molecules such as bilirubin which may bind to plasma proteins [9, 10]. These may displace drugs from binding sites, and at least transiently increase the apparent volume of distribution of the drug. More importantly, the increase in the fraction of free drug, which occurs because of the displacement reaction, may result in a transiently enhanced pharmacological response. However, a clinically important protein binding displacement reaction will only occur if a drug is more than 80 to 90% protein bound. Endogenous molecules may displace drugs from their binding sites, but there are also drugs which can displace endogenous molecules from their binding sites. This may lead to unacceptable high levels of for instance bilirubin with the potential risk of increasing the incidence of kernicterus. Antibiotics that have been shown to significantly displace bilirubin from albumin-binding sites include sulfonamides, moxalactam, cefoperazone and ceftriaxone [11].

Body Water Compartment Sizes

Age dependent changes in the composition of various fluid compartments have recently been reviewed. Total body water comprises nearly 92% of body weight in the young fetus, with the extracellular fluid volume accounting for 65% of body weight, and the intracellular fluid volume responsible for 25% of body weight. Body fat comprises less than 1%. At term total body water falls to approximately 75% of body weight, and the amount of fat increases to approximately 15%. Measurements of extracellular fluid volume ranged from 350 to 440 mL/kg body weight in neonates after a 40 week gestation. As a consequence, the intracellular volume increases from 25% of body weight in the young fetus to 33% at birth.

In addition there is a 8 to 15% reduction of body weight during the first 3 to 5 days after birth. This weight loss is due to mobilization of both intracellular and extracellular fluid through urinary and transepidermal losses, and tissue loss due to low calory intake.

These issues may have important implications for optimal drug use in the tiny infant. Attainment of the same peak serum concentration of drugs which are primarily distributed in the extracellular fluid space may require twice the relative dose, on mg/kg basis, because the very low birth weight preterm infant has an extracellular fluid compartment more than twice the relative size of that of an adult. In contrast, a much smaller apparent volume of distribution would be expected for highly lipophilic compounds in the very low birth weight premature infant. In addition rapid changes in body composition, especially over the first days of life, may complicate pharmacokinetic calculations.

Drug Metabolism

The primary organ for drug metabolism is the liver, but the kidneys, intestines, lungs and skin are also capable of biotransformation. Metabolites of most drugs are generally pharmacologically weak or inactive but parent compounds may be transformed into active metabolites. Furthermore, pharmacologically inactive compounds may be converted to their active moiety. The first step in drug metabolism is uptake of the drug by the metabolizing cell. Ligandin, or Y-protein, is a basic protein that binds bilirubin and organic anions such as drugs. It is present in hepatocytes, as well as in proximal renal tubular cells and nongoblet, small intestinal mucosal cells. The concentration of ligandin in the fetus and neonate is low but appears to approach adult values during the first 5–10 days of postnatal life [12]. Thus it is likely that the hepatic clearance of capacity-limited drugs will be lower in neonates than in older infants and children. Drug biotransformation within the hepatocyte involves two primary enzymatic processes: phase I, or nonsynthetic, and phase II, or synthetic, reactions.

Phase I Reactions

Phase I biotransformation reactions, which include oxidation, reduction, hydrolysis and hydroxylation, transform compounds into more polar, less lipid-soluble molecules that may be more rapidly eliminated in the urine or bile. The hepatic cytochrome P450 oxidase system is responsible for many of the phase I reactions in the human liver. In the newborn the activity of the oxidative enzyme systems is markedly reduced. Although this system matures rapidly after delivery at term, the rapidity of maturation in premature infants is unknown [13]. Hydroxylation is decreased in both preterm and term newborns, and the activities of alcohol dehydrogenase and aromatic nitro reduction pathways are very low in both fetuses and neonates. In addition esterase activity, responsible for hydrolysis of chloramphenicol, is very low in the fetus and the neonate [14].

Phase II Reactions

Phase II reactions, or conjugation reactions, synthesize more water-soluble com-pounds by combining a substance with an endogenous molecule in order to enhance excretion of that substance. Glucuronide, sulfate, and glycine are the common endogenous molecules to which drugs are bound. A drug must possess a specific functional group, such as a carboxyl, hydroxyl, amino, or sulphydryl group, in order to be conjugated. Alternatively, a drug may acquire one of these functional groups by undergoing phase I reactions.

Glucuronidation is the most common conjugation pathway, but it is also the most deficient immediately after birth. In contrast, conjugation to sulfate or glycine does not appear to be decreased in the neonatal period, and methylation reactions, which are generally insignificant in adults, have a prominent role in drug metabolism during the neonatal period [14]. In 2- to 3-day old infants a limited ability to conjugate paracetamol with glucuronide was demonstrated. However this was compensated for by a well developed sulfation pathway [15].

Drug Excretion

Most drugs (aminoglycosides, penicillins, third generation cephalosporins, vancomycin) or their metabolites are excreted from the body by the kidneys. Renal excretion is dependent on glomerular filtration, tubular reabsorption, and tubular secretion. At birth, renal function is limited, because the kidney is anatomically and functionally immature [16–18]. The main factors involved in the development of renal function are the gestational age and the dramatic sequential hemodynamic changes in a situation initially dominated by high vascular resistance and extremely low blood flow. At birth the glomerular filtration rate (GFR) is 2 to 4 mL/min in term neonates and it may be as low as 0.6 to 0.8 mL/min in preterm infants. The increase in GFR after birth is important and usually greater in term than in preterm infants [16,17,19]. The increase is due to the increase in cardiac output which is associated with specific changes in renal vascular resistances resulting in an increase in renal blood flow, changes in renal blood flow distribution, and a higher permeability of the glomerular membrane.

The clinical implications for the maturation of GFR become apparent when one considers drugs that are primarily eliminated by glomerular filtration. Recent studies have investigated the pharmacokinetics of cephalosporins and penicillins in preterm infants [20, 21, 22]. It was shown that the clearance of ceftazidime and amoxicillin increased significantly with increasing gestational age. The clearance was significantly decreased after prenatal exposure to indomethacin [20]. For preterm infants with gestational age of less than 32 weeks the authors recommend dosage adjustments during the first days of life, and additional dosage adjustments are indicated in prematures who are prenatally exposed to indomethacin.

The low GFR may be partially compensated for by a relatively greater reduction in tubular reabsorption. This may be due to the relative immaturity of the renal tubule. Generally, the clearance of drugs such as gentamicin follows the renal maturation [23]. Tubular secretory function is low compared with adults. Reasons for the reduced transport capacity are the low blood flow in peritubular regions, the immaturity of energy-supplying processes, the small mass of working tubular cells, and the small size of as yet undeveloped tubuli. A similarly low capacity has been reported for drugs such as penicillins and sulfonamides.

Conclusion

Available data on drug biodisposition and action in the neonate have increased during the last years, but pharmacokinetic-pharmacodynamic interactions for many commonly used drugs in the neonatal period remain poorly understood. Absorption, distribution, metabolism and excretion of drugs in preterm infants are significantly different from those in fullterm infants and older children. The bioavailability of enterally administered drugs in preterm infants is unreliable and this route of administration should be restricted. The reduced renal elimination in neonates affects the disposition of many drugs. The rapid development of renal clearing capacity during the first month of life therefore requires continuous monitoring and dosage adjustment of drugs that are dependent on renal elimination.

Finally, the development of dosing strategies should at least take into account variables such as gestational age, postnatal age, concomitant pre- or postnatal exposure to different drugs (eg. betamethasone, indomethacin), perinatal asphyxia, and respiratory difficulties.

References

1. Besunder JB, Reed MD, Blumer JL (1988) Principles of drug biodisposition in the neonate: A critical evaluation of the pharmacokinetic-pharmacodynamic interface (Part I). Clin Pharmacokinet 14:189–216.
2. Hyman PE, Feldman EJ, Ament ME, Byrne WJ, Euler AR (1983) Effect of external feeding on the maintenance of gastric acid secretory function. Gastroenterology 84:341–345.
3. Hyman PE, Clarke DD, Everett SL, et al (1983) Gastric acid secretory function in preterm infants. J Pediatr 106:467–471.
4. Cavell B (1981) Gastric emptying in infants fed human milk or infant formula. Acta Paediatr Scand 70:639–641.
5. Paap CM, Nahata MC (1990) Clinical pharmacokinetics of antibacterial drugs in neonates. Clin Pharmacokinet 19:280–318.
6. Prober CG, Stevenson DK, Benitz WE (1990) The use of antibiotics in neonates weighing less than 1200 grams. Pediatr Infect Dis J 9:111–121.
7. Evans NJ, Rutter N, Hadgraft J, Parr G (1985) Percutaneous administration of theophylline in the preterm infant. J Pediatr 107:307–311.
8. Mulhall A (1985) Antibiotic treatment of neonates – does route of administration matter? Dev Pharmacol Ther 8:1–8.
9. Radde IC (1985) Mechanisms of drug absorption and their development. In: MacLeod SM, Radde IC. Textbook of pediatric clinical pharmacology. Littleton, MA: PSG, 17–31.
10. Rane A, Wilson JT (1976) Clinical pharmacokinetics in infants and children. Clin Pharmacokinet 1:2–24.
11. Robertson A, Fink S, Karp W (1988) Effect of cephalosporins on bilirubin–albumin binding. J Pediatr 112:291–294.
12. Boreus LO (1982) Principles of pediatric pharmacology. In Azarnoff DL (Ed.) Monographs in clinical pharmacology, vol 6, pp. 48–49 and p. 106, Churchill Livingstone, New York.
13. Neims AH, Warner M, Loughnan PM, Aranda JV (1976) Developmental aspects of the hepatic cytochrome P450 monooxygenase system. Annu Rev Pharmacol Toxicol 16:427–445.
14. Juchau MR, Chao ST, Omiecinski CJ (1980) Drug metabolism by the human fetus. Clin Pharmacokinet 5:320–339.

15. Levy G, Khanna NN, Soda DM, Tsuzuki O, Stern L (1975) Pharmacokinetics of acetaminophen in the human neonate: formation of acetaminophen glucuronide and sulfate in relation to plasma bilirubin concentartion and D-glucaric acid excretion. Pediatrics 55:818–825.
16. Guignard JP, Torado A, Da Cunha O, Gautier E (1975) Glomerular filtration rate in the first three weeks of life. J Pediatr 87:268–272.
17. Leake RD, Trygstad CW (1977) Glomerular filtration rate during the period of adaptation to extrauterine life. Pediatr Res 11:959–962.
18. Van der Heijden AJ, Grose WF, Ambagtsheer JJ, Provoost AP, Wolff ED, Sauer PJ (1988) Glomerular filtration rate in the preterm infant: the relation to gestational and postnatal age. Eur J Pediatr 148:24–28.
19. Van den Anker JN, Hop WCJ, De Groot R et al (1994) Effects of prenatal exposure to betamethasone and indomethacin on the glomerular filtration rate in the preterm infant. Pediatr Res 36:578–581.
20. Van den Anker JN, Schoemaker RC, Hop WCJ, et al (1995) Ceftazidime pharmacokinetics in preterm infants: effects of renal function and gestational age. Clin Pharmacol Ther 58:650–659.
21. Van den Anker JN, Schoemaker RC, Van der Heijden AJ, Broerse HM, Neijens HJ, De Groot R (1995) Once-daily versus twice-daily administration of ceftazidime in the preterm infant. Antimicrob Agents Chemother 39:2048–2050.
22. Huisman-de Boer JJ, Van den Anker JN, Vogel M, Goessens WHF, Schoemaker RC, De Groot R (1995) Antimicrob Agents Chemother 39:431–434.
23. Koren G, James A, Perlman M (1985) A simple method for the estimation of glomerular filtration rate by gentamicin pharmacokinetics during routine drug monitoring in the newborn. Clin Pharmacol Ther 38:680–685.

Drug Metabolism in the Neonate and Young Infant

G. L. Kearns and J. N. van den Anker

Introduction

Over the past two decades, pharmacokinetic data clearly demonstrate that development can markedly influence the absorption, distribution, excretion and metabolism of xenobiotics. With respect to many of the processes which govern drug metabolism, the underlying pharmacogenetic determinants which may control either the affinity and/or capacity of a drug/toxicant substrate for the enzyme(s) responsible for its biotransformation appear to be altered as a function of development by mechanisms that are, for the most part, not well defined. Nonetheless, for many therapeutic drugs, development *per se* produces a "pattern" for drug metabolism which when characterized, supports the pharmacokinetic properties (ie. drug clearance) reported for many agents across the pediatric age spectrum [1].

During the first year of life, advances in the discipline of clinical pharmacology and in particular, in the application of methods to quantitate the pharmacokinetics and pharmacodynamics of specific drugs, have demonstrated the importance of the concentration vs. effect relationship. In particular, the ability to understand this relationship has produced valuable data which in turn, has enabled the individualization of therapy for many drugs (eg. caffeine, digoxin, phenobarbital, phenytoin, theophylline, aminoglycoside antibiotics, indomethacin, cephalosporin antibiotics) which are commonly used. However, there are countless other therapeutic agents which are often introduced in the neonatal period for which the relationship between dose requirement, plasma or tissue concentration and effect is either incompletely characterized (eg. enalaprilat, captopril, fentanyl, lorazepam, morphine, chloral hydrate, zidovudine, metoclopramide, ranitidine, carbamazepine, acyclovir) or unknown (eg. cisapride, famotidine, carnitine). When these agents are used, the clinician must often integrate basic pharmacologic knowledge about the drug (eg. pharmacokinetic properties in older children and adults) with principles of developmental physiology in order to select an initial dose of the drug and to establish criteria for monitoring therapy. While this approach of "guided empiricism" is always superior to scaling the dose based on body size or weight, it clearly posses more risk to both the patient and practitioner as opposed to having sufficient data to establish a firm understanding of how development influences both drug disposition and action.

Although development represents a continuum of biologic events that enable adaptation, somatic growth and eventually, reproduction, its impact on the metabolism of drugs resides largely with the acquisition of specific organ function via organogenesis (especially in preterm infants) and recruitment of functional "units" within a given organ. With regard to those organs that possess the metabolic machinery necessary to biotransform xenobiotics, the underlying genetic determinants that regulate drug metabolism are influenced by both developmental and environmental (eg. therapeutic and/or non-therapeutic) factors that can alter the expression of activity for a given drug-metabolizing enzyme [2]. As a result of these multifactorial determinants, developmentally-dependent changes in drug metabolism may directly influence therapeutic response to produce either positive or adverse effects which can manifest themselves in an immediate, subacute or delayed fashion [3]. Given the fact that the most dynamic period of human development resides within the first year of life [1], it is imperative that the clinician who treats neonates and young infants develop a firm understanding of the interface between pharmacogenetics and those developmentally-associated events which collectively represent the determinants of the rates and routes for drug metabolism.

The purpose of this review is to acquaint the clinician with the ontogeny of important Phase-I (ie. oxidative) pathways for human drug metabolism during the first year of life by reviewing the interface between pharmacogenetics, developmental physiology and pharmacokinetics. The enzymes which regulate Phase-I metabolism will be highlighted because of fundamental work in molecular pharmacology which has enabled the examination of their ontogeny in humans. This review is not intended to recapitulate the information contained in many excellent recent reviews of pharmacogenetics [2,3–6] which may be consulted for a more comprehensive presentation and discussion of existing work in this field. Finally, the potential clinical importance of this "interface" will be highlighted through the provision of specific examples that represent relevant therapeutic scenarios encountered during the first year of life.

Non-Cytochrome p450 Drug Metabolizing Enzymes

Alcohol Dehydrogenase

Alcohol dehydrogenase (ADH) is the rate-limiting enzyme responsible for the biotransformation of ethanol. Based on work performed over two decades ago, it was demonstrated that ADH activity in human fetal liver exists at approximately 2 months of age but that it is at only 3% of adult activity [7]. As summarized by May [3], the ontogeny of hepatic ADH involves a sequential promoter activation of the corresponding ADH alleles by hepatic nuclear factor 1, CCAAT/enhancer-binding protein, liver activator protein and D-element binding protein.

While the disparity in ADH isoenzyme kinetic constants secondary to genetic polymorphism may contribute to the ethnic differences observed for ethanol metabolism [3], the effect of development on these parameters has not been characterized. However, early pharmacokinetic data for ethanol in neonates [8] clearly support reduced clearance and its accumulation in plasma; findings which corroborate the previously reported developmental immaturity in ADH activity [7]. However, in a case report of acute alcohol intoxication in a 30 month old child [9], the plasma clearance of ethanol was found to be more rapid than previously reported in adults and also, to proceed by a first order process. These data might imply either a much lower Km or higher Vmax value for ADH in young children or alternatively, suggest a quantitative importance for other enzymes (eg. CYP2E1) which contribute to ethanol metabolism. These data were also corroborated by a previous study of chloral hydrate disposition in pediatric patients which reported an elimination half life for trichloroethanol in children between 1 to 13 years of age (ie. mean value 9.7 hr) which was significantly lower than that for preterm (39.8 hr) and term (27.8 hr) neonates [10]. In view of the aforementioned data, it would appear that by 12 to 30 months of postnatal age, ADH activity equal to or greater than that observed in adults is reached. If the activity of ADH (and possibly other enzymes which contribute to ethanol biotransformation such as aldehyde dehydrogenase and CYP2E1) is increased in older infants and young children relative to adults, it is possible that the influence of development may have a protective effect in cases of ethanol intoxication or alternatively, a detrimental effect in cases of other alcohols which are ADH substrates but are biotransformed to potentially toxic metabolic intermediates (eg. isopropanol). In the case of chloral hydrate, the substantial variability noted clinically in the dose vs. duration of effect relationship is readily explained by the pharmacokinetic differences [10] which result from the developmental dependence of ADH activity and perhaps, other enzymes which may be quantitatively important in governing its metabolism as well (eg. CYP2E1).

Epoxide Hydrolase

Microsomal epoxide hydrolase (mEH) is a critical biotransformation enzyme that catalyzes the hydrolysis of a wide variety of xenobiotic epoxides, resulting in the formation of corresponding *trans*-dihydrodiol intermediates [11]. As recently reviewed by Gaedigk et al [12], substrates for mEH include arene oxide intermediates of aromatic anticonvulsant agents (eg. phenytoin, carbamazepine, phenobarbital), epoxide derivatives of valproic acid, polyaromatic hydrocarbons, aromatic amines and benzene. In concert with oxidative metabolism by specific cytochrome P450 isoforms, the hydrolysis of epoxides produced from specific polyaromatic hydrocarbons can lead to the formation of highly electrophilic and mutagenic diol-epoxides. Relative deficiencies in mEH, whether the result of developmental immaturity and/or a genetic polymorphism, has been linked to an increased incidence of birth defects, childhood and adult cancers and serious adverse drug reactions in both children and adults [13].

While several previous studies have examined mEH activity in human fetal livers, only Omiecinski et al [14] have reported data on mEH activity and protein content sufficient to enable examination of its developmental expression. In this study, hepatic mEH activity was found to be directly correlated with both increasing gestational age and protein content and that after 125 days of gestation, fetal activity was approximately 50% of that obtained from 15 adult liver specimens. However, a lack of concordance found between mRNA levels and the activity of mEH in fetal tissue suggested that a post-transcriptional regulatory process participated in directing the developmental acquisition of mEH activity.

In view of the relative importance of mEH in the process of detoxification of a number of substrates, it would appear that the low levels of hepatic activity found before 90 days of gestation [14] may represent a limitation of the early developing fetus to detoxify xenobiotics which produce epoxide intermediates. The potential importance of developmental immaturity in mEH activity has been suggested by Buehler et al [15] who, in four infants identified prospectively with low mEH activity indistinguishable from the poor-metabolizer (PM) phenotype and who were exposed in utero to phenytoin, predicted the occurrence of the fetal hydantoin syndrome. Despite the important caveat residing with this particular example (ie. the assumption that low mEH activity and inability to detoxify phenytoin intermediates have a causal relationship in fetal hydantoin syndrome), it is conceivable that the pharmacogenetic-developmental interface for mEH might place the fetus and perhaps, the premature infant at increased risk for tissue injury produced by reactive epoxide intermediates. This may not be true, however, concerning the role of mEH in adverse drug reactions produced by aromatic anticonvulsant compounds as recent work demonstrated that a genetic defect altering the structure and function of mEH protein was unlikely to be primarily associated with the predisposition to cytotoxic injury produced by these compounds and/or their metabolites [12]. The absence of data which solely examines the function of mEH with increasing age precludes an accurate estimation as to when adult competence with respect to enzyme activity may be reached and also, whether mEH activity in young infants/children may exceed that of adults.

N-acetyltransferase

Among the earliest discovered and most widely recognized genetic polymorphisms is represented by arylamine-N-acetyltransferase 2 (NAT2) activity. With approximately 50% of Caucasians and African Americans residing on the North American continent expressing the poor metabolizer (PM) phenotype for NAT2, the predominance of this polymorphism potentially places a substantial number of individuals at increased risk for the development of adverse drug effects (eg. sulfasalazine-induced hemolysis, hydrazine or arylamine-induced peripheral neuropathy, drug-induced lupus erythematosus associated with procainamide or isoniazid therapy and Steven's-Johnson syndrome or toxic epidermal necrolysis associated with sulfonamide administration) [3, 4]. Given the extensive number of drugs which are subject to polymorphic acetylation in humans (Table 1), this particular genetic polymorphism is of potential clinical importance with regard to the provision of drug therapy.

As summarized by May [3], two enzymes capable of catalyzing N-acetylation are expressed in human liver, NAT1 and NAT2, both of which show selectivity for arylamine substrates. With respect to its activity, NAT2 is polymorphic while NAT1 appears to be monomorphic. It is the allelic variants for NAT2 and its mutations which determine the pharmacogenetic expression of this enzyme and account for the marked ethnic differences in prevalence of the slow acetylator phenotype (eg. 45–50% in Caucasians vs. 6.6% for Japanese) [3, 16]. However, recent work by Cribb et al [17] demonstrated a positive linear correlation in 14 slow acetylators between NAT2 activity and NAT1 activity in peripheral blood mononuclear cells. This work suggested that in NAT2 slow acetylators with high NAT1 activity, NAT2 phenotype determination by the use of a pharmacologic probe (eg. caffeine) may be inaccurate for individuals whose genotype for NAT2 may place them near the antimode, thereby producing a genotype-phenotype discordance. Given the fact that NAT2 exists as allelic variants and that NAT1 activity in man may not be normally distributed [17], it is possible that NAT1 may be polymorphic in its expression; a speculation which requires further confirmation.

With respect to the N-acetyltransferases, only the ontogeny of NAT2 has been examined. In a study of human fetal liver, acetylation of the NAT2 substrate 7-aminoclonazepam was absent at 11 and 14 weeks with some activity being detected by 16 weeks [18]. The impact of development on NAT2 activity was examined by Pariente-Khayat et al [19] in 54 infants from 8 to 447 days of postnatal age using oral caffeine administration and quantitation of the caffeine metabolite ratios (ie. AFMU/1X) in urine. In those infants between 0 and

Table 1. Pharmacologic substrates for NAT2. (Adapted from Kearns [2] and May [3])

Hydrazines
Isoniazed
Hydralazine
Phenelzine
Arylamines
Procainamide
Dapsone
Sulfamethazine
Sulfapyridine
Drugs Metabolized to Amines
Sulfasalazine
Nitrazepam
Clonazepam
Caffeine
Acebutolol

55 days of age, all were phenotypically slow acetylators in contrast to infants between 122–224 and 225–342 days of age where 50% and 62%, respectively where characterized as fast acetylators. These data demonstrated that prior to 15 months of age, developmental regulation of the NAT2 gene product produced profound effects on the expression of the pharmacologic phenotype. These results were also corroborated by previous reports of caffeine plasma clearance [20] and urinary molar ratios of the caffeine metabolite 1-methylxanthine (ie. 1X) [21] which demonstrated marked increases over the first six to ten months of life. However, by three to four years of age, normal European children as well as Caucasian and African Americans have NAT2 phenotypes which correspond to the frequency distributions reported for adults of the same races [2]. Accordingly, it appears that NAT2 activity is fully expressed by three years of age with possible competence (ie. as compared to adult values) reached as early as 10 to 12 months of age.

The Cytochromes P450

As reviewed previously [3–5], the cytochrome P450s are ubiquitous heme-containing enzymes found in both prokaryotes and eukaryotes that exist as a superfamily of closely related isoenzymes. More than 60 distinct forms of these enzymes, each encoded by a separate gene, have been purified from rat and human liver. Cytochrome P450s catalyze the biotransformation of a wide variety of structurally unrelated endogenous (eg. steroid hormones) and exogenous (eg. drugs, environmental chemicals) compounds (Table 2).

They may exhibit broad specificity (ie. several compounds serving as a substrate for a specific isoenzyme) or alternatively, be highly selective. While the regulation of cytochrome P450s which govern the biotransformation of endogenous compounds is largely hormonal, the regulation of those which are involved in the metabolism of xenobiotics is often multifactorial and involves an interface between development and pharmacogenetics. Given the fact that three cytochrome P450 isoenzymes (eg. CYP1A2, 2D6 and 3A4) are collectively responsible for the metabolism of the vast majority of therapeutic drugs (Table 2), our discussion will be limited to their ontogenic expression during the first year of life.

CYP1A2

CYP1A2 is the sole member of the CYP1A subfamily expressed in human liver and is involved in the metabolism of drugs, environmental toxins and presumably, of endogenous substrates such as uroporphyrinogen [2, 3]. As recently summarized by Tang et al [22], CYP1A2 is involved in the biotransformation of several drugs (Table 2). Its activity can be induced by polycyclic aromatic or halogenated hydrocarbons found in cigarette smoke and inhibited by the co-ingestion of estrogen and progestin containing oral contraceptives.

Table 2. Major cytochrome P450 enzymes in humans. (Adapted from Kearns [2])

P450	Example Substrates*
CYP1A1	polycyclic hydrocarbons, benzo[a]pyrene
CYP1A2	caffeine, phenacetin, imipramine, theophylline
CYP2C8	diazepam, tolbutamide, diclofenac
CYP2C9	phenytoin, tolbutamide, ibuprofen, imipramine, S-warfarin, naproxen, losartan
CYP2C19	S-mephenytoin, omeprazole
CYP2D6	dextromethorphan, propafenone, amitriptyline, d-amphetamine, codeine, desipramine, haloperidol, metoprolol, nortriptyline, propranolol, thioridazine, captopril, labetolol, timolol, fluoxetine, mexilitine, diphenhydramine, norfluoxetine, oxprenolol
CYP2E1	chlorzoxazone, ethanol, acetaminophen
CYP3A4	cyclosporine, nifedipine, tacrolimus, erythromycin, lidocaine, rifampin, triacetyloleandomycin, cortisol, dapsone, theophylline, acetaminophen, azole antifungal agents, terfenadine, midazolam, quinidine
CYP3A7	dehydroepiandrosterone, ethynylestradiol, triazolam
CYP4A11	leukotriene receptor antagonists

* Examples represent only substrates for the respective cytochrome P450s and do not imply that a given P450 is quantitatively important for its in vivo biotransformation in man

The pharmacogenetics of CYP1A2 in man have been examined by the use of caffeine as a pharmacologic probe since approximately 95% of the 1-, 3-, and 7-demethylations of the drug by human liver microsomes are catalyzed by CYP1A2 and 90% of systemic caffeine clearance depends on the activity of this isoenzyme [23]. In those individuals where CYP1A2 activity may be low and therefore, the biotransformation of caffeine becomes quantitatively more or less (as is probably the case during the first two months of postnatal life) dependent on other P450s (eg. CYP2E1, CYP2A6, CYP3A4) known to play a role in its metabolism [22], its use as an index of CYP1A2 phenotype or activity has the potential to yield results which do not correctly characterize the genotype-phenotype relationship for this isoform.

The ontogeny of CYP1A2 activity has recently been examined by Cazeneuve et al [24] who examined the biotransformation of caffeine in human liver microsomes obtained from fetuses (n = 10), neonates (n = 10), infants (n = 9) and adults (n = 5). In this study, both N-3 and N-7-demethylation (steps catalyzed by CYP1A2) matured over the postnatal age range of 0 to 300 days while no influence of maturation on N-1-demethylation was detected during this time period. Furthermore, N-3-demethylation correlated with both methoxyresorufin-*O*-demethylase activity (a CYP1A2 pharmacologic probe) and microsomal CYP1A2 content while N-7-demethylation correlated only with microsomal CYP1A2 content. The apparent absence of CYP1A2 in fetal liver lead the authors to conclude that the small extent of caffeine metabolism to paraxanthine

(1-7X) and theophylline (1-3X) by N-3 and N-7-demethylation, respectively, most likely resulted from the contribution of fetal CYP3A activity.

In contrast to neonates who clearly have deficient CYP1A2 activity relative to adults, older infants (ie. 3–6 months of age) and younger children may have increased activity. This assertion is well supported by the developmental pharmacokinetics of both caffeine and theophylline which clearly demonstrate reduced clearance in the first two months of life and increased clearance (relative to adults and post-pubertal adolescents) during infancy and childhood [25]. In conclusion, CYP1A2 activity appears to be both genetically determined and developmentally dependent. Pharmacokinetic data examining the plasma clearance of two commonly used substrates for this isoenzyme (eg. caffeine and theophylline) would support minimal activity during the first weeks of life with a precipitous increase in activity by three to six months of postnatal age for term infants. For premature infants, postnatal adaptation and development would also appear to produce an increase in CYP1A2 activity (ie. as reflected by methylxanthine pharmacokinetics), but at a pattern which is delayed and somewhat discordant from that observed in term infants. At present, no specific information exists on how development *per se* produces the up- or down-regulation in CYP1A2 activity suggested by specific studies of caffeine biotransformation and methylxanthine pharmacokinetics [24, 25].

CYP2D6

Debrisoquine-4-hydroxylase (CYP2D6) represents the best characterized isoform of cytochrome P450 to date. The pharmacogenetics of CYP2D6 and its relevance to human pharmacology have been discussed in several recent reviews [3, 4]. This isoenzyme is variably expressed in human liver and mutations and/or abnormalities of alternative splicing of the CYP2D6 gene product lead to the absence of functional protein in approximately 7% to 10% of whites and 2% of African Americans [2–4]. In Orientals including Japanese, Thai, Malaysian and Chinese populations, the incidence of the PM phenotype appears to be 0 to 2%. Also, the frequency of the PM phenotype for CYP2D6 has also been reported to be low in blacks of African origin, ranging from 0 to 8.6%. Finally, a lower incidence for the PM phenotype has been reported in Greenlanders and American Indians, 3.2% and 0%, respectively; both of which represent groups of Mongolian origin [3]. While there is generally good (ie. >94%) concordance between the CYP2D6 genotype and phenotype determined by the use of pharmacologic probes (eg. dextromethorphan), the metabolic ratio of dextromethorphan/dextrorphan may not reliably discriminate between individuals who are homozygous and heterozygous for the extensive metabolizer (EM) phenotype [26].

CYP2D6 does not appear to be active early in gestation based on the absence of codeine and dextromethorphan oxidation in human fetal liver obtained at 14–24 weeks gestation [27]. However, in an apparent adaptational response to extra-uterine life, an increase in CYP2D6 immunoreactive protein occurs during the first week of postnatal life irrespective of the gestational age. This increase in protein appears to be associated with the onset of dextromethorphan O-demethylation and is preceded by a rise in CYP2D6 mRNA, suggesting that regulation of this isoenzyme early in life is primarily at the transcriptional level (28). It is also interesting to note that in infants (ie. those >30 days of age), the amount of hepatic CYP2D6 protein is approximately 50% of that seen in adults [29]. Since the amount of protein within a given age group has been shown to correlate with the O-demethylation of dextromethorphan [29], it seems reasonable to speculate that CYP2D6 activity may require several months (possibly 3 to 6) to acquire developmental competence and that attempts to phenotype young infants using pharmacologic probes such as dextromethorphan might produce an inaccurate assignment as has been suggested for NAT2 [19]. At present, the biological/biochemical signal(s) responsible for the up-regulation of CYP2D6 during development are not known.

While the adverse consequences of the CYP2D6 phenotype with regard to treatment with beta-blockers and antiarrhythmic agents (eg. propaphenone, encainide, flecainide) in adults are well known as is the potential for lack of efficacy or therapeutic failure from codeine treatment of individuals with the PM phenotype (ie. that reflected by genotype or alternatively, an EM which is converted to a PM by concomitant administration of the CYP2D6 inhibitor quinidine) [3], the therapeutic and/or toxicologic impact of the CYP2D6 polymorphism during the first year of life can only be projected based on adult data. Conceivably, developmental differences in CYP2D6 phenotype/activity in such children would be manifested clinically by unpredictable dose-effect relationships for commonly used drugs (eg. beta blockers, captopril, diphenhydramine) which represent substrates for this isoform (Table 2).

CYP3A4

Cytochromes P450 constituting the CYP3A subfamily account for the majority of P450s present in the adult human liver and small bowel. The pharmacogenetics of this gene subfamily and its biological and pharmacological relevance have been the topic of several recent reviews [2–6]. Although the hepatic enzymes which comprise the 3A subfamily share over 85% amino acid sequence homology, the enzymes have been shown to differ substantially in their catalytic properties and in their regulation [6]. This is illustrated by the examples depicted in Table 2 which reflect both specificity and overlap in the substrates for the 3A subfamily. It is also important to note that the extreme variability reported for the plasma clearance of many CYP3A substrates in adults [4, 8] is supported by the finding of a 10 fold variation in the amount of hepatic CYP3A4 mRNA present in man [2].

As summarized by Watkins [30], CYP3A3, allelic variants of CYP3A4, CYP3A5 and CYP3A7 have been demonstrated to be present in human liver. CYP3A5 is expressed polymorphically in 20–25% of adult human livers, is 83% homologous to CYP3A4 and has overlapping substrate specificity with CYP3A4 for nifedipine and to a lesser degree, with midazolam, progesterone and androstenedione. CYP3A7 was first isolated from human fetal liver where it is the major cytochrome P450 present and preferentially catalyzes the biotransformation of dehydroepiandrosteindione-sulfate (DHEA) [30]. While CYP3A7 mRNA can be detected in approximately 50% of adult human livers, it is unclear if CYP3A7 protein is also present [7]. Unlike the expression of CYP3A in rodents, gender does not appear to alter the expression of prenatal CYP3A5 or 3A7 although it may influence the activity of CYP3A4 in adults [6]. It is also important to note that with the exception of CYP3A7, all of the members of the 3A subfamily have been found in extrahepatic sites which include the jejunum, colon, pancreas and stomach. Given the facts that CYP3A4 and CYP3A5 constitute the largest fraction of drug metabolizing enzymes throughout the human digestive tract, differences in their expression may account for inter-organ differences in the metabolism of 3A substrates (Table 2). Also, in the case of CYP3A isoforms expressed in the intestine, the induction or inhibition of these enzymes by pharmacologic (eg. rifampin, an inducer and ketoconazole, an inhibitor) or dietary (eg. naringenin from grapefruit juice, an inhibitor) compounds may produce significant drug-drug interactions and thereby, alter the extent of pre-systemic clearance (and therefore, the bioavailability) for a variety of CYP3A substrates (eg. cyclosporine A).

The ontogeny of the CYP3A subfamily has been recently examined by both molecular and pharmacologic methods. Initial recognition of the role of CYP3A (most probably, 3A7) in the 16-hydroxylation of DHEA, an estrogen precursor in the placenta [31], demonstrated the functional importance of this enzyme in both homeostasis and fetal development. Subsequent studies reviewed elsewhere [2] have demonstrated the importance of fetal CYP3A in the N-demethylation of caffeine, codeine, dextromethorphan and possibly, in the C-8 oxidation of caffeine. In a study of N-demethylation of dextromethorphan to 3-methoxymorphinan in fetal hepatic microsomes, Jacqz-Aigrain and Cresteil [29] reported a fetal CYP3A which was detectable in large amounts as early as 17 weeks gestation and which by 30 weeks attained 75% of the activity found in adult hepatic microsomes. This was in contrast to the amount of CYP3A protein found in fetal microsomes at 30 weeks gestation which was only one third of that detected in adults. The results from these previous studies suggest that the acquisition of developmental competence in CYP3A activity involves an initial up-regulation of the gene responsible to manufacture a functionally complete isoform critical for the biotransformation of endogenous substances early in gestation (ie. CYP3A7). This is followed by an increase in the synthesis of this particular isoform and then by differential up-regulation of the gene products responsible for the synthesis of other members of the CYP3A subfamily which are required to catalyze the biotransformation of both endogenous and exogenous substrates [2].

A pharmacokinetic example which lends some measure of support for increased CYP3A activity in infants and young children is illustrated by nifedipine, a well characterized CYP3A4 substrate [4, 6]. In a study of nifedipine pharmacokinetics and pharmacodynamics in children with bronchopulmonary dysplasia and pulmonary hypertension, Johnson et al [32] reported a mean elimination half life (ie. 1.8 hr) which was less than previously observed in adults (ie. range 2.4 to 3.4 hr). However, independent analysis of the estimated plasma clearance of nifedipine from this study of nine infants demonstrated no apparent correlation between clearance and the age of patients studied (ie. 8 to 68 months). Therefore, future studies are needed in larger numbers of infants during the first year of life to accurately determine the true relationship between CYP3A activity and development.

The potential adverse consequences of developmental dependence in CYP3A activity must be considered for pharmacologic and environmental substrates (Table 2) that predominate from prenatal life through adulthood. This is especially true for those instances where previous data point towards an area of concern. As reviewed previously [2], specific examples might include the dependence of CYP3A for the biotransformation of the antineoplastic agents vinblastine and taxol, compounds which inhibit CYP3A (eg. ketoconazole, itraconazole, nifedipine, erythromycin, cimetidine, nizatidine, terfenadine) and produce clinically significant drug-drug interactions (eg. terfenadine-erythromycin, ketoconazole-midazolam, itraconazole-erythromycin-midazolam, terfenadine-clarithromycin, ketoconazole-CSA) and also, the importance of CYP3A in the metabolic activation of carcinogens such as Aflatoxin B_1 and of fetal CYP3A isoforms in the bioactivation of environmentally acquired heterocyclic amines that may act as promutagens. Of recent note is the potentially serious (ie. production of cardiac dysrhythmias) drug-drug interaction between the prokinetic agent cisapride and erythromycin, an inhibitor of CYP3A4 activity. Since both of these agents are routinely used in the neonate and young infant who developmentally, may have low CYP3A4 activity, it is quite possible that an exaggeration of this drug-drug interaction could occur. Clearly, if the phenotype for CYP3A isoenzymes is relevant in the production of either efficacy or toxicity produced by substrates of these enzymes (Table 2), the profound influence of development upon its expression must be considered in order to accurately assess the dose-concentration-effect relationship. This is especially true for compounds such as midazolam and cisapride which represent preferential CYP3A substrates, are increasingly being used for long periods of time in sick infants (eg. for continuous IV sedation regimens and treatment of gastroesophageal reflux) and whose pharmacologic action is related to developmentally determined changes in both pharmacokinetics (eg., clearance) and pharmacodynamics (ie., receptor regulation).

The Multiplicity of Drug Metabolizing Enzymes and their Clinical Importance

Based on the information available for important Phase-I drug metabolizing enzymes and their activity during the first year of life, it is clear that the dynamic somatic changes which characterize this period of development are associated with equally dynamic changes in the ability of the body to metabolically

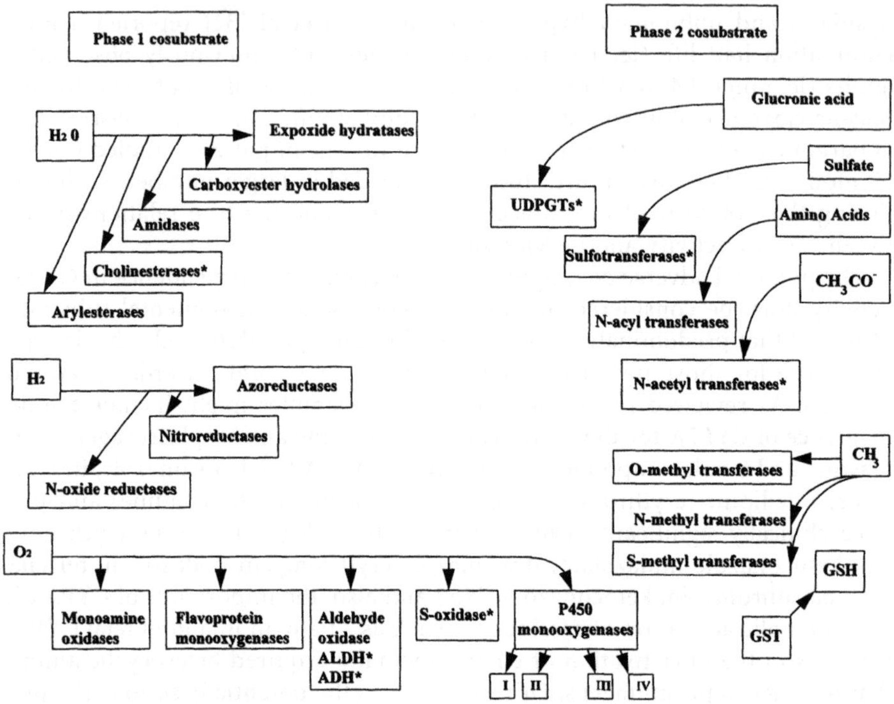

Fig. 1. Multiplicity and polymorphism of xenobiotic metabolizing enzymes. Asterisks indicate classes in which genetic polymorphism occurs. ADH - alcohol dehydrogenase; ALDH-aldehyde dehydrogenase; GSH-glutathione; GST-glutathione-S-transferase; UDPGT-uridine diphosphoglucuronyl transferase. (From Kearns [3] with permission)

process both endogenous and exogenous substrates. Unfortunately, this only represents a mere part of the picture. As illustrated in the Figure, there is a true multiplicity and polymorphism for many drug metabolizing enzymes, many of which represent those responsible for Phase-II biotransformation reactions as well.

While a complete discussion of important Phase-II reactions is outside the scope of this review, it is crucial to recognize that many medications commonly administered to neonates and young infants represent substrates for important enzymes and, in several cases (eg. glucuronyltransferase), their particular isoforms. A representative "list" of such compounds may include agents such as lorazepam, ibuprofen, chloramphenicol and acetaminophen, all substrates for glucuronyltransferase, and epinephrine, salicylates, acetaminophen, all of which represent substrates for human sulfotransferase enzymes [33]. Historically, our inability to appreciate the developmental differences in the activity of important Phase-II enzymes has contributed to therapeutic misadventure (ie. the Gray Baby Syndrome associated with accumulation of chloramphenicol concentrations in the neonate) and also, protection from certain drug-associated toxicities (eg. reduced propensity of acetaminophen overdose to produce hepatotoxicity in young infants as opposed to adults consequent to increased sulfation ability). It must also be recognized that while specific substrate-enzyme combinations for both Phase-I and Phase-II reactions usually result in deactivation or detoxification of a given drug substrate, metabolic activation can also result (eg., the formation of hydroxylamine and nitroso intermediates from cytochrome P450-mediated metabolism of sulfamethoxazole and the formation of certain phenolic and acyl glucuronide conjugates of selected drugs) in the "manufacturing" of intermediates capable of producing or modulating cellular injury. Since many therapeutic drugs represent polyfunctional substrates for Phase-I and/or Phase-II enzymes, the interpretation or prediction of dose-concentration-effect relationships can only be undertaken if the ontogeny of all the pathways involved in the metabolism of a given drug are considered.

Conclusions

An assessment of risk with regard to exposing a developing human to a therapeutic drug or environmental chemical requires a multifactorial approach. This approach must be based on knowledge of the interface between developmental physiology, its impact on the acquisition and expression of activity for drug metabolizing enzymes and the pharmacologic/toxicologic properties of a given xenobiotic. However, the large "information gap" which exists concerning our complete understanding of the ontogenic expression of many important drug metabolizing enzyme requires the clinician to use inductive reasoning which often times is based equally on intuition and science in the selection of drug dosing regimens and/or the development of a therapeutic plan sufficient to monitor the safety and efficacy of a given drug. Until data become available which are sufficient to close this "information gap", clinicians must use scientifically based inference to individualize drug therapy for the neonate and young infant and must not rely on extrapolation which does not consider the impact of development on both the disposition and action of both new and old drugs.

References

1. Kauffman R, Kearns G (1992) Pharmacokinetic Studies in Paediatric Patients: Clinical and Ethical Considerations. Clin Pharmacokinet 1:10–29.
2. Kearns GL (1995) Pharmacogenetics and Development: Are Infants and Children at Increased Risk for Adverse Outcomes? Curr Opin Pediatr 7:220–233.
3. May G (1994) Genetic Differences in Drug Disposition. J Clin Pharmacol 34:881–897.
4. Gonzalez F, Idle J (1994) Pharmacogenetic Phenotyping and Genotyping: Present Status and Future Potential. Clin Pharmacokinet 26:59–70.
5. Beaune PH (1993) Les Cytochromes P450 Humains: Applications en Pharmacologie. Therapie 48:521–526.
6. Wrighton S, Stevens J (1992) The Human Hepatic Cytochromes P450 Involved in Drug Metabolism. Clin Rev Toxicol 22:1–21.

7. Pikkarainen P, Raiha N (1967) Development of Alcohol Dehydrogenase Activity in the Human Liver. Pediatr Res 1:165–168.
8. Idanpaan-Heikkila J, Jouppila P, Akerblom H, Isoaho R, Kauppila E, Koivisto M (1972) Elimination and Metabolic Effects of Ethanol in Mother, Fetus and Newborn Infant. Am J Obstet Gynecol 112:387–393.
9. Lopez G, Yealy D, Krenzelok E (1989) Survival of a Child Despite Unusually High Blood Ethanol Levels. Am J Emerg Med 7:283–285.
10. Mayers D, Hindmarsh K, Sankaran K, Gorecki D, Kasian G (1991) Chloral Hydrate Disposition Following Single-Dose Administration to Critically Ill Neonates and Children. Dev Pharmacol Ther 16:71–77.
11. Guengerich F (1982) Epoxide Hydrolase: Properties and Metabolic Roles. Rev Biochem Toxicol 4:5–30.
12. Gaedigk A, Spielberg S, Grant D (1994) Characterization of the Microsomal Epoxide Hydrolase Gene in Patients with Anticonvulsant Adverse Drug Reactions. Pharmacogenetics 4:142–153.
13. Park B, Pirmohamed M, Kitteringham N (1992) Idiosyncratic Drug Reactions: a Mechanistic Evaluation of Risk Factors. Br J Clin Pharmacol 34:377–395.
14. Omiecinski C, Aicher L, Swenson L (1994) Developmental Expression of Human Microsomal Epoxide Hydrolase. J Pharmacol Exp Ther 269:417–423.
15. Buehler G, Delimont D, van Waes M, Finnell R (1990) Prenatal Prediction of the Risk of the Fetal Hydantoin Syndrome. N Engl J Med 322:1567–1572.
16. Grant DM (1993) Molecular Genetics of the N-acetyltransferases. Pharmacogenetics 3:45–50.
17. Cribb A, Isbrucker R, Levatte T, Tsui B, Gillespie C, Renton K (1994) Acetylator Phenotyping: The Urinary Caffeine Metabolite Ratio in Slow Acetylators Correlates with a Marker of Systemic NAT1 Activity. Pharmacogenetics 4:166–170.
18. Peng D, Birgersson C, von Bahr C, Rane A (1984) Polymorphic Acetylation of 7-aminoclonazepam in Human Liver Cytosol. Pediatr Pharmacol 4:155–159.
19. Pariente-Khayat A, Pons G, Rey E, et al. (1991) Caffeine Acetylator Phenotyping During Maturation in Infants. Pediatr Res 29:492–495.
20. Pons G, Carrier O, Richard M, et al. (1988) Developmental Changes of Caffeine Elimination in Infancy. Dev Pharmacol Ther 11:258–264.
21. Kraus D, Fischer J, Reitz S, et al. (1993) Alterations in Theophylline Metabolism During the First Year of Life. Clin Pharmacol Ther 54:351–359.
22. Tang B, Zhou Y, Kadar D, Kalow W (1994) Caffeine as a Probe for CYP1A2 Activity: Potential Influence of Renal Factors on Urinary Phenotypic Trait Measurements. Pharmacogenetics 4:117–124.
23. Kalow W, Tang B (1993) The Use of Caffeine for Enzyme Assays: A Critical Appraisal. Clin Pharmacol Ther 53:503–514.
25. Aranda J (1984) Maturational Changes in Theophylline and Caffeine Metabolism and Disposition: Clinical Implications. In Lemberger L, Reidenberg M (eds.): Proceedings of the Second World Conference on Clinical Pharmacology and Therapeutics, Bethesda, Maryland: the American Society for Pharmacology and Experimental Therapeutics, pp. 868–877.
26. Evans W, Relling M (1991) Concordance of P450 2D6 (Debrisoquine Hydroxylase) Phenotype and Genotype: Inability of Dextromethorphan Metabolic Ratio to Discriminate Reliably Heterozygous and Homozygous Extensive Metabolizers. Pharmacogenetics 1:143–148.
27. Ladona M, Lindstrom B, Thyr C, Peng D, Rane A (1991) Differential Fetal Development of the O- and N-demethylation of Codeine and Dextromethorphan in Man. Br J Clin Pharmacol 323:295–302.
28. Treluyer J, Jacqz-Aigrain E, Alvarez F, Cresteil T (1991) Expression of CYP2D6 in Developing Human Liver. Eur J Biochem 323:295–302.
29. Jacqz-Aigrain E, Cresteil T (1992) Cytochrome P450-Dependent Metabolism of Dextromethorphan: Fetal and Adult Studies: Dev Pharmacol Ther 18:161–168.
30. Watkins P (1994) Noninvasive Tests of CYP3A Enzymes. Pharmacogenetics 4:171–184.

31. Komori M, Nishio K, Ohi H, Ktada M, Kamataki T (1989) Molecular Cloning and Sequence Analysis of cDNA Containing the Entire Coding Region for Human Fetal Liver Cytochrome P-450. J Biochem 105: 161–163.
32. Johnson C, Beekman R, Kostyshak D, Nguyen R, Oh D, Amidon G (1991) Pharmacokinetics and Pharmacodynamics of Nifedipine in Children with Bronchopulmonary Dysplasia and Pulmonary Hypertension. Pediatr Res 29: 500–503.
33. Conjugation Reactions in Drug Metabolism: An Integrated Approach, Mulder GJ (ed.), 1990, Taylor and Francis, London, pp. 51–106 and 107–162.

Pharmacology of Antimicrobial Agents in Preterm Infants

J. N. van den Anker, G. L. Kearns and R. de Groot

Introduction

Bacterial infections continue to be a major cause of morbidity and mortality in preterm infants admitted to neonatal intensive care units [1]. Nosocomial infections including septicemia, meningitis, pneumonia or urinary tract infection occur in approximately 18% of neonates with a very low (<1500 g) birth weight. Major pathogens responsible for bacterial infections during the first month of life are *Staphylococcus* aureus, coagulase-negative staphylococci, enterococci, group B *streptococcus*, *Escherichia coli*, klebsiella, enterobacter, pseudomonas and other gram-negative bacteria. The combination of prolonged hospitalization, multiple invasive procedures, prolonged positive pressure ventilation, parenteral nutrition, and an impaired host defence is largely responsible for the increased susceptibility of preterm infants for bacterial, viral and fungal infections.

An early diagnosis of invasive infections remains difficult since signs and symptoms are frequently nonspecific. Between 4.4% and 10.5% of all newborn infants therefore receive systemic antibiotic therapy before results of bacterial cultures are known. In preterm infants admitted to a neonatal intensive care unit even more than 60% are treated with antibiotics during the first week of life. The most commonly used drug classes are penicillins, aminoglycosides and cephalosporins (53, 43 and 16%, respectively). The extensive use of antibiotics in infants whose renal and hepatic function are developmentally immature underscores the need to perform pharmacokinetic and pharmacodynamic studies which will contribute to optimal therapy and minimize drug-related toxicity and cost of therapy. The purpose of this review is to summarize the pharmacokinetic data for aminoglycosides, third generation cephalosporins and vancomycin in preterm infants. The current policy not to reduce antibiotic dosage intervals in preterm infants with gestational ages of less than 32 weeks until after the fourth week of life will be discussed. Currently recommended and possible alternate dosing regimens for the different antibacterial agents will be presented. However, additional prospective studies are required for the majority of these alternate dosing regimens.

Disease-specific therapy and pharmacologic principles underlying neonatal drug therapy are beyond the scope of this article since they have recently been addressed in reviews [1, 2, 3].

Aminoglycosides

Gentamicin, tobramycin, netilmicin and amikacin have adequate antibacterial activity against most gram-negative pathogens isolated from preterm infants with nosocomial infections. Renal excretion accounts for the elimination of approximately 90% of the aminoglycoside dose. The risk of toxicity therefore increases when drug elimination is impaired by a reduction in renal function. Nephro- and ototoxicity are the major side effects of aminoglycosides in adults. Two studies on treatment of newborns with aminoglycosides did not demonstrate significant nephrotoxic effects. In contrast, others reported that treatment with amikacin led to a delayed postnatal maturation in the glomerular filtration rate (GFR) of 56 preterm infants. In other studies, reversible increases in serum creatinine were reported, particularly when aminoglycosides were combined with nephrotoxic drugs such as indomethacin. Increases in enzymuria and beta-2-microglobulin excretion were also observed in newborns treated with gentamicin. However, these changes were transient and not predictive of glomerular function impairment.

The differences in nephrotoxicity of aminoglycosides between newborns and adults are similar to those reported in animal models. The lower nephrotoxicity in newborn as compared to adult rats has been attributed to factors such as lower intrarenal perfusion and a reduced uptake by proximal tubular cells. Peak and trough serum concentrations and cumulative dose are factors involved in the ototoxicity of aminoglycosides. Comparative studies in adults did not reveal significant differences in ototoxicity between amikacin, gentamicin, and tobramycin. However, netilmicin was shown in adults to be less ototoxic in comparison with other aminoglycosides. Controversy exists as to whether the aminoglycosides are a significant cause of early onset hearing impairment in infants. Confirmation of the cause of ototoxicity in newborns is confounded by other potentially ototoxic factors such as meningitis, prematurity, intracranial hemorrhage, and otitis media. Nevertheless, several well-conducted studies detected only a few cases (0–3%) of permanent injury in infants treated with high dosages of these drugs. This suggests that the ototoxicity of aminoglycosides is less prevalent in newborns (0–3%) than in adults (2–24%). However, in only one study was auditory function evaluated longitudinally. Long–term follow-up studies are necessary to detect the possible presence of ototoxicity in preterm infants treated with aminoglycosides.

Studies on the pharmacokinetics of aminoglycosides in preterm infants are summarized in Table 1 [4, 5, 6, 7, 8, 9, 10, 11]. Gentamicin is the most extensively studied aminoglycoside in preterm infants. The serum half-life correlates inversely with creatinine clearance, gestational age (GA), birth weight and postnatal age. During the first week of life, serum half-life values up to 14 h have been observed in infants with birth weights between 800 and 1500 g. The serum half-life of gentamicin is significantly lower in term infants, generally ranging between 4 to 5 h. After the first two weeks of life, serum half-life is approximately 3 h irrespective of actual weight. Both perinatal asphyxia and a

Table 1. Pharmacokinetics of aminoglycosides

Reference	Antibiotic	No	GA (weeks)	PNA (days)	Weight (g)	CL (mL/h/kg)	V (mL/kg)	$t_{1/2}$ (h)
Kildoo [4]	Gentamicin	15	<33	<7	<1500	23	530	11.1
		15	<33	8–30	<1500	27	500	10.8
		6	<33	>31	<1500	71	500	4.4
Koren [5]	Gentamicin	12	–	2	<1000	31	350	7.9
		20	<31	2	–	35	–	7.4
Landers [6]	Gentamicin	6	28	–	<1000	32	480	11.4
Nahata [7]	Tobramycin	5	31–32	2–6	1000–1499	74	930	9.5
Nahata [8]	Tobramycin	9	28–30	2–6	–	67	840	9.3
		7	–	2–6	1000–1250	63	1020	11.3
		6	–	2–6	1260–1500	67	740	8.2
Nahata [9]	Tobramycin	8	<30	<7	<1000	41	590	9.9
Kuhn [10]	Netilmicin	12	28–33	<28	770–2050	50	630	8.6
Kenyon [11]	Amikacin	28	31	–	1380	50	570	8.4

Abbreviations: No, number; *GA,* gestational age; *PNA,* postnatal age; *CL,* total body clearance; *V,* apparent volume of distribution; $t_{1/2}$, serum half-life

patent ductus arteriosus are associated with prolongation of the serum half-life values.

Tobramycin serum half-life is also inversely related to birth weight, GA, postnatal age and creatinine clearance. In infants who weigh less than 1500 g at birth and are younger than 1 week of age, serum half-life values may be as long as 9 to 17 h whereas serum half-life values of 3 to 4.5 h are reported in infants larger than 2500 g at birth and 1 to 4 weeks of age. The serum half-life of netilmicin is also inversely related to birth weight, GA and postnatal age. Serum half-life values between 4.6 and 11.5 h were reported in 12 preterm infants (mean weight: 1335 g) [10]. Accumulation of netilmicin has been documented in preterm infants. As with the other aminoglycosides, the serum half-life values of amikacin are inversely related to GA and postnatal age. The mean serum half–life in preterm infants between 1 and 3 days of age ranges between 7 to 8 h. In term infants older than 1 week of age, the mean serum half-life is 4 to 5 h. Serum half-life is also prolonged in hypoxemic newborns. These data suggest that there are only slight differences in pharmacokinetic behavior between the different aminoglycosides with renal function being the primary determinant of drug clearance.

Cerebrospinal fluid (CSF) concentrations of gentamicin in newborn infants with meningitis vary between 0.3 and 3.7 mg/L (mean 1.6 mg/L) after a dose of 2–2.5 mg/kg. Peak values observed 4 to 6 h after the dose directly correlate with the degree of meningeal inflammation and the dosage of gentamicin. CSF concentrations of amikacin measured between 1 and 4 h after a 10 mg/kg dose vary between 0.2 and 2.7 mg/L.

The data on the disposition of aminoglycosides in preterm infants indicate that serum half-life values are inversely related to GA, postnatal age and renal function. There is a rapid GA and postnatal age dependent increase of the GFR which enhances the capacity to eliminate these drugs from the body [12]. GFR values are also significantly lower in preterm infants with GA <28 weeks in comparison to preterm infants with GA between 28 and 32 weeks. In addition GFR values increase rapidly after birth irrespective of GA [12]. Based on these data investigators have proposed to prolong the dosing interval of gentamicin to 24 h in newborns weighing less than 1000 g [5]. Others have recommended tobramycin dosage intervals of 18 to 24 h in infants with GAs of less than 30 weeks [9]. For netilmicin, twice daily administration of 2.5 mg/kg to infants younger than 1 week of age will result in potentially toxic trough levels in 25–50% of preterm infants [10]. These data underscore the need to individualize aminoglycoside therapy in the first week of life.

We conclude that the current policy not to reduce antibiotic dosage intervals in preterm infants with GAs of less than 32 weeks until after the fourth week of life should therefore be revised [3]. Dosage guidelines should be stratified according to GA and postnatal age. We propose a stratification based both on GA (<28 weeks; 28–32 weeks) and on postnatal age (<7 days; 1–4 weeks), which takes into account both GA and postnatal age dependent changes in both renal drug clearance and the apparent volume of distribution (Table 2).

The reduced renal capacity to eliminate aminoglycosides, especially during the first week of life, enables a prolongation of the dosing interval from 18 h to 36 h in preterm infants with GAs of less than 28 weeks and from 18 h to 24 h in preterm infants with GAs between 28 and 32 weeks. The rapid postnatal changes in GFR suggest that an extension of the dosing interval from 18 h to 24 h is only indicated after the first week of life in preterm infants with GAs of less than 28 weeks. The increased apparent volume of distribution of aminoglycosides which corresponds to an increased extracellular fluid pool requires an increase of the dosage from 2.5 mg/kg to 3.5 mg/kg in preterm infants with GAs of less than 28 weeks and from 2.5 mg/kg to 3.0 mg/kg in preterm infants with GAs between 28 and 32 weeks. The dynamic postnatal changes in apparent volume of distribution suggest that a higher dosage is only indicated after the first week of life in preterm infants with GAs of less than 28 weeks. Possible alternate and currently recommended dosing regimens for aminoglycosides are presented in Table 2. However, additional prospective studies are required to validate the majority of these alternate dosing regimens.

Prenatal exposure to indomethacin, perinatal asphyxia, and a patent ductus arteriosus may necessitate prolongation of the dosing intervals. Careful monitoring of renal function is indicated to further adjust these dosing schedules as well as to detect nephrotoxicity. Whether these guidelines need to be changed in the presence of meningitis has not been determined. There is a lack of data on CSF penetration of the aminoglycosides, especially in preterm infants. However, there is some evidence that the transfer across the blood-CSF barrier may be higher in these infants than in fullterm infants. If the penetration is higher the current recommendation to increase drug dosage in patients with meningi-

Table 2. Alternate and currently used dosage schedules for aminoglycosides

Antibiotics	Dosage (mg/kg) and interval of administration			
	GA <28 weeks PNA (days)		GA 28–32 weeks PNA (days)	
	0–7	7–28	0–7	7–28
Gentamicin	3.5 q 36h (2.5 q 18h)	3.0 q 24h (2.5 q 18h)	3.0 q 24h (2.5 q 18h)	2.5 q 18h (2.5 q 18h)
Tobramycin	3.5 q 36h (2.5 q 18h)	3.0 q 24h (2.5 q 18h)	3.0 q 24h (2.5 q 18h)	2.5 q 18h (2.5 q 18h)
Netilmicin	3.5 q 36h (2.5 q 18h)	3.0 q 24h (2.5 q 18h)	3.0 q 24h (2.5 q 18h)	2.5 q 18h (2.5 q 18h)
Amikacin	12 q 24h (7.5 q 12h)	10 q 18h (7.5 q 12h)	10 q 18h (7.5 q 12h)	7.5 q 12h (7.5 q 12h)

Abbreviations: GA, gestational age; *PNA*, postnatal age
Values given between parentheses represent currently recommended dosages

tis should be reconsidered, especially in view of the poor outcome in neonates with gram-negative meningitis treated with intraventricular gentamicin.

Third Generation Cephalosporins

Third generation cephalosporins (cefoperazone, cefotaxime, ceftizoxime, ceftriaxone, ceftazidime) have adequate antibacterial activity against a wide range of gram-positive and gram-negative microorganisms. We will limit this discussion to cefotaxime, ceftazidime and ceftriaxone since neonatal studies on the pharmacokinetics of the other agents are not available.

Approximately 80% of a cefotaxime dose is excreted in the urine. However, only a third is eliminated in unchanged form. Cefotaxime is rapidly metabolized to desacetyl–cefotaxime through the action of esterases in the liver, erythrocytes and other tissues. In preterm infants, approximately 70% of cefotaxime appears to be converted to its active metabolite desacetyl-cefotaxime [13]. This metabolite retains, depending on the pathogen, 10 to 100% of the antimicrobial activity of its parent compound. Seventy to 90% of a ceftazidime dose is eliminated in unchanged form by the kidneys while approximately 70% of a ceftriaxone dose is excreted in unchanged form in the urine. The remainder is eliminated by the liver.

Cephalosporins are frequently used in the empiric treatment of neonatal septicemia and are generally well-tolerated by the newborn. Alterations of the bowel flora are most pronounced with third generation agents, especially ceftriaxone and cefoperazone, which may lead to intestinal colonization by resistant organisms. Subsequent superinfections by drug-resistant pathogens have been described. High biliary concentrations of ceftriaxone have been associated with reversible bile sludging (pseudolithiasis) in children receiving this drug. High doses of ceftazidime may result in neurotoxicity because of interference with cerebral enzyme activity. Bleeding disorders due to hypoprothrombinemia have been observed after therapy with moxalactam and cefamandole but are rare in patients treated with cefotaxime and ceftriaxone as these drugs do not possess the N-methylthiotetrazole substituent.

The data on the pharmacokinetics of cefotaxime, ceftriaxone and ceftazidime in preterm infants are presented in Table 3 [14, 15, 16, 17, 18, 19, 20, 21]. The serum half-life of cefotaxime is inversely correlated with GA and postnatal age [14]. In contrast, the pharmacokinetic parameters of the active metabolite, desacetyl-cefotaxime, were not correlated with postnatal age, GA or birth weight [15], and were not affected by in utero exposure to betamethasone. The serum half-life of ceftazidime is also inversely related to GA and postnatal age [18, 19, 20]. Both perinatal asphyxia and patent ductus arteriosus treated with indomethacin are associated with prolonged serum ceftazidime half-life values [20, 22]. The serum half-life of ceftriaxone is inversely correlated with GA having values which ranged from 8 to 34 h in neonates. In another study, the mean serum half-life for ceftriaxone was 15.5 h.

Table 3. Pharmacokinetics of third generation cephalosporins

Reference	Antibiotic	No	GA (weeks)	PNA (days)	Weight (g)	CL (mL/h/kg)	V (mL/kg)	$t_{1/2}$ (h)
Aujard [14]	Cefotaxime	3	<32	<7	–	65	340	3.5
Kearns [15]	Cefotaxime	18	<32	<8	<1500	50–100	310–790	3.4–6.4
Gouyon [16]	Cefotaxime	10	28–37	3–8	–	36–192	219–636	1.9–6.8
Kearns [15]	Desacetyl-Cefotaxime	17	<32	<8	<1500	–	–	3.1–35.8
McCracken [17]	Ceftriaxone	10	–	1–4	<1500	60	610	7.7
		3	–	6–8	<1500	44	530	8.4
McCracken [18]	Ceftazidime	7	<33	<22	–	59	530	6.7
Anker [9]	Ceftazidime	136	24–37	3	1413	37	350	7.0
Anker [20]	Ceftazidime	11	29	3	1052	31	363	8.7
		11	29	10	1163	42	292	5.0
Anker [21]	Ceftazidime	15	<32	3	1141	31	323	8.2
		13	<32	3	1168	28	305	7.1

Abbreviations: No, number; *GA*, gestational age; *PNA*, postnatal age; *CL*, total body clearance; *V*, apparent volume of distribution; $t_{1/2}$, serum half-life

Cefotaxime and desacetyl-cefotaxime penetrate into the CSF of infants with meningitis. Ceftazidime also penetrates well into the CSF, especially in the presence of meningitis. Penetration into the CSF is apparently independent of meningeal inflammation, which is in agreement with recent data in preterm infants without meningeal inflammation. Penetration of ceftriaxone into the CSF was higher in patients with bacterial meningitis (17%) in comparison with that observed in infants with aseptic meningitis (4.1%). The CSF penetration of ceftriaxone is substantially less in older infants and children with bacterial meningitis (2 to 7%).

We conclude that GA, postnatal age, renal and hepatic function are important determinants for the clinical pharmacokinetics of the three most frequently used cephalosporins. Possible alternate and currently recommended dosing regimens for cefotaxime, ceftriaxone and ceftazidime are presented in Table 4. The reduced capacity to eliminate cephalosporins, especially during the first week of life, enables a prolongation of the dosing interval of cefotaxime and ceftazidime from 12 h to 24 h in preterm infants with GAs of less than 28 weeks, and from 24 h to 36 h for ceftriaxone. The rapid postnatal changes in plasma drug clearance enables a shortening of the dosing interval of cefotaxime from 12 h to 8 h in preterm infants with GAs between 28 and 32 weeks who have a postnatal age of >7 days. For ceftriaxone, a shortening of the dosing interval from 24 h to 18 h seems indicated based on developmental changes in its pharmacokinetics. Once-daily administration of 25 mg/kg of ceftazidime in preterm infants with GAs of less than 32 weeks leads to serum levels well above the minimal inhibitory concentration for major neonatal pathogens during the entire dosing interval [21]. Alternatively this can also be achieved by twice-daily administration of 10 mg/kg of ceftazidime in preterm infants with GAs of less than 28 weeks during the first week, or twice daily dosing of 15 mg/kg in

Table 4. Alternate and currently used dosage schedules for third generation cephalosoporins

	Dosage (mg/kg) and interval of administration			
Antibiotics	GA <28 weeks PNA (days)		GA 28–32 weeks PNA (days)	
	0–7	7–28	0–7	7–28
Cefotaxime	50 q 24h (50 q 12h)	50 q 12h (50 q 12h)	50 q 12h (50 q 12h)	50 q 8h (50 q 12h)
Ceftriaxone	50 q 36h (50 q 24h)	50 q 24h (50 q 24h)	50 q 24h (50 q 24h)	50 q 18h (50 q 24h)
Ceftazidime	25 q 24h 10 q 12h (50 q 12h)	25 q 24h 15 q 12h (50 q 12h)	25 q 24h 15 q 12h (50 q 12h)	25 q 12h 25 q 12h (50 q 12h)

Abbreviations: GA, gestational age; *PNA,* postnatal age

Values given between parentheses represent currently recommended dosages preterm infants with GAs between 28 and 32 weeks [19]. In the second week this should be altered to twice daily doses of 15 mg/kg in preterm infants with GAs of less than 28 weeks, or 25 mg/kg twice daily in preterm infants with GAs between 28 and 32 weeks [20]. Therefore, alteration of both the dose and dosing interval may be required to ensure optimal therapy with ceftazidime. There is a need to obtain more information on desacetyl-cefotaxime and ceftriaxone in order to further specify dosage recommendations for preterm infants.

Vancomycin

Vancomycin has good antibacterial activity against methicillin-resistant staphylococci. This drug is not appreciably metabolized but rather, is excreted primarily unchanged in the urine. Although vancomycin was originally thought to be ototoxic and nephrotoxic, recent animal experimental studies did not show any evidence of toxicity. It is likewise difficult to document that vancomycin is ototoxic or nephrotoxic in humans. Vancomycin is well tolerated and safe, particularly in newborn and young infants. When administered in a less than 30-minute infusion, older patients may develop the Red Man syndrome, a histamine reaction characterized by an erythematous, pruritic rash on the upper part of the body and arms and on the neck and face. Such reactions have not been reported in newborns.

The data on the pharmacokinetics of vancomycin in preterm infants are presented in Table 5 [23, 24, 25, 26, 27, 28]. The serum half-life of vancomycin correlates inversely with GA and postnatal age in neonates during the first week of life [28]. It is also inversely correlated with serum creatinine [26,27,28] and with postconceptional age in older neonates [23, 24, 26, 28]. CSF concentrations of vancomycin vary between 1.2 and 4.8 mg/L and represent 7 to 21% of the corresponding serum concentrations in infants with ventriculo-peritoneal shunt infections.

Table 5. Pharmacokinetics of vancomycin

Reference	Antibiotic	No	GA (weeks)	PNA (days)	Weight (g)	CL (mL/h/kg)	V (mL/kg)	$t_{1/2}$ (h)
Reed [23]	Vancomycin	12	28	21	1069	74	520	6.6
Lisby-Sutch [24]	Vancomycin	5	30–34	13–42	–	43	470	7.8
Gross [25]	Vancomycin	3	24–27	27–32	<1000	66	970	9.9
		6	26–28	26–62	>1000	62	450	5.3
Leonard [26]	Vancomycin	19	24–29	20	<1000	48	680	10.6
Kildoo [27]	Vancomycin	15	29	29	1297	64	480	5.6
James [28]	Vancomycin	17	25–35	–	880	36–78	–	6–17

Abbreviations: No, number; *GA*, gestational age; *PNA*, postnatal age; *CL*, total body clearance; *V*, apparent volume of distribution; $t_{1/2}$, serum half-life

In adults with normal renal function, routine monitoring of serum vancomycin concentrations is generally not required for avoiding toxicity. However, there are a number of clinical settings in which the determination of vancomycin levels in serum or other body fluids is advocated. These include patients who receive vancomycin/aminoglycoside combinations, patients undergoing hemodialysis, patients receiving higher-than-usual-doses, patients with rapidly changing renal function (eg. preterm infants) and in patients with a sensitive organism who fail to respond (ie. clinically or microbiologically). Monitoring to achieve therapeutic and non-toxic concentrations of vancomycin was originally based upon models used to direct aminoglycoside therapy, in which peaks were assumed to be therapeutically important. Current understanding of both agents makes such a comparison inappropriate. Optimal vancomycin therapy requires the maintenance of therapeutic through concentrations and avoidance of unnecessary high peaks. Trough levels should ideally be maintained between 5 and 12 mg/L, and concentrations above 10 mg/L should be thought of as early signs of accumulation. Recent data support that peak vancomycin concentrations do not need to be routinely measured in preterm infants if trough concentrations are below 12 mg/L [29].

Possible alternate and currently recommended dosing regimens for vancomycin are presented in Table 6. The reduced renal capacity to eliminate vancomycin, especially during the first week of life, enables an extension of the dosing interval from 24 h to 36 h in preterm infants with GAs of less than 28 weeks. The rapid postnatal changes in GFR enable a shortening of the dosing interval from 24 h to 18 h in preterm infants with GAs between 28 and 32 weeks. Alternatively, a reduction of the dosage to 5 mg/kg twice daily will probably produce therapeutic serum concentrations whereas high peak values are avoided. However, if the apparent volume of distribution is greater than 0.7 L/kg, which may occasionally occur in the sick neonate, this dose may yield subtherapeutic serum concentrations for the treatment of infections caused by methicillin resistant staphylococci. Prenatal exposure to indomethacin, the concomitant prescription of an aminoglycoside, and asphyxia may necessitate

Table 6. Alternate and currently used dosage schedules for vancomycin

	Dosage (mg/kg) and interval of administration			
Antibiotics	GA <28 weeks PNA (days)		GA 28–32 weeks PNA (days)	
	0–7	7–28	0–7	7–28
Vancomycin	15 q 36h 5 q 12h (15 q 24h)	15 q 24h 7.5 q 12h (15 q 24h)	15 q 24h 7.5 q 12h (15 q 24h)	15 q 18h 10 q 12h (15 q 24h)

Abbreviations: GA, gestational age; *PNA,* postnatal age
Values given between parentheses represent currently recommended dosages

further dosage adjustments and the need to monitor serum vancomycin concentrations.

We conclude that GA, postnatal age, and renal function are major determinants for the disposition of vancomycin and that age-associated pharmacokinetic parameters should be used to individualize doses of this drug in the neonate.

Conclusion

The pharmacokinetics and pharmacodynamics of many antibiotics are insufficiently studied in newborns with GAs of less than 32 weeks. Antibiotic pharmacokinetic data in preterm infants with GAs of less than 28 weeks are almost completely absent. The few available studies show that the absorption, distribution, protein binding, biotransformation and excretion of antibiotics in preterm infants are significantly different from those in older children and adults. The metabolism and renal excretion of several antibiotics are initially severely impaired, but show a rapid improvement in the first month of life. The rapid acquisition of developmental competence in drug clearance in the first month of life has a major impact on the pharmacokinetics and dosing schedules of antibiotics in preterm infants as is illustrated in this review.

Finally, it is important to combine pharmacokinetic studies of antimicrobial agents in the newborn with assessments of both tolerability and pharmacodynamics. This will enable the development of "target" dosing strategies which are both age and disease specific and most importantly of immediate clinical utility.

References

1. Remington JS, Klein JO, eds (1995) Infectious diseases of the fetus & newborn infant. 4th ed. Philadelphia: Saunders.
2. Besunder JB, Reed MD, Blumer JL (1988) Principles of drug biodisposition in the neonate. A critical evaluation of the pharmacokinetic-pharmacodynamic interface (Part 1) Clin Pharmacokinet 14:189–216.
3. Prober CG, Stevenson DK, Benitz WE (1990) The use of antibiotics in neonates weighing less than 1200 grams. Pediatr Infect Dis J 9:111–121.
4. Kildoo C, Modanlou HD, Komatsu G, Harralson A, Hodding J (1984) Developmental pattern of gentamicin kinetics in very low birth weight (VLBW) sick infants. Dev Pharmacol Ther 7:345–356.
5. Koren G, Leeder S, Harding E, Jacques D, MacLeod SM (1985) Optimization of gentamicin therapy in very low birth weight infants. Pediatr Pharmacol (New York) 5:79–87.
6. Landers S, Berry PL, Kearns GL, Kaplan SL, Rudolph AJ (1984) Gentamicin disposition and effect on development of renal function in the very low birth weight infant. Dev Pharmacol Ther 7:285–302.
7. Nahata MC, Powell DA, Gregoire RP, et al (1983) Tobramycin kinetics in newborn infants. J Pediatr 103:136–138.
8. Nahata MC, Powell DA, Durrell DE, Miller MC, Glazer JP (1984) Effect of gestational age and birth weight on tobramycin kinetics in newborn infants. J Antimicrob Chemother 14:59–65.

9. Nahata MC, Powell DA, Durrell DE, Miller MA (1986) Tobramycin pharmacokinetics in very low birth weight infants. Br J Clin Pharmacol 21:325-327.
10. Kuhn RJ, Nahata MC, Powell DA, Bickers RG (1986) Pharmacokinetics of netilmicin in premature infants. Eur J Clin Pharmacol 29:635–637.
11. Kenyon CF, Knoppert DC, Lee SK, Vandenberghe HM, Chance GW (1990) Amikacin pharmacokinetics and suggested dosage modifications for the preterm infant. Antimicrob Agents Chemother 34:265–268.
12. Van den Anker JN, Hop WC, De Groot R, et al (1994) Effects of prenatal exposure to betamethasone and indomethacin on the glomerular filtration rate in the preterm infant. Pediatr Res 36:578–581.
13. Jacobs RF, Kearns GL (1989) Cefotaxime and desacetylcefotaxime in neonates and children: a review of microbiologic, pharmacokinetic, and clinical experience. Diagn Microbiol Infect Dis 12:93–99.
14. Aujard Y, Brion F, Jacqz-Aigrain E, et al (1989) Pharmacokinetics of cefotaxime and desacetyl-cefotaxime in the newborn. Diagn Microbiol Infect Dis 12:87–91.
15. Kearns GL, Jacobs RF, Thomas BR, Darville TL, Trang JM (1989) Cefotaxime and desacetyl-cefotaxime pharmacokinetics in very low birth weight neonates. J Pediatr 114:461–467.
16. Gouyon JB, Pechinot A, Safran C, Chretien P, Sandre D, Kazmierczak A (1990) Pharmacokinetics of cefotaxime in preterm infants. Dev Pharmacol Ther 14:29–34.
17. McCracken GH Jr, Siegel JD, Threlkeld N, Thomas M (1983) Ceftriaxone pharmacokinetics in newborn infants. Antimicrob Agents Chemother 23:341–343.
18. McCracken GH Jr, Threlkeld N, Thomas ML (1984) Pharmacokinetics of ceftazidime in newborn infants. Antimicrob Agents Chemother 26:583–584.
19. Van den Anker JN, Schoemaker RC, Hop WC, et al (1995) Ceftazidime pharmacokinetics in preterm infants: effects of renal function and gestational age. Clin Pharmacol Ther 58:650–659.
20. Van den Anker JN, Hop WC, Schoemaker RC, Van der Heijden AJ, Neijens HJ, De Groot R (1995) Ceftazidime pharmacokinetics in preterm infants: effect of postnatal age and postnatal exposure to indomethacin. Br J Clin Pharmacol 40:439-443.
21. Van den Anker JN, Schoemaker RC, Van der Heijden AJ, Broerse HM, Neijens HJ, De Groot R (1995) Once-daily versus twice-daily administration of ceftazidime in the preterm infant. Antimicrob Agents Chemother 39:2048–2050.
22. Van den Anker JN, Van der Heijden AJ, Hop WC, et al (1995) The effect of asphyxia on the pharmacokinetics of ceftazidime in the term newborn. Pediatr Res 38:808–811.
23. Reed MD, Kliegman RM, Weiner JS, Huang M, Yamashita TS, Blumer JL (1987) The clinical pharmacology of vancomycin in seriously ill preterm infants. Pediatr Res 22:360–363.
24. Lisby-Sutch SM, Nahata MC (1988) Dosage guidelines for the use of vancomycin based on its pharmacokinetics in infants. Eur J Clin Pharmacol 35:637–642.
25. Gross JR, Kaplan SL, Kramer WG, Mason EO Jr (1985) Vancomycin pharmacokinetics in premature infants. Pediatr Pharmacol (New York) 5:17–22.
26. Leonard MB, Koren G, Stevenson DK, Prober CG (1989) Vancomycin pharmacokinetics in very low birth weight neonates. Pediatr Infect Dis J 8:282-286.
27. Kildoo CW, Lin LM, Gabriel MH, Folli HL, Modanlou HD (1990) Vancomycin pharmacokinetics in infants: relationship to postconceptional age and serum creatinine. Dev Pharmacol Ther 14:77–83.
28. James A, Koren G, Milliken J, Soldin S, Prober C (1987) Vancomycin pharmacokinetics and dose recommendations for preterm infants. Antimicrob Agents Chemother 31:52–54.
29. De Hoog M, Mouton JW, Van den Anker JN (1995) Why monitor peak vancomycin concentrations? Lancet 345:646.

Pulmonary Function

Monitoring and Assessment of the Pulmonary Function in Ventilated Infants and Children

Y. Sivan and Chr. J. L. Newth

Introduction

Respiratory monitoring is standard of care of ventilated children with respiratory failure. This by itself may be an indication for admission to a Pediatric Intensive Care Unit (PICU) equipped with modern technology since continuous monitoring has the potential for alerting the clinician for sudden deteriorations and thus allow for timely intervention.

The major goals of respiratory measurements and monitoring are:

1) to measure, continuously, ventilatory indices that enhance our understanding of the underlying pathophysiology, aid in diagnosis, and guide management;
2) to provide alarms that alert caregivers to a significant change in the patient's condition; and
3) to provide trends that assist in the assessment of the severity of the disease and the therapeutic response and prognosis. Hence, all patients with moderate to severe respiratory failure should be monitored for gas exchange and preferably also for respiratory mechanics.

Two main difficulties arise when assessing pulmonary functions in infants and small children:

a) Lack of co-operation: co-operation is required to perform many "adult-type" pulmonary function tests and can be achieved in children only after 6–7 years of age;
b) Small size of young patients: The latter is evident as small volumes and flow rates in absolute terms which necessitate the use of complex equipment and technique.

On the other hand, unique physiological and anatomical characteristics of the infant and the small child make certain methods of evaluation of the respiratory system possible mainly and almost exclusively in this age group (e.g. transcutaneous blood gas measurement, maximal expiratory flow rates, thoracoabdominal asynchrony in some clinical situations).

Therefore, monitoring of pediatric patients requires an individual and careful approach based on physical examination, non-invasive techniques and selective application of invasive measures.

Clinical assessment of cyanosis and alveolar ventilation, and hence arterial oxygen and carbon dioxide tensions, is unreliable [1, 2]. Thus, precise assessment of ventilatory adequacy must be based on both clinical and laboratory studies, and much emphasis has had to be placed on arterial blood gases (or their indirect measurement) for help with both the diagnosis and management of respiratory failure. Recently, the incorporation of high speed microprocessors and personal computers has enabled the application of old, and the development of new, pulmonary function tests suitable for those unable to cooperate (e.g. infants, young children and patients who are under neuromuscular blockade and/or heavily sedated). This has allowed those involved in the care of such patients to make novel measurements of physiologic variables and reach new perspectives in both the assessment and management of respiratory failure.

This chapter reviews the options available today for the clinician in monitoring and evaluation of the function of the respiratory system in ventilated infants and children. Some of the methods, such as continuous non-invasive assessment of oxygen saturation, are standard of care while other techniques might be indicated only for specific patients because they are time consuming and require expensive equipment and skill. We believe that any intervention which provides more understanding of disease processes is expedient and justified, providing there is little or no deleterious effect on the patient.

Assessment of the Respiratory System

Monitoring and evaluation of the respiratory system is based on three major themes:

1) physical examination;
2) invasive monitoring;
3) non-invasive monitoring.

Much effort has been devoted to develop new non-invasive techniques which would replace invasive methods. We emphasize that "invasiveness" is a relative term and that non-invasive techniques may also harm the patient. For example, procedures such as flow-volume loops originated by forced chest compression and chest radiography are not considered invasive; nevertheless, repeated and frequent assessment may harm the patient.

Physical Examination Monitoring

- Respiratory rate
- Breathing pattern
- Breath sounds
- Skin color
- Pulsus paradoxus
- Cerebral function

Respiratory rate is an easy variable to monitor in non-ventilated infants and children. This variable is reliable primarily during sleep and may vary significantly in awake situation. Breathing rate changes significantly with age so normal values for age should be referenced. Breathing pattern, chest retractions and breathing asynchrony may all characterize respiratory status, nevertheless, they are applicable almost exclusively to non-ventilated patients (or those on low ventilator rate and CPAP). Clinical scoring systems based on skin color, breathing pattern, breath sounds and cerebral function have been developed for common acute respiratory failure situations in infants and children including acute asthmatic attack and acute upper airway obstruction (UAO) [3, 4,5]. However, at least for acute UAO these were found to be unreliable, when compared to objective measurements [5].

Invasive Respiratory Monitoring

- Arterial blood gases
- Mixed venous oxygen tension

Arterial Blood Gases

The interpretation of arterial blood gases is beyond the scope of this paper, but comprehensive reviews of the types of arterial blood gas and acid-base disturbances observed in respiratory failure are available [1].

Invasive respiratory monitoring of patients in respiratory failure is based on arterial blood sampling for arterial blood gas (ABG) analysis. Intermittent arterial blood gas analysis is still regarded as the standard diagnostic tool for accurate assessment of pulmonary gas exchange and ventilator management. This is either a painful procedure or requires indwelling arterial catheters which may produce complications. Another major disadvantage is that ABG analysis provides only intermittent data and may miss sudden changes. Oxygenation indices based on arterial pO_2 levels have been used in clinical practice. These include: $(A\text{-}a)DO_2$, PaO_2/PAO_2 (alveolar-arterial pO_2 difference and ratio respectively) and PaO_2/FiO_2.

Recently, *continuous invasive ABG monitoring* has become available for pediatric patients. This allows continuous analysis of pH as well as PaO_2 and $PaCO_2$ by means of an intra-arterial fiberoptic sensor and the results are displayed on a bedside monitor [1]. Clinical studies are still required to prove its usefulness, applicability, reliability and cost effectiveness in infants and children. Potential applications include all clinical conditions with a high probability for cardiorespiratory instability requiring frequent ABG sampling, including intra- and post-operative management of patients undergoing cardiothoracic surgery, weaning from ECMO and HFOV, and ARDS.

Another problem is that ABG is affected also by patient's crying or altered ventilation just prior to ABG sampling. In the sedated ventilated child with indwelling arterial lines, this should not occur. In some more severe situations, mixed venous (pulmonary artery) SvO_2 is also used. This is, however, much less commonly performed in children as it requires pulmonary artery catheterization, a technique seen as being less applicable in children compared with adults.

Technologic advances made noninvasive devices available for continuous monitoring of oxygen (O_2) and carbon dioxide (CO_2). These include end-tidal CO_2, transcutaneous CO_2 and O_2 and pulse oximetry (*vide infra*). If the caregiver is aware of their limitations, they allow a quick feedback on rapidly changing conditions and are helpful in the continuous supervision of respiratory therapy. Detailed descriptions of their operation and limitations are available in recent reviews [8, 9]. Noninvasive blood gas monitoring has the potential to reduce significantly the frequency of ABG sampling (e.g. at the Children's Hospital of Los Angeles a 50% decrease in ABG sampling was recorded during the first three years that pulse oximetry, transcutaneous and end-tidal CO_2 were introduced into the PICU, with similar numbers of patients admitted each year).

Non-Invasive Respiratory Monitoring

- Chest radiography
- Ventilation
- Oxygenation
- Respiratory mechanics
- Lung volumes
- Metabolic Gas Exchange
- Respiratory muscle function

Chest Radiography

Although not unanimously agreed, it appears appropriate to do routine daily chest radiographs in intubated mechanically ventilated children. Out of 538 routine daily chest radiographs in one series of 74 adult ICU patients [10], major findings, defined as those requiring immediate diagnostic or therapeutic intervention, were detected in 13 patients (17.6%). However, the fraction of new major findings determined solely by the chest films as a percentage of total films was small (18/538 or 3.4%). Endotracheal tube (ETT) malposition counted as the most common major finding followed by central venous line malpositioning, pneumothorax and pleural effusion. The clinical value of routine chest radiographs in a pediatric ICU has also been demonstrated [11]. It is reasonable to assume that tube malposition will be encountered more frequently in infants and small children than in adults because of the ETT mobility with head position and thus has less room for error in this age group [12].

Ventilation

Arterial carbon dioxide level is the measurement of alveolar ventilation. Non-invasive techniques for $PaCO_2$ measurement include *capnography* and *transcutaneous CO_2* monitoring.

End-Tidal Carbon Dioxide
End-tidal carbon dioxide (E_TCO_2) is usually measured and monitored by respiratory mass spectrometry or by non-dispersive infrared absorption spectrophotometry. Two techniques are available: side-stream in which gas from the proximal end of the ETT is continuously aspirated and main-stream in which an inline CO_2 sensor is directly connected to the ETT and is thus advantageous in ventilated patients. This allows a continuous display of a breath-by-breath waveform of CO_2 concentration changes during respiration. End-tidal CO_2 pressure ($PetCO_2$), measured as the plateau value of an exhaled CO_2 display, closely approximates the $PaCO_2$ in normal lungs and may be used to measure $PaCO_2$ non-invasively and continuously. Although end-tidal CO_2 monitoring by capnography is routinely used for healthy infants and children in sleep laboratories, its use to assess $PaCO_2$ is limited to following trends in children requiring assisted ventilation for cardiorespiratory diseases that affect gas exchange and ventilation-perfusion (/) matching [13]. In patients with extreme / mismatches such as with ARDS or obstructive lung diseases large alveolar-arterial CO_2 gradients can be observed and E_TCO_2 underestimates $PaCO_2$. It has been shown that E_TCO_2 can be used for $PaCO_2$ estimation in ventilated children with mild to moderate lung disease, but can be used only for detecting trends in children with severe pulmonary impairment and / mismatching [1]. This may explain why capnography has not been so widely used in the pediatric ICU. Several investigators have suggested that $PetCO_2$ is not applicable to children with severe / mismatching and that correction factors should be employed [15]. The gap between $PaCO_2$ and $PetCO_2$ is partly caused by uneven ventilation and nonhomogeneous pulmonary capillary blood distribution. An error in recording may also result from the lack of alveolar plateau (which is necessary for end-tidal recording). The lack of the plateau phase is more likely to occur in small children who breath at relatively high rates and small V_T. In a study of 134 mechanically ventilated infants and children where only end-tidal CO_2 values were used, it was possible to define the limitations of the technique [14]. $PetCO_2$ was found to be a reliable and accurate method for $PaCO_2$ assessment as long as the PaO_2/PAO_2 ratio was greater than 0.3. In ventilated children with PaO_2/PAO_2 less than 0.3, $PetCO_2$ could still be used but only for detecting trends in $PaCO_2$ changes. However, capnography is very useful in the guidance of hyperventilation for intracranial hypertension, detection of endotracheal tube accidents (disconnection, obstruction, accidental extubation, esophageal intubation) and the determination of the patient's progress during weaning from ventilatory support [16–21]. When a sudden drop in $PetCO_2$ occurs and $PaCO_2$ is unchanged one should suspect increased dead space ventilation. This is typical for pulmonary vascular disease or pulmonary embolism. In

this situation, there are alveoli which are not perfused so their $PaCO_2$ stays low resulting in low end-tidal CO_2 levels. During cardiac arrest, circulation ceases and $PetCO_2$ gradually falls (while $PaCO_2$ rises) reappearing as an elevated Pet-CO_2 only when pulmonary circulation is restored by effective resuscitation. Hence, $PetCO_2$ monitoring can be used to assess the extent to which resuscitative measures maintain pulmonary perfusion.

Transcutaneous CO_2 Monitoring

Transcutaneous CO_2 ($P_{tc}CO_2$) monitoring devices measure the CO_2 tension at the surface of the epidermis. Because of the high CO_2 tissue solubility this allows an accurate estimation of $PaCO_2$ in conditions with normal skin perfusion [16, 1,2]. This is especially true for neonates where a thin skin improves the degree of accuracy of $P_{tc}CO_2$ monitoring [24, 25]. However, it is important to emphasize that $P_{tc}CO_2$ is higher than the corresponding $PaCO_2$. This difference is influenced by the higher temperature at which the electrodes operate (43–44°C), local metabolic CO_2 production, capillary blood flow and cardiac output [1]. This leads to an unpredictable overestimation of $PaCO_2$ in conditions with significantly reduced skin perfusion [15]. In a study of 134 children receiving mechanical ventilation, skin perfusion at the site of the transcutaneous electrode was found to significantly influence $TcPCO_2$ accuracy [14]. In infants and children with normal skin perfusion (capillary refill time less than 3 seconds), the mean difference between $TcPCO_2$ and $PaCO_2$ was only 0.2 mmhg (SD = 5.4) compared to 4.1 (SD = 9.9) in patients with decreased skin perfusion. Hence, this technique may not be satisfactory and applicable in patients with low skin perfusion. Further, the long response and lag times of the electrode limit the use to a select group of hemodynamically stable patients [23]. Despite its limitations, $P_{tc}CO_2$ is accurate in neonatal patients and adds valuable information (at the least as a trend monitor) in older infants and children.

Oxygenation

Pulse Oximetry

Pulse oximetry is based on the fact that oxygenated and reduced hemoglobin can be distinguished by their differential absorption of two wavelengths of light. It allows an easy and continuous way to measure and assess oxygen saturation (SaO_2). In addition to the ECG and respiration, most ventilated infants and children are monitored for SaO_2 by pulse oximetry (SpO_2). One concern about pulse oximetry in pediatric ICU patients is the decreased accuracy at low saturation levels resulting in significantly overestimation or underestimation of true SaO_2 when O_2 saturation falls below 75–80% [1, 2]. Pulse oximetry is quite accurate at SaO_2 levels above 85% with 95% confidence limits of approximately + 4% (4). However, because of the shape of the oxygen dissociation curve with its characteristic flat section at PaO_2 levels above 60 mmHg, large discrepant oxygen tensions may be related to a single level of pulse oximetry reading. This may be even more pronounced when the hemoglobin dissociation curve is shifted to the right or left as a result of changes in pH, temperature and 2,3 DPG or from the presence of fetal hemoglobin in small infants. When 14 pulse oximeters were evaluated and their SpO_2 was compared to SaO_2 measured simultaneously with drawn blood samples, it was found that both the error in accuracy (mean $SpO_2 - SaO_2$), and the error in precision (SD of the differences) remained below 3% for $SaO_2 > 83\%$, but were increased to 8% and 5% respectively for deeper hypoxia [1]. Inaccuracies may also occur in the presence of jaundice, elevated carboxyhemoglobin and skin pigmentation [30, 31] and during the loss of a reliable waveform in low perfusion states. The latter may be partially overcome with the new combined pulse oximeters which also simultaneously monitor pulse rate from chest electrodes. This pulse oximeter disregards measurements when peripheral and central pulse rates are not in agreement. Although there is little in the literature, there appears to be only a marginal influence on accuracy due to the presence of fetal rather than adult hemoglobin in neonates and infants in the first 2–3 months of life. Another disadvantage of the pulse oximeter is that it does not alert for hyperoxygenation – a situation which may be dangerous in preterm infants. Thus, infants of this age group need to be monitored by the transcutaneous PO_2 technique which has been found reliable for preterm neonates whose skin is very thin [27]. Despite these limitations, pulse oximetry is very useful in monitoring oxygenation, the detection of hypoxemia and the guidance of cardiorespiratory therapy.

Respiratory Mechanics

The mechanic properties of the lungs are best described by flow-volume loops.

Tidal Breathing Flow-Volume Loops

Tidal breathing flow-volume or pressure-volume loops (TBFV or TBPV loops) are increasingly used in continuous or intermittent monitoring of mechanical ventilation in both Neonatal and Pediatric ICU's. They can be measured on special "stand-alone" equipment, or are increasingly incorporated into modern ventilators. These allow the measurement of tidal volume (V_T), tidal flows and pressures generated during mechanical and spontaneous breaths. Thus, impacts of alteration in ventilator settings or lung physiology on these parameters can be readily detected [32, 33]. Spontaneous tidal volume breaths and ventilator breaths can be compared (especially along the expiratory flow limb where flow-limitation may be readily seen) which enables an estimate of the ventilatory reserve provided by mechanical ventilation (Figures 1 and 2).

Nevertheless, experience showing the usefulness of this variable in clinical practice is scarce. Spontaneous breaths may differ significantly, hence, the TBFV loops vary so that no significant clinical information can be obtained. Ventilator breaths are much more consistent so are the TBFV loops derived. One possible use of TBFV curves is when flow limitation already occurs during

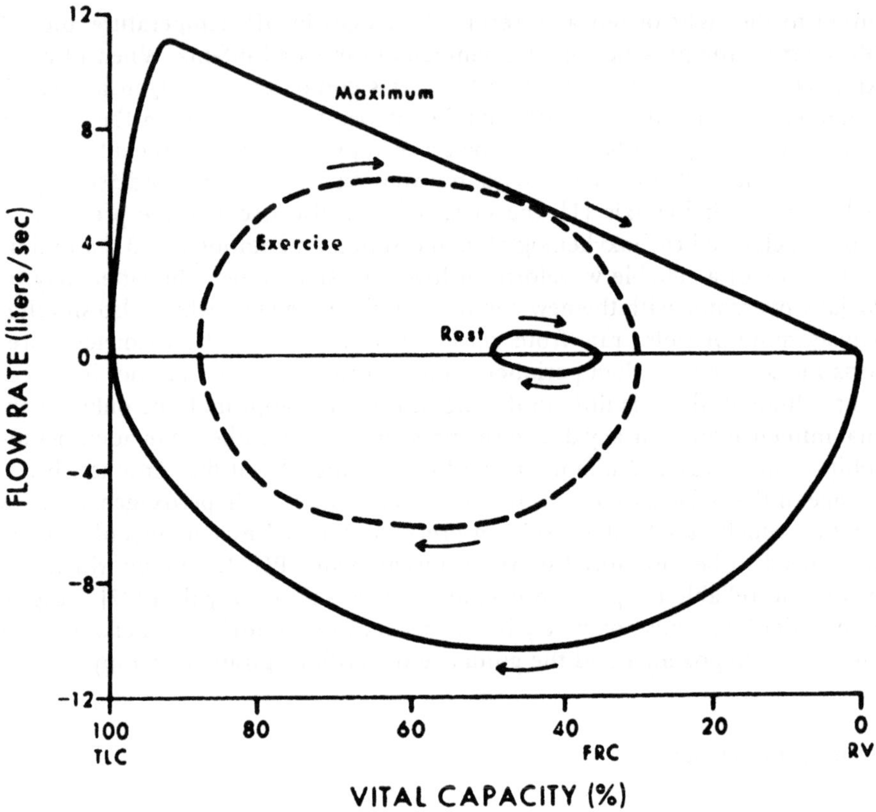

Fig. 1. Superimposed FV-loops demonstrating the concept of flow limitation. Three FV-loops from a tidal breath, a tidal breath during exercise and from a voluntary maximal expiratory maneuver demonstrate that flow limitation can be partly reached during exercise.

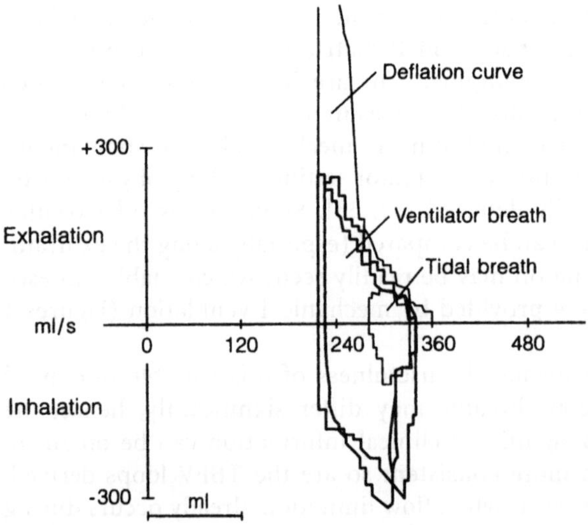

Fig. 2. Superimposed tidal breath, ventilator breath and forced deflation FV-loops of a 9.5 month old infant with BPD illustrate the lack of ventilatory reserve. In this patient airway obstruction is so severe that flow limitation (proven by forced deflation) occurs even during tidal breathing (Reproduced with permission from Hammer J and Newth CJL. Intensive Care Med (1995) 21:744)

tidal breathing indicating lack of respiratory reserve (Figure 2). However, this still requires forced expiratory flow-volume loops for comparison and reference. The shape of the loop may be useful to detect various types of airway pathology or partially obstructed endotracheal tubes [34].

Forced Expiratory Flow-Volume Loops

The measurement of maximal expiratory flows (MEF) is a sensitive test of abnormalities in the tracheobronchial tree and contributes greatly to the diagnosis and treatment of lung disease. Two different techniques have been developed to allow examination of forced expiratory flow-volume loops (FEFV loops) in small children who are unable to generate a voluntary maximal expiratory maneuver: the forced deflation (FD) technique and the rapid thoracoabdominal compression (RTC) technique [1, 2]. These methods are also used to measure maximal flow rate at FRC and flow limitation [36–38]. It is important that techniques measuring MEF rates reach flow limitation for precise interpretation of the acquired data. Unless it is certain that flow is limited (effort independent) at a particular lung volume, changes in flow rates after a therapeutic maneuver (e.g. bronchodilator) may still be attributed to factors other than a simple response to therapy. It has recently been shown that the FD and the RTC techniques are capable of producing forced expiratory flows at flow limitation in intubated animals and infants with normal and obstructed airways [37,38,1]. Nevertheless, it should be noted that the RTC method may be difficult and cumbersome to perform in ventilated infants and small children because it requires wrapping the patient's chest and abdomen interfering with tubes and sensors applied to the trunk which also may prevent satisfactory contact of the jacket onto the body. While RTC can be performed in non-ventilated spontaneously breathing children, the deflation method was developed specifically for intubated infants and children, may be advantageous in this population and may be regarded as the "gold standard" to measure vital capacity (VC) and MEF in intubated or tracheotomized infants and children.

For the FD test procedure, the lungs are inflated by squeezing a breathing bag filled from a continuous compressed O_2 supply to +40 cm H_2O inflation pressure, defined as total lung capacity (TLC). Inflation pressures are held static for at least 3 seconds, after which a sliding valve is activated to expose the airways to a 100-L capacity, constant negative pressure source of -40 cm H_2O deflation pressure. The lungs are deflated until expiratory flow ceases at residual volume (RV) or for at least 3 seconds. VC and MEF at various subdivisions are measured by an interposed pneumotachograph. Throughout the procedure the individual is usually under neuromuscular blockade and/or heavy sedation.

Normal values for VC and MEF at the various subdivisions still need to be defined, but in our laboratory lie in the range of 55–70 $ml \cdot kg^{-1}$ for VC and 24–38 $ml \cdot kg^{-1} \cdot sec^{-1}$ for MEF_{25} and 6–15 $ml \cdot kg^{-1} \cdot sec^{-1}$ for MEF_{10}. Since it has become standard of care to use inhaled bronchodilators on intubated and ventilated patients in a variety of diseases, their effectiveness can easily be documented by the FD technique [1]. Obstructive airways and restrictive lung dis-

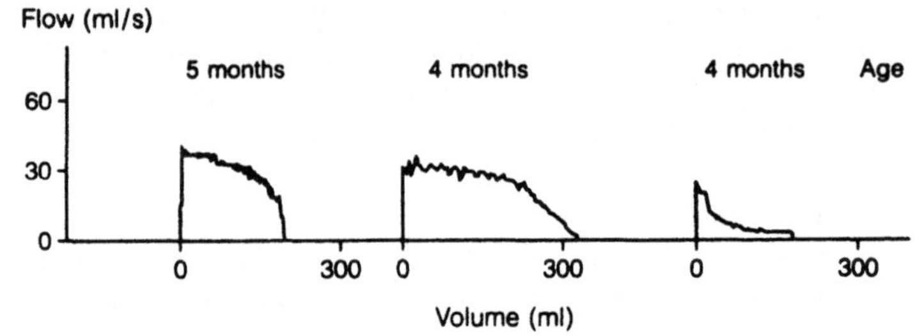

	ARDS (restrictive)	Normal	Bronchiolitis (obstructive)
VC (ml/kg)	30	68	23
MEF_{25} (ml/kg/s)	48	45	3

Fig. 3. Typical forced deflation FV-curves from TLC (+40 cm H_2O) to RV (−40 cm H_2O). Each curve generated from a child with cuffed 3.5 mm I.D. ETT under neuromuscular blockade (Reproduced with permission from Hammer J and Newth CJL. Intensive Care Med (1995) 21:744)

eases produce very characteristic patterns (Figure 3) which are helpful in assessing the underlying pathophysiology (e.g. RSV infection causing bronchiolitis, airway disease in BPD, ARDS or pneumonia).

Serial VC and MEF assessments are helpful in a variety of lung diseases like BPD and ARDS requiring long term mechanical ventilation and document the resolution or progression of the disease process [41]. These measurements are helpful in the evaluation of the response to therapy in a wide range of clinical situations: e.g. the response of a ventilated child with bronchiolitis, viral pneumonia or BPD to aerosolized bronchodilators and the response of patients with cardiogenic pulmonary edema, ARDS, diffuse pneumonia to diuretics.

Resistance and Compliance

Compliance and resistance reflect the mechanical properties of the respiratory system and require the measurement of flow, volume and pressure. Compliance (C) is defined as the change in volume per unit change in pressure:

$$C = \frac{\Delta \text{volume}}{\Delta \text{pressure}} = \frac{\text{ml}}{\text{cm H}_2\text{O}}$$

Monitoring of respiratory compliance and resistance as well as of lung volumes can assist the clinician to: a) obtain better understanding of the physiology of the disease b) indicate the course of the disease; c) optimize ventilator settings; d) assess the effectiveness of treatments modalities and medications. It must be emphasized that compliance reflects the mechanical properties of the respiratory system only if measured value is corrected for the absolute volume of gas in the lungs (*specific compliance*). In other words, the value obtained is different at various lung volumes, dependent on the shape of the pressure-volume curve, which in turn depends on the amount of lung disease and therapeutic maneuvers such as PEEP or surfactant administration. Sudden changes in compliance often reflect the opening and closing of individual lung units rather than changes in lung tissue and surface tension characteristics [42]. Thus, ideally compliance should be corrected for total lung capacity (TLC) and body weight [43].

Resistance (R) is calculated from the equation:

$$R = \frac{\text{pressure}}{\text{flow}} = \frac{\text{cm } H_2O}{\text{ml/sec}}$$

and represents the resistive properties of the airways, lung tissue and chest wall.

Obtaining pulmonary functions in ventilated children has been previously considered experimental and safely and reproducibly accomplished only in a few laboratories. With the incorporation of microprocessors and electronic sensors and the availability of automated systems, this area has developed to the stage of clinical bedside practice. Several methods have been designed to measure compliance and resistance in ventilated infants which has led to a confusing nomenclature for the practitioner. Compliance is referred to as either dynamic compliance (C*dyn*) when it is measured when ventilation is in motion, or as static (passive) compliance (C*rs*) when respiratory muscles are inactive during the test procedure. The same applies to the resistance of the respiratory system, which is referred to as either dynamic (Re) or total respiratory system resistance (R*rs*). C*dyn* can be simply calculated by dividing tidal volume (V_T) by the total change in pressure necessary to deliver that volume. These numbers can be easily extracted from mechanical ventilation. However, it is understood that C*dyn* is related to both elastic and flow resistive characteristics according to the equation of motion of the single compartment model of the respiratory system:

$$P = \frac{V}{C} + RF$$

where P = transpulmonary pressure, V = tidal volume and F = tidal flow. Thus, C*dyn* changes with alteration of mechanical ventilation settings including respiratory frequency, inspiratory and end-expiratory pressure [1].

The respiratory dynamic compliance (C*dyn*) of the lungs and chest wall can be measured using an esophageal balloon and a pneumotachograph placed at the proximal end of the ETT. This allows for pressure-volume curves to be displayed for calculations of C*dyn* and for differentiation of C*dyn* into its components of lung compliance (C_L) and chest wall compliance (C_{CW}). However,

C_{CW} is usually very high in infants and its contribution to total respiratory compliance (C_{TOT}) can often be neglected [45, 46], since C_L and C_{CW} are related as follows:

$$\frac{1}{C_{TOT}} = \frac{1}{C_L} + \frac{1}{C_{CW}}$$

This technique has several limitations [43]. Average pleural pressure necessary for calculations is not always possible to obtain, the technique is highly dependent on accurate placement of the esophageal catheter, compliance results are affected by the respiratory rate and the accuracy of such measurements in intubated infants and children is controversial [1, 2]. Therefore, methods which measure static compliance (C*rs*) and resistance (R*rs*) based on relaxation of both inspiratory and expiratory muscles during brief airway occlusions during exhalation have become more popular, especially in ventilated infants and children.

The most widely used methods are the passive deflation and the multiple occlusion techniques [49–51]. The following discussion concentrates on the passive deflation technique. The reader is referred to recent literature for the other methods [52].

If one measures alveolar pressure at a known lung volume at which no flow occurs, static C*rs* can be determined. If one measures alveolar pressure at a known lung volume at which no flow occurs, static C*rs* can be determined (Δ*volume*/Δ*pressure*). Alveolar pressure can be obtained by measuring pressure at the proximal end of the ETT during relaxation of the respiratory muscles against an occluded ETT (zero gas flow). The concept uses the Hering-Breuer reflex in infants but is easily performed also in older ventilated patients by occluding the expiratory port long enough to allow the airway pressure to reach a constant value and equilibration of alveolar with the proximal ETT pressure. This technique may be especially applicable to infants and children ventilated for acute respiratory failure because they are usually heavily sedated or paralyzed so that their respiratory muscles are not activated and end inspiratory relaxation is easily achieved. Fitting a straight line to the passive expiratory flow-volume curve obtained following release of an expiratory occlusion and measuring the slope, C*rs*, R*rs* and time constant (T*rs*) can be obtained from a single occlusion procedure (slope = time constant) [53, 54]. The expiratory time constant or emptying time of the respiratory system will be entirely dependent on the mechanical properties of the lungs and can be described as follows:

$$Trs = Crs \times Rrs$$

Hence, both C*rs* and R*rs* can be obtained from a single breath. The technique is highly reproducible and requires only transient disruptions of mechanical ventilation [43]. The determination of T*rs* gives some idea of how rapidly the lung empties following a mechanical breath. A single time constant is defined

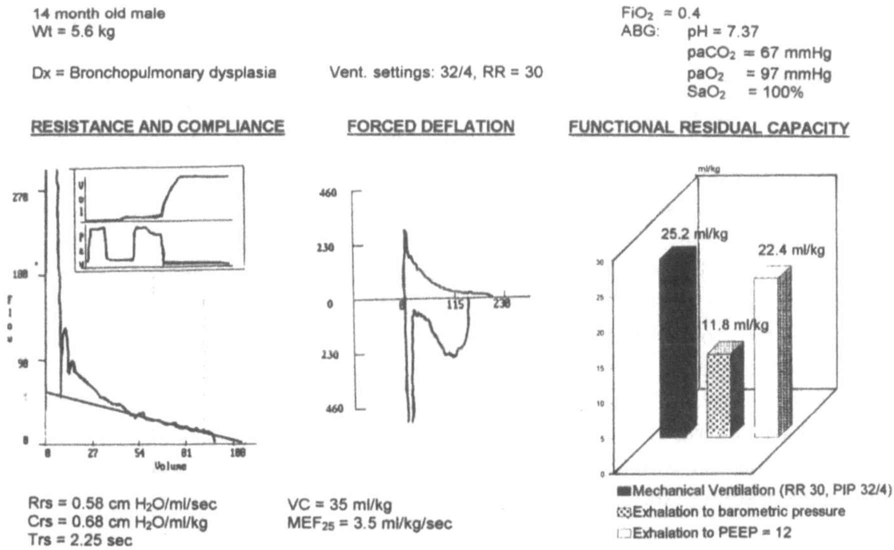

Fig. 4. Passive FV-loop, forced deflation FV-loop and FRC measurements in a 14 month old male with severe BPD demonstrate severe obstructive and restrictive lung disease. There is generation of inadvertent PEEP during mechanical ventilation at a rate of 30 min^{-1} and ventilator pressures of 40/4 cm H_2O comparable to a real PEEP of about 12 cm H_2O.

as the time required to exhale 63% of the tidal volume. Three time constants are needed to exhale 95% of the delivered tidal volume. This permits the determination of respiratory rates allowing complete exhalation or the detection of rate settings which lead to inadvertent PEEP (Figure 4).

The passive deflation technique relies on the assumption that the respiratory system can be regarded as a single compartment model with a linear flow-volume curve (single T*rs*). This occurs only if C*rs* and R*rs* are constant (or changing reciprocally which is unlikely). This is valid in most healthy infants especially over the tidal volume range. However, in the presence of lung disease, the lung may be nonuniform in terms of regional T*rs* so that the respiratory system will not always behave like a single compartment model and a single time constant (single slope) will not adequately describe all the respiratory mechanics [55, 56]. Infants with restrictive lung diseases such as acute ARDS or pulmonary edema or with severe obstructive airway disease may exhibit multiple time constants [57]. In all these circumstances C*rs* and R*rs* are best measured over the longest linear fit of the passive expiratory FV-curve. However, calculation of time constants at different intercepts may give additional information and better describe the respiratory mechanics over the whole expiration phase [58]. Pattern recognition adds valuable information to the interpretation of results obtained by measuring respiratory mechanics. While obstructive lung disease is characterized by a concave slope of the passive expiratory FV curve. Restrictive lung disease often results in convex curve patterns. It is important to note that in the case of intubated patients, C*rs* and

R*rs* measurements include the physical properties of the ETT which may distort the flow-volume relationships. The resistance of the ETT is flow dependent and is related to the internal diameter and length of the tube [59]. The effect of the ETT becomes negligible with ETT sizes of 5.0 mm internal diameter or higher. Therefore, the resistance of the ETT over a range of flow rates should be taken into consideration. Nevertheless, even with small ETTs, the technique can be used to follow disease progress and response to therapy. Unfortunately, there is still a great lack of normal values for C*rs* and R*rs* in intubated infants and children with normal lungs. According to our studies, such normal data lie in the range of 0.8–1.2 $ml \cdot cm\ H_2O^{-1} \cdot kg^{-1}$ for C*rs* and 0.4–0.8 $ml \cdot cm\ H_2O^{-1} \cdot sec$ (up to 1.0 with ETT <3.5mm I.D.) for Rrs (see Table 1).

Alternatively, accurate measurements of volume and flow for a precise numeric characterization of the severity and type of the disease process are easily obtained by the rapid thoracic compression technique or, preferably in intubated patients, the forced deflation technique, because these techniques do not rely upon a single compartment model.

Lung Volumes

Although the most fundamental interest in lung volume measurements in infancy and childhood relates to the assessment of normal and abnormal lung growth, the determination of lung volumes is an important part of the respiratory management of infants and children [1]. Lung volume measurements can help in diagnosing respiratory disorders, in evaluating responses to therapy,

Table 1. Normal values for pulmonary function variables for ventilated infants

	Los Angeles [a]	Lund [d]	Pittsburgh [e]
N	10	20	16
Age (mon)	6.8	8.4	2.9
Weight (kg)	6.5	7.5	5.6
C_{RS} ($ml/cmH_2O/kg$)	0.96		
R_{RS} ($cmH_2O/ml/s$)	0.06		
MEF_{25} (ml/kg/s)	41.1		27.3/39.2 [f]
TLC (ml/kg)	68.9	60.6	
FVC (ml/kg)	57.2		41.8
FRC (ml/kg)	24.4/17.1–25.2 [b]	18.5	
RV (ml/kg)	11.7		
FRC/TLC	0.35	0.31	
RV/TLC	0.17		
Extrathoracic V_D (ml/kg)	1.75–2.5 [c] Age-dependent		
Intrathoracic V_D (ml/kg)	1.03 [c] Not age-dependent		

[a] Hammer et al. [76]; [b] Sivan et al. [63]; [c] Numa A, Newth CJL [1]; [d] Thorsteinsson et al. [65]; [e] Mallory et al. [40]; [f] Mallory et al. [1]

and in finding suitable ventilator settings with respect to rate and ventilating pressures [61–63]. Lung volume is also an important variable when lung mechanics are measured [1] because *specific compliance* and *specific resistance* are normalized by lung volume, i.e., the functional residual capacity (FRC), as are maximal expiratory flow rates in partial FV-loop maneuvers performed using the RTC compression technique.

While in non-intubated infants and small children the only lung volumes that can be accurately, repeatedly, and reliably measured are the FRC and tidal volume (V_T), in intubated patients other lung volumes such as total lung capacity (TLC), vital capacity (VC) and residual volume (RV) can also be obtained.

FRC can be measured by three techniques: plethysmographic (infant body box), helium (He) dilution (a closed-circuit method), and nitrogen (N_2) washout (in its modern form, an open-circuit method). Sulphahexafluoride has recently been used in a promising washin – washout technique [1], but as yet, has been validated only in an animal laboratory [1]. In contrast to the gas dilution techniques which measure only gas volume that is in connection with the mouth and which can be diluted or washed out, the infant body plethysmography measures the thoracic gas volume (TGV) i.e. it measures all gas spaces including lung areas which are not in communication with the airway. At present, this technique is relatively impractical in ventilated infants and children although continuing efforts are being made to apply this technique also to the PICU environment [1, 2].

Helium (He) Dilution

The closed-circuit He dilution method is based on the principle of gas equilibration. Gas which contains a known concentration of He as a marker is equilibrated between an unknown lung volume, V_L (FRC or any other volume to be measured) and a closed system which has a reservoir of known volume (V_{gas}) in line, by rebreathing. After equilibration is achieved, the He concentration is the same in all parts of the system including the reservoir. The total volume of the gas distribution ($V_L + V_{gas}$) can thus be calculated from the initial concentration and volume of distribution of the He and its final concentration. Substructing apparatus volume from total volume gives lung volume. That is, if C_1 = He concentration at start of experiment, and C_2 = the concentration when gas mixing is complete, then:

$$V_{gas} \cdot C_1 = (V_{gas} + V_1) \cdot C_2$$

and

$$V_L = \frac{V_{gas}(C_1 - C_2)}{C_2}$$

The initial He concentration can range between 6% and 15%, although concentrations as low as 3% have been used. Therefore, the He dilution technique can be used on patients with lung disease requiring very high inspired oxygen concentrations ($FiO_2 = 0.97$).

Time of equilibration in healthy infants and young children is usually between 40–60s, but may be considerably longer, and even 3–5 minutes, in the presence of airway disease.

The closed-circuit He dilution method has been adapted to measure FRC on ventilated patients by Heldt et al. [69]. The patient is connected via the ETT and a sliding valve to both a bag (which is situated inside a transparent plexiglass box) and to the ventilator (Figure 5).

In normal pre-test position the patient is ventilated directly by the ventilator through the valve. The bag, which contains a known amount of gas with known He concentration (and thus a known amount of Helium) is sealed and is not connected to the patient. At end-exhalation the valve is switched so that the patient is directly connected only to the He-containing bag while the ventilator ventilates the box surrounding the bag and compresses the bag accordingly. The patient is thus ventilated by the bag which is externally compressed by the ventilator cycle. After several breaths, equilibration of He concentration between the lungs and the bag is achieved and FRC can be calculated in the same way as in non-ventilated subjects.

Lung volume measurement by He dilution is a bedside procedure, but still requires considerable operator training and many technical issues have to be considered. Size and volume of the spirometric system as well as of the circuit

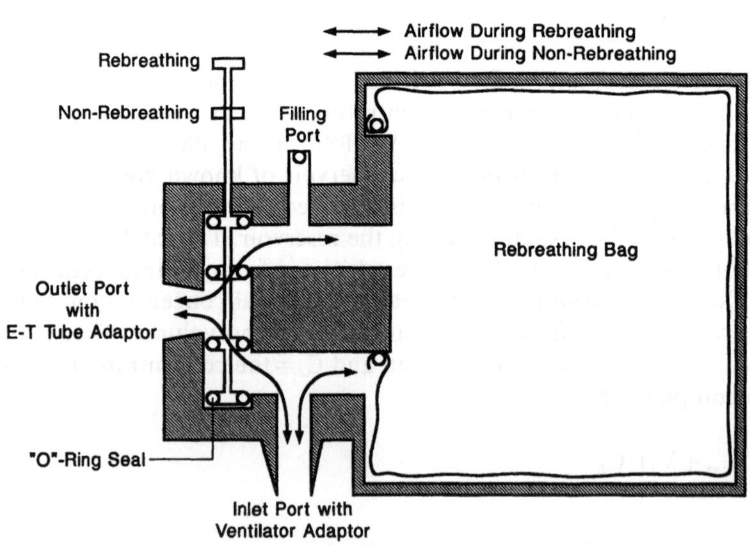

Fig. 5. Schematic diagram for ventilation circuit for FRC measurement in ventilated patients by the He dilution technique (Reproduced with permission from Heldt GP and Peters RM. Chest (1978) 74:492).

need to be adjusted for patient's size. A rapid and accurate He analyzer should be used and its linearity and calibration over a wide range of FiO_2 levels should be carefully evaluated. Moreover, calibration depends on the O_2/He mixture ratio and should be repeated each time. The system must include a CO_2 scrubber and a water absorption system. Because the system is a closed one, during measurements, O_2 must be added at exactly the same rate as CO_2 is absorbed in order to keep the volume of the circuit constant. This can prove to be a technically demanding procedure requiring complex valving which may affect the reliability of the technique.

Leak-free connections in intubated infants are more difficult to achieve in this age group, where cuffed tubes are rarely used. If the leak is minimal, it may be eliminated by gentle tracheal pressure during the recording period. Although a method for correcting leaks during FRC_{He} measurements has been described [1] and is currently incorporated into some automated systems, this has not been fully evaluated nor validated and may result in significant errors.

Nitrogen (N_2) Washout

The technique is based on washing out the N_2 from the lungs by giving the subject 100% O_2 to breathe. If the amount of N_2 washed out is measured and the initial alveolar N_2 concentration is known, then the lung volume from which point the washout started can be derived. Hence, when washout starts at FRC:

$$FRC = \frac{VN_2}{\text{initial lung } [N_2]}$$

In this open circuit method, the patient is switched to breathing 100% O_2 and from this point the volume of N_2 exhaled is determined by integration with respect to time of the instantaneous N_2 concentration flowing in the exhalation circuit multiplied by the instantaneous flow.

$$VN_2 = \int \dot{V}\,[N_2] \cdot dt$$

In 1985, Gerhardt and co-workers [71] devised an open washout system to which a constant background O_2 flow was delivered. The patient inhaled from and exhaled to that circuit with background flow. Although the instantaneous flow rate of the washout circuit changes continuously as the subject breathes, the average flow leaving the system over time remains unchanged because the volume of gas subtracted during inspiration is added back to the system during exhalation (this is true as long as the temperature and humidity of the inhaled and exhaled gas are equal – a condition which is easy to meet by using a humidifier). Hence, if flow is a constant value the equation can be simplified. This holds for both test and calibration procedures:

$$VN_{2\,test} = \dot{V}_{test} \int [N_2]_{test} \cdot dt$$

and the volume of the washed out N_2 is obtained from dividing these equations to provide

$$VN_{2\,cal} = \dot{V}_{cal} \int [N_2]_{cal} \cdot dt$$

the basic equation for the nitrogen washout technique.

$$VN_{2\,test} = \frac{\dot{V}_{test}}{\dot{V}_{cal}} X \frac{VN_{2\,cal}}{\int [N_2]_{cal} \cdot dt} X \int [N_2]_{test} \cdot dt$$

If the constant flow is kept unchanged during both calibration and test procedures ($\dot{V}_{cal} = \dot{V}_{test}$), the equation can be simplified:

$$VN_{2\,test} = \frac{VN_{2\,cal}}{\int [N_2]_{cal} \cdot dt} X \int [N_2]_{test} \cdot dt$$

The integrated N_2 concentration (measured during the test) is related to N_2 volume by the calibration factor: $VN_{2\,cal}/\int [N_2]_{cal}\,dt$ which is defined during calibration procedure ($VN_{2\,cal}$ is the preset calibration volume and $\int [N_2]_{cal}\,dt$ is measured during calibration).

Calibration is performed by washing out a preset amount of room air from a precision syringe connected to the washout circuit and the piston is pushed back and forth analogous to breathing.

Because the method ignored the instantaneous change in flow and used only the average constant flow for calculation, it was essential that sampling of N_2 for concentration measurements would "see" a continuous decrease of N_2 concentration as the washout proceeds, without the effect of the respiratory phase (Figure 6).

This was achieved by incorporating a mixing chamber in the exhalation circuit before the sampling port from which mixed expired gas was sampled for N_2 analysis (Figure 7).

The technique developed by Gerhardt et al for spontaneously breathing infants and children [72] is not immediately applicable to ventilated children

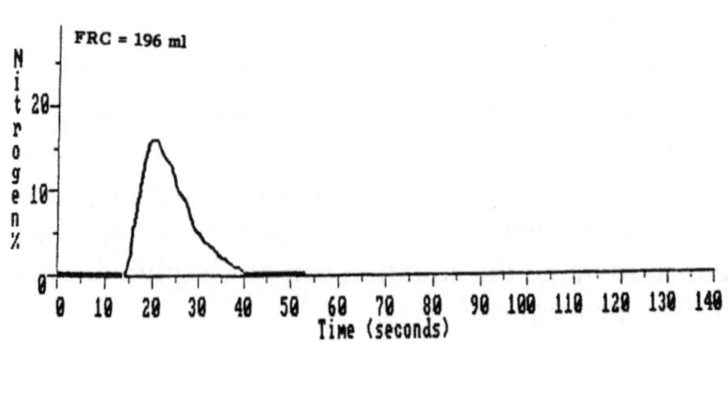

Fig. 6. N_2 washout curve during lung volume measurement by the N_2 washout technique.

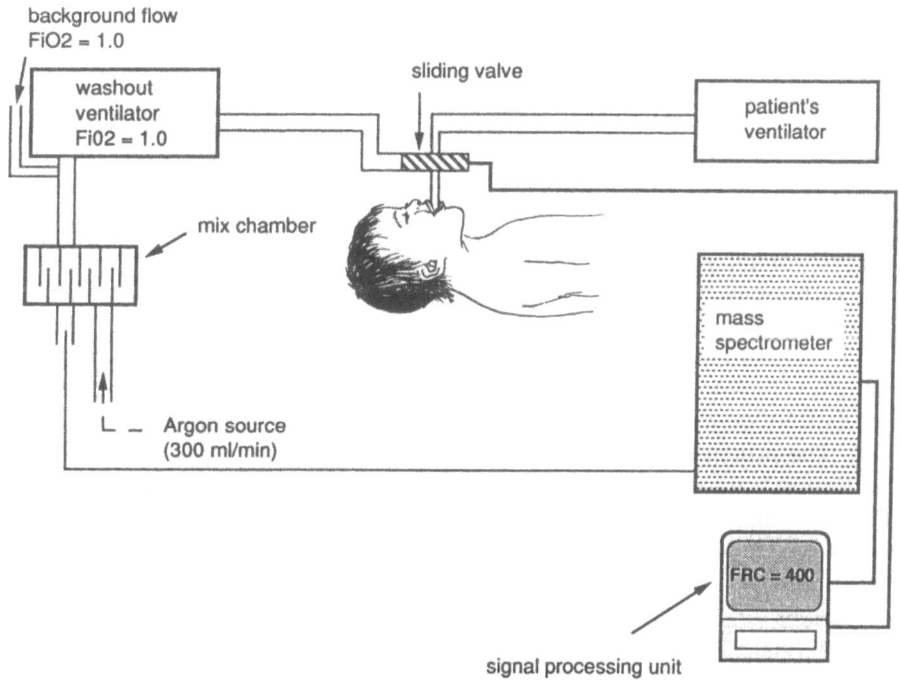

Fig. 7. Schematic diagram for the N_2 washout system for lung volume determinati on in ventilated patients (Reproduced with permission from Sivan Y, Deakers TW and Newth CJL. Pediatri Res (1990) 28:446).

mainly because the gas flow during calibration does not equal the flow during the test so the simplified equation is not valid. In order to overcome this difficulty, we used the respiratory mass spectrometer already "in-line" for measuring the instantaneous N_2 concentration [73], to record the minute ventilation (flow per time) by the argon dilution technique [74]. This is performed during both calibration and test and their ratio ($\dot{V}_{test}/\dot{V}_{cal}$) is calculated for use in the basic equation. At FRC the patient is switched to a second ventilator delivering 100% O_2 (washout ventilator) and washout starts.

This N_2 washout technique (which unlike the He dilution method is limited to patients at $FiO_2 < 0.65$) in our PICU allows accurate determination of FRC during mechanical ventilation and correlates well with those values produced using the Douglas bag technique [73]. In other studies of patients with restrictive lung disease, including a group with ARDS [57], FRC measured at clinically chosen levels of PEEP (4–10 cm H_2O) was 45% below predicted FRC for nonintubated normal children and 60% below that of ventilated children with normal lungs at physiological levels of PEEP (2–4 cm H_2O). The use of progressively greater levels of PEEP produced increases in FRC towards predicted normal values [63]. However, these observations suggest that in ARDS at least, normalization of FRC would require sufficient PEEP to contribute to barotrauma or to compromise of cardiac output and systemic oxygen transport. In spontaneously breathing infants and children, FRC is the same whether determined by He dilution or N_2 washout methods [75], and is in the range of 17.1–25.2 $ml.kg^{-1}$ (mean = 20.4 $ml \cdot kg^{-1}$). Only limited data has been reported for FRC in ventilated infants and children with normal lungs [63] [76]. Sivan et al [63] showed values which were up to 50% more than the normal values for spontaneously breathing children on PEEP's of 2–4 cm H_2O. (See Table I).

As already mentioned, measurement of FRC is required for calculation of *specific compliance* and for V_{max}FRC during forced deflation procedures. The N_2 washout technique has also been shown to measure also lung volumes above FRC accurately [77].

The measurement of oxygen consumption, carbon dioxide production and minute ventilation ($\dot{V}_E$, $\dot{V}_{O_2}$ and $\dot{V}_{CO_2}$) can be done by a number of techniques. A relatively easy method is performed by respiratory mass spectrometry alone [74]. The principle is that a known mass flow of a marker gas of known concentration is injected into the patient's expirate upstream of a mixing box, and the resulting gas composition downstream is used to deduce the mass flows of all its components. A major problem with this technique is that it requires a very stable O_2 concentration with variation of no more than 0.2%. This may necessitate very accurate and stable O_2 supply systems other than the ICU wall. This problem becomes greater when the FiO_2 is increased. Nonetheless, these measurements can be performed reproducibly at $FiO_2 < 0.8$, without difficulty.

Respiratory Muscle Function

The evaluation of the performance of the respiratory muscles is divided into the measurement of two components:

a) *muscle strength* which is a function of muscle bulk is assessed by the instantaneous development of pressure during a contraction and is clinically represented by diaphragmatic weakness – failure of the diaphragm to generate force; and
b) *muscle endurance* which is defined as the ability of the diaphragm to sustain a previously targeted force output during repetitive contraction. Muscle endurance is a function of muscle fiber type, integrity of contractile elements, number of muscle mitochondria, oxidative enzymes and capillary blood supply. Diaphragmatic fatigue represents a failure of this ability to sustain force output and is reversible with rest [78].

Inspiratory and expiratory *muscle strength* can be evaluated by monitoring maximum respiratory pressures: maximum inspiratory pressure (Pi_{max}) and maximum expiratory pressure (Pe_{max}) obtained during inspiratory or expiratory maneuvers against an occluded airway. Proper performance of these exercises requires patient cooperation. In ventilated children Pi_{max} or its more common term NIF (negative inspiratory force) may be used in the evaluation of patient ability to be weaned from assisted ventilation where values of NIF more negative than 30 cm H_2O usually predict successful weaning. Pi_{max} is measured after exhalation to residual volume and Pe_{max} is measured from total lung capacity. Inspiratory muscle strength can also be assessed by measuring the pressure across the diaphragm (transdiaphragmatic pressure; Pdi). This is obtained by inserting a balloon catheter into the esophagus and the stomach simultaneously to measure pleural and abdominal pressures respectively. Pdi is the difference *abdominal pressure – esophageal pressure* measured during a maximal inspiratory effort against closed airways.

Another test for evaluation of respiratory muscle strength is the measurement of vital capacity (VC). VC greater than 10–15 mL/kg has been suggested to predict successful weaning.

The major problem with all these tests is that they are effort dependent and therefore are applicable mainly to older cooperative children. Serial measurements of these indices in children with neuromuscular disorders such as Guillain-Barré syndrome and other causes of diaphragmatic failure are useful in the assessment of disease progress.

Respiratory *muscle endurance* is quantified by relating the level of ventilation to the time it can be sustained. This may be assessed by measuring Pdi response to phrenic nerve stimulation, electromyography of the diaphragm, relaxation rate of respiratory pressures and maximum sustained ventilation [1]. These tests are of limited clinical value because they are invasive, require patient cooperation and they have not been proven useful in clinical practice. A relative simple and non-invasive way to assess diaphragmatic fatigue is by measuring the paradoxical inward motion of the diaphragm on inspiration. This may be quantitated by measuring the chest wall to abdominal asynchrony which easily done by the phase angle technique (the abdomen lags behind the chest motion). Although breathing asynchrony on CPAP prior to extubation has been showed to predict successful weaning in adults, preliminary results in infants and children are not promising [1]. More studies are needed to see whether this technique may be used to follow progression and response to therapy.

Although breathing asynchrony in increasingly used in infants and children with a variety of respiratory disorders including in the PICU environment [1], its use in ventilated patients is limited because chest wall-abdominal asynchrony may be observed only on spontaneous patient breaths.

Summary

Today, modern technology allows for bedside assessment of many physiologic variables of the respiratory system in infants and children requiring assisted ventilation. Miniaturization of equipment and the application of technology based on the personal computer with rapid data acquisition and processing has made the evaluation of the respiratory status in ventilated patients possible. Moreover, it has allowed for monitoring and assessment of the respiratory system even in ventilated, uncooperative infants and small children in whom some of the variables measured are very small in absolute terms to make any measurement difficult. Hence, these developments open up new possibilities for monitoring changes in disease processes affecting the respiratory system, and improved medical management of infants and children with lung and heart diseases in particular.

The challenges of measuring resistance, compliance, forced expiratory flows, diffusion, functional residual capacity, metabolic gas exchange and thoracoabdominal asynchrony has led recently to the development of a number of ingenious techniques.

However, all of these techniques are limited by implicit assumptions, by the physiology of the respiratory system they intend to assess, and to differing degrees by the invasiveness required for measurement. It is most important to be aware of the limitations of each of the techniques and to use each method within its limitations. For example lung volume measurement by the N_2 washout technique is limited to $FiO_2 \leq 0.70$. Any measurement of lung volume in an infant or child ventilated at a higher FiO_2 requires the use of another method (e.g. helium dilution) or decreasing the FiO_2 momentarily for the test period (if clinically possible). Several techniques (measurement of lung volumes, R*rs*, C*rs*, forced deflation, rapid thoracic compression, O_2 consumption and CO_2 production) require that there be no leak around the endotracheal tube. Therefore, they are applicable only to infants and children with cuffed endotracheal tubes or with uncuffed tubes with pharyngeal packing, where leaks of gas (or pressure) can be prevented. Cuffed ETT are not recommended for use in children under the age of 8 years [1], but in a recent prospective study involving 250 infants and children, using cuffed ETT one-half size smaller than the calculated uncuffed ETT for age, no greater incidence of complications either short-term (post-extubation stridor) or long-term (tracheostomy) were observed [83].

Some techniques such as measurement of thoracoabdominal asynchrony by the phase angle technique and transcutaneous O_2 and CO_2 measurements are age limited. Other are limited by the respiratory disease itself, e.g. pulse oximetry and CO_2 assessment by capnography. RTC, FD, R*rs*, C*rs*, lung volumes by gas dilution techniques and metabolic gas exchange measurements are not possible in the presence of a draining pneumothorax. Arterial CO_2 assessment by capnography is inaccurate in the presence of severe $\dot{V}/\dot{Q}$ mismatch and transcutaneous O_2 and CO_2 measurements are severely affected by low skin perfusion. Flow-volume relationships may be distorted in the presence of a small ETT and this effect should be corrected for, and assessment of respiratory mechanics from passive deflation flow-volume curves assumes a single-compartment model which is not always true, e.g. severe restrictive and obstructive diseases.

In this review, only the basic concepts of the various techniques are presented. For a more detailed description of the technical aspects of the pulmonary function measurements and for a step-by-step "how to do it" guide the reader is referred to the new textbook of Infant Pulmonary Function Testing – A Practical Guide [84] where the limitations and reference normal values for each technique are also presented.

Nevertheless, when applied with meticulous care and within these limitations, these novel techniques bring new insights and awareness, but also new responsibilities in the management of infants and children with respiratory compromise. Not all of these techniques need to be applied to all infants in the ICU. Not all the assumptions upon which some of these techniques we have described are based will prove true. Any such methods which do not withstand solid scientific testing must be quickly discarded and replaced with better and (hopefully) easier methods.

References

1. Comroe JHJ, Botelho S (1947) The unreliability of cyanosis in the recognition of arterial hypoxemia. Am J Med Sci 214:1–6.
2. Mithoefer JC, Bossman OG, Thibeault DW, Mead GD (1968) The clinical estimation of alveolar ventilation. Am Rev Respir Dis 98:868–871.
3. Heiser MS, Downs JJ (1984) Acute respiratory failure in infants and children due to lower respiratory tract obstructive disorders. In: Shoemaker WC, Thompson WL, Holkbrook PR (eds) Textbook of Critical Care. WB Saunders, Philadelphia, 1984.
4. Kilham H, Gillis J, Benjamin B (1987) Severe upper airway obstruction. Pediatr Clin N Am 34:1–14.
5. Sivan Y, Deakers TW, Newth CJL (1990) Thoraco-abdominal asynchrony in acute upper airway obstruction in small children. Am Rev Respir Dis 142:540–544.
6. Newth CJL (1979) Recognition and management of respiratory failure. In: Levison H (ed) Pediatr Clin North Am. WB Saunders, Philadelphia, pp 617–644.
7. Newth CJL (1986) Respiratory disease in respiratory failure: Implications for the young and old. Brit J Dis Chest 80:209–216.
8. Clark JS, Votteri B, Ariagno RL, Cheung P, Eichhorn JH, Fallat RJ, Lee SE, Newth CJL, Rotman H, Sue DY (1992) Noninvasive assessment of blood gases. Rev Respir Dis 145:220–232.
9. Tobin MJ, Grenvik A (1991) Contemporary management in critical care: Respiratory Monitoring. Volume 1, Number 4. Churchill Livingstone, New York, pp 3–136.
10. Hall JB, White SR, Karrison T (1991) Efficacy of daily routine chest radiographs in intubated, mechanically ventilated patients. Crit Care Med 19:689–693.
11. Hauser GJ, Pollack MM, Sivit CJ, Taylor GA, Bulas DI, Guion CJ (1989) Routine chest radiographs in pediatric intensive care: A prospective study. Pediatrics 83:465–470.
12. Bosman YK, Foster PA. (1977) Endotracheal intubation and head posture in infants. S Afr Med J 52:71–73.
13. Luft WC, Loeppy JA, Mostyn DM (1979) Mean alveolar gases and alveolar-arterial gradients in pulmonary patients. J Appl Physiol 46:534–540.
14. Sivan Y, Eldadah MK, Cheah T, Newth CJL (1992) Estimation of arterial carbon dioxide by end-tidal and transcutaneous PCO_2 measurements in ventilated children. Pediatr Pulmonol 12:153–157.
15. Epstein MF, Cohen AR, Feldman HA, Raemer DB (1985) Estimation of $PaCO_2$ by two noninvasive methods in the critically ill newborn infant. J Pediatr 106:282–286.
16. Mc Aslan TC (1976) Automated respiratory gas monitoring of critically injured patients. Crit Care Med 4:255–260.
17. Murray IP, Modell JH (1983) Early detection of endotracheal tube accidents by monitoring carbon dioxide concentration in respiratory gas. Anesthesiology 59:344–346.
18. Linko K, Paloheimo M, Tammisto T (1983) Capnography for detection of accidental oesophageal intubation. Acta Anesthesiol Scand 27:199–346.

19. Hoffman RA, Krieger BP, Kramer MR et al (1989) End-tidal carbon dioxide in critically ill patients during changes in mechanical ventilation. Am Rev Respir Dis 140:1265–1268.
20. Healey CJ, Fedullo AJ, Swinburne AJ, Wahl GW (1987) Comparison of noninvasive measurements of carbon dioxide tension during withdrawal from mechanical ventilation. Crit Care Med 15:764–768.
21. Potter WA (1976) Mass spectrometry for innovative techniques of respirator care, ventilator weaning and differential ventilation in an intensive care unit. Crit Care Med 4:235–238.
22. Greenspan GH, Block AJ, Halderman LW, Lindsay S, Martin CS (1981) Transcuta neous noninvasive monitoring of carbon dioxide tension. Chest 80:442–446.
23. Monaco F, Nickerson BG, McQuitty JC (1982) Continuous transcutaneous oxygen and carbon dioxide monitoring in the pediatric ICU. Crit Care Med 11:765–766.
24. Martin RJ, Beoglos A, Miller MJ, DiFiore JM, Robertson SS, Carlo WA (1988) Increasing arterial carbon dioxide tension: influence on transcutaneous carbon dioxide tension measurements. Pediatrics 81:684–687.
25. Bucher HU, Fanconi S, Fallenstein F, Duc G (1986) Transcutaneous carbon dioxide tension in newborn infants: reliability and safety of continuous 24 hour measurement at 42°C. Pediatrics 78:631–635 .
26. Tremper KK, Mentelos RA, Shoemaker WC (1980) Effect of hypercarbia and shock on transcutaneous carbon dioxide at different electrode temperatures. Crit Care Med 8:608–612.
27. Fanconi S, Doherty P, Edmonds JF, Barker GA, Bohn DJ (1985) Pulse oximetry in pediatric intensive care: Comparison with measured saturations and transcutaneous tension. J Pediatr 107:362–366.
28. Severinghaus JW, Naifeh KH (1987) Accuracy of response of six pulse oximeters to profound hypoxemia. Anesthesiology 67:551–.
29. Hannhart B, Haberer JP, Saunier C, Laxenaire MC (1991) Accuracy and precision of fourteen pulse oximeters. Eur Respir J 4:115–119.
30. Jubran A, Tobin MJ (1990) Reliability of pulse oximetry in titrating supplemental therapy in ventilator-dependent patients. Chest 97:1420–1425.
31. Lawson D, Norely I, Korbon G, Loeb R, Ellis J (1987) Blood flow limits and pulse oximeter signal detection. Anesthesiology 67:599–603.
32. Milner AD, Saunders RA, Hopkin IE (1978) Tidal pressure volume and flow volume respiratory loop patterns in human neonates. Clin Sci Molec Med 54:257–264.
33. Stocks J, Thomson A, Wong C, Silverman M (1985) Pressure-flow curves in infancy. Pediatr Pulmonol 1:33–40.
34. Abramson AL, Goldstein MN, Stenzler A, Steele A (1982) The use of the tidal breathing flow volume loop in laryngotracheal disease of neonates and infants. Laryngoscope 92:922–926.
35. Motoyama EK (1977) Pulmonary mechanics during early postnatal years. Pediatr Res 11:220–223.
36. Taussig LM (1977) Maximal expiratory flows at functional residual capacity: a test of lung function for young children. Am Rev Respir Dis 116:1031–1038.
37. Newth CJL, Amsler B, Anderson GP, Morley J (1991) The effects of varying inflation and deflation pressures on the maximal expiratory deflation flow-volume relationship in anesthetized rhesus monkeys. Am Rev Respir Dis 144:807–813.
38. Hammer J, Sivan Y, Deakers TW, Newth CJL. (1995) Flow limitation in anesthetized rhesus monkeys: a comparison of rapid thoracoabdominal compression and forced deflation techniques. Pediatr Res. In Press.
39. Hammer J, Deakers TW, Newth CJL (1993) The achievement of flow limitation in intubated infants with normal lungs and obstructive airways disease. Am Rev Respir Dis 147:A222.
40. Mallory GB, Motoyama AK, Koumbourlis AC, Mutich RL, Nakayama DK (1989) Bronchial reactivity in infants in acute respiratory failure with viral bronchiolitis. Pediatr Pulmonol 6:253–259.

41. Motoyama EK, Fort MD, Klesh KW, Mutich RL, Guthrie RD (1987) Early onset of airway reactivity in premature infants with bronchopulmonary dysplasia. Am Rev Respir Dis 136:50–57.
42. Ratjen F, Zinman R, Stark S, Lesczczynski LE, Wohl MEB (1989) Effect of changes in lung volume on respiratory system compliance in newborn infants. J Appl Physiol 67:1192–1197.
43. England SJ (1988) Current techniques for assessing pulmonary function on the newborn and infant: advantages and limitations. Pediatr Pulmonol 4:48–53.
44. Sly PD, Brown KA, Bates JHT, Spier S, Milic-Emili J (1988) Noninvasive determination of respiratory mechanics during mechanical ventilation of neonates: a review of current and future techniques. Pediatr Pulmonol 4:39–47.
45. Davis GM, Coates AL, Papageorgiou A, Bureau MA (1988) Direct measurement of static chest wall compliance in animal and human neonates. J Appl Physiol 65:1093–1098.
46. Gerhardt T, Bancalari E (1980) Chest wall compliance in fullterm and premature infants. Acta Paediatr Scand 69:359–364.
47. LeSouëf PN, Lopes JM, England SJ, Bryan MH, Bryan AC (1983) Influence of chest wall distortion on esophageal pressure. J Appl Physiol 55:353–358.
48. Heaf DP, Turner H, Stocks J, Helms P (1986) The accuracy of esophageal pressure measurements in convalescent and sick intubated infants. Pediatr Pulmonol 2:5–8.
49. Zin WA, Pengelly LD, Milic-Emili J (1982) Single-breath method for measurement of respiratory mechanics in anesthetized animals. J Appl Physiol 52:1266–1271.
50. Olinsky A, Bryan MH, Bryan AC (1976) A simple method of measuring total respiratory system compliance in newborn infants. S Afr Med J 50:128–130.
51. Guslits BG, Wilkie RA, England SJ, Bryan AC (1987) Comparison of methods of measurement of compliance of the respiratory system in children. Am Rev Respir Dis 136:727–729.
52. American Thoracic Society/European Respiratory Society (1993) Respiratory mechanics in infants: physiologic evaluation in health and disease. Am Rev Respir Dis 147:474–496.
53. Mortola JP, Fisher JT, Smith B, Fox G, Weeks S (1982) Dynamics of breathing in infants. J Appl Physiol 52:1209–1215
54. LeSouëf PN, England SJ, Bryan AC (1984) Passive respiratory mechanics in newborns and children. Am Rev Respir Dis 129:727–729.
55. Richardson P, Scott J, Hansen TN (1989) Mechanics of the respiratory system during passive exhalation on preterm lambs. Pediatr Res 26:425–428.
56. Davies CJ, Cooper SG, Fletcher ME et al (1990) Total respiratory compliance in infants and young children with congenital heart disease. Pediatr Pulmonol 8:155–161.
57. Stretton M, Deakers TW, Newth CJL (1992) Spirometry, lung mechanics and volumes during the acute phase of ARDS in pediatric patients. Am Rev Respir Dis 143:A248.
58. Similowski T, Bates JHT (1991) Two-compartment modelling of respiratory system mechanics at low frequencies: gas redistribution or tissue rheology? Eur Respir J 4:353–358.
59. Wall MA (1980) Infant endotracheal tube resistance: Effect of changing length, diameter, and gas density. Crit Care Med 8:38–40.
60. Shannon DC (1989) Rational monitoring of respiratory function during mechanical ventilation of infants and children. Intensive Care Med 15:13–16.
61. Richardson CP, Jung AL (1978) Effects of continuous positive airway pressure on pulmonary function and blood gases of infants with respiratory distress syndrome. Pediatr Res 12:771–774.
62. East TD, in't Veen JC, Pace NL, McJames S (1988) Functional residual capacity as a noninvasive indicator of optimal positive end-expiratory pressure. J Clin Monit 4:91–98.
63. Sivan Y, Deakers TW, Newth CJ (1990) Functional residual capacity in ventilated infants and children. Pediatr Res 28:446–450.
64. Sivan Y, Deakers TW, Newth CJ (1991) Effect of positive end-expiratory pressure on respiratory compliance in children with acute respiratory failure. Pediatr Pulmonol 11:103–107.

65. Thorsteinsson A, Larsson A, Jonmarker C, Werner O. (1994) Pressure-volume relations of the respiratory system in healthy children. Am J Respir Crit Care Med 150:421–430.
66. Schulze A, Schaller P, Töpfer A, Kirpalani H (1994) Measurement of functional residual capacity by sulfur hexafluoride in small-volume lungs during spontaneous breathing and mechanical ventilation. Pediatr Res 35:494–499.
67. Edberg KE, Sandberg K, Silberberg A, Ekstrom-Jodal B, Hjalmarson O (1991) Lung volume, gas mixing, and mechanics of breathing in mechanically ventilated very low birth weight infants with idiopathic respiratory distress syndrome. Pediatr Res 30:496–500.
68. Edberg KE, Sandberg K, Silberberg A, Sjöqvist BA, Ekström-Jodal B, Hjalmarson O (1991) A plethysmographic method for assessment of lung function in mechanically ventilated very low birth weight infants. Pediatr Res 30:501–504.
69. Heldt GP, Peters RM (1978) A simplified method to determine functional residual capacity during mechanical ventilation. Chest 74:492–496.
70. Fox WW, Schwartz JG, Shaffer TH (1979) Effects of endotracheal tube leaks on functional residual capacity determination in intubated neonates. Pediatr Res 13:60–64.
71. Gerhardt T, Hehre D, Bancalari E, Watson H (1985) A simple method for measuring functional residual capacity by N_2 washout in small animals and newborn infants. Pediatr Res 19:1165–1169.
72. Gerhardt T, Reifenberg L, Hehre D, Feller R, Bancalari E (1986) Functional residual capacity in normal neonates and children up to 5 years of age determined by a N_2 washout method. Pediatr Res 20:668–671.
73. Sivan Y, Deakers TW, Newth CJ (1990) An automated bedside method for measuring functional residual capacity by N_2 washout in mechnically ventilated children. Pediatr Res 28:446–450.
74. Davies NJH, Denison DM (1979) The measurement of metabolic gas exchange and minute volume by mass spectrometry alone. Respir Physiol 36:261–267.
75. Tepper RS, Asdell S (1992) Comparison of helium dilution and nitrogen washout measurements of functional residual capacity in infants and very young children. Pediatr Pulmonol 13:250–254.
76. Hammer J, Numa A, Newth CJ. (1995) Albuterol responsiveness in infants with respiratory failure caused by respiratory syncytial virus infection. J Pediatr 127:485–490.
77. Sivan Y, Hammer J, Newth CJL (1994) Measurement of high lung volume by the N_2 washout method. J Appl Physiol 77:1562–1564.
78. Nichols DG (1991) Respiratory muscle performance in infants and children. J Pediatr 118:493–502.
79. Rochester DF (1988) Test of respiratory muscle function. Clin Chest Med 10:199–214.
80. Sivan Y, Deakers T, Newth CJL (1990) Thoraco-abdominal asynchrony during weaning from mechanical ventilation in infants and small children. Pediatr Res 25:44A.
81. Allen JL, Sivan Y (in press) Measurement of chest wall Function. In: Stocks J, Sly P, Tepper R, Morgan Y (eds) Infant pulmonary function testing – A practical guide. Wiley-Liss.
82. Scheien CL, Kuluz JW, Shaffner DH, Rogers MC (1992) Cardiopulmonary resuscitation in infants and children. In: Rogers MC (ed) Textbook of Pediatric Intensive Care. 2nd edn. Williams & Wilkins, Baltimore, pp 3–51.
83. Deakers TW, Reynolds G, Stretton M, Newth CJL (1994) Cuffed endotracheal tubes in pediatric intensive care. J Pediatr 125:57–62.
84. Stocks J, Sly P, Tepper R, Morgan Y (eds) (in press) Infant pulmonary function testing – A practical guide. Wiley-Liss.
85. Numa A, Newth CJL. (1994) Oropharyngeal deadspace in children. Am J Respir Crit Care Med 149(4):A693.
86. Mallory GB, Jr., Chaney H, Mutich RL, Motoyama EK. (1991) Longitudinal changes in lung function during the first three years of premature infants with moderate to severe bronchopulmonary dysplasia. Pediatr Pulmonol 11:8–14.

Pulmonary Function Testing in Sick, Preterm Infants

K. E. Edberg

Introduction

Infants with very low birth weight (VLBW) and respiratory disease have dominated neonatal intensive care units during recent decades. However, the pattern of morbidity has changed lately, and both the severity of the lung disorders and the number of sick neonates are decreasing. Improved pre- and postnatal care with increased use of prenatal maternal steroid treatment, exogenous surfactant, improved ventilatory techniques and methods for extracorporeal gas exchange are factors that might contribute to the change in both morbidity and mortality of newborn infants.

Infantile respiratory distress syndrome (IRDS) is still the main reason for intensive care of the preterm infant. Other common reasons are meconium aspiration syndrome (MAS) and group B streptococcal septicemia. The etiology of these respiratory disorders are not completely known but includes both structural and functional changes of the lungs. The introduction of positive end-expiratory airway pressure, different modes of mechanical ventilation and techniques for gas exchange into the arsenal of treatment over the last twenty years has meant considerable improvement in survival for the most affected infants [1]. On the other hand, associated disorders such as pneumothorax, cerebral hemorrhage, patent ductus arteriosus and bronchopulmonary dysplasia (BPD) are still common, especially in the most immature infants [2]. Particularly, BPD has been a feared complication to prematurity, lung disease and mechanical ventilation. With improved ventilatory techniques, however, a changing pattern of chronic lung disease has been observed, with a number of less severe and reversible pulmonary sequels with a less poor prognosis [3, 4].

Despite the fact that mechanically ventilated infants have such a conspicuous status in neonatal intensive care, research on lung function in this particular group has been limited. The main reason for this is the absence of suitable methods. Examples of important fields to penetrate are functional properties in the very immature lung, pathophysiology of respiratory insufficiency, how mechanical ventilation and other means of treatment affect the respiratory system, and how such treatment can be optimized in order to avoid injury to the sick and fragile lung tissue and prevent development of chronic lung disease.

A natural first step towards a better understanding of lung physiology and pathophysiology in immature infants would be to develop applicable methods for pulmonary function assessment.

Methods

Approaching the very sick, preterm baby for lung function studies has been a challenge, because of the fragility of the infant and also because comprehensive intensive care must remain in progress throughout the examination. Especially in the very preterm infant, one of the aims of intensive care is minimized handling of the baby to prevent hypothermia and stress-induced alterations of blood pressure and oxygenation. This is an obstacle to any investigative procedure, and it is important to develop techniques which are as little invasive as possible. In both sick and healthy newborns, however, it is also a prerequisite to use methods for measurements of ventilation, mechanics of the respiratory system and lung volumes that do not require the cooperation of the infants. A variety of such methods has been developed over the years in methodological work that is still in progress.

Information about the mechanical properties of the lung and respiratory system is based on measurements of airway pressure and ventilatory flow. For proper interpretation of this information, it is also necessary to know the actual lung volume, on which the mechanical properties are strongly dependent. Other qualities of interest are distribution of ventilation and the efficiency of gas mixing in terminal airspaces. Another important parameter of lung function is the effective lung blood flow which has a major impact on the gas exchange.

Some of the techniques used for providing information on pulmonary function will be reviewed here.

Mechanics of Breathing

Measurement of the mechanical properties of the respiratory system provides information about both the airways and the pulmonary tissue. Accurate measurement of ventilatory flow and airway pressure is a prerequisite for calculating the mechanics of breathing.

A commonly used linear model to characterize the mechanical properties of the respiratory system is based on the following algorithm:

$$P(t) = 1/C \cdot V(t) + R \cdot F(t) + I \cdot dF(t)/dt + e(t)$$

This model shows the opposing elastic, resistive and inertial components of the respiratory system to the applied driving pressure and the residual term (e) which describes the deviation between the measured driving pressure and the pressure predicted by the model. Compliance (C), resistance (R) and inertia (I) are defined in the equation. The inertia is very low at normal breathing and the inertial term may then be omitted [5]. This simple model characterizes the mechanical properties of the respiratory system well in spontaneously breathing infants [6]. It can also be used in mechanically ventilated infants and the mechanical properties may be estimated in a part or over the whole breath [7].

Based on the same model, Olinski et al. [8] described in 1976 a method of measuring static compliance of the respiratory system in spontaneously breathing, newborn infants. The airway was occluded at end-inspiration, tidal volumes were measured by spirometry, and as the Hering-Breuer reflex caused respiratory muscle relaxation, airway pressure corresponding to elastic forces at the actual lung volume could be measured.

Mortola et al. [9] used multiple occlusions of the airway at different lung volumes during expiration and calculated passive compliance of the respiratory system. By analysis of the expiratory flow-volume loop, they also calculated the time constant, and from that, resistance of the respiratory system. LeSouef et al. [10] developed this technique further for use in sick and healthy, term and preterm, spontaneously breathing or paralyzed infants. They introduced one single end-inspiratory occlusion to relax the respiratory muscles and measure occlusion pressure. Compliance and resistance of the respiratory system could then be calculated from the subsequent passive expiration.

Even further modifications of the airway occlusion technique have been developed later, and are now widely used to assess lung function in many neonatal intensive care units in commercially available, computerized systems.

Measurement of airway pressure. Transpulmonary pressure is needed to evaluate the mechanical properties of the lung. This is the pressure difference between the airway and the pleural space. Airway pressure can be measured by means of a catheter close to the airway opening. As direct measurement of pleural pressure cannot easily be performed, it has been estimated by measuring oesophageal pressure by means of an oesophageal balloon or a water-filled catheter placed in the lower third of the oesophagus. However, there are several reports on unreliable estimates of mean pleural pressure achieved by measuring oesophageal pressure in preterm infants with pulmonary disease [11, 12, 13]. Measuring the properties of the whole respiratory system makes it possible to avoid problems with oesophageal pressure measurements. Usually there is no need to distinguish between the elastic properties of the lung and the respiratory system in this particular group of infants. Chest wall compliance contributes very little to the total compliance of the respiratory system, which then appears as a good estimate of the lung compliance in the relaxed, preterm baby [14].

Similarly, airway resistance is the major contributor to the total resistance of the respiratory system, and resistive tissue forces in lung and chest wall are very small. Thus, resistance of the respiratory system can also be regarded as a good estimate of airway resistance [15].

In intubated infants, airway pressure is usually recorded at the outer end of the endotracheal tube, in which case the calculated resistance includes the endotracheal tube. The resistances of endotracheal tubes of certain measures and at different gas flows can be measured in vitro [16]. Attempts have been made to estimate the resistance of the infant's respiratory system without the contribution of the endotracheal tube, but this cannot be made simply by retracting the in vitro values from the total resistance of the respiratory system. Introduction of an artificial airway with a small inner diameter may add resistance, but the outer diameter may exceed the diameter of narrow parts of the natural airway and thus reduce the difference in resistance between the intubated and non-intubated infant, especially if nasal intubation is performed.

Measurement of respiratory flow. Respiratory flow in mechanically ventilated infants is usually measured directly in the airway by means of a pneumotachograph. By integrating the measured flow, tidal volumes and minute ventilation can be achieved. Flow meters for use in infants must be designed to stay linear over a certain range, and the resistance of the device must be low. These demands, however, tend to increase the dead space, which must be kept as small as possible to prevent rebreathing. Pneumotachographs with low mass, low dead space and low resistance have been specially designed for use in very low birth weight infants [17]. Problems with condensation or collection of contents from inspired or expired gas in the pneumotachograph may still occur, and this may alter the linearity and make the measurements inaccurate. The composition of the breathing gas also influences the flow measurements, and proper calibration with a similar gas mixture as during the recording procedure has to be made. The use of pneumotachographs in a pressurized system, as the ventilator circuit, may also give inaccurate information about the respiratory flow [18].

Another source of error in direct flow measurements in the airway is air leakage around the endotracheal tube bypassing the flow meter, meaning that the respiratory flow may be either over- or underestimated depending on the mode of ventilation. Such leakage is also difficult to detect or predict and may be very variable over time. Because of the vulnerability of the airway in newborn infants, mechanical methods for eliminating an existing leakage might bring a risk of airway complications for the infant. Of similar reasons, when non-cuffed endotracheal tubes are used, the size is often chosen to permit some leakage and the ventilator settings are adjusted to compensate for a leakage. A sudden elimination of the leakage for the purpose of a pulmonary function measurement, for example by laryngeal pressure, also changes the state of ventilation radically, and thus does not reflect the steady state present prior to the investigation. However, a recent report on the use of cuffed endotracheal tubes in mechanically ventilated infants and children has not shown any increased incidence of airway complications, neither short- nor long-term [19]. Thus, the use of at least temporarily cuffed endotracheal tubes might be a means of avoiding airway leakage and provide more accurate direct airway flow measurements.

There are also other flow meters for direct airflow measurements. Hot wire anemometry has been shown to give accurate measurements of airway flow [20]. The devices used for this technique can usually be made of lighter weight and smaller dead space than pneumotachographs.

Airway flow can also be measured indirectly by means of a jacket plethysmograph or face out plethysmography. Milner described the use of a soft, inflatable latex rubber jacket for measuring changes of tidal thoracic volume in 1970 [21]. Duffty et al. [22] described tidal volume measurements using induction plethysmography in infants in 1981. In 1974, Hjalmarson et al. [6] described a system with face out, whole body plethysmography and a computerized technique for least mean square analyses of the mechanics of breathing in spontaneously breathing newborn infants with pulmonary disease. A similar system for measurement of pulmonary mechanics extended with facilities for measuring breathing gas nitrogen concentration was described by Sandberg et al. [23] in 1984, and these techniques were also later modified for use in mechanically ventilated preterm infants [24].

Measurement of Lung Volumes

The lung volume at the end of a normal expiration is called the functional residual capacity (FRC). FRC is related to pulmonary gas exchange, and the mechanical properties of the respiratory system are firmly dependant on the actual lung volume. A lot of commonly used therapeutic interventions during assisted ventilation aim at restoring or increasing FRC. The advantageous effect of exogenous surfactant in infants with IRDS seems to be related to an increased FRC. Thus, measurement of FRC is important for a better understanding of neonatal pulmonary pathophysiology.

The most commonly used techniques for determination of FRC are the helium dilution technique, the nitrogen washout technique and the sulfur hexafluoride washout technique.

The helium dilution technique. This technique is based on the introduction of a tracer gas, such as helium, into the lungs of the infant from a closed system where helium concentrations can be measured after an equilibrium is achieved. Thus, the lung volume added to the closed system can be estimated.[25] The helium rebreathing technique has been modified for use in intubated neonates [26].

The nitrogen washout technique. This technique is based on analysis of the washout of nitrogen from the lungs during breathing with a nitrogen-free breathing gas. By measuring breathing flow and nitrogen concentration of the expired gas, both the nitrogen volume in the lungs prior to the washout and the functional residual capacity, can be calculated. In 1984, Sjöqvist et al. [27] described a computer-assisted method for multiple breath nitrogen washout analysis, which later has been modified for use in mechanically ventilated infants [28].

The sulfur-hexafluoride washout technique. Measurement of FRC with this technique is also based on the washout pattern of the tracing gas, sulfur hexafluoride [29]. As the amount of this tracer gas is so small, high concentrations of inspired oxygen during the mechanical ventilation is of little or no concern, and only one ventilator has to be used.

The washout pattern of the different tracer gas techniques provides more information than only about the lung volume. Different indices for gas mixing efficiency have been calculated from the elimination pattern and the respiratory flow [30].

Lung Blood Flow and Diffusion Capacity

The importance of the pulmonary blood flow for the lung function has so far attracted little attention compared with the airways and lung tissue. Undoubtedly, impaired pulmonary blood flow might as well be a part of the etiology as a contributing mechanism in many severe pulmonary disorders in the neonate. The effect of different conventional and non-conventional mechanical ventilation, as high positive end-expiratory pressure and high frequency oscillatory ventilation, on pulmonary blood flow is not fully described. With the possibility of selective treatment of increased pulmonary vascular resistance and decreased blood flow with nitric oxide, methods for estimating lung blood flow have gained enhanced interest. Flow velocity measurement with Doppler technique is widely used to estimate tissue blood flow [31]. A multiple gas, rebreathing technique provides accurate measurements of FRC, effective pulmonary capillary blood flow and diffusing capacity of the lung [32].

Conclusion

Pulmonary function testing in sick, preterm infants is still used to a very little extent in the daily neonatal intensive care. Lack of accurate, simple and noninvasive methods for lung function assessment contributes to an incomplete knowledge about important physiological mechanisms in the diseased and healthy neonate. The methods described in this chapter are to the main part used in specific investigative procedures. Ideally, pulmonary function testing should be used as a diagnostic aid and as a tool for guiding different therapeutic interventions in the neonate with respiratory failure. Further intensive efforts must be made to develop lung function measuring techniques to be used in routine care.

References

1. Greenough A, Roberton NRC (1985) Morbidity and survival in neonates ventilated for the respiratory distress syndrome. Br Med J 290:597–600.
2. Wariyar U, Richmond S, Hey E (1989) Pregnancy outcome at 24–31 weeks' gestation: neonatal survivors. Arch Dis Child 64:678–686.
3. Hyde I, English RE, Williams JD (1989) The changing pattern of chronic lung disease in prematurity. Arch Dis Child 64:448–451.

4. Van Lierde S, Cornelis A, Devlieger H, Moerman Ph, Lauweryns J, Eggermont E (1991) Different pattern of pulmonary sequelae after hyaline membrane disease: Heterogeneity of bronchopulmonary dysplasia? A clinicopathologic study. Biol Neonate 60:152–162.
5. Rodarte J R, Rehder K (1986) Dynamics of respiration. In "Handbook of Physiology. Section 3: The Respiratory System." (Ed. Fishman AP) III:131–144 American Physiological Society, Bethesda, MD 1986.
6. Hjalmarson O (1974) Mechanics of breathing in newborn infants with pulmonary disease. II. Theoretical considerations and methods. Acta Paediatr Scand [Suppl] 247:6–25.
7. Silberberg A R, Edberg K E, Sandberg K, Hjalmarson O (1991) Respiratory System Mechanics in Ventilated Newborn Infants: Evaluation of single compartment models. Technical Report 6:91 (1991), Laboratory of Medical Electronics, Chalmers University of Technology, Göteborg, Sweden.
8. Olinsky A, Bryan A C, Bryan MH (1976) A simple method of measuring total respiratory system compliance in newborn infants. S Afr Med J 50:128–130.
9. Mortola J, Fisher J T, Smith B, Fox G, Weeks S (1982) Dynamics of breathing in infants. J Appl Physiol 52(5):1209–1215.
10. LeSouef PN, England SJ Bryan CA (1984) Passive respiratory mechanics in newborns and children. Am Rev Respir Dis 129:552–556.
11. LeSouef PN, Lopez JM, England SJ, Bryan HM, Bryan CA (1983) Influence of chest wall distortion on esophageal pressure. J Appl Physiol 55:353–358.
12. Thomson A, Elliot J, Silverman M (1983) Pulmonary compliance in sick low birthweight infants. How reliable is the measurement of oesophageal pressure? Arch Dis Child 58:891–896.
13. Beardsmore CS, Stocks J, Silverman M (1983) Esophageal pressure in infants at elevated lung volumes and positive airway pressure. J Appl Physiol 55:377–382.
14. Gerhardt T, Bancalari E (1980) Chestwall compliance in full-term and premature infants. Acta Paediatr Scand 69:359–364.
15. Helms P (1982) Problems with plethysmographic estimation of lung volume in infants and young children J Appl Physiol 53:698–702.
16. Hatch DJ (1978) Tracheal tubes and connectors used in neonates – dimensions and resistance to breathing. Br J Anaesth 50:959–964.
17. Brady JP, Deming DD, McCann EM (1985) Neonatal endotracheal flowmeter for tidal volume, airway pressure and end-tidal gas. J Appl Physiol 58:1023–1025.
18. Deakers TW, Reynolds G, Stretton M, Newth CJL (1994) Cuffed endotracheal tubes in pediatric intensive care. J Pediatr 125:57–62.
19. Baboolal R, Kirpalani H (1990) Measuring on-line compliance in ventilated infants using hot wire anemometry. Crit Care Med 18:1070–1072.
20. Milner AD (1970) The respiratory jacket. A new method for measuring respiration. Lancet 2:80–81.
21. Duffty P, Spriet L, Bryan MH, Bryan AC (1981) Respiratory induction plethysmography (Respitrace): an evaluation of its use in the infant. Am Rev Respir Dis 123:542–546.
22. Sandberg K, Sjöqvist BA, Hjalmarson O, Olsson T (1984) Analysis of alveolar ventilation in the newborn. Arch Dis Child 59:542–547.
23. Edberg KE, Sandberg K, Silberberg A, Sjöqvist BA, Hjalmarson O (1991) A plethysmographic method for assessment of lung function in mechanically ventilated very low birth weight infants. Pediatr Res 30:501–504.
24. Schwartz JG, Fox WW, Shaffer TH (1978) A method for evaluation of functional residual capacity (FRC) in neonates with endotracheal tubes. IEEE Trans Biomed Eng 25:304–307.
25. Heldt GP, Peters RM (1978) A simplified method to determine functional residual capacity during mechanical ventilation. Chest 74:492–496.
26. Sjöqvist BA, Sandberg K, Hjalmarson O, Olsson T (1984) Calculation of lung volume in newborn infants by means of a computer-assisted nitrogen washout method. Pediatr Res 18:1160–1164.

27. Edberg KE, Sandberg K, Silberberg A, Ekström-Jodal B, Hjalmarson O (1991) Lung volume, gas mixing and mechanics of breathing in mechanically ventilated very low birth weight infants with idiopathic respiratory distress syndrome. Pediatr Res 30:496–500.
28. Schulze A, Schaller P, Topfer A, Kirpalani H (1994) Measurement of functional residual capacity by sulfur hexafluoride in small-volume lungs during spontaneous breathing and mechanical ventilation. Pediatr Res 35:494–499.
29. Sjöqvist BA, Sandberg K, Hjalmarson O, Olsson T (1986) Method for analyzing multiple breath nitrogen washouts. Med Biol Eng Comput 24:83–90.
30. Walther FJ, Benders MJ, Leighton JO (1992) Persistent pulmonary hypertension in premature neonates with with severe respiratory distress syndrome. Pediatrics 90:899–904.
31. Bose CL, Lawson EE, Greene A, Mentz W, Friedman M (1986) Measurement of cardiopulmonary function in ventilated neonates with respiratory distress syndrome using rebreathing methodology. Pediat Res 20:316–320.

Cardiac Surgery

Long-Term Outcome After Surgery for Congenital Heart Disease

F. J. Meijboom, A. J. J. C. Bogers, E. M. W. J. Utens and J. Hess

Introduction

Before the era of cardiac surgery about half of the patients born with a congenital heart defect died within the first year of life [1, 2]. Survival until adulthood was very rare for patients with transposition of the great arteries (20 years survival $<1\%$) [3], rare with tetralogy of Fallot (20 years survival $<10\%$)[4] and although survival beyond two decades was more common for patients with atrial septal defect, ventricular septal defect and pulmonary stenosis, also their life expectancy was considerably reduced [5,6,7,8,9]. Cardiac surgery changed the natural history dramatically.

History

It started in 1939, when Gross ligated a patent ductus arteriosus in a 7 year old girl. In 1941 Crafoord was the first to treat a patient with aortic coarctation surgically [10] and in 1945 Blalock sutured the subclavian artery end-to-side on the pulmonary artery of a patient with tetralogy of Fallot, establishing the Blalock-Taussig shunt [11]. Brock introduced the blind valvulotomy for pulmonary stenosis in 1948 [12]. Lewis became the first surgeon to do open-heart surgery by closing an atrial septal defect with the use of total body hypothermia and inflow occlusion in 1953 [13]. In the following years this technique was successfully used in patients who needed cardiac surgery for atrial septal defect, isolated valvular aortic or valvular pulmonary stenosis. However, failure was uniform when applied in patients with a more complex congenital heart defect. Lillehei was the first to perform successful open-heart surgery in patients with more complex intracardiac defects, such as ventricular septal defect, atrioventricular septal defect or tetralogy of Fallot [14]. He used cross-circulation as a technique for extracorporal oxygenation. This technique implicated that the circulation of a healthy volunteer, who was lying next to the patient in the operation theatre, was used during the surgical procedure to support the patient's circulation. Partly because of the potential dangers for the "donors" this technique was abandoned soon in favor of extracorporal circulation with a membrane oxygenator, which would become the standard for the subsequent decades [15, 16]. Extracorporal oxygenation, or cardiopulmonary bypass, provided the surgeon sufficient time to visualize the structures in the non-beating heart to permit corrective measures [17], and so even complex cardiac malformations became eligible for surgery. In these same early postwar years cardiac catheterization was proved to be feasible, for which the pioneers Cournand, Richards and Forssman were awarded the Nobel prize in 1956. These developments both in the medical and in the surgical field were the start of one of the most impressive changes in modern medicine: instead of a *mortality* of 85% in the first two decades, the 20-years *survival* has become 85% or more nowadays [18]. This change took two or three decades, and was the result of a gradual decline of number of patients who were considered inoperable (see Figure 1), and, due to improvements in surgical techniques and peri-operative care, a substantial reduction of hospital mortality of operated patients. Enthusiasm about this accomplishment was understandable and justified, but was sometimes carried too far. This is represented by the language that is commonly used for surgical procedures; if these are not evidently palliative, they are often called corrective.

Perloff, one of the pioneers in the field of long-term care for patients who underwent cardiac surgery for congenital heart disease, stated in 1973 in his article "Pediatric congenital becomes a postoperative adult; the changing population of congenital heart disease" [19] :"whether we are dealing with correction of congenital cardiac defects or developing rockets to the moon, we must not let the brilliant glare of technologic success obscure our long-term objective to promote the quality of life". He stressed the fact that in the important field of follow-up after cardiac surgery "more is unknown than known". Maron remarked in 1977 that "limited attention has been focused on the ultimate fate of patients many years after their apparently successful operations." In 1987, in the chapter "The fate of survivors of surgery for congenital heart disease" in the first edition of the textbook on Pediatric Cardiology edited by Anderson, Macartney and Tynan, is stated: "Cardiac surgery was born of hope and thrived on the tide of enthusiasm which flooded from the recognition that all but the most severe defects were amenable to surgical repair. The last thirty years have been like a breathless tour of the Himalayas, with one 'last great problem' after another succumbing to the surgeon's knife. Now we must address the irritating question of what has been achieved. What kind of life can be offered to these blue and breathless mites, snatched from the jaws of death." It was emphasized that, even after 30 years, there were very few long-term follow-up studies which could provide data on this subject.

The Assessment of the Long-Term Results of Cardiac Surgery; Why Are Solid Follow-Up Studies Lacking?

In 1988, Stark mentioned in his famous lecture "Do we really correct congenital heart defects?" [20] that only 4 follow-up studies had been published with a duration of follow-up of more than 8 years in the leading journal in the field of cardiac surgery in the preceding two years. What is the reason that, although the necessity to acquire more information about the fate of survivors of surgery for congenital heart disease was so obvious, there had been so little comprehensive follow-up studies.

Some explanations may be considered in this regard. Prospective follow-up studies, the best (although slow) way for systematic evaluation of the results of any kind of treatment, were not conducted. This might be explained by lack of manpower: the number of staff members of departments Pediatric Cardiology and Cardiac Surgery until the 1970's was in general very small according to modern standards. Most physicians were simply too busy doing their actual (short-term) job to be able to do meticulous long-term follow-up of all operated patients. Another probable explanation is that there was a tremendous optimism about the outlook for these patients. Compared with what the outlook would have been without surgery, something that most physicians remembered only too well, the outlook for patients, once operated, was incomparably better. It must have felt as a kind of blasphemy to question whether the achieved result was actually good enough. So, many patients were discharged from routine outpatient check-up when there were no symptoms or obvious sequelae.

When the years went by, the optimism of the early years gradually wore out. More and more patients who had undergone supposedly "corrective" surgery developed symptoms and presented with sequelae. This created a new problem: to whom could you present these problems?

The Need for Specialized GUCH-Doctors

As long as patients were still children, a pediatric cardiologist would take care, but who would take care of these patients when they outgrew the pediatric age group? Adult cardiologists are generally trained in acquired, not in congenital heart disease and pediatric cardiologists are in general not trained to deal with adult patients, and coping with problems specific for adults. Some recognized this dilemma early and became the pioneers of a new subspeciality: congenital heart disease in adults, or grown-ups with congenital heart disease (GUCH). The example was set in Toronto, where the first specialized medical facility for the care of adults with congenital heart disease was started in the 1960's. Dr. Jane Somerville, who would become one of the most ardent advocates of specialized care for this patients group, developed a similar facility in the National Heart Hospital in London in 1975. Perloff and Child started the Adult Congenital Heart Center in Los Angeles in 1978. Only a few more centers followed. A recent informal survey among members of the Association of European Pediatric Cardiologists (AEPC) confirmed that there were less than 10 centers in Europe in which there was a well organized adult congenital heart disease unit with all hospital and outpatient facilities. One of these centers is the Sophia Children's Hospital/Dijkzigt Hospital in Rotterdam. Patient care would benefit by more of these centers, but not too many. Although a growing population, the GUCH-group still comprises relatively few patients, and dilution of facilities by too many centers would lead to dissipation of experience, which is not in the patient's interest [21].

Concentration of care for all patients with congenital heart disease, explicitly including GUCH, was a matter of debate in The Netherlands in the past few years. Both the Dutch Health Council and the professional groups (cardiac surgeons, pediatric cardiologists and adult cardiologists) recognized the need for concentration. Because, as Somerville stated in the lecture "The problem-an overview" during the First International Symposium on Congenital Heart Disease in Adolescents and Adults in Rotterdam in May 1990: "the welfare and the needs of the patient (not status and wishes of individuals, physicians or organizations) must be first consideration", this centralization will hopefully take place in the coming years.

One of the major problems in the GUCH patient group – late symptoms and sequelae that will have to be detected and treated – will be managed optimally by good quality, centralized care. Other important problems of this patient group, which cannot be solved by the medical profession (alone), are the uncertain employment prospects and poor insurability of patients after cardiac surgery for congenital heart disease. This might be understandable for patients with evident symptoms, such as decreased exercise capacity or symptomatic arrhythmia, but is hard to accept for patients who feel healthy. Because there is an understandable time lag between medical developments and acceptance of their impact on late survival, follow-up studies are needed which can provide data on the prevalence and clinical relevance of sequelae. These data would be of value not only for patients and physicians, but also for occupational health advisors and medical advisors of insurance companies. However, apart from the earlier mentioned lack of prospective follow-up studies, there are also amazingly few retrospective follow-up studies of nonselected series of patients who were actually examined at follow-up. There are several studies in which follow-up data were acquired by means of telephonic interviews or written interviews with the patients or their relatives, [22,23,24,25] but since patients were not examined, many sequelae will remain undetected. A positive exception in this respect was the large American multi-center study, the Joint Study on the Natural History Study of Congenital Heart Defects, of which the first report was published in 1977 [26] and the second in 1993 [27]. Apart from these data, confined to the long-term health status of patients with ventricular septal defect, aortic stenosis and pulmonary stenosis, it is difficult to find information on the health status of patients operated upon for any type of congenital cardiac malformation. It was the lack of this kind of information that prompted the initiation of the Rotterdam Quality of Life study.

The Rotterdam Quality of Life Study

This long-term follow up study, which started in Rotterdam in 1989, focused both on the medical and the psychological aspects long-term after surgery. The study was based on a consecutive series of 734 patients: all patients who underwent open heart surgery for a congenital cardiac malformation in Rotterdam between 1968 and 1980 and who were younger than 15 years of age at the time of the operation. Of all patients who were alive at the time of the start of the follow-up study, and who could be traced, over 80% participated in the psychological part of the study, and 70% participated in the medical part. Because all patients were traced uniformly, and because there were no differences in baseline characteristics between the patients who did participate in the follow-up study and those who did not, we presume that there was no intentional selection bias. Because a representative sample of the entire study population was thoroughly examined, we think that we can comment on the prevalence of sequelae, and the clinical importance of these sequelae in this particular patient group. Because it is a one center experience, and in some subgroups even a one-surgeon experience (Mustard-group), one should refrain from generalization of these results. One should also realize that studies on long-term results of cardiac surgery with a really long period of follow-up, like in this study up to 22 years, unavoidably concern surgical techniques and patient groups selected for surgery that represent the state of the art many years ago. Surgical techniques have been changed constantly over the past 20 years and also the group of patients who are considered to be eligible for surgical repair changed substantially. The optimal age for surgery has become younger and younger, and patients with complex congenital cardiac malformations, who were considered to be inoperable 20 years ago are now candidates for surgical repair. Many changes have already proved to be improvements in terms of improved short-term outcome. Many think that these changes will also have a beneficial effect on the long-term outcome, but, of course, this will have to be proven by new long-term follow-up studies.

The most important conclusions from the medical part of the Rotterdam Quality of Life study were that survival was good (Mustard, surgical repair of tetralogy of Fallot and ventricular septal defect; all between 80 and 90% 20 years survival) to excellent (ASD II and isolated valvular pulmonary stenosis) (Figure 1), that personal health assessment was similar to that of the normal population with no differences between the diagnosis groups (Table 1), that exercise capacity was normal in a large majority of the patients (Table 2), and that the proportion of symptomatic patients – with substantially decreased exercise capacity or symptomatic arrhythmia – was small.

However, the prevalence of arrhythmia and severe right ventricular dilatation, present throughout the entire study population, was high [28,29,30,31,32]. Apart from the positive qualities of this study in providing data of prevalence of sequelae, it is self evident that it has many limitations, especially in the interpretation of the clinical relevance of the findings.

What is the clinical significance of the arrhythmias? This seems to be clear for the small minority of symptomatic arrhythmias: these represent a definite pathological condition and even with treatment these arrhythmias remain potentially life-threatening. The key question is: what is the significance of asymptomatic arrhythmias? Does ventricular arrhythmia represent damage of the myocardium, such as scarring and loss of electrophysiologic integrity? Do

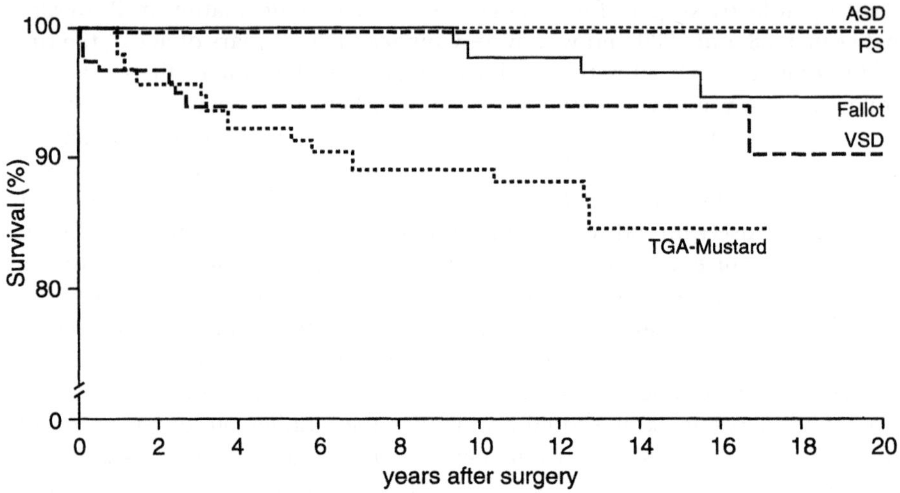

Fig. 1. Kaplan-Meier survival curve of all hospital survivors of open heart surgery for a congenital cardiac malformation before the age of 15 years

Table 1. Personal health assessment of 388 study patients and of 1510 persons of the normal Dutch population <35 years

	ASD n=104	VSD n=109	Fallot n=77	TGA-Mustard n=58	PS n=40	Dutch population n=1510
Excellent	20 (19%)	24 (22%)	13 (27%)	12 (21%)	10 (25%)	611 (40%)
Good	70 (67%)	68 (62%)	50 (65%)	39 (67%)	26 (65%)	755 (50%)
Fair	14 (13%)	16 (15%)	11 (14%)	7 (12%)	4 (10%)	127 (9%)
Not good	0	1 (1%)	3 (4%)	0 (0%)	0 (0%)	17 (1%)
Bad	0	0 (0%)	0 (0%)	0 (0%)	0 (0%)	0 (0%)

ASD=atrial septal defect; *VSD*=ventricular septal defect; *Fallot*=tetralogy of Fallot; *TGA-Mustard*=transposition of the great arteries after Mustard repair; *PS*=pulmonary stenosis

supraventricular arrhythmias, which we defined as signs of sinus node dysfunction on the basis of the criteria as proposed by Kugler [33], indeed represent damage to the sinus node, or are these criteria too unspecific and is the prevalence of sinus node dysfunction overestimated? Longer follow-up, and meticulously executed follow-up studies, will reveal whether or not these asymptomatic arrhythmias are predictors of symptomatic arrhythmia later.

Right ventricular dilatation definitely reflects a pathological situation. Although it seemed to be tolerated fairly well for the duration of follow-up of this study, there was an association with decreased exercise capacity, in particular in the group of patients after surgical repair of tetralogy of Fallot. Therefore, concern remains whether longer duration of severe dilatation will not unavoid-

Table 2. Maximal exercise capacity assessed by bicycle exercise test

	ASD n=100	VSD n=102	Fallot n=71	TGA-Mustard n=49	PS n=37
Maximal exercise capacity[1]	104±17%	100±17%	90±18%*	84±16%*	106±19%
Number of patients with					
– exercise capacity >120%	18 (18%)	13 (13%)	0 (0%)	1 (2%)	8 (22%)
– exercise capacity 80–120%	70 (70%)	72 (70%)	56 (79%)	29 (59%)	25 (68%)
– exercise capacity 50–80%	12 (12%)	17 (17%)	13 (18%)	18 (37%)	4 (11%)
– exercise capacity <50%	0 (0%)	0 (0%)	2 (3%)	1 (2%)	0 (0%)

[1] = relative to predicted value ± SD; *ASD* = atrial septal defect; *VSD* = ventricular septal defect; *Fallot* = tetralogy of Fallot; *TGA-Mustard* = transposition of the great arteries after Mustard repair; *PS* = pulmonary stenosis; * significantly lower than normal

ably lead to right ventricular failure. Longer follow-up of these patients will be mandatory to assess right ventricular function. For this, a diagnostic tool to assess right ventricular size reliably and, ideally, predict impending right ventricular failure would be of enormous value.

The most important outcome of the psychological part of the study was that, irrespective of the cardiac diagnosis, many children and adolescents had social problems, attention problems at school and complaints of anxiety and depressions [34]. In contrast, adult patients compared favorably with a reference group in terms of daily activities, in leisure-time activities and emotional functioning [35]. An effective denial mechanism is the probable explanation for this positive outcome, possibly in combination with the fact that most patients were very achievement-oriented to prove that they were "no less than anybody else".

Conclusion

We are convinced that the interpretation and treatment of the problems encountered in the group of grown-ups with congenital heart disease (GUCH) requires specific knowledge. The care for these patients should be concentrated in specialized centers for grown-ups with congenital heart disease, with doctors specially trained in this difficult field. Only then good patient care can be achieved.

Until know, little is known about prevalence of sequelae, but data on this subject are essential in the judgement of long-term results of cardiac surgery.

Apart from its use as technology assessment, such data could provide a basis for guidelines for insurance doctors and occupational physicians in the difficult process of judging employability and insurability of this group of patients. Apart from good quality patient care for the individual patient, optimal integration of this patient group as a whole in the social and professional life should be one of the goals of the treating GUCH-doctors.

References

1. Engle MA, Adams FH, Betson C, DuShane JW, Elliott LT, McNamara DG, Rashkind WJ, Talner S (1971) Resources for the optimal acute care of patients with congenital heart disease. Circulation 43:A–123.
2. Perloff JK (1973) Pediatric congenital cardiac becomes a postoperative adult. Circulation 42:606–619.
3. Liebman J, Cullum L, Belloc NB (1969) The natural history of transposition of the great arteries. Circulation 40:237–241.
4. Bertranou EG, Blackstone EH, Hazelrig JB, Turner ME, Kirklin JW (1978) Life expectancy without surgery in tetralogy of Fallot. Am J Cardiol 42:458–465.
5. Campbell M. (1970) Natural history of atrial septal defect. Br Heart J 32:820–826.
6. Campbell M. (1971) Natural History of ventricular septal defect. Br Heart J 33:246-257.
7. Corone P, Doyon F, Gaudeau S, Guerin F, Vernant P, Ducam H, Rumeau-Roquette C, Gaudeul P. (1977) Natural history of ventricular septal defect; a study involving 790 cases. Circulation 55 no 6:908–915.
8. Weidman WH, Blount SG, DuShane JW, Gersony WM, Hayes CJ, Nadas AS. (1977) Clinical course in ventricular septal defect. Circulation 56(suppl I):56–69.
9. Mody MR. (1975) The natural history of uncomplicated valvular pulmonic stenosis. Am Heart J 90:317–321.
10. Crafoord C, Nylin G. (1945) Congenital coarctation and its surgical treatment. J Thorac Surg 14:347–61.
11. Blalock A, Taussig HB. (1945) Surgical treatment of malformations of the heart in which there is pulmonary stenosis or pulmonary atresia. JAMA 128:189–202.
12. Brock R. (1961) The surgical treatment of pulmonary stenosis. Br Heart J 23:337–356.
13. Lewis FJ, Tauffic M. (1953) Closure of atrial septal defect with the aid of hypothermia: experimental accomplishments and the report of one successful case. Surgery 33:52–59.
14. Lillehei CW, Varco RL, Cohen M, Warden HE, Patton C, Moller JH. (1986) The first open-heart repairs of ventricular septal defect, atrioventricular communis, and tetralogy of Fallot using extracorporal circulation by cross-circulation: a 30 year follow-up. Ann Thorac Surg 41:4–21.
15. Gibbon JH, Miller BJ, Fineberg C. (1953) An improved heart and lung apparatus: its use during open cardiotomy in experimental animals. Med Clin North Am 37:1603–1609.
16. Hill JD, Gibbon Jonh H Jr. (1982) Part I. The development of the first successful heart-lung machine. Ann Thorac Surg 34:337–339.
17. Kirklin JW, DuShane JW, Patrick RT, Donald DE, Hetzel PS, Harshbarger HD, Wood EH. (1955) Intracardiac surgery with the aid of a mechanical pump-oxygenator (Gibbon-type): report of eight cases. Proc. Staff Meet. Mayo Clin. 30:201–213.
18. Perloff JK. (1991) Congenital heart disease in adults. Circulation 84:1881–1890.
19. Perloff JK. (1993) Pediatric congenital becomes postoperative adult; the changing population of congenital heart disease. Circulation 47:606–619.
20. Stark J. (1989) Do we really correct congenital heart defects? J Thorac Cardiovasc Surg 97:1–9.
21. Somerville J. (1992) The problem-an overview. In Congenital heart disease in adolescents and adults. editors J.Hess and G.R.Sutherland. Kluwer Academic Press, Dordrecht/Boston/London 1–13.

22. Murphy JG, Gersh BJ, McGoon MD, Mair DD, Porter J, Ilstrup DM, McGoon DC, Puga FJ, Kirklin JW, Danielson GK. (1990) Long-term outcome after surgical repair of isolated atrial septal defect. New Engl J Med 323:1645–1650.
23. Murphy JG, Gersh BJ, Mair DD, Fuster V, McGoon MD, Ilstrup DM, McGoon DC, Kirklin JW, Danielson GK. (1993) Long-term outcome in patients undergoing surgical repair of tetralogy of Fallot. New Eng J Med 329:593–599.
24. Fuster V, McGoon DC, Kennedy MA, Ritter DG, Kirklin JW. (1980) Long-term evaluation (12–22 years) of open heart surgery for tetralogy of Fallot. Am J Cardiol 46:635–42.
25. Chen D, Moller JH. (1987) Comparison of late clinical status between patients with different hemodynamic findings after repair of tetralogy of Fallot. Am Heart Journal 113:767–772.
26. Nadas A, Ellison RC, Weidman HC. (1977) Pulmonary stenosis, aortic stenosis, ventricular septal defect: clinical course and indirect assessment. Report from the Joint Study on the Natural History of Congenital Heart Defects. Circulation 56 suppl I:I-1–I-87.
27. O'Fallon MW and Weidman WH eds. (1993) Long-term follow-up of congenital aortic stenosis, pulmonary stenosis, and ventricular septal defect. Report from the second joint study on the natural history of congenital heart defects (NHS-2). Circulation 87 suppl.2:1-126.
28. Meijboom F, Hess J, Szatmari A, Utens EMWJ, McGhie J, Deckers JW, Roelandt JRTC, Bos E. (1993) Long-term follow-up (9 to 20 years) after surgical closure of atrial septal defect at a young age. Am J Cardiol 72:1431–1434.
29. Meijboom F, Szatmari A, Utens EMWJ, Deckers JW, Roelandt JRTC, Bos E, Hess J. (1994) Long-term follow-up after surgical closure of ventricular septal defect in infancy and childhood. J Am Coll Cardiol 24:1358–64.
30. Meijboom F, Szatmari A, Deckers JW, Utens EMWJ, Roelandt JRTC, Bos E, Hess J. (1995) Cardiac status and health related quality of life long-term after surgical repair of tetralogy of Fallot in infancy and childhood. J Thorac Cardiovasc Surg.
31. Meijboom F, Szatmari A, Deckers JW, Utens EMWJ, Roelandt JRTC, Bos E, Hess J. (1996) Long-term follow-up after Mustard repair for transposition of the great arteries. J Thorac Cardiovasc Surg: in press.
32. Meijboom F, Bos E, Szatmari A, Deckers JW, Utens EMWJ, Roelandt JRTC, Hess J. Long-term results of surgery for valvular pulmonary stenosis in infancy and childhood. submitted.
33. Kugler JD. (1990) Sinus node dysfunction. In A.Garson, J.T.Bricker, D.G.McNamara, eds. The science and practice of pediatric cardiology, 1st ed. Philadelphia/London. Lea & Febiger 1751–1785.
34. Utens EMWJ, Verhulst FC, Meijboom FJ, Duivenvoorden HJ, Erdman RAM, Bos E, Roelandt JRTC, Hess J. (1993) Behavioral and emotional problems in children and adolescents with congenital heart disease. Psychological Med 23:415–424.
35. Utens EMWJ, Verhulst FC, Meijboom FJ, Duivenvoorden HJ, Erdman RAM, Bos E, Roelandt JRTC, Hess J. (1994) Psychosocial functioning of young adults after surgical correction for congenital heart disease in childhood: a follow-up study. J Psychosomatic Res 38:745–758.

Curative Repair in Pediatric Cardiac Surgery is Increasingly Feasible

A. J. J. C. Bogers and F. J. Meijboom

Introduction

As demonstrated almost every month in the relevant journals, curative surgical repair for congenital anomalies of the heart and the thoracic vessels is increasingly feasible and can be accomplished at a very young age as well. Most likely the trend towards repair of these anomalies very early in life will continue. In this regard, even fetal surgery may sometime in the future become part of the cardiac surgical practice [1, 2]. However, to put the concept of "curative surgery" into the right perspective, it should be realized that there is also an increase in the number of adolescents and adults coming for surgical repair of congenital anomalies of the heart and thoracic vessels [3, 4, 5]. For some of these older patients this is the first operation, because they have been asymptomatic or because the risk of surgery decreased below the gradually increasing risk of ongoing conservative treatment. For an increasing number of these older patients, however, this means a reoperation, the patient being a survivor of surgical therapy performed in infancy and childhood [3, 4, 5]. The specific problems of this older patient group will not further be addressed to in this chapter. Also issues concerning cardiac and cardiopulmonary transplantation will not be discussed.

Regardless the age of the subject to be treated invasively for an anomaly of the heart or thoracic vessels, the result will always depend on the accuracy of the preoperative analysis, on the efficacy of the surgical intervention, on the quality of the perioperative care and on the successful neutralization of the numerous risks in all stages of treatment. In addition, it is very important to have an adequate data registry of all stages of treatment, in particular on long-term follow up [4]. In other words, It should be clear that successful repair in pediatric cardiac surgery is interrelated with and dependant on accurate preoperative analysis and adequate perioperative care.

Although it might be tempting just to refer to and to comment on the recent literature on the surgical treatment of congenital cardiovascular anomalies at very young age, it is more challenging not to discuss surgical results per se, but to try and discuss some of the aspects of pediatric cardiac surgery on which the discussion is not closed or even just opened. Such a discussion can only be put into perspective if it is adequately appreciated that a neonate is a rapidly changing physiologic entity [6]. These rapid changes are the result of the continuation of the maturation of the different organ systems and of the adjustments to postnatal existence [6]. The neonate responds differently to artificial ventilation and cardiopulmonary bypass as compared to older individuals. Knowledge of these specific responses is mandatory for successful surgical and overall management.

Preoperative Care

It is essential to get as accurate as possible an anatomic and physiologic diagnosis of the anomaly to be able to make a realistic plan of management. Whether the diagnostic assessment uses derived (using ultrasound methods) or measured (using cardiac catheterization) data is not relevant as long as the diagnostic process leads to an accurate diagnosis and does not increase the risk of the eventual outcome. From a practical point of view, ultrasound diagnostics can be performed almost instantly and can be repeatedly applied. If cardiac catheterization is indicated, this can be planned taken into account the condition of the patient.

An optimal preoperative condition will allow a better outcome of surgical therapy. Although some congenital cardiac anomalies do not allow postponement of surgical therapy for more than 24 hours (for example total anomalous pulmonary venous return), in others (for example transposition of the great arteries with intact ventricular septum) the preoperative condition may be optimalized on prostaglandin treatment for up to several weeks if necessary. On exceptional indication, it is even feasible to apply this regimen for some months (for example to allow growth from a low birth weight of below 1.5 kg to over 2.2 kg in pulmonary atresia with intact ventricular septum in order to construct successfully a modified Blalockshunt). It is therefore important to pay a great deal of attention to improvement of the preoperative condition instead of rushing into surgery. If possible, the neonate should be stabilized and allowed to accommodate to neonatal life [6] and the consequences of hemodynamic deteriorization at initial presentation should be treated adequately [7]. Prostaglandin treatment, diuretics, tube feeding and artificial ventilation, are important tools to allow improvement of condition before cardiac surgical treatment [7]. This line of management allows good results with decreased risks in regard to outcome.

Extracorporal Circulation

Improvements in the technology of extracorporal circulation have been instrumental in the increasing feasibility of surgical repair of congenital cardiovascular anomalies. It provides the surgeon adequate time to operate on even complex cardiac anomalies. It should be clear that cardiopulmonary bypass is an essential asset to pediatric cardiac surgery. However its side effects should be regarded as damaging [7, 8]. This is the more true for circulatory arrest, even at appropriate low body temperature. In fact, one should seriously consider to avoid this methodology at all, except for aortic reconstructions, that cannot be done otherwise with the present day technology.

The damage of cardiopulmonary bypass is due to altered perfusion patterns as well as to (micro)emboli, resulting in ischemic injury, endothelial damage, systemic presence of cytokines and leukocyte activation [2, 7,8]. For the young patient this will result in postoperative organ dysfunction on one hand, like seizures, renal dysfunction or lung injury resulting in diminished pulmonary gas exchange, and generalized capillary leak syndrome on the other hand.

Despite an increased knowledge on cardiopulmonary bypass in general as well as in neonates more specifically, numerous questions remain to be answered on possible interactions between the extracorporeal circuit and the patient [2, 7, 8], before the optimal feasibility and results of curative repair of congenital cardiovascular anomalies will be realized.

Intensive Care

Improvement in existing intensive care techniques and implementation of new techniques, is continuously providing a sound base for further allowing an increase in the feasibility of surgical repair in congenital cardiovascular anomalies. However some of these features still leave room for improvement.

Despite the fact that in the treatment of acute lung injury in general as well as more specifically lung injury resulting from cardiopulmonary bypass, opinions seem to be gradually converging, there is still no firm consensus regarding the appropriate ventilatory management of acute lung injury [9]. Especially in patients, who also show pulmonary hypertension and pulmonary vascular reactivity, ventilation with nitric oxide has shown to be a valuable asset, but certainly not a universally successful treatment modality. The same holds for the different methods of extracorporeal membrane oxygenation or carbondioxide extraction. The newest tool in this regard is liquid ventilation, being introduced as partial liquid ventilation with perfluorochemicals installed in the major airways [9]. It has to be kept in mind that these treatment modalities are not frequently indicated, but may be of great support in individualized situations.

An important factor in the improving results of curative repair of congenital cardiovascular anomalies is the awareness of the metabolic state of the operated patient [7]. The evolving idea is that the metabolic state not only should be adequate, but can also be modulated positively in order to diminish postoperative septic events and shorten the stay in the intensive care. This concept has already been called "Immunonutrition" [10]. In this regard metabolic monitoring of operated patients with an expected longer intensive care stay, deserves adequate attention. Changing concepts on cardiovascular function also have contributed to an increase in feasibility of pediatric cardiac surgery. It is well known that heart rate plays an important role in the cardiac output of the neonate and that postoperatively preload and afterload should be optimalized.

Especially in univentricular parallel circulations, as after the Norwood reconstruction for the hypoplastic left heart syndrome, it is however much more important to manipulate the vascular resistance of the pulmonary and systemic vascular bed in order to achieve an optimal balance between pulmonary and systemic circulation [11].

Generation of Knowledge from Data

In considering the increasing possibilities of any treatment, there are conceptually two possible causes of failure of treatment in general and pediatric cardiac surgery more specifically, being lack of scientific progress and human error [8]. Lack of scientific progress is gradually overcome by the continuous generation of new knowledge [8]. Human error is gradually brought down in frequency by recognition that the commission of suboptimal performance is part of human activity and can be minimized by techniques of reducing errors from professional areas other than cardiac surgery [8]. Accurate collection of data is a prerequisite for any reliable analysis, whether it is to support health care management or to serve the purpose of research. Independent of the computersystem chosen, accurate data collection may be a bottle neck for any reliable analysis. In considering to combine data from multiple centers, it should be made perfectly clear what the purpose of database is, where the legal ownership of the database resides, what the initial and yearly expenses of the contributants will be. Agreement on the data to be included and on the methods of analysis and presentation is essential. In addition, a data-base should be relational to allow internal checkup of data, should be perfect in any legal aspect concerning privacy of the patients, should be user-friendly, should be user-motivating by simply providing or allowing tabular and graphical display and should provide a perfect help-function or an adequate help-desk. By now commercially available systems are readily filling the market, but all of them have their limitations. Locally developed, noncommercial systems, built by and maintained by institutional professionals, may provide better quality and more support to the customer. However, for these systems it may be more difficult to be implemented elsewhere.

Regardless the database and its management, there is a need for defining not only the more or less clear points of outcome, for example hospital readmission, reintervention, and death, but very importantly also the quality of life after an intervention [4]. Furthermore, an assessment should be designed of the quality of life with and without a possible treatment in order to define the so called "quality adjusted life years". In this regard there is an important role for medical technology assessment.

Molecular Biology

It is only since recently that the practice of pediatric cardiac surgery is being supported by molecular biological data concerning the myocardium. At present this has still more the nature of an inventory, but already signal induction and manipulation at RNA level is being investigated in animal studies [12]. At present studies of human right ventricular myocardium in tetralogy of Fallot at several stages of disease and surgical treatment is being investigated. Fetal gene reprogramming, switches in contractile proteins, myocardial angiogenesis and fibrosis, as well as messengers of extracellular matrix building and break down are being investigated. It may be speculated that given time, detailed molecular genetic manipulation can be applied [12], for instance to restimulate an involuted left ventricle at late presentation in transposition of the great arteries with intact ventricular septum without banding of the pulmonary artery or to close multiple muscular defects in the ventricular septum without banding of the pulmonary artery.

Fetal Cardiac Surgery

Although it has been stated that the ability to diagnose fetal cardiac anomalies early in pregnancy presents us with the possibility to intervene for these anomalies before birth, there is at present no yet a realistic view on solving the many remaining problems before fetal open heart surgery becomes a clinical reality [2]. Even if arguments may be constructed to support the concept of fetal intervention for certain congenital cardiac defects, practical realities dictate that the development of successful interventional approaches to fetal cardiac disease will demand a thorough grasp of a wide range of unique issues [1]. Safe and reliable fetal extracorporeal circulatory support and a thorough understanding of its pathophysiologic responses in the fetomaternal unit has not yet been achieved [1].

Conclusion

As continuously demonstrated in the relevant literature, curative surgery for congenital cardiovascular anomalies is increasingly feasible at young age. However there is still ample room for improvement. Accurate diagnosis and adequate preoperative care should be regarded as ongoing items of attention. Much improvement of the understanding of the molecular genetics of the myocardium in congenital heart disease is to be expected and one can speculate molecular tools to be derived from this area to influence the perioperative myocardial condition of the patient. Apart from improvements in actual pediatric cardiac surgery, the understanding of the effect of cardiopulmonary bypass on the patient may be further improved. Further innovations in the intensive care are to be expected, specifically on respiratory and metabolic care. Last but not least the construction of databases and their use should not be underestimated and deserves professional support, especially with regard to long-term follow up.

References

1. Hanley FL (1994) Fetal cardiac surgery: steady progress in the laboratory (editorial). Ann Thor Surg 57:279–280
2. Jonas R, Elliot M (1994) Current practice and research directions – a review. In: Jonas RA, Elliot MJ (eds) Cardiopulmonary bypass in neonates, infants and young children. Butterworth-Heinemann, Oxford pp 285–293
3. Bogers AJJC (1992) Surgery for congenital heart disease in adults. In: Hess J, Sutherland GR (eds) Congenital heart disease in adolescents and adults. Kluwer, Dordrecht pp171–174
4. Meyboom FJ (1995) Longterm outcome after surgery for congenital heart disease in infancy and childhood. Thesis, Rotterdam
5. Stark J (1989) Do we really correct congenital heart defects? J Thorac Cardiovasc Surg 97:1–9
6. Hanley FL (1994) Organ development and maturation. In: Jonas RA, Elliot MJ (eds) Cardiopulmonary bypass in neonates, infants and young children. Butterworth–Heinemann, Oxford pp 5–26
7. Castaneda AR, Jonas RA, Mayer JE jr, Hanley FL (1994) Cardiac surgery of the neonate and the infant. Saunders, Philadelphia
8. Kirklin JW, Barratt-Boyes BG (1993) Cardiac surgery, 2nd edition. Churchill Livingstone, New York
9. Marini JJ (1995) Down side up – a prone and partial liquid asset (editorial). Int Care Med 21:963–965
10. Koretz RL (1993) Immunonutrition? (editorial) Gastroenterol 104:936–938
11. Rossi AF, Sommer RJ, Lotvin A et al (1994) Usefulness of intermittent monitoring of mixed venous oxygen saturation after stage I palliation for hypoplastic left heart syndrome. Am J Cardiol 73:1118–1123
12. Van Bilzen M, Chien KR (1993) Growth and hypertrophy of the heart: towards an understanding of cardiac specific and inducible gene expression. Cardiovasc Res 27:1140–1149

Ethics

Ethics

R. Truog, J. Burns and M. C. Rogers

Introduction

The competent practice of critical care medicine today requires more than a knowledge of the relevant medical science. At least some understanding of medical ethics and related law is required, and perhaps in no area of medicine is this more true than in the care of critically ill patients. During the past century dramatic changes have occurred in physicians' ability to prolong life. The ethical dilemmas associated with the advances in medical technology and the evolution of the physician-patient relationship have become the subject of wide public concern. As we enter into an era of medicine where the cost of care and the utilization of limited resources are increasingly debated, critical care physicians, with expertise in life and death decisions and with responsibility for caring for patients who require life-sustaining treatments, must possess a clear ethical framework for decision making. This chapter focuses on the key foundations of medical ethics and practical approaches to ethical decision making in the pediatric intensive care unit.

The Development of Medical Ethics

The terms "ethics" and "morality" are often used interchangeably, but most philosophers draw a subtle distinction between the two. Morality consists of social norms of behavior, and often varies dramatically between cultures. The discipline of ethics, on the other hand, involves the development of philosophical reasons for or against a set of moral judgments. Usually the latter effort attempts to articulate and justify principles which form the foundation for rules of conduct and decision making for competing moral claims.

Medical ethics is the discipline devoted to the identification, analysis, and resolution of problems which arise in the care of patients. It is a special kind of ethics only insofar as it relates to the peculiar dilemmas that arise in medicine, and not because it embodies or appeals to some special moral principles or methodology. The term "bioethics" is often used interchangeably with "medical ethics", although the former has a slightly broader meaning, including ethical problems that arise outside the area of medicine (such as issues surrounding research on animals, for example). In summary, the practice of medical ethics seeks to identify and resolve competing moral claims among patients, their families, health care professionals, health care institutions, and society at large.

Concern for ethical issues in medicine dates back at least to the time of Hippocrates. Nevertheless, until the middle of this century, little additional thought was given to the unique problems that arise in the context of clinical practice and medical research. The exposure of the Nazi atrocities after World War II lead to the reaffirmation of the importance of ethics in medicine and research, and was directly responsible for the formulation of codes of ethics pertaining to research on human subjects (e.g., the Nuremberg Code in the late 1940's, followed by the declaration of Helsinki in 1964) [1, 2].

In the decades following World War II, the introduction of antibiotics, vaccines and effective diagnostic therapeutic technologies transformed medicine from a profession focused on caring to one focused on curing. The expectations of physicians and patients have grown considerably, yet, medical advances have brought with them ethical dilemmas that increasingly find their way into public and professional consciousness.

A 1962 Life Magazine article entitled "They Decide Who Lives, Who Dies" marked such an event [3]. The article described the efforts of a committee of ordinary citizens in Seattle, not physicians, charged with the task of allocating access to hemodialysis, then a scare resource, for critically ill patients who would die without this therapy. The committee disbanded itself after it realized that its selection process was influenced by its own middle class values, rather than by an objectively fair allocation procedure. Public and then Congressional outrage at the reality of scarce but effective medical technology lead to passage in 1973 of the end stage renal disease program. Under this legislation, the Federal Medicare Program assumed responsibility for anyone in need of chronic dialysis, regardless of socioeconomic status. Like many federal initiatives in the 1960's and 1970's, this program has proven to be far more costly than initially expected [4].

The medical profession's attention to these issues was further heightened by a 1973 article in the New England Journal of Medicine which described the decision by physicians and parents to withhold treatment from 43 critically ill infants in the neonatal intensive care unit at Yale-New Haven Hospital [5]. This account was among the first to bring attention to the fact that medical technology had reached a point where the decision to end life had to be taken deliberately by physicians and families.

But perhaps no event captured public and professional attention to these difficult issues more than the 1976 New Jersey Supreme Court Decision on patient Karen Ann Quinlan. On the night of April 15, 1973, this 21 year old woman experienced a respiratory arrest that left her in a persistent vegetative state. Her father petitioned the court for authority to be named her guardian and for permission to discontinue the ventilator. His request was opposed by her doctors, the hospital, and prosecutors for the local county and the State of New Jersey. The New Jersey Supreme Court ruled that she had a constitutional "right to privacy" to be removed from the ventilator if the family, the physicians, and the hospital ethics committee agreed. Despite the prevailing opinion of her doctors, she did not die when removed from the ventilator, but lived for almost another decade. This was the first of many cases that helped to shape to our current views about the withdrawal of life-sustaining treatments.

Ethical Theory

Broadly speaking, two dominant ethical theories have developed in the Western intellectual tradition. Both attempt to provide a set of "first principles" for approaching ethical conflict.

The Utilitarian Theory

One is the Utilitarian Philosophy, as developed by English philosophers Jeremy Bentham and John Stuart Mill [6]. Utilitarianism is rooted in the thesis that an action or practice is right (when compared to any alternative action or practice) if it leads to the greatest possible balance of good consequences or the least possible balance of bad consequences, in the world as a whole. According to this view, moral codes and traditions are designed to promote human welfare by maximizing benefits and minimizing harms.

The other dominant ethical theory, deontology, was heavily influenced by the writings of philosopher Immanuel Kant [7]. According to this approach, certain actions or practices are always wrong, regardless of the consequences.

The current debate about euthanasia illustrates the differences between these approaches. Utilitarians may argue, for example, that when a terminally ill patient requests to be killed, the consequences of complying with that request are favorable for everyone concerned. The patient's desires are satisfied, the physician can rest assured that the act was in the patient's best interest (as defined by the patient), and even society may benefit by not incurring the expenses associated with a prolonged dying process. Deontologists, on the other hand, feel differently. For a deontologist, the prohibition against killing should stop us from taking the life of another, regardless of the consequences. Under this approach, euthanasia is always wrong, even if we are convinced that doing so does not harm anyone's interest. Some deontologists base their beliefs upon a religious perspective (the Ten Commandments are a typical list of deontologic principles), whereas others derive a set of duties and obligations by theoretical analysis. Even utilitarians often agree that rules have an important place in ethics, if only because of the inherent difficulties involved in predicting the consequences of our actions. To use the euthanasia example again, a deontologist might claim that even when performing euthanasia does not appear to harm anyone's interest, the long-term consequences of permitting this act might be to diminish our respect for human life, and could eventually work to erode the core values of the medical profession. This would be a reason to oppose euthanasia, even by the utilitarian standard.

Ethical Principles

In reality, few people are pure deontologists or consequentialists. Most of us blend these two perspectives in our reasoning about ethical issues. In the search for practical guidance to moral dilemmas, therefore, leading ethical theorists over the last twenty years have turned instead to the so called "principles approach" to moral reasoning. For example, in what is widely regarded as the classic textbook on modern medical ethics, Tom Beauchamp and James Childress advocate four principles on which to ground ethical analysis [8]. They are respect for autonomy (self-determination), beneficence (doing good), nonmaleficence (avoiding harm), and justice (fair distribution).

Beauchamp and Childress have outlined the process of moral justification using the principles approach in terms of three levels:

Principles
↓
Rules
↓
Particular Judgments

When one is faced with a moral dilemma, the task is to identify the relevant ethical principles that should be brought to bear on the case. These principles will suggest a set of rules that are pertinent to the situation. From these rules, one should be able to discern the proper judgment regarding the particular case.

The obvious problem with this approach is that different principles will give rise to different sets of rules, which will in turn produce conflicting judgments. Assigning priority to one moral principle over another depends on the situation, since none of the principles always trumps any of the others. Analysis of ethical dilemmas in terms of these four principles is therefore seldom sufficient for determining the "correct" answer, but is often very useful in helping to identify the salient issues that are at stake.

Criticisms of Principles

More recently, several alternatives to the principle-based mode of analysis have been proposed and developed. Proponents of "case-based reasoning", or casuistic analysis, argue that the four principles of Beauchamp and Childress are too indeterminate and abstract to be of much help with real-life dilemmas [9, 10]. They advocate instead for the use of "paradigmatic cases", that is, real cases about which there is currently a consensus. As new cases arise, they are analyzed in terms of the ways that they are similar to, or different from, the paradigmatic cases. This has been referred to as "moral triangulation." For example, since the "Baby Doe" episode in 1984, there is general agreement in medicine, law, and ethics that babies with Down Syndrome and correctable surgical anomalies should undergo surgical repair of their conditions, and not be allowed to die from them [11]. Similarly, there is also general agreement that babies with Trisomy 13 or 18 who have potentially lethal congenital defects need not be offered life-prolonging therapies, but may ethically be treated with only comfort care. When faced with the problem of how to treat a newborn with congenital anomalies intermediate between those of Trisomy 21 and 13/18, a proponent of the case-based approach might attempt to address the question by first exploring the ways in which the child is more like an infant with Down Syndrome, or more like an infant with Trisomy 13/18. In combination with factors such as the severity of the defects and the preferences of the family, this approach would attempt to "triangulate" toward the most reasonable solution.

As the field of bioethics has continued to develop, still other ways of thinking about difficult cases have emerged. An alternative which has arisen from the feminist movement is an approach based upon the primacy of "caring" [12]. In its more radical form, this perspective minimizes the importance of ethical theory and principles, and seeks resolutions to difficult cases that best preserve the relationships involved. As opposed to a principle-based approach, this perspective is less concerned with maintaining internal consistency and with the observance of formal rules. When confronted with a case about whether to allow a small child to donate a kidney to a sibling, for example, a proponent of the "caring" approach would ask which of the alternative options would best promote the well-being of the relationships between the family and others involved.

Finally, a perspective that has developed within the fields of literature and the humanities focuses on the value of "narrative" [13]. Unlike the terse case-histories that tend to be favored in the busy hospital setting, this approach emphasizes the importance of understanding cases in all of their detail and complexity. Rather than attempting to "shrink" cases to their essential elements, and then applying a specific "rule" or "principle," the proponent of the narrative approach will insist that only by analyzing cases in all of their richness and texture can we hope to arrive at solutions that are sufficiently nuanced and sophisticated. Indeed, this approach hearkens back to the admonitions of many of the great medical clinicians who emphasized the overriding importance of careful history taking. These giants of medicine would undoubtedly be just as critical of our over-reliance on invasive technology and imaging studies as the proponent of narrative is critical of "principles."

Ethics and the Law

Physicians generally have one of two attitudes toward the law. Either they claim to be unconcerned about legal precedent and only interested in practicing "good medicine", or they are fearful of making any decision or taking any action without first finding out if it is "legal". Both extreme views could lead to naive or imprudent decisions about difficult ethical dilemmas in clinical practice.

First, when considering legal precedents in ethical decision making it is important to keep in mind that there is no single, monolithic statement that can be made about that the "law" in most ethical controversies. The body of law supporting the American legal system is actually the product of many factors. For example, legislative mandates or court decisions in one state do not hold as precedent or law in any other state. Superimposed on state law and legislation is the federal system with its own jurisdictions, which can also disagree over key points.

Second, while both ethics and the law are concerned with identifying which actions are acceptable within a given society, they remain fundamentally distinct. Acting in accordance with the law is no guarantee that one is acting ethically, as emphasized by the Nuremberg Court in evaluating the actions of the Nazi concentration camp guards. Law, as it relates to morality, usually represents the minimum requirements regarding moral duties and rights for a given society. Law represents the floor, and not the ceiling, for standards about morality.

Ethics and Informed Consent

Ethical and Legal Basis of Consent

One of the fundamental tenets of contemporary medical ethics and American law is that a competent adult is the master of his or her own body, and that a physician must obtain the free and informed consent of a patient, or a patient's surrogate if the patient is incompetent, before medical care is provided.

For thousands of years this was not the case in medical decision-making. Dating from the age of Hippocrates until the very recent past, most decisions were the sole prerogative of the physician. This approach to medical care can no longer be justified, however, since it fails to respect the fundamental importance of the patient's values and goals by placing the clinician's value structure ahead of that of the patient [14].

The ascendancy of respect for patient autonomy and the right to self-determination has become paramount only in the last several decades, yet the roots of this transformation are much deeper. The philosophical and ethical basis for self-determination can be found in the Medieval and Renaissance thinkers who so greatly influenced the framers of the American Constitution and Bill of Rights. Philosophers such as John Locke, Edmund Burke, and Immanuel Kant, among others, articulated the intellectual foundation for the notion that it is not the State but the individual who is sovereign.

The legal basis for an individual's right to self-determination arose from a series of landmark cases [15]. In an early case from 1914, Justice Cardozo made his celebrated observation that "Every human being of adult years and sound mind has a right to determine what shall be done with his own body, and a surgeon who performs an operation without his patient's consent commits an assault, for which he is liable in damages". For many years, courts held physicians to what is known as the "professional standard" of informed consent, where physicians are expected to disclose only that information which is customarily disclosed by their colleagues. In the 1972 case of *Canterbury* v. *Spence*, however, the Federal Appeals Court in Washington broke away from the traditional application of a professional standard in favor of a patient-oriented standard that required physicians to disclose all information that might be relevant to the patient in making an informed decision, regardless of whether such information is "customarily" provided by other physicians in the community.

Exceptions to Informed Consent

Two exceptions to "informed consent" have traditionally been recognized. The first, and least controversial, is the emergency exception, which allows a physician to treat a patient when significant harm is imminent, when the patient is incapable of consenting, and when no surrogate is immediately available.

More controversial is the second traditional exception to informed consent, the therapeutic privilege exception. Under this exception, physicians may forego attempts to obtain informed consent when they believe that the patient will experience more harm than benefit from the disclosure. Recently, there has been a tendency in law and ethics to constrain this exception because it assumes that the physician knows what is best for the patient. This assumption violates the general view that patients themselves provide the most reliable information about what is in their best interest, as well as a body of empirical evidence indicating that physicians systematically underestimate the desire of patients to know their diagnosis and to be involved in decision-making [16, 17].

Consent for Research on Human Subjects

Informed consent is especially important when patients are given innovative therapies or are recruited for research. Intensivists are often tempted to try new therapies on critically ill patients who are desperate for a cure. Despite the perceived urgency of the situation, physicians must respect the safeguards that have been developed to protect patients from therapies that are potentially harmful. Physicians who skirt the requirements for approval by institutional review boards and informed consent under the guise being "compassionate" threaten the very future of the innovation they are trying to promote. Finally, children should never receive innovative therapies solely because future patients might benefit from them. In keeping with the fiduciary relationship between doctor and patients, there must be some reasonable expectation that the patient may benefit, regardless of the potential for benefit to future patients [18].

Consent for Practicing Procedures on Newly Deceased Patients

The use of dead patients to teach procedures has been a source of controversy dating at least to the Middle Ages. Some have argued that it is ethically justifiable to perform practice procedures on the newly dead without permission from the family because these procedures cannot harm the deceased, there is substantial social benefit to be gained, and families could not realistically be expected to discuss consent at such a difficult time [19]. Indeed, a recent study showed that 39% of training programs in emergency and critical care medicine use newly dead patients to teach various resuscitation procedures (for example, endotracheal intubation, central line placement, and pericardiocentesis). Few of these programs obtain either verbal or written consent from the families [20].

Despite the frequency of this practice without consent, some have argued that teaching procedures on newly deceased patients is ethical only when permission is first obtained from the family. In addition, given its sensitive nature, this teaching technique should be reserved only for those who truly need to master the skills and only as the culmination of a structured learning sequence, and not a haphazard event [20].

Informed Consent: Inducement for a Therapeutic Alliance

Although the doctrine of informed consent has become standard medical practice, many physicians still view it as a burden imposed by lawyers. In this context, the communication process is reduced to the physicians' effort to avoid a lawsuit. A more constructive view is that the informed consent process can actually help strengthen the communication in the patient-physician relationship. As noted by Gutheil and colleagues, "Informed consent is not an empty gesture toward liability reduction, but an interaction between physician and patient, a dialogue intended not only to satisfy their legal requirements, but to do more as well. The real clinical opportunity offered by informed consent is that of transforming uncertainty from a threat into the very basis on which an alliance can be formed "[21]

Medical Decision-Making

Competency and Decision-Making Capacity

The distinction between competency and decision-making capacity is often misunderstood. All adults over the age of majority (18 years in most states) are presumed to be legally competent. This legal presumption can only be overridden in a court of law. A separate concept is "decision-making capacity". A person can be legally competent and yet not have the capacity to make decisions on their own behalf (an acute trauma victim, for example). Conversely, even patients who are considered legally incompetent may have the decision-making capacity to determine whether they want certain medical interventions (most adolescents, for example). As a President's Commission observed, "Determining whether a patient lacks capacity to make a particular health care decision requires assessing the patient's capability to understand information relevant to the decision, to communicate with care givers about it, and to reason about relevant alternatives against a background of reasonably stable personal values and life goals." [22] Patients with decisional capacity have the right to direct their medical therapy, while those without decisional capacity do not.

Advance Directives

Several mechanisms exist to enable patients to retain some control over health care decisions after they have lost the capacity to participate directly in decision making. Most states now have legislation which recognizes the legality of certain advanced directives. Written and oral instructions, usually called a "living will", contain treatment directives to be followed if and when a patient becomes incapable of making treatment decisions [23]. These documents have been criticized as being too ambiguous in many critical decisions, for no one could possibly anticipate every potential occurrence that might confront them [24].

Over the last decade, the health care durable power of attorney, or "proxy", has emerged as another form of advance directive designed to overcome the limitations presented by living wills. Unlike living wills, which specify treatment decisions in advance, the health care proxy establishes a decision making process. Health care proxy laws permit patients to delegate the authority to make medical treatment decisions for them in the event of incapacity. The Patient Self Determination Act, passed by Congress in 1991, requires that all Medicare-participating institutions inform patients of their rights to formulate advance directives upon admission [25].

In making decisions for patients who no longer have decisional capacity, surrogate decision-makers should base their decisions, in descending order of preference, on the subjective standard, the substituted judgment standard, and the best interests standard [26, 27]. The subjective standard is the preferred guide for decision making. This requires that any relevant statements made by the patient while decisionally capable should guide all decisions. If there is not any firm evidence of what the patient specifically desired, then the surrogate should apply the substituted judgment standard. This requires the surrogate to apply the patient's own values, religious beliefs and preferences in arriving at the treatment decision. When this information is not available, or when the patient never obtained the capacity to espouse such preferences, the next step in the decision-making hierarchy is the best interests standard. Unlike the substituted judgment standard, which focuses on the patient's known preferences to guide decision making, the best interests standard attempts to rely on "objectively" weighing the benefits and burdens of the proposed treatment alternatives.

The Role of Parents in Decision-Making

There is broad societal consensus that parents are the preferred decision makers for their children [27, 28]. When a child is too young to have formed any clear preferences regarding treatment, it is left to the parents, most of whom unquestionably have a profound love and commitment to their children, to decide what is in the best interests of the child based on an assessment of the benefits and burdens of proposed treatment.

Although parents will bear much of the hardship of future therapies, and therefore have legitimate concerns about the effect of treatment decisions on themselves and their other children, these concerns cannot be used exclusively to justify the denial of clearly beneficial therapy. To quote a recent expert panel of pediatricians, "When a child would clearly benefit from available treatment, such as appendectomy for appendicitis, or chemotherapy for acute lymphoblastic leukemia, his or her interests must be given precedence" [29].

When parents deny treatment that is *not* clearly beneficial, however, the burden shifts to the health care team to justify the need to override the parents wishes. For example, in a 1991 Delaware case, Christian Science parents' were permitted the right to refuse treatment for their child suffering from Burkitt's lymphoma after expert testimony was introduced stating that the proposed therapy had the potential for significant risk and offered only a 40 percent chance of success [30]. As in all cases of conflict over medical decision making between patients, families, and providers, resort to legal mechanisms should always be a last step after exhausting all other avenues of resolution, including the use of consultants and institutional ethics committees.

Special Considerations for the Adolescent

While parents generally take full responsibility for decision-making for newborns and young children, this should not be the case for older children and adolescents. The legal age of majority is an oversimplification of the maturational and developmental process in children. Children as young as six or seven are often able to have reasoned opinions about certain aspects of their care, and most adolescents have views and perspectives that deserve serious consideration. The fact that parents must give legal consent for medical treatments performed on minor children does not mean that the opinions of the children and adolescents should be considered irrelevant or ignored.

Many states have recognized this developmental continuum in the form o. emancipated minor or mature minor statutes. An emancipated minor, in most jurisdictions, is someone under the age of majority who lives independent from their parents, is the parent of a child, or is in the military. In most states, these patients can legally consent to their own medical treatment [31].

Recognizing that some adolescents do not meet the criteria for emancipated minor and yet are mature enough to make decisions about medical therapy for themselves, many jurisdictions now recognize the concept of a "mature minor" [32]. While the legal requirements may vary, a generally accepted ethical principle is that children should always, at the very least, be evaluated for their ability to "assent" to treatment. In other words, while children may not have the cognitive or emotional skills to fully understand all of the implications of various treatment choices, even young children will often have the capacity for a general understanding of the proposed course of treatment and what they should expect. Furthermore, children should be given the opportunity to "assent" to this treatment ("consent" being reserved for those situations in which the patient can fully understand the benefits, risks, and alternatives for the proposed treatment). If the child refuses to assent, considerable effort should be made to explore the child's feelings and to seek strategies for accommodating these views and preferences. Only in unusual circumstances should children not be apprised of a proposed plan of treatment, or should their refusal to assent be categorically overridden.

Religious Beliefs in the Decision Making Process

While the courts have acknowledged the virtually unlimited right of competent adults to refuse medical treatments, they have been much more protective of children. The threshold for overriding the parents' wishes depends upon an objective assessment of the risks to the child. In general, if the circumstances do not involve life-threatening choices, and there are no certain risks of substantial harm to the child, physicians are obligated to respect the decisions of the parents, even when the physicians strongly disagree with the choice. In some jurisdictions, for example, parents are permitted the right to refuse standard immunizations for religious reasons [28].

It is only as the threat to the child increases, and the benefits of treatment are more certain, that actions to override parental choices are not only legally supportable, but in most jurisdictions required. Numerous court opinions have upheld the notion, first articulated in the famous 1944 case of *Prince* v. *Massachusetts*, that a parent may make a martyr of himself because of religious convictions, "but he is not free to make a martyr of his child" [33]. In numerous decisions since then, courts have upheld the right of physicians to override parental refusal of transfusions or other accepted therapy when the child's life is at risk [28].

Limitations of Life-Sustaining Treatments

The concept of doing anything less than everything possible to preserve the life of the patient is both old and new. The Hippocratic corpus admonishes physicians "to refuse to treat those who are overmastered by their diseases, realizing that in such cases medicine is powerless."[34] Nevertheless, as the specialty of critical care medicine developed and as the capability to prolong life evolved, the mere ability to use life-sustaining technology was transformed into a virtual imperative. Beginning with the Cruzan case in the mid–1970s, the pendulum has begun to swing back toward a more rational use of this technology. Over the past twenty years, clinicians, ethicists, lawyers, theologians and others have sought to articulate and define the conditions under which limitations in life-sustaining treatments are legitimate and justified.

DNR Orders

Until 1976, no hospital in the United States publicly acknowledged that they ever provided care that was not solely intended to prolong and preserve life. In that year, both the Massachusetts General Hospital and Boston's Beth Israel Hospital acknowledged their use of "do-not-resuscitate" orders in the New England Journal of Medicine [35, 36]. Over the past 20 years, DNR orders have become increasingly accepted and have undergone numerous modifications. More recently, however, there is evidence that the complexity of decision-making around terminally ill patients has progressed to the point where the philosophy behind DNR orders is no longer sufficient. Alternatives to the traditional DNR order will be discussed below.

Procedure-Specific DNR Orders

In most hospitals, DNR orders are written by the attending physician in the Doctor's Orders Sheets. These orders are often vague, and may leave substantial opportunity for miscommunication and error. Does "resuscitation" refer to treatment of an acute cardiac arrest (intubation and ventilation, chest compressions, cardioversion, and medications), or does it also mean "do-not-intubate" for conditions like respiratory failure from a pneumonia? Should patients with DNR orders receive suctioning for airway secretions, be treated with antibiotics, or be given tube feedings? Should they be excluded from the ICU, or denied palliative surgery? The answers to these questions are almost never clear in the interpretation of a simple "DNR order".

In response to these concerns, many institutions have now adopted "Procedure-Specific DNR Orders". This approach is intended to reduce much of the ambiguity surrounding these orders. This page appears at the beginning the "Doctor's Orders" section of the patient's chart, so that it is readily available at all times in a place easily identified by physicians and other caregivers who may not be familiar with the details of the patient's care at the time of an arrest. The form first specifies whether a "code blue" should be called in the event of a cardiorespiratory arrest, and then provides a checklist of exactly which procedures are to be performed or withheld. There is a section for identifying special instructions, and then lines for the signatures of both the attending physician and the bedside nurse, with a requirement for renewal every 7 days. Finally, there is a section to be completed if the patient or family rescind the DNR order. A recent study showed that use of procedure-specific DNR forms reduces the uncertainty and confusion that often accompanies the decision not to resuscitate [37].

"CPR-Not-Indicated" Orders

Is it necessary for the patient or family to consent to a DNR order?[38–42] Some states (e.g., New York) have laws that generally require the consent of the patient or family before a DNR order is written, and many hospitals have this requirement in their internal policies [43]. Recently, however, some hospitals have adopted policies that permit physicians to write DNR orders without the permission (or sometimes, without even the knowledge) of the patient or family. The presumption behind this approach is the view that CPR is a medical therapy, and that physicians are uniquely qualified to determine whether and when a medical therapy is indicated. These policies are therefore often referred to as "CPR-not-indicated" policies [44].

The belief of many physicians that they should have the authority to determine when CPR is appropriate is understandable. Many patients and families are unable to accept the fact that they or a loved one is terminally ill and about to die. In these situations, patients or families may maintain an irrational belief that CPR can offer them a meaningful extension in the quality or duration of their life. Under these circumstances, caregivers often feel that they are doing CPR to "treat the family," and that performing this procedure when it can offer no real benefit to the patient is a violation of their professional integrity.

On the other hand, this development in DNR orders should be viewed with great caution. As noted in the discussion of informed consent, physicians have a long history of seeing complex situations from a uniquely medical perspective, ignoring important factors related to the patient's values and preferences. Rarely is the question of whether or not to do CPR purely a medical issue. Often the patient's or family's denial of impending death can be overcome by proper counseling, whereas simply using the physician's authority to overrule the family's wishes can be profoundly destructive to the patient/physician relationship. While this debate over the legitimacy of "CPR-not-indicated" orders is far from resolved, there is little doubt that this approach should be used only under the most conservative and well-defined circumstances [44].

Redirection of Care / Comfort Policies

DNR orders are unique. They are the only physician's order that is focused exclusively upon what will *not* be done, rather than what *will* be done. Not surprisingly, patients with DNR orders often feel that they have been abandoned by their caregivers. Indeed, studies have shown that physicians do in fact spend less time caring for patients who have DNR orders. This is not always appropriate, because patients with DNR orders often need more attention in terms of aggressive palliative care than patients who are not imminently dying.

In addition, DNR orders tend to be concerned with only a small fraction of the issues that arise with dying patients. Often the question of whether or not a patient should be resuscitated is actually peripheral to the more important questions surrounding the use of less dramatic interventions. Should the patient be intubated and ventilated for the next episode of pneumonia? Should he receive antibiotics? Should he receive opioids to relieve the sensation of dyspnea, even though the respiratory depression from the opioids could hasten his death? Should the patient be fed only as much as he wants, realizing that this could lead to death from gradual dehydration and malnutrition, or should he be given a gastrostomy tube to optimize nutrition and hydration?

These questions are not adequately addressed by the traditional DNR order. Hospitals are therefore increasingly developing more global policies that are more responsive to the variety of issues posed by end-of-life decision-making than narrow DNR policies. The Joint Commission on Accreditation of Hospitals Organization (JCAHO) has indicated that it will soon require hospitals to have policies of this type.

Withdrawing Life-Sustaining Treatments

There is a clear ethical and legal consensus in the United States which supports the right of patients or their surrogates to refuse or remove unwanted medical treatment, even if such a decision involves life-sustaining therapy. This right has been supported by the United States Supreme Court; a special Presidential Commission; and in policy statements by the American Medical Association; the Society for Critical Care Medicine; and the American Thoracic Society [22,45–49].

In discussions about whether or not to provide life-sustaining therapies, several issues arise commonly. Among them are the distinction between ordinary and extraordinary treatments, the distinction between withholding a treatment and withdrawing a treatment, the appropriate role of sedatives and analgesics in the care of the dying, and whether artificial nutrition and hydration ("tube" feedings) may ever be foregone. These issues are discussed below.

The Ordinary/Extraordinary Distinction

One of the most commonly used justifications for withholding "high-tech" therapy from patients is the belief that "extraordinary" treatments are not ethically mandatory. For example, a recent survey showed that 74% of physicians and nurses think that the ordinary/extraordinary distinction is helpful in resolving ethical dilemmas [50]. Although this terminology is still used in the writings of some religious traditions, clinicians should understand that the distinction between ordinary and extraordinary treatments is not considered to be helpful when trying to reason about the ethical aspects of difficult decisions.

To illustrate why this is so, consider two alternative interpretations of the ordinary/extraordinary distinction. One interpretation would be that ordinary treatments are *customarily* performed, whereas extraordinary treatments are not. Clearly, however, a simple appeal to what is customary cannot suffice as a justification for what is morally required. In addition, from a legal perspective, the courts have explicitly rejected the view that there is any relationship between what is "customary" and what is "legal."

Another interpretation of the ordinary/extraordinary distinction would hold that ordinary treatments are morally required, whereas extraordinary treatments are morally optional. But this is essentially a circular argument, since it claims that ordinary treatments are morally required because they are ordinary, and extraordinary treatments are morally optional because they are extraordinary. Words cannot substitute for moral reasoning.

As an example of this fallacy in the literature, pediatricians were asked about their views on repair of duodenal atresia in healthy babies and in babies with Down Syndrome [51]. Most pediatricians said that duodenal atresia was an "ordinary" procedure in the case of healthy infants, but an "extraordinary" procedure in the case of babies with Down Syndrome. Since the procedure was the same in each case, the use of the terms "ordinary" and "extraordinary" served to mask the ethical judgments that were being made about the nature of the clinical condition.

A much more legitimate and useful approach to thinking about whether a procedure is ethically required is to inquire about the balance of the benefits versus the burdens for a particular procedure in a particular patient. In other words, instead of relying on terminology like ordinary and extraordinary to decide whether a treatment should be offered, consider instead whether the proposed benefits exceed the burdens. If, for example, a child with a malignancy is very unlikely to survive even with the administration of highly toxic chemotherapy, then the burdens of that therapy clearly exceed the benefits. On the other hand, physicians and society now generally agree that the benefits of repairing duodenal atresia in patients with Down Syndrome exceed the burdens, and thus the procedure is morally required.

The Withholding/Withdrawing Distinction

Is there a difference between stopping a treatment once it is started, and not starting it in the first place? In other words, is there an ethical difference between deciding not to intubate a patient because we do not think that he will recover, and extubating a patient who has failed to recover despite a period of ventilation? Surveys have repeatedly shown that physicians do believe there is a difference. For example, one recent study reported that 66% of physicians and nurses think that there is an ethical difference between withdrawing and withholding a treatment, and nearly half agreed with the statement "there is an emerging consensus that withdrawing a treatment is ethically different from withholding or not starting it."[50] In another survey of 360 attendings, housestaff, and medical students, 73% felt that withdrawing is different from withholding [52]. These reports all indicate that physicians are much more comfortable in withholding treatments than in withdrawing them.

This issue is particularly interesting in light of the fact that this opinion among clinicians is strikingly at odds with the prevailing views among ethicists and lawyers. Legal scholars and ethicists have been quite consistent in expressing the opinion that doctors should not differentiate between decisions to withhold or withdraw medical treatments. In the landmark *Cruzan* case, for example, justices from the US Supreme Court wrote that doctors should consider decisions to withhold and withdraw as equivalent in order to assure that patients receive adequate trials of therapy [45,53,54]. A typical example occurs in the delivery room, when the viability of premature babies is often difficult to assess in the moments immediately after birth. The Supreme Court's decision implies that physicians should deal with this uncertainty by proceeding with the resuscitation, but that the physicians should be willing to withdraw the life-sustaining treatment if, after a trial of therapy, further support is no longer justified.

Despite these opinions from law and philosophy, clinicians persist in believing that there is a difference between these two actions. Part of the reason in clearly psychological. Physicians feel more responsible for the death of a patient when it results from the withdrawal of a therapy than they do when it results from the withholding of a therapy. This psychological distinction is important, and cannot be made to disappear by legal or philosophical reasoning, no matter how persuasive. Nevertheless, when confronted with these situations, physicians should consider the perspectives from law and philosophy, since in many cases adoption of these views will lead to better clinical decision-making.

Another reason that clinicians are reluctant to withdraw life-sustaining therapy is their fear of legal liability, both civil and criminal. In this case, however, many clinicians are simply misinformed. In a review by David Orentlicher from the American Medical Association's Council on Judicial and Ethical Affairs, he concludes that "No person has ever been found liable for withdrawing life sustaining treatment without court permission."[53] This is a strong statement, and should be very reassuring to physicians who are concerned about this issue.

On the other hand, physicians often believe that they have no legal liability if they refuse to terminate life-sustaining treatments at the request of a patient or family, as long as they always act to preserve life. This is also a serious misconception. Orentlicher notes that "The risk of liability may be significant" when a physician refuses to honor a request to have life-sustaining treatment withdrawn."[53] He cites 2 successful suits against physicians who refused to withdraw care at the request of a patient or surrogate. In other words, the commonly held view among physicians that they may be at legal risk if they withdraw life-support but are legally immune if they always act to prolong life can be seen to be exactly backwards!

Sedatives and Analgesics in the Care of the Dying

Unfortunately, physicians who care for patients in a pediatric intensive care unit will frequently be called upon to discontinue life-support from a dying patient. In these often tragic circumstances, the question then becomes how best to manage the patient during the dying process. Some erroneously believe that no sedatives or analgesics should be given in these situations, since they believe that it is important both ethically and legally that the patient die from his underlying disease, without any contribution from the respiratory or cardiac depression that are frequent side-effects of these medications.

This reluctance of many physicians to aggressively treat the pain and suffering often experienced by the terminally ill has been one of the most powerful forces driving the movement in favor of euthanasia and physician-assisted suicide over the last several years [55–57]. Individuals who have watched loved ones die without adequate pain relief have spearheaded this movement with the belief that patients should have the opportunity to commit suicide if their suffering is unbearable, particularly since physicians seem unwilling to do whatever is necessary to control that suffering. This is unfortunate, particularly since there is nothing in the law, ethics, or any of the major religious traditions that should preclude physicians from aggressively treating the pain and suffering of the terminally ill, even when such treatment may hasten a patient's demise. Nevertheless, a recent survey showed that as many as 40% of doctors and nurses give inadequate pain medication most often out of fear of hastening a patient's death [50].

The ethical principle that is relevant to this question is the Doctrine of Double Effect, originally developed within the Catholic tradition but now widely acknowledged in other religious traditions as well as in law and philosophy [8]. The doctrine states that when an action has two effects, one of which is inherently good and the other of which is inherently bad, it can be justified if certain conditions are met. For example, the administration of morphine to a dying patient has both a good effect (relief of pain and suffering) and the potential for a bad effect (hastening the patient's death through respiratory depression). The conditions which must be satisfied in order for the action to be justified are:

1) *The action in itself must be good or at least morally indifferent.* (Administration of the morphine itself is morally indifferent)
2) *The agent must intend only the good effect and not the evil effect. The evil effect is foreseen, not intended. It is allowed, not sought.* (In the case of administering morphine to a terminally ill patient, the physician must intend only the relief of the patient's pain and suffering. Respiratory depression and the potential for an earlier death is a foreseen complication, but is not sought.)

3) *The evil effect cannot be a means to the good effect.* (If the physician administers a bolus of potassium chloride instead of morphine, this condition would be violated. By administering potassium chloride, the evil effect (death) becomes the means to the good effect (relief from suffering). By contrast, morphine does not depend upon the side effect of death in order to effectively relieve pain.)
4) *The good intended must outweigh the evil permitted.* (In the case of an imminently dying patient, the benefit of pain relief clearly outweighs the risk of death. This would not be true if the patient were not terminally ill. For example, if an otherwise healthy patient required so much morphine for pain control that he developed serious respiratory depression, he should be placed on a ventilator, not allowed to die.)

In summary, despite the beliefs of many clinicians, there are no moral, legal, or religious reasons for withholding adequate pain relief from dying patients. Pain and suffering should always be adequately treated, even if the treatment results in a foreseen but unintended hastening of death.

What is the difference between currently accepted practice and the performance of euthanasia? The key difference lies in the *intention* of the physician. As long as the physician's intention is treatment of the patient's pain and suffering, the administration of analgesics and sedatives is noncontroversial. When the physician's intention is to kill the patient, then the line between accepted practice and euthanasia has been crossed. This distinction is observed within the law as well as within ethics. Physicians should be reassured that as long as they act with the intention of relieving a patient's pain and suffering, the risk of legal liability is exceedingly small. In a recent review by Larry Gostin, then the Executive Director of the American Society of Law and Medicine, he wrote that "In a search of reported decisions, *no case* was found in which a health care professional was convicted of causing, inducing, or assisting in the death of her patient" [58].

Medical Nutrition and Hydration

Should techniques for providing medical nutrition and hydration (IV fluids, parenteral nutrition, tube feedings, etc.) be considered medical treatments? If so, can they then be ethically withdrawn by the same process and criteria that are used for other types of medical treatment? In other words, if it is ethically acceptable to withdraw a ventilator from a terminally ill patient, is it also ethically acceptable to withdraw medically provided nutrition and hydration? (Note that this question does not propose withholding oral feedings from patients who want to eat or drink.)

The last decade has seen a gradually emerging consensus in both law and ethics that answers the questions posed above in the affirmative [59, 60]. A large number of court decisions, including the decision of the US Supreme Court in *Cruzan*, have now concluded that medically provided nutrition and hydration should be considered medical treatments, and that patients or their surrogates should have the right to refuse them [45,53,54]. The decision of whether or not to administer this therapy should be based upon the same criteria outlined above for other treatments, that is, an analysis of the balance between the benefits and burdens of providing the therapy.

Many clinicians have been reluctant to accept this approach, at least in part because "feeding" seems to be such a basic and fundamental aspect of the care they provide to their patients. In the terminology of the distinction discussed above, it seems so "ordinary". This provides yet another example of the inadequacies of the ordinary/extraordinary distinction, however, since for certain patients, particularly those who are permanently unconscious or imminently dying, medically administered feedings can no longer provide any benefit.

Pediatricians have been particularly slow to acknowledge this emerging consensus [61]. The reasons for this reluctance are several. First, prognoses are often more uncertain in children, given their remarkable ability to recover from injury. Second, even normal newborns need assistance with feedings, so pediatricians are less likely to see artificial feedings as a "medical" treatment. Third, whereas the hospice experience shows that refusal of food and water is frequently seen in elderly patients dying a natural death, the death of a child is never a "natural" event, and there is a reluctance to accept it with apparent passivity. Nevertheless, the principles that have evolved governing the administration or withdrawal of medically provided feedings in adults are equally applicable in children, and there is no justifiable reason to treat the pediatric population any differently.

How are Decisions Made?

Relatively little is known about the manner, reasons, and circumstances under which life support is withheld or withdrawn in the intensive care unit. Much of what is known comes from observational studies or surveys of practices. Despite the wide agreement on the principles discussed above, many studies have noted considerable variation in the practices of critical care physicians [62–66]. Faber-Langendoen noted that among 308 randomly selected intensivists responding to a survey, 15% almost never withdrew ventilators from patients [67]. Asch found that among adult intensivists responding to survey, 34% reported continuing life-sustaining treatment despite patient or surrogate wishes that it be discontinued, while approximately 80% admitted to unilaterally withholding or withdrawing life-sustaining treatment they judged to be futile [68].

Descriptive studies of the practices of pediatric intensivists are also limited. Levetown and colleagues reported that 38% of all deaths in 16 PICUs had some form of limitation of life-sustaining treatment [69]. Among those patients with some "restriction" in medical care, the precipitating event was most often an acute illness, and the most common justification for the restriction was the imminent death of the patient (not poor quality of life or excessive burden).

Ryan and colleagues examined the modes of death in a neonatal and pediatric intensive care unit in Alberta, Canada and found that the majority of deaths in both units occurred either as a result of withdrawal of treatment or after a no-CPR decision [70].

Finally, a recent study by Cook et al found that while ICU health care workers identified common factors important to decision making in withdrawing care (likelihood of long-term survival, premorbid cognitive function, and age of the patient), there was extreme variability in the level of care that was chosen for various patient scenarios [71]. This study suggests that ICU providers demonstrate wide variability in values and belief systems in how they approach such decisions.

Breaking Bad News

Doctors receive limited training in learning to talk easily with patients. The difficulties of physicians' problems with communication are especially exposed when dealing with critically ill patients and their families. Studies show that patients, their families, nurses, social workers and chaplains often complain of the brevity and poor choice of words doctors use in these settings [72–74].

Obviously, patients and their families will react differently to bad news depending on their preparedness, culture, and coping skills. There are several strategies, however, that may prove helpful for the pediatric intensivist:

1) Prepare in advance. Know who will be in the meeting and their relationship to the patient before entering the room. Anticipate questions and prepare answers that will be clear, direct and understandable from the families viewpoint.
2) Have everyone be seated. Studies show that families like to be seated near the door when receiving bad news so as to reduce the feeling of being trapped. Do not stand during the conversation. Families find this particularly offensive and studies show that people consistently think the doctor spent less time with them when the physician was standing during the conversation. Introduce yourself and all your colleagues by title and name. Although many families cannot remember anyone's name after hearing tragic news, they appreciate the personal connection the formal introduction establishes.
3) Avoid jargon. Doctors and nurses easily slip into the jargon associated with the intensive care culture, but these loose terms only confuse families or lead to misconceptions that can be difficult to retract.
4) Show caring. Although most physicians believe they really care, families consistently believe the opposite after these events. Many want to hear an expression of sorrow by the healthcare team as an affirmation of their grief. They also wish time to talk and express their feelings.
5) Avoid distractions. As far as possible, make a real effort to establish a therapeutic environment for the sensitive information to be shared. Leave the beeper outside the room, position someone near the door to avoid interrup-

tions, ensure follow-up both immediately and in the days and weeks thereafter with appropriate counselors [75–79].

These are important issues; and physicians, especially critical care physicians, need to spend as much time mastering these skills as they do some of the more technical aspects of the practice. The damage borne by families when this is done poorly can last a lifetime.

This manuscript was derived with permission from the Textbook of Pediatric Intensive Care – Third Edition – Williams & Wilkins Publisher.

References

1. The Nuremberg Code, in Beauchamp TL, Walters L (eds): Contemporary Issues in Bioethics. Belmont, California, Wadsworth Publishing Company; 1989:420.
2. World Medical Association: Declaration of Helsinki, in Beauchamp TL, Walters L (eds): Contemporary Issues in Bioethics. Belmont, California, Wadsworth Publishing Company; 1989:421–423.
3. Alexander S. They decide who lives, who dies, in Hunt R, Arras J (eds): Ethical Issues in Modern Medicine. Palo Alto, California, Mayfield; 1977:409–424.
4. Iglehart JK (1993) The American health care system. The End Stage Renal Disease Program [see comments]. N Engl J Med 328:366–371.
5. Duff RS, Campbell AG (1973) Moral and ethical dilemmas in the special-care nursery. N Engl J Med 289:890–894.
6. Mill and Utilitarian Theories, in Beauchamp TL (ed): Philosophical Ethics: An Introduction to Moral Philosophy. New York, McGraw-Hill, Inc. 1991:127–168.
7. Kant and Deontological Theories, in Beauchamp TL (ed): Philosophical Ethics: An Introduction to Moral Philosophy. New York, McGraw-Hill, Inc. 1991:169–208.
8. Beauchamp TL, Childress JF: Principles of Biomedical Ethics, New York, Oxford University Press; 1994.
9. Jonsen AR, Toulmin S: The Abuse of Casuistry, University of California Press, Los Angeles, 1988.
10. Toulmin S (1981) The tyranny of principles. Hastings Cent Rep 11:31–39.
11. Lantos JD (1987) Baby Doe five years later. Implications for child health. N Engl J Med 317:444–447.
12. Carse AL (1991) The "voice of care": Implications for bioethical education. J Med Philos 16:5–28.
13. Coles R: The call of stories: Teaching and the moral imagination, Boston, Houghton Mifflin; 1989.
14. Katz J: The Silent World of Doctor and Patient, New York, Free Press; 1984.
15. Faden RR, Beauchamp TL: A History and Theory of Informed Consent, New York, Oxford University Press; 1986.
16. Novack DH et al. (1979) Changes in physician's attitudes toward telling the cancer patient. JAMA 241:897.
17. Annas GJ (1994) Informed consent, cancer, and truth in prognosis. N Engl J Med 330:223–225.
18. Abramson NS (1981) Meisel A, Safar P. Informed consent in resuscitation research. JAMA 246:2828–2830.
19. Orlowski JP, Kanoti GA, Mehlman MJ (1988) The ethics of using newly dead patients for teaching and practicing intubation techniques. N Engl J Med 319:439–441.
20. Burns JP, Reardon FE, Truog RD (1994) Using newly deceased patients to teach resuscitation procedures. N Engl J Med 331:1652–1655.

21. Gutheil TG, Bursztajn H, Brodsky A (1984) Malpractice prevention through the sharing of uncertainty. Informed consent and the therapeutic alliance. N Engl J Med 311:49–51.
22. President's Commission for the Study of Ethical Problems in Medicine and Biomedical and Behavioral Research: Deciding to Forego Life-Sustaining Treatment: Ethical, Medical, and Legal Issues in Treatment Decisions, Washington, D.C. U.S. Government Printing Office; 1983:121.
23. Emanuel LL, Emanuel EJ (1989) The Medical Directive. A new comprehensive advance care document [see comments]. JAMA 261:3288–3293.
24. Brett AS (1991) Limitations of listing specific medical interventions in advance directives. JAMA 266:825–828.
25. La Puma J, Orentlicher D, Moss RJ (1991) Advance directives on admission. Clinical implications and analysis of the Patient Self-Determination Act of 1990 [Review]. JAMA 266:402–405.
26. Steinbrook R, Lo B (1984) Decision making for incompetent patients by designated proxy. California's new law. N Engl J Med 310:1598–1601.
27. Buchanan AE, Brock DW: Deciding for Others: The Ethics of Surrogate Decision Making, Cambridge, Cambridge University Press; 1989.
28. Holder AR: Legal Issues in Pediatrics and Adolescent Medicine, New Haven, Yale University Press; 1985.
29. Fleischman AR, Nolan K, Dubler NN, et al. (1994) Caring for gravely ill children. Pediatrics 94:433–439.
30. Newark v. Williams. 588 A.2d. 1108 (Del.1991).
31. Holder AR (1987) Minors' rights to consent to medical care. JAMA 257:3400–3402.
32. Sigman GS, O'Connor C (1991) Exploration for physicians of the mature minor doctrine. J Pediatr 119:520–525.
33. Prince v. Commonwealth of Massachusetts. 321 U.S. 158 (1944).
34. Hippocrates: Art, in Reiser SJ, Dyck AJ, Curran WJ (eds): Ethics in Medicine: Historical Perspectives and Contemporary Concerns. Cambridge, MA, MIT Press; 1977:6.
35. Rabkin MT, Gillerman G, Rice NR (1976) Orders not to resuscitate. N Engl J Med 295:364–366.
36. Optimum care for hopelessly ill patients. A report of the Clinical Care Committee of the Massachusetts General Hospital. N Engl J Med. 1976;295:362–364.
37. Mittelberger JA, Lo B, Martin D, Uhlmann RF (1993) Impact of a procedure-specific do not resuscitate order form on documentation of do not resuscitate orders. Arch Intern Med 153:228–232.
38. Murphy DJ, Finucane TE (1993) New do-not-resuscitate policies: A first step in cost control. Arch Intern Med 153:1641–1648.
39. Snider GL (1991) The do-not-resuscitate order: Ethical and legal imperative or medical decision. Am Rev Respir Dis 143:665–674.
40. Hackler JC, Hiller FC (1990) Family consent to orders not to resuscitate: reconsidering hospital policy. JAMA 264:1281–1283.
41. Tomlinson T, Brody H (1990) Futility and the ethics of resuscitation. JAMA 264:1276–1280.
42. Blackhall LJ (1987) Must we always use CPR? N Engl J Med 317:1281–1285.
43. McClung JA, Kamer RS (1990) Legislating ethics: Implications of New York's do-not-resuscitate law. N Engl J Med 323:270–272.
44. Waisel DB, Truog RD (1995) The cardiopulmonary resuscitation-not-indicated order: Futility revisited. Ann Intern Med 122:304–308.
45. Annas GJ (1990) Nancy Cruzan and the right to die. N Engl J Med 323:670–673.
46. Orentlicher D (1990) The right to die after Cruzan. JAMA 264:2444–2446.
47. Council on Ethical and Judicial Affairs; American Medical Association. Decisions near the end of life. JAMA. 1992;267:2229–2233.
48. Society of Critical Care Medicine Ethics Committee. Consensus report on the ethics of foregoing life-sustaining treatments in the critically ill. Crit Care Med. 1990;18:1435–1439.

49. American Thoracic Society. Withholding and withdrawing life-sustaining therapy. Ann Intern Med. 1991;115:478–485.
50. Solomon MZ, O'Donnell L, Jennings B, et al. (1993) Decisions near the end of life: professional views on life-sustaining treatments. Am J Public Health 83:14–23.
51. Shaw A, Randolph JG, Manard B (1977) Ethical issues in pediatric surgery: a national survey of pediatricians and pediatric surgeons. Pediatrics 60:588–599.
52. Caralis PV, Hammond JS (1992) Attitudes of medical students, housestaff, and faculty physicians toward euthanasia and termination of life-sustaining treatment. Crit Care Med 20:683–690.
53. Orentlicher D (1989) From the Office of the General Counsel. Cruzan v Director of Missouri Department of Health: an ethical and legal perspective. JAMA 262:2928–2930.
54. Bioethicists' statement on the U.S. Supreme Court's Cruzan decision. N Engl J Med. 1990;323:686–687.
55. Angell M (1982) The quality of mercy. N Engl J Med 306:98–99.
56. Foley KM (1991) The relationship of pain and symptom management to patient requests for physician-assisted suicide. J Pain Symptom Manage 6:289–297.
57. Truog RD, Berde CB (1993) Pain, euthanasia, and anesthesiologists. Anesthesiology 78:353–360.
58. Gostin LO (1993) Drawing a line between killing and letting die: The law, and law reform, on medically assisted dying. Journal of Law, Medicine, and Ethics 21:94–101.
59. McCann RM, Hall WJ, Groth-Juncker A (1994) Comfort care for terminally ill patients: The appropriate use of nutrition and hydration. JAMA 272:1263–1266.
60. Lynn J, ed. By No Extraordinary Means: The Choice to Forgo Life-Sustaining Food and Water. Bloomington, Indiana University Press; 1989.
61. Frader J: Forgoing life-sustaining food and water: Newborns, in Lynn J (ed): By No Extraordinary Means: The Choice to Forgo Life-Sustaining Food and Water. Bloomington, Indiana University Press; 1989:180–185.
62. Smedira NG, Evans BH, Grais LS, et al. (1990) Withholding and withdrawal of life support from the critically ill. N Engl J Med 322:309–315.
63. Wilson WC, Smedira NG, Fink C, McDowell JA, Luce JM (1992) Ordering and administration of sedatives and analgesics during the withholding and withdrawal of life support from critically ill patients. JAMA 267:949–953.
64. Lee DKP, Swinburne AJ, Fedullo AJ, Wahl GW (1994) Withdrawing care: Experience in a medical intensive care unit. JAMA 271:1358–1361.
65. Jayes RL, Zimmerman JE, Wagner DP, et al. (1993) Do-not-resuscitate orders in intensive care units: Current practices and recent changes. JAMA 270:2213–2217.
66. Christakis NA, Asch DA (1993) Biases in how physicians choose to withdraw life support. Lancet 342:642–646.
67. Faber Langendoen K (1994) The clinical management of dying patients receiving mechanical ventilation: A survey of physician practice. Chest 106:880–888.
68. Asch DA, Hansen-Flaschen J, Lanken PN (1995) Decisions to limit or continue life-sustaining treatment by critical care physicians in the United States: conflicts between physicians' practices and patients' wishes. American Journal of Respiratory & Critical Care Medicine 151:288–292.
69. Levetown M, Pollack MM, Cuerdon TT et al. (1994) Limitations and withdrawals of medical intervention in pediatric critical care. JAMA 272:1271–1275.
70. Ryan CA, Byrne P, Kuhn S, Tyebkhan J (1993) No resuscitation and withdrawal of therapy in a neonatal and a pediatric intensive care unit in Canada. J Pediatr 123:534–538.
71. Cook DJ, Guyatt GH, Jaeschke R, et al. (1995) Determinants in Canadian health care workers of the decision to withdraw life support from the critically ill. Canadian Critical Care Trials Group. JAMA 273:703–708.
72. Cassileth BR, Zupkis RV, Sutton-Smith K et al. (1980) Information and participation preferences among cancer patients. Ann Intern Med 92:832–836.
73. Greenberg LW, Jewett LS, Gluck RS, et al. (1984) Giving information for a life-threatening diagnosis. Parents' and oncologists' perceptions. American Journal of Diseases of Children 138:649–653.

74. Tolle SW, Elliot DL, Hickam DH (1984) Physician attitudes and practices at the time of patient death. Arch Intern Med 144:2389–2391.
75. Sharp MC, Strauss RP, Lorch SC (1992) Communicating medical bad news: parents' experiences and preferences. J Pediatr 121:539–546.
76. Krahn GL, Hallum A, Kime C (1993) Are there good ways to give 'bad news'? Pediatrics 91:578–582.
77. Campbell ML (1994) Breaking bad news to patients. JAMA 271:1052.
78. Quill TE, Townsend P (1991) Bad news: delivery, dialogue, and dilemmas. Arch Intern Med 151:463–468.
79. Lindemann E (1994) Symptomatology and management of acute grief. 1944 [classical article]. American Journal of Psychiatry 151:155–160.

'Good' Medicine: Ethics and Pediatric Critical Care

F. A. Carnevale

Introduction

In a recent study of 16 pediatric intensive care units (PICU), in the United States, Levetown and her associates reported that every unit systematically restricted medical intervention for particular groups of patients [1]. In their examination of 5415 consecutive PICU admissions, the care of 119 patients was restricted; 79% of these patients subsequently died in the PICU. This group of 'restriction' patients that died represented 38% of all deaths in the study settings.

It was clear that these settings did not view 'life- support' as an absolute commitment. Clinicians within these units believed that it was permissible to withdraw life-sustaining treatment under certain circumstances. The most common justification for restricting intervention was, by far, the imminence of death (not quality of life nor the excessive burden of intervention).

Writing a paper on the 'State of the Art' of ethics in pediatric critical care is a difficult task. I find it difficult because there is a considerable controversy over what is 'good' (ie. ethical) medical care. Ethical viewpoints vary significantly across cultures as well as within cultures. Finally, there exist a wide diversity of ways of analyzing ethical problems, making it difficult to engage in a comparative discussion of different approaches to problems.

Therefore, in this attempt to map out the State of the Art of ethics in pediatric critical care, I have organized my paper into two principal sections. In the first section, I will outline some of the prominent controversies surrounding 'theoretical' models for discussing ethics in medicine. This is necessary for establishing a framework for the second section, wherein I will review some of the leading ethical controversies in pediatric critical care practice.

In addressing an international audience, I am particularly conscious of how my discussion may express ideas that are bound in the 'North American medical culture' within which I practice. In particular, this is a culture wherein a scientific, 'biological' model of medicine (biomedicine) is an established and largely accepted system. I recognize that other cultures may value traditional medical systems more highly, and others may concurrently rely on a diversity of 'medicines.' Each culture, in a particular time in its history, will form its own views of health, sickness, and healing that will inescapably shape what would be considered ethical medical practice within that society. For the purposes of this paper, directed to a critical care audience, I am deliberately restricting my discussion of ethics to the biomedical context. As well, I am using the term 'medicine' in a generic sense; intending to address the variety of disciplines that practice within the biomedical framework: physicians, nurses, and technologists, among others.

Theoretical Controversies

It is not uncommon in many medical papers to see a practical problem, such as cessation of treatment, to be discussed as a controversy over conflicting moral duties. Such 'practical' discussions frequently fail to recognize that the duties discussed are themselves a matter of controversy. The duties that are relevant to a bioethical discourse, as well as the reliance on duties itself, is an unsettled controversy in bioethics.

Within the Western traditions, this relates to a fundamental question in moral philosophy (from Socrates to the present) about 'how do we determine what is morally good?' For example, a dominant manner of framing this debate runs like this: Is ethical conduct a matter of the consequences of that action (consequentialism) or is it a matter of fulfilling moral duties regardless of the consequences (deontological)? In turn, these viewpoints have been criticized in favor of other moral frameworks, such as virtue ethics, casuistry, feminist ethics, and hermeneutics (among others).

Within the midst of these philosophical debates, the field of bioethics emerged as an organized professional and academic endeavor within a diversity of disciplines, to analyze ethical problems in modern biomedicine (for further historical background regarding the emergence of bioethics, see [2] and [3]).

Given the controversies over how to frame ethical discourse, bioethics has struggled with establishing a cohesive 'theoretical' framework; many bioethics commentators are speaking from highly divergent (typically unarticulated) philosophical positions.

Principlism (or the principled approach) has emerged as a dominant framework for bioethics in North America [4]. This approach asserts that ethical problems should be analyzed in terms of fundamental moral principles. Beauchamp and Childress [5] are regarded as authors of the most cited model of principlism, sometimes referred to as the four-principles approach. They have argued that ethical medical practice should respect the following moral principles [5]:

(a) respect for autonomy – the practitioner recognizes a person as free and capable of intentional action; a patient is free to choose what is best for him/her;
(b) beneficence – the practitioner has a moral obligation to act for the benefit of others;
(c) nonmaleficence – the practitioner has an obligation not to inflict harm intentionally;

(d) justice – the practitioner recognizes that persons are due benefits or burdens because of their particular properties or circumstances.

The reader may note that a large proportion of bioethics papers interpret ethical problems as a conflict between principles. For example, the euthanasia debate could be framed as a conflict between a respect for the patient's autonomous choice and the physician's duties of beneficence and nonmaleficence. A major problem for principlism has been to deal with how to resolve conflicts between principles (for a thorough critique of principlism see [6] and [7]).

A scanning of the bioethics literature also reveals a significant reliance on legal ideology. Many discourses tend to ultimately refer to law and court judgments as a 'final word' on what is ethically permissible. This is probably reflective of the central status law has attained within many Western societies. This typically shapes ethical discussion in terms of 'rights' and whose rights should prevail. Some critics of this trend have argued that law serves merely as a system for social regulation [8]. Law upholds a minimalist view of ethics, even in the most 'legally-oriented' societies; respecting the law may be necessary in ensuring an absolute minimal standard of ethics – but does not promote a sufficient conception of the full richness of ethics within a society.

So, although principlism and legalism are dominant frameworks within bioethics (and will therefore be used for parts of this paper), they are also problematic and are far from being settled upon as ideal models. It is beyond the scope of this short paper to outline additional controversies within bioethical theory.

Practical Controversies

In this section, I will discuss a number of ethical dilemmas that are relevant to pediatric critical care practice. I will outline the central arguments that have been documented regarding these dilemmas and offer my own analytic comments.

Who Decides?

Before moving into a discussion of what practices are ethically acceptable, we need to determine who (ultimately) decides what is 'good.' The American Academy of Pediatrics (AAP) Committee on Bioethics recently published guidelines on forgoing life-sustaining treatment in children [9]. These guidelines clearly recognize that the authority over treatment decisions rests ultimately with 'competent' patients, or with their surrogates when the patient is 'incompetent.'

This is congruent with the quasi-absolute status of self-determination (freedom to choose what can be done to one's person/body) in many Western na-tions [5]. Court rulings have consistently recognized a (competent) person's right to refuse treatment (including a Jehovah's Witness right to refuse a blood transfusion), regardless of the outcome for the patient. In many settings, the deployment of interventions against the competent patient's will, is liable for battery.

This viewpoint involves an elaboration of the 'respect for the autonomy of persons' principle described above. Many Western societies have developed a doctrine of 'informed consent' in order to operationalize this moral principle into a practical form [10]. The practice of informed consent involves a recognition that a person (patient) is self-governing, and chooses what is to be done to him/her. Informed consent consists of a free and informed choice. This obliges practitioners to provide patients with all information (full disclosure) that is relevant to making decisions and refrain from applying any coercion toward particular choices. Informed consent has become legally obligatory in most North European and North American countries – societies that have particularly embraced individualism as a moral ideal.

Indeed, many of these countries have extended this doctrine toward children, "the gravity of decisions about life-sustaining medical treatment requires careful, explicit attention to the wishes and feelings of the children, regardless of the legal status of the patients" [9, p.535]. Conscious and alert children have been recognized as self-governing, in some legal doctrine, through the notions of mature minor (typically above the age of 14 years) or emancipated minor [9, p.535]. These children are required to consent to treatment and are entitled to refuse treatment, on whatever personal grounds they choose.

Finally, a child may be judged to be incompetent or incapable of medical treatment decisions on the grounds of relevant 'mental dysfunction' or non-fulfillment of the local legal definition of maturity. In these cases, decisions are made by a surrogate, typically the child's parents. As with adult patients, in societies that have adopted this practice of informed consent, the surrogate is required to infer from the patient's previously expressed preferences and choose as the patient would have chosen (substituted judgment standard); or, when such preferences are unknown (eg. infants) the surrogate is required to choose on the basis of the child's best interests (best interests standard).

Informed consent has emerged, in part, to counter potential domination of vulnerable patients, by physicians as well as other agents. There is much that is admirable in the aims of this doctrine to ensure a respect of (sick) persons. Yet, the practice of informed consent encounters some difficulties in the clinical context.

First, surrogate decision-making (which is necessarily prevalent in pediatric settings) is highly problematic within the framework described above. Deciding for previously competent patients, on the basis of what the patient would have chosen (substituted judgment), has questionable validity. Several empirical studies comparing patient preferences with surrogate 'guesses' have reported high rates of disagreement, wherein the latter tend to favor more treatment than patients would have preferred [11, 12]. As well, physician estimates of their patients' preferences were not more predictive than flipping a coin [12].

Therefore, the practice of substituted judgment may not be fulfilling the respect for patient autonomy it is premised upon.

The capacity of surrogates to make decisions that are primarily in the patient's best interests also needs to be examined. First, it is difficult to determine what the sick child's interests are: how do we then determine if treatments are 'good' for a child. Robert Veatch [13] has argued that the interests of the incompetent patient should be judged on the basis of the proportionality of the benefits in relation to the burdens of an intervention; this is a view that is highly supported [9].

However, how do we judge the benefits and burdens? How much benefit (of which kind) is good enough? How much burden (of which kind) is too much? The decision makers are caught with a struggle to resolve these questions. This is further complicated by altered states of consciousness [14] and in children in a persistent-vegetative-state [15]: how do these states affect the construal of benefit and burden?

One element of burdens that has received particular attention is suffering. Eric Casell has argued that biomedicine needs to deepen the way suffering is conceived [16]. There has been a tendency to equate suffering with pain. Whereas pain is typically viewed as a psychophysiological phenomenon, associated with nociception, that can usually be minimized with analgesics, suffering is a complex 'existential' phenomenon that is not directly related to nociception and not necessarily relieved with analgesics [17]. The suffering experience of children is a particularly abstract phenomenon to work with [18].

A second difficulty with surrogate decision making is: can a parent truly choose what is best for a child, without significant implication of the parent's interests? [19, 20] Indeed, some anthropology work has suggested that, even in the (individualistic) West, persons are socially interdependent – persons view themselves in interconnection with others [21].

Third, are the interests of others necessarily secondary to those of the patient? Practitioners working within the informed consent tradition would have great difficulty disregarding the interests of the family, when these may conflict with what appears to be best for the patient [22]. Along the same line, many elderly persons state that they would refuse heroic measures that may cause them to become a burden to their family.

Deciding in the patient's best interests seems pragmatically dubious and perhaps morally limited (although it may be the 'best' model available for now). A framework for reconciling the interests of others with those of the incompetent patient will need to be developed.

Empirical studies of informed consent suggest this process involves therapeutic phenomena beyond a legal respect for the person's autonomy. In her examination of physician disclosure of breast biopsy results, Kathryn Taylor [23] has reported that physicians structured the process in a way that made 'the news' most bearable for patients. The physician's work was more complex than simply providing information to enable the patient to make 'free' decisions. Rather, the physicians also tried to help their patients adjust to the implications of the biopsy.

In their study of informed consent among Aboriginal (Native) Canadians, Kaufert and O'Neil reported that practitioners and Natives conceived the nature of the encounter in very different ways. Whereas the physicians were trying to establish a contractual agreement, Natives were preoccupied with establishing trusting relationships [24].

Cross-cultural studies of medical disclosure and consent reveal that these practices are very much related to broader social and cultural factors. Gordon has reported that nondisclosure of cancer diagnoses was prevalent in a North Italian setting [25]. At first glance this seems simply unethical; a blatant example of medical paternalism. However, this study relates nondisclosure to a protection of the patient in a society wherein cancer is strongly associated with death and hopelessness; protection of the patient from a social condemnation.

In Japan, it is widely held among medical practitioners that a grave diagnosis should be withheld from a patient. The former argue that it is their burden to deal with this difficult information and that it would be disrespectful to subject a patient to a pessimistic view of their future. On the other hand, the benevolence of this view has been challenged in terms of the power imbalance it maintains between patients and practitioners [26].

Thus, the doctrine of informed consent is not universally practiced. As a moral ideal, it is intertwined with how a society regards a patient: on one end of a continuum, as a free, autonomous agent versus, on the other end, as an afflicted, dependent requiring beneficent protection. The (cross-cultural) empirical studies I have cited suggest that this dilemma is a fundamental tension in the physician-patient relationship.

Whereas my discussion in this section has examined some central controversies within clinical bioethics, I will now review specific problems that are prevalent in pediatric critical care.

Withholding and Withdrawal of Treatment

It is widely held within bioethics that a medical intervention is ethical if the patient has consented (freely) to it or, where this is not possible, a recognized surrogate has judged the treatment to be in the patient's best interests [4, 5, 10, 13]. Therefore, it can be ethically permissible to withhold or withdraw an intervention if a competent patient or surrogate refuses such intervention – regardless of the outcome [9]. The following sections will examine some particular controversies in this area.

Medical Futility

Recent discussions of life-support interventions in the medical and bioethical literature have increasingly involved the notion of 'medical futility' in arguments that assert: If life support is determined to be futile for a certain population, then it should not be offered, saving needless suffering and costs [27, 28]. Although this has a surface appeal, this argument is highly problematic when examined more closely [29, 30, 31].

I performed a Medline database search on the keyword 'futility,' from 1965 to 1994. I discovered two group of reports. The first group refers to the futility of very specific interventions that do not involve life-support. These relate directly to efficacy, "does a technique do what it is expected to do?" For example, one title was "All vulvar lesions should be biopsied. Basal cell carcinoma – an example of the futility of diagnosis by gross appearance." Another was, "Fiber implantation for pattern baldness." The abstract stated, "Examination of 20 patients who had fiber implantation for the treatment of pattern baldness showed that nearly all of the fibers had fallen out by ten weeks." One to ten such publications were reported each year. A second set of reports discussed the futility of life-supports. There were no such papers prior to 1985. Following one paper in each of 1985 and 1986, there was a veritable explosion in the number of articles published on this topic from 1988 onward (3 in 1988, 1 in 1989, 9 in 1990, 5 in 1991, 26 in 1992, 38 in 1993, and 34 in 1994). Given that life-support technology has been in practice since the 1960s, why are published discussions of futility arising now?

This pattern could be interpreted in a number of ways. First, can the rise in the popularity of futility arguments be related to a rise in cost constraints (indeed a number of reports focused on cost-savings realized by withholding life supports from some 'high-risk' groups)?

Second, the rise in futility arguments may be related to the rise in patient self-determination initiatives (policies and laws that enhance the authority of patients in decision-making). For example, one law that received a great deal of attention was a 1987 New York State statute requiring patient (or surrogate) consent for the withholding of resuscitation (1987 is remarkably close to the 1988 emergence of futility publications). Regardless of how the futility debate gained prominence, a final observation addresses how the term 'futility' is used. The life-support futility literature discusses whether or not it is appropriate for physicians to 'declare' an intervention futile and then unilaterally withhold/withdraw it. A striking problem in this debate on futility is that there is little explicit discussion of the desired utility and clearly no agreed upon outcome against which to evaluate life-supports: eg. short-term survival, intermediate-term survival, long-term survival, survival with no/mild/moderate/severe disabilities, survival to discharge – different authors have adopted different criteria.

The futility controversy has represented the central problem as a quasi-scientific debate over the prediction of 'good' and 'bad' outcomes, without significantly addressing the more fundamental dilemma: what is a good-enough life?

Determining whether or not an intervention can be withheld by a physician, without patient consent, seems to be more a matter of 'standard of practice' than futility. Many treatments are routinely not offered because they do not conform with current standards of practice. For example, for a newborn delivered at 20 weeks gestation, it is generally accepted as good practice, by the medical community, not to attempt resuscitation. For situations like these, norms of good practice are relatively clear. On the other hand, the types of cases raised as ethical dilemmas involve uncertainties about outcome and treatment efficacy (such as resuscitating a 23-week gestation newborn). The best-interests standard for decision-making (which I described earlier) seems to offer a pragmatic framework (in spite of its many limits): Is life-support disproportionately burdensome?

Do-Not-Resuscitate (DNR) Orders

In a survey of 300 deaths in a PICU, a DNR order was the 'mode' of death in 26% of these [32]. In a study of 17,440 ICU admissions in 40 American hospitals, Jayes and associates [33] found that physicians wrote DNR orders for 9% of these. They also found that the trend over recent years was toward more frequent and earlier utilization of DNR orders.

Several organizations in the United States recommend that every hospital adopt a DNR policy in order to ensure that such orders are practiced ethically [34, 35]. Such a policy should explicitly distinguish a DNR order from decisions about other aspects of treatment; a frequent confusion surrounding DNR orders is a slide toward diminution of all therapy at times when this was not intended.

A central controversy surrounding DNR orders involves who should make DNR decisions – the patient/surrogate or the physician. I have addressed this debate indirectly in my previous discussion of futility. Boosters of futility argue that resuscitation involves medical judgment of futility whereas critics assert that resuscitation decisions are inescapably about what type of life is worthwhile – decisions that should be within the control of patients/surrogates. The New York State legislation I previously described, which requires consent for a DNR, suggests that (Western) law will likely favor patient choice in countries that have adopted informed consent practices.

Withholding Food and Water

In light of ethical arguments that have supported the withholding of medical treatments, in certain circumstances, some discussion has emerged regarding the status of nutrition and hydration. If medical intervention is withdrawn/withheld from a patient, because they (or a surrogate) have so chosen, would it also be acceptable to withhold food and water, particularly if these are administered by artificial means? Some writers have argued against this on the basis of the special significance of food and water [36] and the risks that this method (which definitively ends life) will systematically become popular as an easy means of terminating the devalued lives of the unproductive of a society [37]. However, the dominant trend in the bioethics literature, and in court decisions in the United States and United Kingdom, regards artificial feeding as a medical intervention [13]. Therefore, it is argued that artificial feeding can be withheld in the same manner as other treatments [38].

Euthanasia

The preceding discussion on withholding and withdrawing life-sustaining therapy refers to measures (sometimes) referred to as passive euthanasia. With a growing recognition of the permissibility of these practices, there has been a tendency to no longer refer to this as euthanasia. Euthanasia has come to refer, more particularly, to assisted-suicide.

The Netherlands are well known for their open practice of voluntary euthanasia. Although this is technically a crime (according to legal statutes), Dutch legal jurisprudence has accepted the practice of euthanasia as long as the conditions of voluntariness, unbearable suffering, and consultation are respected [39].

In 1995, the Northern Territory in Australia became the first state in the world to legalize voluntary euthanasia [40]. In the American state of Oregon, the public supported a physician-assisted-suicide reform through a referendum. However, this has not been implemented (at the time this paper was written) because its constitutionality is being challenged [40]. On the other hand, remaining countries that have a legal position on euthanasia (through statute law and case jurisprudence) have regarded (and charged) physician-assisted-suicide as a criminal offence. Finally, no state has legally recognized involuntary euthanasia.

Euthanasia remains one of the most intensely contested issues in bioethics. Physician-assisted-suicide has significant support in countries that strongly recognize self-determination. Respect for autonomy and the relief of suffering are argued to outweigh the sanctity of human life. This has consequently excluded (incompetent) children from the debate.

On the other hand, critics have argued that it is wrong to mandate physicians, whom societies have traditionally trusted to save life, to practice the purposeful shortening of life [41]. It has also been asserted that legal permissibility of voluntary euthanasia in the Netherlands, has resulted in a wide unreported practice of involuntary euthanasia [42]. This raises concerns that the undervalued members of a society will be systematically eliminated. The acceptance of euthanasia has also been criticized by some palliative care societies [43]. The latter have argued that the call for assisted-suicide is rooted in the way modern biomedicine has shaped end-stage illness into an experience of alienation, suffering, and indignity. The acceptance of euthanasia prevents significant (and attainable) reform in the care of the terminally ill and dying.

Brain Death and Organ Transplantation

Although organ transplantation is highly practiced, there is significant controversy about the criteria for declaring death prior to organ procurement. The most widely reported criteria for declaring a person dead and a candidate for organ donation are variations of the Harvard criteria for determining irreversible coma [44]; commonly referred to as brain death (or whole-brain death).

Some critics of whole-brain death criteria have argued that neo-cortical death should be a sufficient condition for declaring brain-death, asserting that the cortex is the seat of conscious and relational life [45]. A variation of this argument has been extended to examine the suitability of anencephalic infants as organ donors [46].

In response to an insufficient supply of organs, one setting in the United States has developed a policy wherein non-heart-beating cadavers could be used as organ donors [47]. 'Consenting' patients that are judged terminally ill, and from whom treatments will be withdrawn, are brought to an operating room for removal of life support. When the heart stops beating, the patient is declared dead and organs are subsequently removed. This raises some concerns about the pressures this can exert on the process of discontinuing therapy on the basis of the patient's best interests or 'letting nature take its course.'

Another approach toward increasing the supply of organs, has been the adoption of presumed-consent legislation by some countries [48]. This approach raises some concern about the autonomy of persons that are not aware of such local legislation. For over two decades many societies have recognized brain death as an acceptable definition of the end of life (through law or accepted standards of medical practice). On the other hand, this has been a matter of significant controversy in other countries. For example, Denmark was one of the 'latest' Western countries to legally recognize brain death as the end of life, in 1990, following significant public debate. The Danish Council of Ethics, established by the Danish parliament, had asserted that a public consensus was required in order to redefine death [48, 49].

In Japan, brain death has been highly controversial. Although the Japanese legislature adopted a bill in 1992 which permits the recognition of death on the basis of brain death criteria [50], no heart transplants have been subsequently performed. Indeed, as a result of an ongoing debate over how to define death, only one heart transplant has ever been performed (in 1968) in Japan (although opinion polls suggest a rising support for a recognition of brain death and transplantation [51]). The Japanese 'resistance' to brain death has been extensively analyzed and may be attributable to: (a) the Japanese conception of human life is not as centered on the brain, as it is in Western societies [26]; (b) traditions that value 'the natural' [26]; (c) the complex significance of gift-exchange within Japanese culture [51]; or (d) distrust toward the medical profession in a society where informed consent is not practiced (the physician that performed the only heart transplant in Japanese history was arrested and charged for murder for removing a heart from a person that was not brain dead; he was acquitted six years later) [26, 52].

Concluding Remarks: Medicine, Ethics, and Culture

The brain death controversies that I have outlined highlight that ethics is enmeshed within a culture's way of construing life, 'good' conduct, and who is entrusted to judge these. The acceptance of brain death in many Western countries says as much about their valuation of cerebral life, free choice, trust in biomedicine to save life, a view of the body as a property, and reliance on law to regulate abuses as it says about what is ethical. Indeed, this comment can be extended to the wider range of topics I have discussed in this paper.

Some cross-cultural studies of medical ethics have suggested that ethical practice is shaped by how a culture views life, health, sickness, healing, and healers [53, 54]. In this paper, I have attempted to illustrate this complex cultural dimension of ethics. As we reviewed the various controversies, we uncovered constellations of cultural views and practices that articulate what is 'good' in a particular society at a particular time.

Discussions about ethical dilemmas are by definition controversial - conflicts between moral ideals without an obvious course of resolution. We rarely take time to discuss morals that are largely agreed upon and widely practiced.

Some practitioners are frustrated with the uncertainties and indecision that typically surround bioethical debates. Some of these debates do seem to go on endlessly. Yet, uncertainty is as central to ethics, as conflict is central to law, and certainty is central to science.

Discussions about ethics in biomedicine have arisen as the ideals of scientific medicine have challenged broader moral ideals of human life. What is 'good' medicine should be determined largely on the basis of what a particular society values (in dialogue with international views) about human life - and how this life can be served by medicine.

References

1. Levetown M, Pollack MM, Cuerdon TT, Ruttiman UE, Glover JJ (1994) Limitations and withdrawals of medical intervention in pediatric critical care. Journal of the American Medical Association 272:1271–1275.
2. Fox RC (1994) The entry of U.S. bioethics into the 1990s: A sociological analysis. In: DuBose ER, Hamel RP, O'Connell LJ (eds) A matter of principles? Ferment in US bioethics. Trinity Press International, Valley Forge, Pennsylvania, pp.21–71.
3. Fox RC (1990) The evolution of American bioethics: A sociological perspective. In: Weisz G (ed), Social science perspectives on Medical Ethics. Kluwer Academic, Boston, pp. 201–217.
4. Engelhardt HT (1986) The foundations of bioethics. Oxford University Press, New York.
5. Beauchamp TL, Childress JF (1994) Principles of biomedical ethics, 4th edn. Oxford University Press, New York.
6. DuBose ER, Hamel RP, O'Connell LJ (eds) (1994) A matter of principles? Ferment in US bioethics. Trinity Press International, Valley Forge, Pennsylvania.
7. Kennedy Institute of Ethics Journal: Special issue (1995) Theories and methods in bioethics: Principlism and its critics. Kennedy Institute of Ethics Journal 5:181–286.

8. Schneider CE (1994) Bioethics and the language of the law. Hastings Center Report 24:16–22.
9. American Academy of Pediatrics – Committee on Bioethics (1994) Guidelines on forgoing life-sustaining medical treatment. Pediatrics 93:532–536.
10. Faden RR, Beauchamp TL (1986) A history and theory of informed consent. Oxford University Press, New York.
11. Pearlman RA, Miles SH, Arnold RM (1993) Contributions of empirical research to medical ethics. Theoretical Medicine 14;197–210.
12. Uhlmann RF, Pearlman RA, Cain KC (1988) Ability of physicians and spouses to predict resuscitation preferences of elderly patients. Journal of Gerontology 43:115–121.
13. Veatch RM (1989) Death, dying, and the biological revolution. Yale University Press, New Haven.
14. Gillett G (1990) Consciousness, the brain and what matters. Bioethics 4:181–198.
15. Ashwal S, Cranford R, Bernat JL et al (The Multi-Society Task Force on Persistent Vegetative State) (1994) Medical aspects of the persistant vegetative state. The New England Journal of Medicine 330:1499–1508; & 330:1572–1579.
16. Cassell EJ (1991) The nature of suffering and the goals of medicine. Oxford University Press, New York.
17. Carnevale FA (1991) High technology and humanity in intensive care: finding a balance. Intensive Care Nursing 7: 23–27.
18. Carnevale FA (1995) The experience of critically ill children. L'infirmiere du Quebec 3:21 (abst).
19. Carnevale FA (1995) The experience of families of critically ill children: Family system transitions. Canadian Psychology 36:233 (abst).
20. Carnevale FA (1990) A description of stressors and coping strategies among parents of critically ill children – a preliminary study. Intensive Care Nursing 6:4–11.
21. Spiro ME (1993) Is the Western conception of the self 'peculiar' within the context of the world cultures? Ethos 21:107–153.
22. Carnevale FA (1995) "I want to help people:" Ethics, nursing, and critical care. Official Journal of the Canadian Association of Critical Care Nurses 6:10–11.
23. Taylor KM (1988) Physicians and the disclosure of undesirable information. In: Lock M, Gordon D (eds) Biomedicine examined. Kluwer Academic Publishers, Dordrecht, 441–463.
24. Kaufert JM, O'Neil JD (1990) Biomedical rituals and informed consent: Native Canadians and the negotiation of clinical trust. In: Weisz G (ed), Social science perspectives on Medical Ethics. Kluwer Academic, Boston, 41–63.
25. Gordon DR (1990) Embodying illness, embodying cancer. Culture, Medicine, and Psychiatry 14:275–297.
26. Lock M (1995) Contesting the natural in Japan: Moral dilemmas and technologies of dying. Culture, Medicine and Psychiatry 19:1–38.
27. Taffet GE, Teasdale TA, Luchi RJ (1988) In-hospital cardiopulmonary resuscitation. Journal of The American Medical Association 260:2069–2072.
28. Murphy DJ (1988) Do-not-resuscitate orders: Time for reappraisal in long-term-care institutions. Journal of The American Medical Association 260:2098–2101.
29. Schiedermayer DL (1988) The decision to forgo CPR in the elderly patient. Journal of The American Medical Association 260:2096–2097.
30. Youngner SJ (1988) Who defines futility? Journal of The American Medical Association 260:2094–2095.
31. Weijer C, Elliott C (1995) Pulling the plug on futility. British Medical Journal 310:683–684.
32. Vernon DD, Dean JM, Timmons OD, Banner W, Allen-Webb EM (1993) Modes of death in the pediatric intensive care unit: Withdrawal and limitation of supportive care. Critical Care Medicine 21:1798–1802.
33. Jayes RL, Zimmerman JE, Wagner DP, Draper EA, Knaus WA (1993) Do-not-resuscitate orders in the intensive care units. Journal of The American Medical Association 270:2213–2217.

34. American Medical Association (1991) Guidelines for the appropriate use of do-not-resuscitate orders. Journal of The American Medical Association 265:1868–1871.
35. American Hospital Association. (1994) Values in conflict: Resolving ethical issues in health care. American Hospital Association, Chicago.
36. Callahan D (1983) On feeding the dying. Hastings Center Report 13:22.
37. Seigler M, Weisbard AJ (1985) Against the emerging stream: Should fluids and nutritional support be discontinued? Archives of Internal Medicine 145:129–131.
38. Lynn J, Childress JF (1983) Must patients always be given food and water? Hastings Center Report 13:17–21.
39. de Wachter MAM (1992) Euthanasia in the Netherlands. Hastings Center Report 22:23–30.
40. Singer P (1995) A report from Australia: The legalisation of voluntary euthanasia in the northern territory. Bioethics 9:419–436.
41. Callahan D (1992) When self-determination runs amok. Hastings Center Report 22:52–55.
42. Capron AM (1992) Euthanasia in the Netherlands: American observations. Hastings Center Report 22:30–33.
43. Moulin DE, Latimer EJ, Macdonald N, et al (1994) Statement on euthanasia and physician-assisted suicide. Journal of Palliative Care 10:80–81.
44. Ad Hoc Committee of the Harvard Medical School (to Examine the Definition of Brain Death) (1968) A definition of irreversible coma. Journal of The American Medical Association 205:85–88.
45. Veatch RM (1993) The impending collapse of the whole-brain definition of death. Hastings Center Report 23:18–24.
46. Walters JW (1991) Anencephalic infants as organ sources. Bioethics 5:326–341.
47. Arnold RM, Youngner SJ (eds) (1993) Ethical, psychosocial, and public policy implications of procuring organs from non-heart-beating cadavers (special issue). Kennedy Institute of Ethics Journal 3:103–278.
48. Teo B (1991) Organs for transplantation: The Singapore experience. Hastings Center Report 21:10–13.
49. Rix BA (1990) The importance of knowledge and trust in the definition of death. Bioethics 4:232–236.
50. Cushman R, Holm S. (1990) Death, democracy and public ethical choice. Bioethics 4:237–252.
51. Hoshino K (1993) Legal status of brain death in Japan: Why many Japanese do not accept 'brain death' as a definition of death. Bioethics 7:234–238.
52. Ohnuki-Tierney E (1994) Brain death and organ transplantation: Cultural bases of medical technology. Current Anthropology 35:233–254.
53. Lock M, Honde C (1990) Reaching consensus about death: Heart transplants and cultural identity in Japan. In: Weisz G (ed) Social science perspectives on medical ethics. Kluwer Academic Publishers, Dordrecht, p.99–119.
54. Fabrega H (1990) An ethnomedical perspective of medical ethics. Journal of Medicine and Philosophy 15:593–625.
55. Fox RC, Swazey JP (1984) Medical morality is not bioethics – Medical ethics in China and the United States. Perspectives in Biology and Medicine 27:336–360.

Pain

Developmental Neurobiology of Pain in Neonatal and Pediatric I.C.U. Patients

K. J. S. Anand

Introduction

The development of biological processes in the pain system occurs mainly during the second and third trimesters of human gestation, although maturational changes continue during the first two years of postnatal life. Following these maturational changes, it is likely that "perception" of pain changes very little, although major changes may occur in:
(a) the emotional aspects of painful experiences,
(b) interpretations of the meaning of pain, and
(c) the repertoire of behavioral and cognitive expressions in response to pain and stress.

Current controversies in the treatment of pain in critically ill neonatal and pediatric patients may be partly rooted in varied interpretations of the definition of pain, and its applicability to the neonate and older infant.

Definition of Pain and its Implications

The current definition of pain states that pain is *"an unpleasant sensory and emotional experience associated with actual or potential tissue damage, or described in terms of such damage"*. This definition further states that *"pain is always subjective. Each individual learns the application of the word through experiences related to injury in early life"* [1].

Widespread acceptance of a definition of pain that focuses on pain perception has led, directly or indirectly, to many recent advances [2, 3]. However, the current definition of pain does not apply to organisms that are incapable of self-report, including newborn and older infants, small children, mentally retarded, comatose, demented, or verbally handicapped patients. Thus, acute distress experienced by infants undergoing tissue injury as a part of routine medical care is often discounted, denied, and undertreated as compared to older children or adults [4, 5]. Underdevelopment of the pain system was traditionally presumed because neonates or non-verbal infants were incapable of describing the subjective experience of pain. By default, it was concluded that these age groups were incapable of pain perception.

Although self-report is a component of the "efferent response" to pain, it must be preceded by its "afferent component" or the actual experience of pain. Feeling pain and reporting pain are related and sequential events, although their congruence cannot be guaranteed for any individual pain experience because of response biases and situational influences. Relationships between feeling pain and reporting pain are highly context-dependent, resulting in major discrepancies between self-report, nonverbal expression, and the manifest evidence of tissue damage [6, 7].

This definition further states that use of the word "pain" needs to be learned through experiences in early life. We submit that the perception of pain (whether associated with tissue damage or not) is an inherent quality of life itself, is expressed in all viable living organisms, and, while subject to influence by life experiences, does not require prior experience in the first instance. As the primary sensation that guards against damage to the organism from its external or internal environment, the experience of pain would not require any prior experience of it. The first experience of tissue injury is painful, in much the same way that touch, smell, vision, or hearing need not be learned in order to occur in the human organism. The interpretation and meaning of these sensations will develop with experience through positive, negative, and contextual associations.

Darwin (1872) argued that those emotions that are most necessary for survival are the first to appear in development and evolution [8]. Signalling hunger and tissue damage would be the most necessary for newborn survival, and therefore would appear earlier than other adaptational behaviors during development. This ontogenetic adaptation also implies that each stage in developmental process is an essential whole (a form of completeness) in itself, rather than a series of successive approximations of the final adult form. This contrasts with the traditional view that developmental traits are primarily precursors of adult characteristics [9]. Basing the existence of pain on the ability of self-report (strictly defined within the capabilities of adult interpretation), would only serve to deny the important biological and behavioral roles for the modality of pain, as well as similar roles for the pain system within the living organism.

The behavioral reactions of newborns and infants on the occasion of a first heelprick or needle injection are strikingly evident to parents and clinicians [10], although this evidence may be denied or misinterpreted. That the neonate's expression of unpleasantness does not fit within the strict definition of pain contributes to the failure to recognize and aggressively treat pain in infancy and early childhood. Conversely, behavioral alterations caused by pain are the infantile forms of self-report and should not be discounted as "surrogate measures" of pain. These specific behaviors depend on the repertoire associated with each developmental stage, and have meaning within the biobehavioral milieu during all epochs of life. The communicational specificity of these biobehavioral response patterns is evident and should reduce the barriers to optimal pain management in infants and young children [11]. Management of pain would then be the consequence of actually recognizing its presence rather than based on compassionate feelings or ethical arguments [5]. Support for these arguments may be obtained from a brief description of the developing pain system, which appears to be functional even in the most premature neonates.

Neurobiology of the Pain System

The neuroanatomy of pain-related pathways may be traced from sensory receptors in the skin to the cerebral cortex and the development of each of these components provides a framework to study the development of the peripheral pain system, the dorsal horn of the spinal cord, and supra-spinal centers (Table 1). Much of these data were obtained from studies in the newborn rat, because of neurobiological similarities between the human and rodent species and because the newborn rat's neurological maturity corresponds to that of the human fetus at 24 weeks gestation. Immature somatosensory mechanisms in the newborn rat or human may account for the poor stimulus-response coupling and imprecise somatic localization noted in both species, although their behavioral and physiologic responses leave no doubt about the noxious character of any experience associated with tissue injury [12].

Table 1. Components of the pain system

Anatomical Division	Primary Components	Presumed Biological Function
The peripheral pain system	High-threshold mechanoceptors, polymodal nociceptors, C-fibres, silent C-fibres, A-d fibres, lymphocytes	Registering the initial noxious stimulus, local pain reactions (vasomotor, inflammatory), conduction to the spinal cord
Dorsal horn of the spinal cord	Dorsal root ganglion cells, substantia gelatinosa, inhibitory interneurons, lamina V neurons, projection neurons, descending inhibitory fibres, ascending pain tracts	Integration of pain and other sensory stimuli, sensory hyperexcitability, or 'windup phenomenon', gate-control mechanisms, modulation of pain, chronic pain mechanisms, sympathetic input
Supra-spinal centers	Raphe magnus, periaqueductal gray, reticular activating system, locus coeruleus, inferior olivary nucleus, paraventricular nucleus & other hypothalamic centers, thalamic nuclei, limbic system: amygdala, hippocampus, cingulate gyrus, insula, post-central gyrus, frontal and parieto-occipital cortex	Integration and processing of painful information, localization and identification of pain characteristics, emotional reactions, matching with memories of pain, cognitive interpretation, arousal and attention, modulation of pain preception, stimulation of the systemic responses to pain

The Peripheral Pain System

Previous histological studies found that the density of nociceptive nerve endings in newborn skin was similar to that of adult skin, whereas recent microneurographic investigations have shown that the neurophysiologic properties of the earliest nociceptors are similar to those of adult skin [13]. Rapid adapting pressure receptors are the first to appear during fetal life, followed by the development of slowly adapting pressure receptors, rapidly adapting mechanoceptors, and occasional muscle afferents. The depolarization responses of these receptors to mechanical injury, chemical irritants, and inflammatory mediators are similar to those of adult receptors well before they establish synaptic connections with neurons in the dorsal horn [14, 15]. Signal transduction mechanisms via linkage to G-protein complexes appear to be mature in these early receptors [16].

Fetal sensory receptors are located on or close to the skin surface soon after development and gradually become sub-epidermal with the development of the stratum corneum. Studies in the 1940s noted reflexes to cutaneous sensory stimulation from the perioral area of the human fetus in the 7th week of gestation; from the rest of the face, palms of the hands and the soles of the feet by the 11th week; from the trunk and proximal parts of arms and legs by the 15th week, and from all cutaneous surfaces by the 20th week [17]. The development of sensory reflexes was somatotopically preceded by synaptogenesis between afferent fibers and sensory neurons in the dorsal horn of the spinal cord [18, 19]. Thicker myelinated fibers are the first to grow into the developing spinal cord and form connections with deeper layers of the dorsal horn, with collaterals to neurons in the substantia gelatinosa. Following the ingrowth of unmyelinated C-fibers and synaptogenesis with superficial dorsal horn neurons, these collaterals undergo a gradual developmental degeneration [20]. It is likely that nociceptive stimuli in during fetal life may be conducted by myelinated A-b and A-d fibers, until the maturation of C-fibre connections in the substantia gelatinosa.

Dorsal Horn of the Spinal Cord

Development of the dorsal horn begins with the closure of the neural canal in the first trimester of pregnancy. Sequential electron microscopic and immunocytochemical studies during the second trimester found that the development of the various neuronal cell types in the dorsal horn, together with their laminar arrangement, interneuronal connections, and the expression of their specific neurotransmitters and receptors begins before 13 weeks gestation and is completed by 30–32 weeks [21]. Initially the receptive fields of dorsal horn neurons are very large with much overlap between the receptive fields of adjacent neurons. As maturation occurs, the receptive fields of individual dorsal horn cells progressively decrease and can be more precisely defined [22].

The transmission of nociceptive impulses through the dorsal horn of the spinal cord is mediated via the release of excitatory neurotransmitters, mainly including substance P, glutamate, calcitonin-gene-related peptide (CGRP), vasoactive intestinal polypeptide (VIP), neuropeptide Y, and somatostatin. Modulation of this nociceptive transmission occurs primarily by the release of met-enkephalin from local interneurons, and norepinephrine, dopamine and serotonin from descending inhibitory axons [3,20,23]. These descending inhibitory axons originate from supra–spinal centers and terminate at all levels of the spinal cord and brainstem that are involved in sensory processing. Of the nociceptive neurotransmitters, substance P, CGRP and somatostatin are expressed in the dorsal horn of 8–10 week-old human fetuses, whereas glutamate, VIP, and neuropeptide Y appear at about 12–16 weeks of human gestation [23]. Modulation of incoming noxious or non-noxious sensory stimuli in extremely premature infants may occur by the local release of met-enkephalin which is first expressed at 12–16 weeks of gestation. Descending inhibitory control from supra-spinal centers develops and matures in the third trimester, with the expression and release of dopamine and norepinephrine. These neurotransmitters are first expressed in late human gestation, followed by the expression of serotonin in the descending inhibitory fibers after birth [24].

Descending inhibitory mechanisms are responsible for modulating the behavioral responses to pain, thus mediating the effects of attention, context-dependence, degree of arousal, behavioral state, and the presence of other sensory stimuli. Selective modulation or enhancement of painful stimuli occurs at various levels in the CNS, and forms the physiologic basis for the Gate-Control theory of Pain. Other phenomena that are dependent on these mechanisms include habituation to non-noxious stimuli, the hypersensitivity and resting joint positions that occur following severe injury or inflammation, the summation of noxious stimuli with close anatomical proximity, and other clinical phenomena associated with pain.

Supra-spinal Centers

Conduction of nociceptive impulses to the supra-spinal centers occurs via the spinothalamic, spinoreticular and spinomesencephalic tracts located mainly in the anterolateral and lateral white matter of the spinal cord. Lack of myelination in these nerve tracts was proposed as an index of immaturity in the neonatal CNS and was used to support the argument that neonates cannot feel pain. However, quantitative neuroanatomical data from the Collaborative Perinatal Project showed that nociceptive nerve tracts to the brain stem and thalamus were completely myelinated by 30 weeks of human gestation, and the thalamo-cortical pain fibers were myelinated by 37 weeks [25].

The timing of the thalamocortical connection is of crucial importance for cortical perception, since most sensory pathways to the neocortex have synapses in the thalamus. In the primate fetus, thalamic neurons produce axons that arrive in the cerebrum before mid-gestation. These fibers then “wait” just below the neocortex until migration and dendritic arborization of cortical neurons are complete and finally establish synaptic connections at 20–24 weeks of gestation. Functional maturity of the cerebral cortex is suggested by fetal and neonatal electroencephalographic patterns and the cortical components of somatosensory, auditory and visual evoked potentials recorded in preterm babies from 26 weeks of gestation [26]. In addition, several forms of behavior imply cortical function during fetal life. These include well-defined periods of quiet sleep, active sleep, and wakefulness *in utero* from 28 weeks of gestation, specific behavioral responses to pain, or the cognitive and associative capabilities in response to visual and auditory stimuli [27]. These data help to support the concept that the pain system is functional even in premature neonates. In fact, recent data suggest that the pain threshold may be lower in preterm neonates, as compared term neonates or older infants.

The Gate-Control Theory of Pain

Pain was previously described as a process in which specific nociceptive receptors were stimulated and produced standard responses within dorsal horn neurons in the spinal cord, with well-defined patterns of conduction to the brainstem, thalamus, and other subcortical centers. Such 'hardwired' concepts of the pain system, and other simple explanations of pain mechanisms, were abandoned as accumulating clinical and experimental evidence described the phenomenon of pain as characterized by remarkably adaptive neuronal and neurochemical processes, within neuronal networks whose elements may increase or decrease in number. Such adaptive processes were noted to be dependent on the characteristics of the noxious stimulus, the context in which it was applied, the behavioral state at the time of application, and various other factors, all of which produced significant alterations in the form or degree of pain experienced. Within this framework proposed by Wall and Melzack in 1965, the experience of pain was likened to a 'need state' which elicited a complex neuronal response with regulatory outflows at various levels of the central nervous system, produced in order to modulate the intensity of pain or respond to it.

Traditional classifications of nociceptive neurons were also challenged by these novel concepts. Since there were no fixed relationships between excitation of peripheral fibers and sensory or behavioral outcome, or between the input and output of individual dorsal horn neurons, it was proposed that input-output schemes within the pain system were context- dependent. For example, strong or repeated nociceptive stimuli triggered widespread increases of neural excitability within the spinal cord, with changes in the sensitivity of dorsal horn neurons and expansion of their cutaneous receptive fields [28].

It is now known that the integration of afferent signals occurs in multiple time frames at each level of sensory processing through both excitatory and inhibitory inputs, and is interwoven with efferent output from higher centers which may accentuate or control or modify the cascade of neurochemical events triggered by nociception. This elaborate system provides a plasticity characteristic of the nervous system, and may form the basis for memory and learning from nociceptive experiences. It also produces exquisitely variable responses to the multiplicity of nociceptive experiences within the environment; responses which may initiate or influence widespread processes such as awareness, cardiovascular activation, respiratory adaptation, hormonal stimulation, metabolic alterations, changes in immune function, and a host of other bodily functions. The pain system coordinates these widespread responses within the CNS in neuronal networks that are particularly dense loci for the processing, transmission and integration of painful stimuli.

Evidence for Increased Sensitivity to Pain in Neonates

Developmental changes occur in the expression of pain (crying or facial expressions) which differentiate preterm from term or older infants; however, these findings illustrate a communicational specificity and not changes in pain threshold during development [29, 30].

a) *The cutaneous flexor reflex* has a lower threshold in preterm neonates than in term neonates, or adults [31]. Thresholds for the flexor withdrawal reflex were further decreased ('sensitization') following repeated stimulation or local tissue injury in preterm neonates, this prolonged hypersensitivity was abolished by topical analgesia [32]. Sensitization of this reflex may result from immature descending inhibition in the spinal cord, the immaturity of other spinal or supraspinal mechanisms [33], or factors associated with intensive care [34, 35].
b) *Neurotransmitter development in the dorsal horn of the spinal cord* has demonstrated the early and abundant expression of putative neurotransmitters mediating nociception (substance P, L-glutamate, V.I.P., C.G.R.P.) and increased somatosensory excitability in the premature spinal cord. In contrast, the neurotransmitters contained in descending inhibitory fibers from supraspinal centers (5-HT, norepinephrine, dopamine) were expressed postnatally, implying poorly developed gate-control mechanisms for pain in preterm neonates [3,20,23].
c) *Opioid receptor labelling in the fetal brain stem* demonstrated very high densities in multiple supraspinal centers associated with sensory perception [36]. Theoretically, these inhibitory opioid receptors may protect developing neuronal systems from constant over-stimulation, given the underdeveloped gate-control mechanisms in the substantia gelatinosa.
d) *The magnitude of endocrine-metabolic and other stress responses* to invasive procedures or surgical operations was much greater in neonates as compared to adults; neonatal catecholamine and metabolic responses were upto 3–5 times those of adult patients undergoing similar surgery [37].
e) *Pharmacokinetic studies* of anesthetic drugs have shown that higher plasma concentrations were required to maintain effective surgical anesthesia in preterm neonates as compared to older age groups [38, 39].

These data indicate a lower pain threshold in preterm neonates and the occurrence of further decreases in pain threshold ('windup' phenomenon) following exposure to a painful stimulus or experience [40]. During these prolonged periods of hypersensitivity, even non-noxious stimuli (such as those produced by handling, physical examination, checking vital signs, etc.) will be perceived as noxious stimuli, and stimulate the systemic physiologic responses to this stress [37]. Although the assessment and treatment of acute painful stimuli have received much greater attention in the past, it is likely that *chronic* noxious stimulation resulting from this hypersensitivity has substantially greater biologic and clinical importance in the management of critically ill neonates and children [41].

References

1. Merskey H (1991) The definition of pain. European Journal of Psychiatry, 6:153–159.
2. Abram SE (1993) The 1992 Bonica Lecture: Advances in chronic pain management since gate control. Reg Anesth., 18:66–81.
3. Anand KJS, Carr DB (1989) The neuroanatomy, neurophysiology and neurochemistry of pain, stress, and analgesia in newborns, infants, and children. Pediatic Clinics of North America 36:795–822.
4. Anand KJS, McGrath PJ (1993) An overview of current issues and their historical background. In: Anand KJS, McGrath PJ (eds) *Pain in Neonates*, Elsevier Science Publishers, Amsterdam, pp.1–18.
5. Walco GA, Cassidy RC, Schechter NL (1994) Pain, hurt, and harm. The ethics of pain control in infants and children. New Engl J Med., 331:541–544.
6. Manne SL, Jacobsen PB, Redd WH (1992) Assessment of acute pediatric pain:do child self-report, parent ratings, and nurse ratings measure the same phenomenon? Pain, 48:45–52.
7. Doherty E, Yanni G, Conroy RM, Bresan B (1993) A comparison of child and parent ratings of disability and pain in juvenile chronic arthritis. J Rheumatol., 20:1563–1566.
8. Darwin C (1872) *The Expression of the Emotions in Man and Animals*, London, John Murray.
9. Oppenheim RW (1984) Cell death of motoneurons in the chick embryo spinal cord:7. Motoneurons prevented from dying in the embryo persist after hatching. Dev Biol., 101:35–59.
10. Hadjistavropoulos HD, Craig KD, Grunau RVE, Johnston CC (1994) Judging pain in newborns:facial and cry determinants. J Pediatr Psychol., 19:485–491.
11. Craig KD, Lilley CM, Gilbert CA (1996) Social barriers to optimal pain management in infants and children. Clin J Pain (in press)
12. Craig KD, Whitfield MF, Grunau RVE, Linton J, Hadjistavropoulos HD (1993) Pain in the preterm neonate:behavioral and physiological indices. Pain, 52:287–299.
13. Fitzgerald M, Fulton BP (1992) The physiological properties of developing sensory neurons. In: Scott (ed): Sensory Neurons: Diversity, Development & Plasticity. Oxford: Oxford University Press.
14. Fitzgerald M (1987) Spontaneous and evoked activity of foetal primary afferents "in vivo". *Nature* 326:603–605.
15. Fitzgerald M (1987) Functional plasticity in the somatosensory system. In W Winlow (ed):*Growth and Plasticity of Neural Connections*. MUP, pp. 192–232.
16. McGuirk SM, Dolphin AC (1992) G-protein mediation in nociceptive signal transduction:an investigation into the excitatory action of bradykinin in a subpopulation of rat sensory neurons. Neuroscience 49:117–128.

17. Anand KJS, Hickey PR (1987) Pain and its effects in the human neonate and fetus. N Engl J Med., 317:1321–1329.
18. Okado N (1981) Onset of synapse formatin in the human spinal cord. J Comp Neurol, 201:211–219.
19. Pignatelli, D, A Ribeiro-da-Silva, A Coimbra (1989) Postnatal maturation of primary afferent terminations in the substantia gelatinosa of the rat spinal cord. An electron microscopic study. Brain Res, 491:33–44.
20. Fitzgerald M (1994) Neurobiology of fetal and neonatal pain. In P.D. Wall and R. Melzack (eds):*The Textbook of Pain.* Edinburgh:Churchill Livingstone, pp. 153–163.
21. Rizvi T, Wadhwa S, Bijlani V (1987) Deverlopment of spinal substrate for nociception. Pain [suppl.], 4:195.
22. Shortland P, Fitzgerald M (1994) Neonatal sciatic nerve section results in a rearrangement of the central terminals of saphenous and axotomized sciatic nerve afferents in the dorsal horn of the spinal cord of the adult rat. *Eur J Neurosci* 6:75–86.
23. Marti E, Gibson SJ, Polak JM, Facer P, Springall DR, van Aswegen G, Aitchison M, Koltzenburg M (1987) Ontogeny of peptide- and amine-containing neurones in motor, sensory and autonomic regions of rat and human spinal cord, dorsal root ganglia and rat skin. *J Comp Neurol* 266:332–359.
24. Hughes HE, Barr GA (1988) Analgesic effects of intrathecally applied noradrenergic compounds in the developing rat:differences due to thermal vs. mechanical nociception. Dev Brain Res, 41:109–120.
25. Gilles FJ, Shankle W, Dooling EC (1983) Myelinated tracts:growth patterns. In:(Gilles FJ, Leviton A, Dooling EC) The Developing Human Brain:growth and epidemiologic neuropathology. Boston:John Wright, pp. 117–183.
26. Klimach VJ, Cooke RWI (1988) Maturation of the neonatal somatosensory evoked response in preterm infants. *Dev Med & Child Neurol* 30:208–214.
27. Bushnell IWR, Sai F, Mullin JT (1983) Neonatal recognition of mother's face. Br J Dev Psychol., 7:3–15.
28. Woolf CJ, Wall PD (1986) The relative effectiveness of C primary afferent fibres of different origins in evoking a prolonged facilitation of the flexor reflex in the rat. *J Neurosci* 6:1433–1443.
29. Johnston CC, Stevens B, Craig KD, Grunau RVE (1993) Developmental changes in pain expression in premature, full-term, two- and four-month-old infants. Pain, 52:201–208.
30. Stevens BJ, Johnston CC, Horton L (1994) Factors that influence the behavioral pain responses in premature infants. Pain, 59:101–109.
31. Fitzgerald M, Shaw A, MacIntosh N (1988) The postnatal development of the cutaneous flexor reflex:a comparative study in premature infants and newborn rat pups. *Dev Med & Child Neurol* 30:520–526.
32. Fitzgerald M, Millard C, McIntosh N (1989) Cutaneous hypersensitivity following peripheral tissue damage in newborn infants and its reversal with topical anaesthesia. Pain, 39:31–36.
33. Andrews KA, Fitzgerald M (1994) The cutaneous withdrawal reflex in human neonates:sensitization, receptive fields and the effects of contralateral stimulation. *Pain,* 56:95–101.
34. Philbin MK, Ballweg DD, Gray L (1994) The effect of an intensive care unit sound environment on the development of habituation in health avian neonates. Developmental Psychobiol 27:11–21.
35. Wiertelak EP, Smith KP, Furness L, Mooney-Heiberger K, Mayr T, Maier SF, Watkins LR (1994) Acute and conditioned hyperalgesic responses to illness Pain 56:227–34.
36. Kinney HC, Ottoson CK, White WF (1990) Three-dimensional distribution of H3–naloxone binding to opiate receptors in the human fetal and infant brainstem. J Comp Neurol, 291:55–78
37. Anand KJS (1993) Relationships between stress responses and clinical outcome in newborns, infants, and children. Crit Care Med, 21:S358–S359.
38. Yaster M (1987) The dose response of fentanyl in neonatal anesthesia. Anesthesiology, 66:433–435.

39. Greeley WJ, de Bruijn NP (1988) Changes in sufentanil pharmacokinetics within the neonatal period. Anesth Analg, 67:86–90.
40. Fitzgerald M, Millard C, MacIntosh N (1989) Cutaneous hypersensitivity following peripheral tissue damage in newborn infants and its reversal with topical anaesthesia. *Pain*, 39:31–36.
41. Anand KJS, McGrath PJ (1993) Future directions. In: Anand KJS, McGrath PJ (eds) *Pain in Neonates*, Elsevier Science Publishers, Amsterdam, pp.321–333.

Pain in Children: A State of the Art

H. Huijer Abu-Saad

Introduction

The last two decades have witnessed a surge in interest among health professionals for the topic pain in children. The work conducted by researchers and clinicians in this area has led to an increase in knowledge regarding pain mechanisms, pain pathways and pain perception. In addition, pain assessment and pain management strategies have been developed and in some cases rigorously subjected to scientific testing. As a result of these developments, the number of myths which have haunted this area of practice have been partially dispelled. The notion that children are less capable of feeling, remembering, and reporting pain has been questioned by researchers. Evidence is as a result accumulating that pain perception in infants is not dependent on the degree of myelination and that pain pathways are formed before birth (Fitzgerald, 1993; Fitzgerald & Anand, 1994). In addition a number of studies have shown beginning evidence that neonates and infants can remember pain. Finally, the child's ability to report pain as early as three years of age has been supported by numerous research studies (Abu-Saad et al, 1994, Beyer et al, 1990; Hamers et al, 1996; McGrath, 1990).

Misconceptions of health professionals, on the other hand, have continued to influence practice and as such the use of appropriate pain relief in this area. Recent reports of physicians ratings of pain in children and neonates have shown that there is a tendency to rate the ability to experience pain lower in younger children (Campbell et al, 1989; McLaughlin et al, 1993). Selbst and Clark (1990) have found in addition, a discrepancy in the type and amount of analgesics given to children and adults suffering from similar clinical conditions or upon admission to the emergency room.

Withholding analgesics from children may be commonly related to the fear that clinicians have that children can easily become addicted and that they are more sensitive to the respiratory depressant of narcotics. There is no evidence yet found however, which confirms the assumption that children can become more easily addicted (Schechter and Allen, 1986). In addition, there is growing evidence that older children have essentially adult-like morphine pharmacodynamics (Yaster and Deshpande, 1988; Yaster and Maxwell, 1994) when compared to neonates and very small infants who have different pharmacokinetics and pharmacodynamics (Koren and Jacobsen, 1993).

Based on the above, one may be led to believe that pain in children is less consequential than pain in adults (Johnston, 1993). Undoubtedly, all children experience pain after surgery or when ill. Unclear, however, is whether this pain is "undertreated". In addition, the consequences of this pain may not be well understood by many health professionals. This may be related to factors that influence the professionals decisions to relieve pain in children.

Long-term consequences of pain in children have not yet been unfortunately, systematically studied. There is evidence to suggest, however, that changes may occur in the peripheral structures in premature infants subjected to repeated injuries (Fitzgerald and Anand, 1993). Children with recurrent pain syndromes or chronic pain have been shown to exhibit more behavioral manifestations of distress (McGrath, 1990), some become more socially isolated and have poor performance at school. Grunau et al (1994) compared premature babies who were exposed to numerous nociceptive events during hospitalization with full-term, healthy ones. The researchers found significantly higher somatization, i.e. somatic complaints of unknown origin, at 4 years of age among premature infants when compared to full-term healthy ones. The finding of higher somatization could suggest that prior pain experience may contribute to pain syndromes.

These and other reasons make it imperative that nurses be more alert and concerned with the pain that children experience in the course of their illness and do their utmost best to alleviate it and prevent it.

These and other points will be further elaborated in the sections that follow.

Are Children Undermedicated?

A number of studies are commonly cited in the literature which support the assumption that children are given insufficient medication when compared to adults (Beyer et al, 1983; Eland and Anderson, 1977; Mather and Mackie, 1983; Schechter et al, 1986). Eland and Anderson (1977) and Foster and Hester (1990) found a discrepancy between prescribed and administered medication, with children receiving less medication than prescribed. Beyer et al (1983) and Schechter et al (1986) upon comparing prescription and administration of analgesics between children and adults with the same medical conditions, came to the conclusion that children are given less opiates than adults. These results were also confirmed by Elander and Hellstrom (1992). Whether these studies provide evidence that children are insufficiently medicated remains however, based on these results, questionable. The children in the above cited studies were not asked to assess their pain or to give an adequate picture if their pain was adequately relieved.

Mather and Mackie (1983) and Johnston et al (1992) on the other hand, examined the incidence and effectiveness of pain and pain relief by asking for the children's input. The researchers concluded that the incidence of pain was very high and that the analgesics administered were not sufficient to relieve pain.

Whether the prescribed analgesics dose was adequate and whether the dose was sufficiently administered by the nurses were questions the authors raised when interpreting their research results. The interpretation of pro-re-nata (PRN) medication, to mean as little as possible, may have influenced, according to the authors, the nurses decisions to relieve a child's pain.

Attitudes of health professionals are known to influence their practice. Surgeons were found to be hesitant in prescribing opiates for postoperative pain relief (Schechter and Allen, 1986). Pain expectations after surgery seemed to differ among different health professionals (Kokke et al 1993) and as a result it is not uncommon that pain prescription practices also widely differ. Nurses knowledge, beliefs, and attitudes, in addition, influence how they practice. In the Netherlands, we have found that nurses see pain as essential and hence should not be relieved completely (Arkestyn et al 1990; Hamers et al 1993) and as a result postpone the administration of a PRN medication as long as possible.

Based on the above, one may still question whether enough evidence is available at the present to support the notion that children in general are undermedicated. There are notions that the expectations of health professionals may differ and as such may lead to insufficient pain prescription. More evidence is available that PRN prescriptions in addition to nurses attitudes and beliefs may influence how nurses administer analgesics to manage pain. Research is as result warranted to disentangle the factors which determine how pain in children is assessed and managed by nurses.

Decision-Making and Pain-Relief in Nursing

The role that nurses play in pain relief in children is becoming increasingly important. Nurses knowledge and experience are constantly taken into consideration in developing pain policies and in implementing these policies in the practice setting. In addition pediatric nurses have the opportunity to specialize as pain consultants and in this capacity are actively involved in pain teams and pain clinics. Research conducted by nurses during the last two decades has provided us with the knowledge on how children experience and respond to pain. This knowledge was instrumental in developing pain assessment tools which are currently used in research and practice.

Although nurses have been since time immortal involved in pain relief, little is known on, for instance, how they decide that a child is in pain?, which information do they use in coming to a decision?, and which factors influence their decisions? Clinical decision making in nursing with regard to pain assessment and management has been receiving as a result a great deal of attention. A number of studies conducted recently show that a number of factors can influence nurses' pain assessments and interventions in children (Hamers et al 1994). These factors include the severity of the medical diagnosis, the child's expression of pain, the age of the child, the information obtained from the parents, as well as the nurses' knowledge, experience, attitude, and workload.

The medical diagnosis seems to justify the presence of pain (Arkesteyn et al, 1990; Burokas, 1985, Hamers et al, 1994). Vocal and verbal expressions of pain (Hamer et al, 1994; Wallace, 1989), the child's behavior (Koolen and Perduijn, 1991), and facial expression (Dick, 1993) seem to be the most determining factors for the presence of pain. Conflicting results have been found regarding the influence of age on pain relief in children. Elander and Hellstrom (1992) report more narcotic use in older children, Gonzales and Gadish (1990) suggest that younger children receive more non-narcotics, and Hamers et al (1994) found that younger children receive non-narcotics sooner than older children.

Nurses characteristics such as knowledge and experience have been often reported in the literature. Hamers et al (1995) found that expertise does not influence pain assessment, however it does have an impact on the administration of non-narcotic analgesics. Experienced nurses were more inclined to administer analgesics than first and fourth year nursing students. In general, one is inclined to assume that education and practical experience increase the accuracy in decision-making, in particular the more years of experience one has the more accurate is the diagnosis. This, however, needs to be further researched.

Strategies for Effective Pain Relief

Two strategies are imperative if pain in children is to be relieved effectively. The first has to do with the establishment of accurate methods for the assessment of pain, and the second concerns the institution of pain management protocols and policies.

Methods for Pain Assessment

The importance of pain assessment in children is based on the premise that if pain is not assessed regularly and accurately, children will continue to suffer inadequate pain relief. Numerous articles attest to the fact that nurses underestimate children's pain, that they question the child's expressions of pain, and that their knowledge about pain management strategies is not always up to date. It is important to mention at this point that the assessment of pain is not always easy. The nurse is in most cases dependent on what the child says, on her observations of the behavior of the child, and in some cases on physiological determinants.

The child's report of pain, although the most reliable, is often very difficult to interpret because it is related to the context in which the child's pain is assessed. The child may feel reluctant to report severe pain because of fear of injections and/or having to stay longer in the hospital. Reassuring the child that pain is legitimate, that many other children in a similar situation have pain, and that something will be done to relieve it, are strategies that can be used by nurses to help children communicate and express their pain. Just as important is the child who will show no indications of pain inspite of the presence of pain. Such a child has learned to cope with pain using distraction strategies such as playing cards or watching TV. Quite often this apparent calmness can be interpreted by nurses that pain is not present and thus pain relief will not be administered. These facts speak as a result, to the importance of using standard assessment methods in nursing practice.

Several pain assessment methods have been reported in the literature. These can be grouped into self-report, behavioral, and physiological measures. Self-report measures are restricted for use by children who have the necessary verbal and cognitive communication skills. Behavioral and physiological methods are used when self-report can not be obtained. They do have the disadvantage further for not being specific to pain. All three methods are used separately or in combination to assess and measure pain in children. The measurement of pain denotes the assessment of one dimension of the pain experience such as intensity, whereas assessment involves a thorough assessment of all the facets of pain as experienced by the child such as intensity, frequency, duration, quality, among others.

There are currently numerous measures developed to measure and assess pain in children. A number of these methods have been extensively validated while others are still in the development phase. A full description of all instruments is surely beyond the scope of this article. An attempt will be made, however, to highlight the tools most commonly used and most rigorously validated.

Self-Report Measures: These measures are either unidimensional or multidimensional in nature. Unidimensional methods include visual analogue scales and their variations (Abu–Saad, 1984) poker chips (Hester 1979), photos (Beyer et al, 1984, 1989, 1990), and faces scales (Bieri et al 1990). The unidimensional methods have been used successfully in children as young as three years of age. Multidimensional methods require more developed communication skills and abstract thinking and hence are suited for children six years of age or older. These measures include the Abu-Saad Pediatric Pain Assessment Tool (Abu-Saad et al, 1990, 1991a, 1991b, 1994) and the children's form of the McGill Pain Questionnaire (Savedra et al, 1993).

Behavioral Methods: These methods are of specific significance when children are unable to speak such as neonates, infants, and intubated children, when they are tool ill, or when they are under the influence of anesthesia. Indicators using crying (Johnston et al, 1988, 1990), body movement (Franck, 1986), and facial expressions (Grunau and Craig, 1987) have been commonly used to assess pediatric pain. Based on these indicators, a number of observational tools have been developed and tested. For a complete overview of these tools see Bours et al (1996).

Physiological Methods: A number of physiological indicators have been used to measure pain in children among them are measures of the variability in heart rate, respiratory rate, blood pressure, intracranial pressure, oxygen saturation, and stress hormones. For a complete overview of these measures in the neonate see Bours et al (1996).

All methods mentioned thus far can be used alone or in combination. Intensity scales are best suited to assess acute pain and pain of short duration. Behavioral and physiological measures when used together can provide a more accurate picture of pain in neonates and very young infants. Multidimensional methods of pain are most appropriate to assess chronic and recurrent pain in children. When choosing a method one should take into consideration first, the appropriateness of the measure for the age group and the clinical situation. Second, if the measure is valid and reliable, the psychometric properties should be known. Lastly, the clinical utility of the measure should be checked such as its length, clarity, ease of use and time needed to use it.

Management of Pediatric Pain

Many methods are cited in the literature to manage pediatric pain and are commonly grouped under the headings pharmacological and non-pharmacological methods. Although pharmacological methods are quite effective, their use in the practice setting is still hampered with a number of misconceptions as well as lack of knowledge with regard to their effectiveness in the treatment of pain in children. This can be illustrated by the differences found in the prescription of pain analgesics among physicians (Kokke et al, 1993). Berde (1989) and Mather and Mackie (1983) in addition, reported that the doses of analgesics prescribed for children are often too small and the frequency of administration too little. This is an example of how misconceptions can stay on for a long time if no measures are taken to remedy them.

Based on research results, it is without any doubt that the management of pain in children should be no different than that of adults. Lynn and Slattery (1987) and Yaster and Deshpande (1988) have shown for instance, that children over 6 weeks of age, with no liver damage, have the ability to clear their opiates at the same rate as adults. It remains however unclear which analgesic type and which dose will produce the most pain relief in children. A number of studies testing the effectiveness of different analgesics after adenotonsillectomies, for example, have failed to give an answer to this question (Hamers et al 1996; Watters et al, 1988). This and others stress the importance of studying the efficacy of analgesics use in children.

Non-Pharmacological Methods have been found to be effective among children. In addition to pharmacological methods children can be taught to use other strategies to help reduce their pain. Psychological and cognitive strategies such as distraction (music, watching tv, playing cards, reading a book) imagery, and self-hypnosis have been found to be effective in reducing pain of short duration (Fowler-Kerry and Ramsay-Lander 1990; McGrath et al, 1993; Kuttner et al, 1988, 1993). Patient education, relaxation training and self-help programs have been found to be effective in relieving headaches in children (McGrath et al , 1988). The effective use of massage, and cold and warm compresses is also frequently cited. Trans electrocutane nerve stimulation (TENS) and acupressure are techniques that the nurse can get skilled in for use in the practice setting.

The different pharmacological and non-pharmacological methods which are currently at the disposition of the nurse for use in clinical practice do not guarantee however the effective relief of pain in children. The knowledge that one has gives no assurance that it will be applied. In other words, what scientists find out through research has a long way to go before it finds its way to the practicc setting. The gap between science and practice does not seem to get smaller. Practices which have been carried out based on experience and tradition and not on research seem to have the overhand. Research conducted by Halfens et al (1994) showed a great discrepancy between what nurses know and what they apply when it comes to pain interventions. These practices are mostly influenced by the motivation of the nurse, time needed to apply the intervention, workload, ward policy, support from colleagues and superiors among others.

Conclusions

The field of pain in children has witnessed a great deal of developments in the last two decades. Successes have been made in almost all areas of pain ranging from the neonate to the adolescent, and covering almost all clinical populations from acute and chronic to recurrent pain episodes in children. Strides have been made in addition, in the areas of pain pathways and pain perception, in developing and testing tools to assess and measure pain, and in testing the effectiveness of specific pain intervention strategies to relieve and prevent pain in children.

Inspite all these accomplishments the field is still hampered by a number of problems which stand in the way of effective pain relief. The remedies for these problems are in my opinion only achievable when the institution together with the health care professionals share the same commitment and goal and that involves the eradication of all unnecessary pain among all children. This would specifically mean the following:

- Develop a clear pain policy for the institution.
- Translate this policy into workable guidelines and protocols for the different health care professionals.
- Ensure the availability of continuing education and refresher courses in the areas of pediatric pain.
- Develop clear lines of responsibility and accountability for pain relief.
- Ensure that the guidelines are implemented at the unit level.
- Introduce standard pain assessment using tools appropriate for age and clinical population.

- Develop and use pain management protocols for adequate analgesic pain relief.
- Avoid the use of PRN medications as much as possible and certainly never the first few days postoperatively.
- Facilitate and encourage the use of non-pharmacological techniques as adjuvants for pain relief.
- Assure a good line of communication and continuity of care through appropriate charting and reporting of pain.
- Encourage staff to question pain policies and to raise issues amenable for further research and inquiry.

References

1. Abu-Saad H (1984) Assessing children's responses to pain. Pain 19:163–171.
2. Abu-Saad HH (1990a) Toward the development of an instrument to assess pain in children: Dutch study. In D.C. Tyler, E.J. Krane (Eds.). Advances in Pain Research and Therapy. Pediatric Pain 15:101–107, Raven Press, New York.
3. Abu-Saad HH, Kroonen EK, Halfens RJS (1990b) On the development of a multidimensional Dutch pain assessment tool for children. Pain 43:249–256.
4. Abu-Saad HH, Pool H, Tulkens B (1994) Further validity testing of the Abu-Saad pediatric pain assessment tool. Journal of Advanced Nursing 19:1063–1071.
5. Arkesteyn S, Huijer Abu-Saad H, Halfens R (1990) De attitude van Verpleegkundigen (Nurses' attitudes). Tijdschrift voor Ziekenverpleging (Journal of Nursing Care) 100:396–398.
6. Berde CB (1989) Pediatric postoperative pain management. Pediatrics Clinics of North America 36:921–940.
7. Beyer JE, DeGood DE, Ashley LC, Russel GA (1983) Patterns of postoperative analgesic use with adults and children following cardiac surgery. Pain 17:71–81.
8. Beyer JE, McGrath PJ, Berde CB (1990) Discordance between self-report and behavior pain measures in children aged 3–7 years after surgery, Journal of Pain and Symptom Management 5:350–356.
9. Bieri D, Reeve RA, Champion GD, Addicoat L, Ziegler JB (1990) The faces pain scale for the self assessment of the severity of pain experienced by children: development, initial validation, and preliminary investigation for ratio scale properties. Pain 41:139–150.
10. Bours G, Huijer Abu-Saad H, Hamers JPS, van Dongen N (1996) Pain in Neonates: A State of the Art Study. University Press, Rijksuniversiteit Limburg, Maastricht.
11. Burokas L (1985) Factors affecting nurses' decisions to medicate pediatric patients after surgery. Heart and Lung 14:373–379.
12. Campbell NN, Reynolds GJ, Perkins G (1989) Postoperative analgesis in neonates: an Australia-wide survey. Anesth.Intensive Care 17:487–491.
13. Eland JM, Anderson JE (1977) The experience of pain in children. In A. Jacox (Ed.). Pain: A Source book for Nurses and other Health Professionals. Little Brown, Boston, pp. 453–473.
14. Elander G, Hellstrom G (1992) Analgesic administration in children and adults following open heart surgery. Scandinavian Journal of Caring Sciences 6:17–21.
15. Fitzgerald M (1993) Development of pain pathways and mechanisms. In K.J.S. Anand, and P.C. McGrath (eds.). Pain in Neonates. Elsevier, Amsterdam, pp. 19-37.
16. Fitzgerald M, Anand KJS (1994) Developmental neuroanatomy and neurophysiology of pain. In N.L. Schechter, C.B. Berde and M. Yaster (eds.). Pain in Infants, Children, and Adolescents. Williams and Wilkins, Baltimore, pp. 11–31.
17. Foster RL, Hester NO (1990) The relationship between pain ratings and pharmacologic interventions for children in pain. In D.C. Tyler and E.J. Krane. Pediatric Pain. Advances in Pain Research and Therapy, Raven Press, New York, 15, pp. 31–35.

18. Franck L (1986) A new method to quantitatively describe pain behavior in infants. Nursing Research 35:28–31.
19. Fowler-Kerry S, Ramsay-Lander J (1990) Using cognitive strategies to relieve pain in young children. In D.C. Tyler and E.J. Krane (Eds.). Advances in Pain Research and Therapy. Pediatric Pain. Raven Press, New York, pp. 247–253.
20. Gonzales J, Gadish H (1990) Nurses decisions in medicating children postoperatively. In D.C. Tyler and E.J. Krane (eds.). Advances in Pain Research and Therapy. Pediatric Pain. Raven Press, New York, pp. 37–41.
21. Grunau VE, Whitfield MF & Petrie JH (1994) Pain sensitivity and temperament in extremely low-birth weight premature toddlers and pre-term and full-term controls. Pain 58:341–346.
22. Grunau RVE, Craig KD (1987) Pain expression in neonates facial expression and cry. Pain 28:395–410.
23. Halfens RJG, Derks WAM, Huijer Abu-Saad H (1994) Verpleegkundige pijninterventies in Nederlandse ziekenhuizen; een inventarisatie van opvattingen en praktijk (Pain interventions in nursing in Dutch hospitals; An inventory on views and practice). Verpleegkunde (Nursing), 4:243–251.
24. Hamers JPH, Huijer Abu-Saad H, van den Hout MA, Halfens RJG, Schumacher JNM (1994) Factors influencing pain assessment and intervention in children. Journal of Advanced Nursing 20:853–860.
25. Hamers JPH, Huijer Abu-Saad H, Geisler FEA, van den Hout MA, Schouten JA, Halfens RJG, van Suijlekom JA. The effects of paracetamol, fentanyl, and systematic assessments on children's pain following (adeno)tonsillectomy. (Submitted).
26. Hamers JPH, van de Hout MA, Halfens RJG, Huijer Abu-Saad H, Heijltjes AEG. Differences in pain assessment and decisions regarding the administration of analgesics between novices, intermediates, and experts in pediatric nursing. (Submitted).
27. Hester NKO (1979) The preoperational child's reaction to immunization. Nursing Research 28:250–255.
28. Johnston CC, O'Shaughnessy D (1988) Acoustical attributes of pain cries: Distinguishing features. In R. Dubner, G.F. Gebhart, and M.R. Bond (Eds.). Advances in Pain Research and Therapy. Raven Press, New York, pp. 336–340.
29. Johnston CC (1993) Pain in Children. refresher Course Syllabus, 7th World Congress on Pain. International Association for the Study of pain, pp.185- 190.
30. Johnston CC, Abbott FV, Gray-Donald K, Jeans ME (1992) A survey of pain in hospitalized patients aged 4–14 years. Clinical Journal of Pain 8:154–163.
31. Kokke FTM, Van der Heide DH, Boelen van de Loo WJC (1993) Postoperatieve pijnbestrijding in drie Nederlandse ziekenhuizen: een pilotstudie (Postoperative pain management in three Dutch hospitals: a pilot study). Tijdschrift voor Kindergeneeskunde (Journal of Pediatric Medicine) 61:48–51.
32. Koolen YHE, Perduijn MD (1991) Clinical judgement. Acutely and chronically ill patients in pain. Rijksuniversiteit Limburg, Maastricht. (Unpublished Masters Thesis)
33. Koren G, Jacobson S (1993) Developmental considerations in the clinical pharmacology of analgesics. In N.L. Schechter, C.B. Berde and M. Yaster (Eds.). Pain in Infants, Children, and Adolescents, Williams and Wilkins, Baltimore, pp. 33–38.
34. Kuttner L (1988) Favourite stories. A hypnotic pain-reduction technique for children in acute pain. American Journal of Clinical Hypnosis 30:289–295.
35. Kuttner L (1993) Hypnotic interventions for children in pain. In N.L. Schechter, C.B. Berde and M. Yaster (Eds.). Pain in Infants, Children, and Adolescents. Williams and Wilkins, Baltimore, pp. 229–236.
36. Lynn AM, Slattery JT (1987) Morphine pharmacokinetics in early infancy. Anesthesiology 66:136–139.
37. Mather L, MacKie J (1983) The incidence of postoperative pain in children. Pain 15:271–282.
38. McGrath PA (1990) Pain in Children: Nature, Assessment and Management. Guilford Press, New York.

39. McGrath PJ, Humphreys P, Goodman JT (1988) Relaxation prophylaxis for childhood migraine: a randomized placebo-controlled trial, Developmental Medicine and Child Neurology 30:626–631.
40. McGrath PJ, Unruh AM (1993) Psychological treatment of pain in children and adolescents.. In N.L. Schechter, C.B. Berde and M. Yaster (Eds.). Pain in Infants, Children and Adolescents. Williams and Wilkins, Baltimore, pp. 219–228.
41. McLaughlin CR, Hull JG, Edwards WH, Cramer CP, Dewey WL (1993) Neonatal pain: a comprehensive survey of attitudes and practices, Journal of Pain and Symptom management 8:–16.
42. Savedra MC, Holzemer WL, Tesler MD, Wilkie DJ (1993) Assessment of postoperative pain in children and adolescents using the adolescent pediatric pain tool. Nursing Research 42:5–9.
43. Schechter NL, Allen D (1986) Physicians' attitudes towards pain in children. Developmental and behavioral Pediatrics 7:350–354.
44. Selbst SM, Clark M (1990) Analgesic use in the emergency department. Annals of Emergency medicine 19:1010–1013.
45. Wallace MR (1989) Temperament: a variable in children's pain management. pediatric Nursing 15:118–121.
46. Watters CH, Patterson CC, Mathews HML, Campbell W (1988) Diclofenac sodium for posttonsillectomy pain in children, Anaesthesia 43 :641–643.
47. Yaster M, Deshpande JK (1988) Management of pediatric pain with opioid analgesics. Journal of Pediatrics 113:421–429.
48. Yaster M, Maxwell LG (1994) Opioid agonists and antagonists. In N.L. Schechter, C.B. Berde and M. Yaster (Eds.). Pain in Infants, Children, and Adolescents, Williams and Wilkins, Baltimore, pp. 145–171.

Perspectives on Pediatric Pain Control

A. R. Lloyd-Thomas

Introduction

It is only in the last ten years that attention has been focused on pain control for children both after operations and during critical care [1]. Unnecessary suffering has occurred as a result of inadequate and ineffective therapy [2] and there is ample evidence in the literature to support this contention [3–7]. There are many reasons for the undertreatment of these children but at the forefront was the perception that, through their immaturity, neonates and infants were incapable of perceiving pain [8]. But the explosion of interest which has occurred during the last ten years in the developmental neurobiology of pain has resulted in considerable changes in the way in which the children are managed [9]. The key word here is developmental, unlike adult practice pediatric critical care specialists have to deal with a developing being, which means that a uniform approach cannot be applied and treatment requires tailoring to the age of the patient.

The Age Perspective

Whilst it is possible to formulate a treatment plan for the older child that can be readily applied across a wide age range (four years to adolescents) it is the infant – especially the neonate – who present the greatest challenge through their inability to communicate, their immature physiology and their developing nervous system.

Pain Control in the Neonate

In considering these patients the first question that springs to mind is do neonates feel pain? The International Association of the Study of Pain (IASP) defines pain as 'an unpleasant sensory and emotional experience associated with actual or potential tissue damage', going on to emphasize the importance of experience relating to past injury. This implies that the brain needs to have achieved a certain level of neural connectivity, as well as having prior experience, before pain is appreciated. But this rather behavioural approach ignores the fact that there is well recognized neuronal activity in the pathways and nuclei involved in sensory processing, [10] which can be identified from about twenty-four weeks post conceptual age. Moreover the neonate mounts a clear stress response to noxious stimulation [11]. Furthermore, it has been suggested that an uncontrolled stress response may result in an adverse outcome, [12, 13] but these suggestions are derived from only small series of patients.

Neonatal spinal cord sensory neurones have larger receptive fields than in adults, whilst ordinary sensory receptors (non-nociceptive) synapse in the neonate with cells that are reserved exclusively for pain input in adults [14]. These factors suggest that the newborn has weak spatial localization of stimuli, whilst discrimination between nociceptive and non-nociceptive inputs will be poor. Finally, descending inhibitory control of the dorsal horn is absent, leading to the exaggerated reflex responses seen in both the fetus and newborn [10]. So whilst the newborn may not 'feel pain', with all the emotional and psychological overtones that is implied by our adult understanding of this concept, they do respond to tissue damaging noxious stimulation. Failure to treat this response may result in alteration in the development of the newborn nervous system with subsequent clinical consequences [15–17]. The suggestion that a rampant stress response, may lead to an adverse outcome, combined with data suggesting that development may be altered by early pain experience, require the clinician to consider their methods of pain control in newborn children.

Neonatal Analgesic Pharmacology
The newborn nociceptive system not only differs in its pattern of neurological connections, but also has wide differences in receptor populations. Many receptors are present in high density whilst others are diffusely spread and in some cases inhibitory neurotransmitters (in the adult) may be excitatory in the newborn [14]. Therefore conventional understanding of opioid receptor binding may need rethinking, whilst the wide difference in pharmacokinetics of the opioids in neonates also mean that the newborn requires special consideration in clinical pain management [18].

Systemic Opioid Analgesics in the Neonate

Pharmacokinetic and Pharmacodynamic Considerations

Morphine remains a popular choice in neonatal analgesia. The principal excretion pathway, glucuronidation to morphine-3-glucuronide (M-3-G) and morphine-6-glucuronide (M-6-G), is present in newborns, but there may be a reduced capacity for biotransformation, possibly related to birth weight and gestational age [19]. Furthermore, adult glucuronidation pathways result in a ratio of 10:1 / M-3-G to M-6-G [20], whilst in the neonate this ratio may be 3:1 [21, 19]. Animal data suggests that M-3-G and M-6-G have opposing clinical actions (M-3-G stimulant and ant-analgesic versus M-6-G depressant and potent analgesic),[22–24] thus immature metabolism may have important therapeutic consequences going some way to explain the unpredictable 'sensitivity' seen in neonates [18]. Further factors contributing to 'sensitivity' come from the prolonged half life [25] and reduced clearance [26] of morphine seen in neonates.

By contrast the synthetic opioids (fentanyl, alfentanil and sufentanil) are metabolized by cytochrome P450 enzymes to more polar and readily excreted compounds, which in comparison with the parent compound have such significantly reduced potency, that they can be regarded as inactive [18]. But these opioids are also subject to a prolonged half-life and reduced clearance - fentanyl [27], alfentanil [28], sufentanil [29]. Whilst metabolism of these drugs will not produce active products, they will have longer and more profound activity due to low clearance and long half-life.

Remifentanil is a most interesting synthetic opioid which has been recently developed. Unlike fentanyl, alfentanil and sufentanil it is structurally unique by virtue of its ester linkage. Because of this, it is susceptible to hydrolysis by non-specific esterases and is therefore rapidly digradated [30]. The elimination half-life is as little as 10 - 20 minutes with a clearance of 3–4 liters/min, but this data is from adults. Because of its rapid clearance by plasma esterases, irrespective of dose or duration of infusion there is little influence on the half-life and recovery is therefore very rapid. Within the context of critical care these pharmacokinetic data suggest that the agent may be titrated rapidly to clinical requirements and equally rapidly terminated. The results of phase two and phase three trials are awaited with interest.

Clinical Choice of Opioids for Critical Care in Neonates

How does this data influence the clinical choice of the 'right' opioid? Nather (1990) [31] has suggested that 'they are all equal after potency and pharmacokinetics have been considered'. As such morphine is the most widely studied and in clinical practice a loading infusion of 100 mcg/kg followed by 20–25 mcg/kg/hr will provide a target plasma concentration of 200 nanograms/ml allowing accommodation with ventilatory support. This will also avoid some of the unwanted effects of high doses, namely convulsions [32]. The loading dose should be infused over thirty minutes, thereby avoiding unwanted hypotension seen when administration is too rapid [18]. Because of the prolonged half-life opioid weaning should begin well in advance of any reduction in ventilatory support [18]. By contrast in self-ventilating post-surgical neonates, our regime of continuous infusions of 2–4 mcg/kg/hr with nurse activated supplementary boluses of 5–10 mcg/kg (maximum of one or two supplements in any one hour), has been successful with a low incidence of complications [33]. For fentanyl a loading dose of 10–20 mcg/kg with an infusion of 1–10 mcg/kg/hr [34] has been successful, whilst for alfentanil a loading dose of 8–20 mcg/kg with an infusion of 5–10 mcg/kg/hr [35] has been described. But none of these regimens will abolish the stress response in the manner described by Anand (1992) [36] when using high dose sufentanil for cardiac surgery patients.

Pain and the Stress Response

Surgery and trauma in children results in a biochemical and metabolic response characterized by increased concentrations of circulating hormones (glucagon, epinephrine, nor-epinephrine, cortisol, cytokines) and local tissue factors, leading to a metabolic response which if uncontrolled results in hyper metabolism, increased oxygen consumption, raised temperature, increased protein turnover, increased cardiac output, impaired hepatic and renal function [37]. In adults many believe that this stress response leads to a greater risk of complications [38]. By contrast, others argue that the fuel requirements of traumatized tissue need to be met by these metabolic changes. Hyperglycemia increases tissue glucose supply [39], whilst protein breakdown affords the amino acid residues required for tissue repair. Lipolysis and ketogenesis may be beneficial by providing an alternative source of fuel for various tissues [37]. Profound anesthesia may modify these responses, but can they be directly equated with pain?

Uncontrolled nociception results in a stress response [12]. Numerous studies have shown that general anesthesia, especially opioid analgesia, can reduce this response [37]. Moreover, local anesthesia when applied as an extradural block, will also obtund the glycemic response to surgery [40]. However, studies in adults have shown that oxygen consumption, nitrogen excretion, cortisol and catecholamines are little diminished by effective epidural analgesia [41, 42], casting doubt on the direct relationship between pain and stress response. Furthermore, is it always necessary to obtund the stress response? Few will have forgotten the suppression of cortisol secretion by etomidate [43] in critically ill patients, which resulted in a higher mortality through inability to mount a stress response. Further investigation in this area is needed especially in the pediatric field where data is sadly lacking.

Local Anesthesia for Neonates

Is there an option which avoids systemic opioids in neonates? For patients requiring mechanical ventilation after surgery, there is little to be gained by the complexity of extradural infusions. But in those self-ventilating, extradural local anesthesia provides good pain relief with little chance of respiratory depression and may avoid the necessity for mechanical ventilation. This is especially true in general surgical cases returning to neonatal intensive care – for example repair of tracheoesophageal fistula through a thoracotomy – in which extradural analgesia with local anesthetics may be the optimal way of managing postoperative pain relief. Thanks to advances in the equipment available to pediatric anesthetists extradural catheterization and infusion of local anesthetics are now possible with many propriety sets. Identification of the extradural space should be by a loss of resistance techniques (LOR) although the approach via the caudal route does not necessary need LOR methodology. There are advocates for using both air and saline as a marker for LOR in children but saline is probably the safest. There have been two case reports of venous air embolism [44, 45] and also a French retrospective multi-centre survey of major accidents following extradural analgesia [46] all of which are testaments to the potential hazards of loss of resistance to air in children. The American experience supports the use of LOR to saline as described by Sethna and Berde (1993) [47] who strongly advocate its use in children.

For satisfactory analgesia when using local anesthetics alone, the tip of the extradural catheter must be sited adjacent to the spinal levels innovating the dermatomes involved in surgery [48]. If the catheter is not adjacent to the dermatomes required, the dilute solutions of local anesthetics which are used in post-operative analgesia for neonates will not afford adequate analgesia. It is hazardous to increase the rate of the bupivacaine infusion - to compensate for an inadequately placed catheter - as this can result in local anesthetic toxicity manifesting either as convulsions [49, 50] or as cardiac dysrhythmias [51]. Berde [52] has recommended a maximum loading dose of 1.5–2 mg/kg followed by an infusion of 0.2–0.25 mg/kg of bupivacaine for post-operative analgesia using the extradural route in neonates. If satisfactory analgesia cannot be achieved with a maximal bupivacaine infusion, an opioid should be added to the infusate and the rate of bupivacaine infusion reduced [48].

The choice of opioid for extradural usage in neonates is also influenced by the site of catheter placement. Lipophilic opioids (e.g. fentanyl) injected at an extradural level away from the spinal dermatomes to be blocked will not result in effective segmental analgesia [53] and will be just like giving an intravenous injection. Therefore these agents should only be chosen when the anesthetist is confident that the catheter is near the site requiring block. By contrast hydrophilic opioids injected at a remote extradural site will provide segmental analgesia [54, 55], of these morphine is the best example. It is clear however that it is preferable to avoid the use of opioid in neonates preferring instead to manage with local anesthetics alone which can be supplemented if required by paracetamol or even intermittent codeine (0.5–1 mg/kg).

Having considered the options for neonates with their special requirements - pharmacokinetics and pharmacodynamics - attention should now be drawn to the older child receiving critical care.

Infants and Older Children

Much that has been discussed above is appropriate to the management of the older child. Clearly in critically ill infants and children considerations of drug clearance are important especially when organ systems are compromised. Morphine remains a popular choice for sedation in the intensive care setting and it should be remembered that the glucuronides are virtually exclusively dependent upon renal excretion for clearance and in those patients who develop renal failure significant accumulation of M-6-G may be seen.

Delivery Systems for Analgesia

Whilst there has not been a significant change in the drugs used to provide analgesia for the older child, the advent of patient controlled analgesia (PCA) infusion pumps has afforded their use in children above the age of five years. Whilst this form of analgesia is not appropriate to those requiring intense sedation during critical care, in the process of recovery and weaning we have found the use of PCA in intensive care to be very acceptable to patients [33]. Patients undergoing heart and lung transplantation have found PCA to be particularly helpful during their some-what prolonged recovery. Adult PCA regimens (no background infusion, bolus dose only) do not translate well into pediatric practice. Instead a background infusion should be used - optimally 4 mcg/kg/hr - which results in better pain scores than no infusion and a lower incidence of side effects [56]. Small bolus doses (less than 10 mcg/kg) are associated with poor pain control during movement. Bolus doses should be 20 mcg/kg with a lockout interval of 5 minutes [57]. Especially in older children it is important to remember that post-operative nausea and vomiting is seen in over fifty percent of children above the age of ten years [33] and this may be a source of distress to the critically ill patient, who may have difficulty in communicating this side effect to his or her carers. Most anti-emetics have a rather dismal record of efficacy but ondansetron 100 – 150 mcg/kg may be considerably more effective and trials are progressing in the area of post-operative nausea and vomiting to see if this results in better relief.

Summary

It is becoming clear that with careful attention to the pharmacology of analgesics, effective pain control can be provided for children requiring critical care. As our understanding of pain pathways improves there will be further treatment possibilities using agents that are active at other transmitters associated with pain control - for example NMDA, antagonists and alpha agonists.

References

1. Aynsley-Green A, Lloyd-Thomas AR, Ward-Platt MP (1995) In: Aynsley-Green A, Ward-Platt MP, Lloyd-Thomas AR (eds) Clinical Paediatrics: Stress and Pain in Infancy and Childhood. Balliere, London, pp ix–xi.
2. Liebeskind JC, Melzak R (1987) The International Pain Foundation:meeting a need for education in pain management. Pain 39:1–2.

3. Eland JM, Anderson JE The experience of pain in children. In: Jacox AK (ed) Pain: A source book for nurses and other health professionals. Little Brown, Boston, Mass, pp 453–473.
4. Beyer JE, De Good DE, Ashley LC, Russ GA (1983) Patterns of postoperative analgesic use with adults and children following cardiac surgery. Pain 17:71–81.
5. Schechter NL, Allen DA, Hanson K (1986) The status of pediatric pain control: A comparison of hospital analgesic usage in children and adults. Pediatrics 77:11–15.
6. Anand KJS, Aynsley-Green A (1985) Metabolic and endocrine effects of surgical ligation of patent ductus arteriosus in the human pre-term neonate: Are there implications for further improvement of postoperative outcome? Modern Prob Paed 23:143–157.
7. Hatch DJ (1987) Analgesia in the neonate. BMJ 294:920.
8. Purcell-Jones G, Doorman F, Sumner E (1988) Paediatric anaesthetists' perceptions of neonatal and infant pain. Pain 33:181–187
9. Abajian JC, Mellish RW, Brown AF, Perkins FM, Lambert DH, Mazuzan JE (1984) Spinal anesthesia for surgery in the high risk infant. Anesth Analg 63:359–362.
10. Fitzgerald M, Anand KJS (1993) Developmental neuro-anatomy and neurophysiology of pain. In: Schechter, Berde, Yaster (eds) Pain in infants, children and adolescents. Williams and Wilkins, Baltimore pp 11–32.
11. Anand KJS, Hickey PR (1987) Pain and its effects in the human neonate and fetus. New Eng J Med 3:1321–1329.
12. Anand KJS, Sippell WG, Aynsley-Green A (1987) Randomised trial of fentanyl in preterm babies undergoing surgery: Effects on the stress response. Lancet I:62–66.
13. Anand KJS, Hickey PR (1992) Halothane, morphine compared with high dose sufentanil for anaesthesia and postoperative analgesia in neonatal cardiac surgery. New Eng J Med 326:1–9.
14. Fitzgerald M (1994) The neurobiology of foetal pain. In: Wall P, Melzak R (eds) The textbook of pain, 3rd edn. Churchill Livingston, Edinburgh pp 153–163.
15. Grunau RVE, Whitfield MR, Petrie JH, Fryer EL (1994) Early pain experience, child and family factors, has procurers of somatization: A prospective study of extremely premature and full term children. Pain 56:353–359.
16. Taddio A, Goldback M, Ipp M, Stevens B, Corren G (1995) Effect of neonatal circumcision on pain responses during vaccination in boys. Lancet 344:291–2.
17. Stevenson J, Aynsley-Green A (1995) The long-term behavioural sequelae of surgery studied in young twins. Proc Br Psy Soc 3:59 (Abst)
18. Hartley R, Levene MI (1995) Opioid pharmacology in the newborn. In: Aynsley-Green A, Ward-Platt M, Lloyd-Thomas AR (eds) Clinical Paediatrics: Stress and Pain in Infancy and Childhood. Balliere, London, pp 467–493.
19. Hartley R, Green M, Quinn MW, Rushforth JA, Levene MI (1994) Development of morphine glucuronidation in premature neonates. Biol Neonate 66:1–9.
20. Venn RF, Michalkiewicz A, Hardy P, Wells C (1990) Concentrations of morphine, morphine metabolites and peptides in human CSF and plasma. Pain (supplement) 5:S188.
21. Choonara IA, Lawrence A, Michalkiewicz A, Bowhay A, Ratcliffe J (1992) Morphine metabolism in neonates and infants. Br J Clin Pharmacol 34:434–437.
22. Smith MT, Watt JA, Crammond T (1990) Morphine-3-glucuronide – a potent antagonist of morphine analgesia. Life Sci 47:579–585.
23. Watt JA, Crammond T, Smith MT (1990) Morphine-6-Glucuronide: Analgesia effects antagonised by morphine-3-glucuronide. Clin Exp Pharmacol Physiol 17 (supplement):83.
24. Gong QL, Headner T, Headner J, Bjorkman R, Nordberg G (1991) Anti-nociceptive and ventilatory effects of the morphine metabolites: morphine-6-glucuronide and morphine-3-glucuronide. Eur J Pharmacol 193:47–56.
25. Hartley R, Green M, Quinn M, Levene MI (1993) Pharmacokinetics of morphine infusion in premature neonates. Arch Dis Child 69:55–58.
26. Bhatt R, Chari G, Gulatt A, Aldana O, Velamati R, Bhargava H (1990) Pharmacokinetics of a single dose of morphine in preterm infants during the first week of life. J Pediatr 117:477–481.

27. Gaunlett IS, Fisher DM, Hertzkar E (1988) Pharmacokinetics of fentanyl in neonatal humans and lambs: effects of age. Anaesthesiology 69:683–687.
28. Wiest DB, Ohning BL, Garner SS (1991) The disposition of alfentanil in neonates with respiratory distress. Pharmacology 11:308–311.
29. Greeley WJ, de Bruijn NP (1998) Changes in sufentanil pharmacokinetics within the neonatal period. Anesth Analg 67:86–90.
30. Durcan T, Philpot G (1996) The metabolic fate of newer anaesthetic drugs. In: Kauffman L, Ginsberg R (eds) Anaesthesia Review 12. Churchill Livinstone, London, pp 165–180.
31. Nather LE (1990) Pharmacokinetic and pharmacodynamic profiles of opioid analgesics: a sameness amongst equals? Pain 43:3–6.
32. Koren G, Butt W, Chinyonga H, Soldis S, Tan YK, Pape K (1985) Post-operative morphine infusion in newborn infants: assessment of disposition characteristics and safety. J Pediatr 107:963–967.
33. Lloyd-Thomas AR, Howard RF (1994) A pain service for children. Paediatric Anaesthesia 4:3–15.
34. Roth B, Schlunder C, Houben F (1991) Analgesia and sedation in neonatal intensive care using fentanyl by continuous infusion. Dev Pharmacol Ther 17:121–127.
35. Marlow N, Weindling AM, van Peer A, Heykants J (1990) Alfentanil pharmacokinetics in preterm infants. Arch Dis Child 65:349–351.
36. Anand KJS, Hickey PR (1992) Halothane, morphine compared with high dose sufentanil for anaesthesia and postoperative analgesia in neonatal cardiac surgery. New Eng J Med 326:1–9.
37. Aynsley-Green A, Ward-Platt MP (1995) The biology of pain and stress:a conspectus. In: Aynsley-Green A, Ward-Platt MP, Lloyd-Thomas AR (eds) Clinical Paediatrics: Stress and Pain in Infancy and Childhood. Balliere, London, pp 449–466.
38. Kehlet H (1995) Does analgesia benefit post-injury outcome? In: Parker MM, Shapero MJ, Porembka DT (eds) Critical0 Care: State of the art. Society of Critical Care Medicine, pp 213–229.
39. Im MJC, Hooper JE (1970) Energy metabolism in healing skin wounds. J Surg Res 10:459–464.
40. Bromage PR, Shiloata HR, Willoughby HW (1975) Influence of prolonged epidural blockade on blood sugar and cortisol responses to operations upon the upper part of the abdomen and thorax. Surg Gyn Obs 132:1051–1056.
41. Hakanson E, Rutberg H, Jorfeldt L, Martensson J (1985) Effects of the extradural administration of morphine or bupivacaine on the metabolic response to upper abdominal surgery. Br J Anaesth 57:394–399.
42. Hjortso NC, Christensen NJ, Andersen T, Kehlet H (1985) Effects of the extradural administration of local anaesthetic agents and morphine on the urinary excretion of cortisol, catecalamines and nitrogen following abdominal surgery. Br J Anaesth 57:400–406.
43. Watt I, Ledingham IM (1984) Mortality amongst multiple traumatic patients admitted to an intensive therapy unit. Anesthesia 39:973–981.
44. Guinard JP, Borboen (1993) Probable venous air embolism during caudal anaesthesia in a child. Anesth Analg 76:1134–5.
45. Schwartz N, Eisenkraft J (1993) Probable venous air embolism during epidural placement in an infant. Anesth Analg 76:1136–8.
46. Flandin-Blety C, Barrier G (1995) Accidents following extradural analgesia in children. The results of a retrospective study. Paediatric Anaesthesia 5:41–46.
47. Sethna N, Berde C (1993) Venous air embolism during identification of the epidural space in children. Anesth Analg 76:925–7.
48. Berde C (1994) Epidural analgesia in children. Can J Anaesth 41:555–560.
49. Agrawal R, Gutlobe D, Lockhart C (1992) Seizures occuring in pediatric patients receiving continuous infusions of bupivacaine. Anesth Analg 75:284–6.
50. McCloskey J, Haun S, Deshbande J (1992) Bupivacaine toxicity secondary to continuous caudal epidural infusion in children. Anesth Analg 75:287–290.
51. Maxwell L, Martin L, Yaster M (1994) Bupivacaine induced cardiac toxicity in neonates:successful treatment with intravenous phenytoin. Anesthesiology 80:682–686.

52. Berde C (1992) Convulsions associated with pediatric regional anesthesia. Anesth Analg 75:164–6.
53. Campbell F, Yentis S, Fear D, Bissonette B (1992) Analgesic efficacy and safety of a caudal bupivacaine fentanyl mixture in children. Can J Anaesth 39:661–664.
54. Krane EJ, Jacobson LE, Lynn AM, Parrot C, Tyler DC (1987) Caudal morphine for postoperative analgesia in children: a comparison with caudal bupivacaine and intravenous morphine. Anesth Analg 66:647–653.
55. Wolf A, Hughes D, Wade A, Mkather S, Prys-Roberts C (1990) Postoperative analgesia after orchidopexy: evaluation of a bupivacaine morphine mixture. Br J Anaesth 64:430–435.
56. Doyle E, Harper I, Morton NS (1993) Patient controlled analgesia with low dose background infusions after lower abdominal surgery in children. Br J Anaesth 71:818–822.
57. Doyle E, Mottart K, Marshall C, Morton N (1994) Comparison of different bolus doses of morphine for patient controlled analgesia in children. Br J Anaesth 72:160–163.

Emergency

Management of Liver Failure Secondary to Mushroom Poisoning in Children

S. Clément de Cléty and D. Moulin

Introduction

A little less than one hundred species of mushrooms, distributed worldwide, are poisonous to humans. The most famous of them in Europe and the United States is the *Amanita phalloides*, which, in these countries , accounts for more than 90 percent of the fatalities [1, 2]. However other species may cause severe poisoning and are found in the genera *Amanita, Galerina* and *Lepiota*, all being grouped under the name of cyclopeptide mushrooms [3, 4].

The toxicity of these mushrooms is mainly related to the amatoxins they produce. The amatoxins (cyclic octapeptides) interfere with DNA transcription by inhibiting RNA polymerase II. Synthesis of messenger RNA and protein is interrupted. All cells are damaged but those with the most active protein synthesis are more affected, particularly in the liver and kidney [2, 4].

Acute hepatitis occurs and may progress, in severe cases, to fulminant hepatic failure with renal failure and shock. In a study of 205 *Amanita phalloides* intoxications, hepatitis was present in 198 (96%). Twenty-six percent of these patients developed hepatic coma and the overall mortality was 22.4% [1]. The mortality is higher in children than in adults, mainly because the amount of amatoxins ingested is higher [1]. One cap of *Amanita phalloides* can kill an adult.

The mainstay in the management is early and aggressive supportive care. Several drugs and antidotes have been tried, but, despite of these, orthotopic liver transplantation (OLT) may finally be the only therapy able to save the patient [2]. Patient selection criteria and timing for transplantation are however not clearly defined in children.

This review discusses shortly the clinical presentation and the most interesting laboratory investigations, and more broadly the different kinds of treatment presently available.

Clinical Presentation

The course of *Amanita phalloides* and other cyclopeptic mushrooms poisoning shows 4 chronological phases. The first is a quiescent period lasting 6 to 24 hours (mean 12.3 hours). The second begins with digestive symptoms: nausea, vomiting, abdominal pain and profuse diarrhea responsible for dehydration, hypovolemia, electrolytes and acid-base disorders. This phase may last 2 to 3 days and its magnitude depends on the quantity of ingested toxins, sex, age and prior health status [4, 5]. Unless circulatory collapse occurs, a third period of well-being (12 to 24 hours) may follow these acute symptoms. Laboratory data at this stage usually demonstrate subclinical evidence of hepatic injury. Transition into the fourth phase can occur quite suddenly. The acute hepatitis becomes clinically evident with the onset of jaundice on the third to the fourth day after ingestion. In severe cases, a clinical picture of fulminant hepatic failure (FHF) appears and, if the liver damage is irreversible, death occurs within 6 to 16 days (mean 8 days) [1].

A functional renal failure is frequent during the gastrointestinal phase and may reappear later, secondary to hemorrhagic shock or to hepatorenal syndrome observed with FHF. A direct nephrotoxic effect of amatoxins has not been proven in human intoxications. Neurologic symptoms are related to hepatic failure but amatoxins might also be responsible for some of the changes revealed by microscopic examination of the brain [2].

Laboratory Investigations

Thirty-six to 48 hours after ingestion of the mushroom, an increase of the serum aspartate aminotransferase (SGOT), alanine aminotransferase (SGPT) and bilirubin levels gives evidence of a beginning liver damage. Hepatic enzymes usually reach a peak between the 60th and the 72nd hour. In our experience as well as that of other teams involved in pediatric liver transplantation, prothrombin time, coagulation factor V and lactic acid levels are the best indicators of severity of hepatocellular failure [6]. Glucose and fibrinogen should also be monitored.

Numerous toxins are synthesized by the cyclopeptide mushrooms. The phallotoxins might be partially responsible for the initial symptoms of gastroenteritis [2, 7]. Their dosage is useless. Of the various amatoxins, α and β amanitins are the most toxic and account for the deleterious effects on the gastrointestinal cells and the hepatocytes. Amatoxins may be detected in biologic fluids by radioimmunoassay or high performance liquid chromatography but these methods are generally not available. If the dosage of the amatoxins in the serum and/or urine truly may help to identify the etiology of acute hepatitis, it should not be forgotten that amatoxins may not be detected in some patients, especially when the measurements are made in the serum [7, 8] or more than 96 hours after the ingestion [7]. In the study of Jaeger et al, amatoxins were detected in only 28 of the 45 patients studied and never after day 5. Fantozzi et al however found amanitin in the urine up to 20 days after ingestion [9]. The persistence of amatoxins in the body might have some therapeutic implication if an OLT has to be performed.

All studies agree with the fact that there is no correlation between amatoxins concentrations and symptoms or outcome [2, 7].

Management

Supportive Therapy
Immediate and vigorous correction of hypovolemia and rehydration have decreased the mortality during the gastrointestinal phase. If hepatic failure occurs, supportive therapy should also be instituted or maintained. Fluid restriction may be necessary on account of the multiple organ failure (MOF) observed at this stage but a careful monitoring of the blood glucose level is mandatory.

Toxins Removal
Amatoxins kinetics studies provided interesting information with therapeutic implications. First, gastric lavage is useless in most cases because of the delay of admission. Second, gastroduodenal fluid aspiration, previously proposed, removes only a little amount of toxins and is therefore not indicated. Third, oral activated charcoal, repeated every 4 hours for 48 hours, may enhance total body clearance and elimination. Fourth, forced diuresis for 3 to 4 days is probably the most efficient way to eliminate toxins and improve outcome. Finally, since amatoxins are present in the plasma only at the early phase of the poisoning and at low concentration, extracorporeal elimination of amatoxins is ineffective unless if a patient with previous chronic renal failure develops *Amanita* intoxication [2, 5, 7, 8].

Specific Antidotes
Several drugs and antidotes have been tried in the management of anatoxin poisoning. In the absence of control studies, it is difficult to prove the efficacy or the superiority of one of them. However penicillin and silibinin (or silymarin) have apparently some antitoxic effects in vitro and have shown, when used in combination, to improve survival rate [1, 5].

They notably act by inhibiting the liver uptake of amatoxins [5]. A high dose of penicillin G is recommended: 300,000 to 1,000,000 units/kilogram/day divided in 4 intravenous injections. The doses of silibinin are 20 to 50 milligrams/kilogram/day and are administered by slow infusion (2 hours) every 6 hours [5]. Both should be continued for 48 to 96 hours. Other drugs such as thioctic acid, cimetidine, ascorbic acid and N-acetylcysteine have been proposed but cannot be recommended [2, 5, 7].

Hepatic Failure
In acute hepatic failure, supportive measures are essential and increase the chance of survival [10]. If the hepatocellular necrosis is severe, multiple organ failure (MOF) is the rule and death may occur even when the liver has begun to recover [11]. The indications of intracranial pressure and cerebral blood flow monitoring, the therapeutic value of flumazenil and the role of plasma exchange and hemofiltration in children with FHF were recently reviewed by Devictor et al [10].

We reserve infusion of fresh-frozen plasma (FFP) and/or coagulation factors when hemorrhage has occurred, before invasive procedures or when liver transplantation has been decided. Otherwise, this transfusion leads to the loss of an important prognosis indication: coagulation factors value. The nephrotoxicity of each medication (e.g. antibiotics and H_2-receptor blockers) should be evaluated in order to avoid further compromise of the renal function. Mechanical ventilation is frequently necessary and its indication should be anticipated since the progression of hepatic encephalopathy in children is particularly explosive [10]. This should not be forgotten before transferring a young patient to a liver transplant unit.

The indications for intubation and ventilation are in our experience: Glasgow coma scale score less than 9; hepatic encephalopathy of grade 3 or more according to the classification of Bicêtre and Cochin Hospitals [6]; clinical signs of intracranial hypertension; cerebral edema; respiratory or cardiovascular failure; significant gastrointestinal hemorrhage; persistent metabolic or lactic acidosis.

In mushroom poisoning, one can reasonably hope that the toxins removal techniques and the specific antidotes, if both are prescribed early after ingestion, may decrease the risk of acute hepatitis. However, there is no scientific proof in the absence of controlled and prospective clinical trials.

We maintain the toxicological management for 4 days after ingestion. If a liver transplantation has been performed, prolongation of this therapy might be indicated, as discussed below.

If the liver function improves with only a medical treatment, a close follow-up of the liver enzymes is requested since cases of chronic active hepatitis has been described. Fantozzi et al for instance reported a 20% incidence of chronic active hepatitis in 40 survivors of *Amanita phalloides* intoxication. Patients with severe hepatocellular necrosis (SGPT above 2,000 UI/L) had the higher risk [9].

Orthotopic Liver Transplantation

Despite extensive experiences of OLT for patients with FHF, there is no consensus on the indications of OLT. The basic problem is deciding on the right time to transplant, which must be nor too soon, when the patient's hepatic insufficiency may be reversible with conservative measures [12, 13], nor too late, when MOF has already occurred [6, 10]. However that may be, emergency liver transplantation is certainly an effective treatment for children with FHF with a survival rate superior to 70% and may avoid death of otherwise condemned patients [6].

Based on the analysis of the factors that most likely indicate a poor prognosis in *Amanita* poisoning, the following criteria for liver transplantation were proposed in the literature [2, 14, 15, 16]: stage II encephalopathy or beyond, prolongation of prothrombin time greater than two times normal, factor V below 10%, lactic acidosis, hypofibrinogenemia, gastrointestinal bleeding, hypoglycemia, marked elevation in serum aminotransferase levels, serum bilirubin level higher than 25 mg/dl (420 mmol/L), oliguria, age less than 12 years.

However all these criteria do not have the same importance when the decision of an OLT has to be made. In FHF of other etiologies, the three first quoted ones are generally accepted as major criteria [10] but it is unknown if there were of an equal importance in the reported cases of mushroom poisoning. Other criteria are disputed because too late or inconstant. Finally, if age is really a major criteria, almost all children should be transplanted after their admission in a pediatric intensive care unit.

Between August 1989 and August 1991, we admitted 3 children for liver transplantation after *Amanita phalloides* poisoning.

Their hepatic function and outcome are reported in Table 1 (patients 1, 2 and 3). All of them had clinical, biological and electroencephalographic signs of severe hepatocellular necrosis and failure. They were transplanted between day 3 to 5. Two of them died, one from cerebral edema and brain death on day 1 post OLT, the other in MOF on day 77 post OLT. The third one is doing well but it is unknown if a spontaneous recovery should have been possible without a liver transplantation.

In 1991, the experience of OLT for mushroom poisoning was very limited, especially in children [17, 18]. At this time, only two children had been transplanted, one unfortunately with neurological sequelae [17]. Basing ourselves on this short experience, as well as our personal experience in liver transplantation and after reviewing the literature, we decided to define major and minor criteria for OLT after mushroom poisoning. They are reported in Table 2.

Two major criteria or 1 major associated with three minor, present at the same time, are enough to register the patient on a liver transplantation list. These criteria are not very different from those we followed in FHF of other etiologies. They do not include the bilirubin and the renal function previously proposed in mushroom poisoning. The age and the levels of hepatic enzymes are considered as minor criteria.

After these criteria had been established, we admitted three other patients for severe mushroom poisoning between July 1992 and October 1994 (Table 1, patients 4, 5 and 6). None of them fulfilled our criteria for OLT. Patient 6 for instance never had 2 major criteria at the same time, despite a severe hepatic failure. He was in hepatic encephalopathy for 6 days and spontaneously recovered. The two others also recovered without OLT.

This experience is certainly limited but can help us to improve the management of these severely ill patients. Up to now and to our knowledge, 23 patients have been transplanted for liver failure secondary to mushroom poisoning (literature and personal communications) [2, 4, 14, 15, 16, 17, 18, 19, 20, 21, 22]. Eight of them are children, 5 are doing well. The analysis of the available parameters of the hepatic function in the reported cases show that the majority of them fulfilled our suggested criteria.

According to the postoperative evolution of these patients and to some kinetics studies [8], there seems to be no risk for the transplanted liver to be intoxicated by some circulating amatoxins. However, in the study reported by Fantozzi et al [9], amanitin was found in the urine of 4 severely affected patients up to 20 days after ingestion. Likely, in our patient 2 transplanted on day 5,

Table 1. Evaluation of the hepatic function (peak values) and outcome

Patient Nr	Patient age (years)	EEG	PT (normal: 70–110%)	Factor V (normal: 70–110%)	Lactate (normal: <2 mmol/L)	SGPT (normal: 4–32 UI/L)	OLT (day post ingestion)	Evolution
1	7	4	<10	ND	6.0	13850	Yes (day 5)	Brain death Day 1 post OLT
2	4	3–4	12%	ND	6.0	10700	Yes (day 5)	Primary poor function; OLT 2 on day 6; Death from MOF on day 77 post OLT
3	4.5	3	14%	ND	1.9	5100	Yes (day 3)	Doing well
4	5.0	2	26%	ND	1.0	7860	No	Doing well
5	4.0	1	20%	33%	1.4	4000	No	Doing well
6	4.0	3	<10%	5%	4.4	4800	No	Doing well

Abbreviations: EEG = worse encephalogram, classification according to reference 6; *PT* = prothrombin time; *SGPT* = serum alanine aminotransferase; *OLT* = orthotopic liver transplantation; *ND* = not done; *MOF* = multiple organ failure

Table 2. Suggested criteria for olt in children after mushroom poisoning

Major
- Hepatic encephalopathy >Grade 2
- PT <20% and/or factor V <20%
- Serum lactate >2 mmol/L

Minor
- Gastrointestinal hemorrhage
- Hypofibrinogenemia (<100 mg/dl)
- Hypoglycemia
- Age <10 years
- GPT >2000 UI/L

The association of 2 major criteria or 1 major plus 3 minor at the same time indicates the need for an OLT

amanitin was still present 33 days after ingestion. It is unknown if this has contributed to his poor postoperative hepatic function and if penicillin, for instance, has to be maintained after the OLT. It would therefore be very interesting to measure urine amanitin concentration after each future OLT to really be sure that there is no risk for intoxication of the transplanted liver, especially if this transplantation is performed within 5 days post ingestion.

Auxiliary Partial Heterotopic Liver Transplantation

Auxiliary partial heterotopic liver transplantations have been performed in emergency situations with reasonably good results [10, 11]. In the case of FHF secondary to mushroom poisoning, a full recovery of the liver function can be expected once all toxins have been eliminated [3, 12, 13]. The auxiliary liver can be removed and the immunosuppressive therapy stopped.

This technique therefore constitutes a very interesting alternative to OLT. A follow-up of the liver enzymes levels is still necessary because of the risks of chronic active hepatitis of the native liver [9].

Other methods of temporary liver support have been reported [10, 11] but have to be developed before to be routinely proposed.

Conclusion

Acute hepatitis is a common complication after cyclopeptide mushroom poisoning. It may progress to fulminant hepatic failure, despite aggressive supportive care and toxicological management. Emergency OLT may, with the present experience, reasonably be considered. Criteria for OLT are proposed to help the clinician in this difficult decision. Auxiliary partial heterotopic liver transplantation is a promising alternative to OLT in the next future.

Since the progression of hepatic encephalopathy is particularly explosive in children and since the interval between the onset of encephalopathy and death is usually only 4 days [9], it is recommended to transfer children who ingested toxic mushroom to a liver transplant unit as soon as marked hepatocellular necrosis (SGPT > 2,000 UI/L) or dysfunction (prothrombin time or factor V below 50% of normal values) has been found, especially in children less than 10 years old.

References

1. Floersheim GL, Weber O, Tschumi P, Ulbrich M (1982) Clinical death-cap (Amanita phalloides) poisoning: prognostic factors and therapeutic measures. Analysis of 205 cases. Schweiz Med Wschr 112:1164–1177.
2. Klein AS, Hart J, Brems JJ, Goldstein L, Lewin K, Busuttil RW (1989) Amanita poisoning: treatment and the role of liver transplantation. Am J Med 86:187–193.
3. Ramirez P, Parilla P, Sanchez Bueno F, et al (1993) Fulminant hepatic failure after Lepiota mushroom poisoning. J Hepatol 19:51–54.
4. Meunier BC, Camus CM, Houssin DP, Messner MJM, Gerault AM, Launois BG (1995) Liver transplantation after severe poisoning due to amatoxin-containing Lepiota – Report of three cases. Clin Toxicol 33(2):165–171.
5. Floersheim GL (1987) Treatment of human amatoxin mushroom poisoning – Myths and advances in therapy. Med Toxicol 2:1–9.
6. Devictor D., Desplanques L, Debray D et al (1992) Emergency liver transplantation for fulminant liver failure in infants and children. Hepatology 16 (5):1156–1162.
7. Jaeger A, Jehl F, Flesch F, Sauder P, Kopferschmitt J (1993) Kinetics of amatoxins in human poisoning: therapeutic implications. Clin Toxicol 31(1):63–80.
8. Vesconi S, Langer M, Iapichino G, Costantino D, Busi C, Fiume L (1985) Therapy for cytotoxic mushroom intoxication. Crit Care Med 13(5):402–406.
9. Fantozzi R, Ledda F, Caramelli L, et al (1986) Clinical findings and follow-up evaluation of an outbreak of mushroom poisoning: survey of Amanita phalloides poisoning. Klin Wochenschr 64:38–43.
10. Devictor D, Yandza T, Soubrane O (1995) Controversies in managing children with fulminant liver failure. In: Vincent JL (ed) Yearbook of intensive care and emergency medicine. Springer Verlag, Berlin, pp 817–824.
11. Lee WM (1993) Acute liver failure. N Engl J Med 329 (25):1862–1872.
12. Lopez A, Jerez V, Rebollo J, Lombardo AG, Julia JA (1988) Fulminant hepatitis and liver transplantation. Ann Intern Med 108:769.
13. Castiella A, Lopez Dominguez L, Txoperena G, Cosme A, Aramburu V, Arenas JI (1993) Indication de la transplantation du foie en cas d'intoxication par amanite phalloïde. Presse Méd 22 (4):177.
14. Pinson CW, Daya MR, Benner KG, et al (1990) Liver transplantation for severe Amanita phalloides mushroom poisoning. Am J Surg 159:493–499.
15. Pouyet M, Caillon P, Ducerf C, et al (1991) Transplantation orthotopique du foie pour intoxication grave par amanite phalloïde. Presse Med 20:2095–2098.
16. Galler GW, Weisenberg E, Brasitus TA (1992) Mushroom poisoning: the role of liver transplantation. J Clin Gastroenterol 15:229–232.
17. Woodle ES, Moody RR, Cox KL, Cannon RA, Ward RE (1985) Orthotopic liver transplantation in a patient with Amanita poisoning. JAMA 253:69–70.
18. Boudjema K, Wolf P, Burtscher A et al (1989) Hépatite fulminante par intoxication phalloïdienne. Une indication d'allotransplantation hépatique. Presse Med 18:937.
19. Doepel M, Isoniemi H, Salmela K, Penttilä K, Höckerstedt K (1994) Liver transplantation in a patient with Amanita poisoning. Transplant Proc 26 (3):1801–1802.
20. Neumann U, Knoop M, Langrehr JM et al (1995) Graft- vs -host reaction: a severe complication after orthotopic liver transplantation. Zentralbl Chir 120 (6):478–481.

21. Schiodt FV, Ott P, Bondesen S (1995) Poisoning by green and white mushrooms at a special hepatology unit, 1989–1994. Ugeskr Laeger 157 (31):4350–4354.
22. Scheurlen C, Spannbrucker N, Spengler U et al (1994) Amanita phalloides intoxications in a family of russian immigrants. Case reports and review of the literature with a focus on orthotopic liver transplantation. Z Gastroenterol 32 (7):399–404.

Subject Index

Acetyl salicylic acid 371
Active immunization 355
Acute hepatitis 539
- hypoxemic respiratory failure 322
- lung injury 460
- pulmonary hypertensive crises 333
- respiratory distress syndrome (ARDS) 271, 323
- respiratory failure (ARF) 277, 294, 312
Air leak syndrome (ALS) 300
- medical physiology 152
Airflow obstruction 337
Airway epithelium 338
- inflammation 337
- pressure 440
- resistance 339
Albuterol 357
Alcohol dehydrogenase 386
Alfentanil 529
Alpha-tocopherol 56
Alveolar capillary membrane 271
- epithelium 271
Amikacin 402
Aminoglycosides 400, 401
Amiodarone 368
Analgesics 517
Anemia 40
Antenatal diagnosis 369
Antiarrhythmic drugs 368
Antimicrobial therapy 223
Antioxyenzymes 42
Arterial blood gases (ABG) 414
Asphyxia 408
Aspirin 372, 373
Asthma 344, 359

Barbiturates 214
Barotrauma 56, 273, 284, 315
Basal ganglia 187
Beta-adrenergics 349
Beta-$_2$-agonists 341, 349
Betamethasone 66
Blood-brain barrier function 187
Blood pressure monitoring 155
Body water compartment sizes 380
Brain damage 188
- death 499
- injury 46, 175, 206
Bronchial hyperresponsiveness 338
- responsiveness 338
Bronchiolitis 354
Bronchodilators 340, 344, 355
Bronchopulmonary dysplasia (BPD) 36, 53, 302, 332, 345
Bronchospasm 345

Calcium entry blockers 190
Cardiac muscle hypertrophy 67
Cardiac catheterization 459
- surgery 449, 458
Cardiopulmonary bypass (CPB) 294
- resuscitation 187
Cardiovascular dysfunction 221
- function 255
Cefotaxime 404
Ceftazidime 404
Ceftriaxone 404
Cell-cell adhesion 266
Cell migration 266
Cerebral autoregulation 207
- blood flow 187, 211
- edema 187
- energy metabolism 187
- hyperemia 206
- hypertension 210
- hypoperfusion 188
- metabolic rate for oxygen ($CMRO_2$) 189
- metabolism 189
- oxygen delivery 212
- perfusion 187
- - pressure (CPP) 212
- pressure 176
Cessation of treatment 492
Chemotaxis 266
Chimerism 4
Chronic neonatal lung injury 53

- lung disease (CLD) 66, 105, 332, 439
- pulmonary disorders 344
Clearance 376, 377
Clinical pharmacokinetics 376, 400,
- risk index for babies (CRIB) 122, 233
Clonazepam 198
Compliance (C) 422, 440
Computerized tomography (CT) 109, 212
Concussion 208
Congenital adrenal hyperplasia (CAH) 370
- cardiac malformations 453
- cardiovascular anomalies 458
- diaphragmatic hernia (CDH) 90, 100, 300, 326
- heart disease 449
- hypothyroidism 371
- toxoplasmosis 369
Continuous invasive ABG monitoring 415
Contusion 208
Conventional mechanical ventilation (CMV) 302
Convulsion 193
Coronary blood flow 257
Corticoids 349
Corticosteroid 66, 96, 341, 344, 355, 358
Cost-benefit 137
C-Reactive protein (CRP) 222
Cutaneous flexor reflex 513
Cytidylyltransferase (CT) 78
Cytochromes P450 367, 390
Cytokines 3, 176, 230, 239

Decision making 467, 494
Developmental biology 6
- physiology 378, 385, 386
Dexamethasone 66, 371
Diazepam 196
Digoxin 368
Dipyridamole 373
Dobutamine 259
Do-not resuscitate orders (DNR orders) 478 , 498
Dopamine 259
Drug absorption 378
- disposition 378
- distribution 379
- excretion 382
- metabolism 381, 385

Effectiveness 117, 133
Efficiency 117, 133
Endothelial damage 241
Endothelium-derived relaxing factor (EDRF;1) 322
Endotoxin 257
Endotracheal intubation 153
End-tidal carbon dioxide (E_TCO_2) 416, 417
Enterococci 224
Epidural hematoma 209
Epinephrine 259, 341, 357
Epoxide hydrolase 387
Ethics 467, 491
- and the law 471
Euthanasia 483, 493, 499
Excitatory amino acid (EAA) 188
Exercise capacity 453
Exogenous surfactant 75
Expiratory flow-volume loops (FEFV loops) 421
Extracorporeal circulation 459
- CO_2 Removal ($ECCO_2R$) 319
- membrane oxygenation (ECMO) 3, 102, 104, 110, 294, 297, 312, 326

Febrile convulsions 195
Fentanyl 529
Fetal cardiac surgery 462
- diagnosis 365
- dysthyroidism 371
- pharmacology and therapy 365
- supraventricular tachyarrhythmias 368
- therapy 366, 367
- toxoplasmosis 368
Fibronectin 263
Flecainide 368
Flow-volume loops 419
Fluid resuscitation 258
Focal brain ischemia 175
Follow-up 453
Fulminant hepatic failure (FHF) 540
Functional residual capacity (FRC) 443
Free radicals 36, 188
Fresh frozen plasma 226

Gastric acid production 378
- aspirate 222
- emptying 378
Gastric intramucosal pH 235
Gastro-intestinal perforations 67
Gate-control theory of pain 512
Gentamicin 401
Global brain ischemia 175
Glomerular filtration rate (GFR) 382
Glutathione peroxidase (GPx) 56
Granulocyte-colony stimulating factor (G-CSF) 241
Group B streptococci 224

Half-life 376, 377
Halothane 352
Head-injured children 206
Helium (He) 349

- dilution 427
- - technique 443
Hepatic coma 539
Hepatitis failure 539
High-frequency
- flow interruption (HFFI) 289
- jet ventilation (HFJV) 284, 285
- oscillation (HFO) 284, 285
- - ventilation (HFOV) 102
- positive pressure ventilation (HFPPV) 285
- ventilation (HFV) 284, 299, 302, 312
Hydroxyl radical 38
Hyperbilirubinemia 41
Hyperglycemia 68
Hyperoxia 37
Hypoglycemia 197
Hypotension 231
Hypothermia 189
Hypoxanthine-xanthine oxidase 38
Hypoxemic newborns 402
Hypoxia-reoxygenation injury 37
Hypoxic-ischemic brain injury 107
- encephalopathy 108
- injury 188

Immunoglobulins 226, 359
Immunomodulatory treatment 239, 247
Inertia (I) 440
Informed consent 472, 494
Inotropic 259
Inspiratory airway pressures 284
- peak pressures 285
Interleukin-6 (IL-6) 241
Intracranial hypertension 206
- pressure (ICP) 187, 212
Intrahospital transfers 156
Intravenous immunoglobulins (IVIG) 359
- prostacyclin (PgI_2) 325
Intraventricular hemorrhage (IVH) 302
Intrinsic PEEP 275
Ipratropium bromide 349, 350, 357
Irreversible lung disease 320
Ischemia-reperfusion injury 175
Isoproterenol 350

Ketamine 352

Lactic acidosis 230
L-arginine 322
Leukocytes 175
Lipid peroxidation 188
Liquid ventilation 102, 276, 299, 305
Listeria monocytogenes 224
Liver failure 539
Local anesthesia 530
Lorazepam 198
Lung compliance 279
- hypoplasia 326
- volume 440
- - measurements 426

Magnetic resonance imaging (MRI) 109
Mean airway pressure 277, 285
Mechanical ventilation 351
Meconium aspiration syndrome (MAS) 300, 327
Medical technology 467
Meningitis 196
Methemoglobinemia 326
Midazolam 198
Mixed venous SvO_2 416
Molecular biology 1, 461
- genetics 2
Monitoring 151, 413
Monoclonal antibodies 226
Morbidity 104
Morphine 528
Multi-organ system failure (MOSF) 314
Multiple organ dysfunction syndrome 231
Multiple organ failure (MOF) 242, 271
Mushroom poisoning 539
Myocardial depression 256

N-acetyltransferase 388
Necrotizing enterocolitis 36
- tracheobronchitis (NTB) 289
Neonatal pharmacology 375
- pulmonary circulation 11
- respiratory distress syndrome (RDS) 75
- seizures 197
- sepsis 219
Nephrotoxicity 401
Netilmicin 402
Neurobiology of the pain system 509
Neurodevelopmental 71
- outcome 104
Neurological sequelae 71
Neuronal damage 199
- depolarization 187
Nitric oxide (NO) 2, 47, 102, 176, 182, 199, 290, 299, 304, 312, 322
Nitrogen (N_2) washout 429, 443
N-methyl-D-aspartate (NMDA) 188
Nociceptive transmission 511
Non-cardiogenic pulmonary edema 271
Non-invasive monitoring 414
- respiratory monitoring 416
No-reflow phenomenon 176
Norepinephrine 259
Nosocomial infections 227, 233
NO synthase 322

- toxicity 329
Nurse-parent relationships 159
- communication 162
Nursing mutual participation model of care (NMPMC) 159
- research 168

Opioid analgesics 528
Opsonin 266
Orthotopic liver transplantation (OLT) 539
Ototoxicity 401
Outcome 5, 104, 134, 146, 234, 235, 449
- assessment 117
Oxygen 36, 344, 348
- consumption 256
- delivery 256
- paradox 36
- radical disease 36
- radicals 36, 176
- toxicity 315
- utilization 256
Oxygenator 296

Pain 507, 517, 527
- assessment 517
- control 527
- management 508, 517, 528
- pathways 517
- perception 517
- relief 517
Parental participation 165
- stress 159
Parent-child connection 163
- relationship 104
Partial liquid ventilation (PLV) 281, 306
Passive immunization 355
Patent ductus arteriosus 402, 403, 405
Patient controlled analgesia (PCA) 532
PEEP 275
Peak inspiratory pressures 274
Pediatric ECMO programs 316
- risk of mortality (PRISM) 122, 137, 233
Pentobarbital 200
Peptide growth factors 30
Perflubron 305
Perfluorocarbon 272, 328
Perfluorocarbon-associated gas exchange (PAGE) 306
Perfluorooctylbromide 305
Perinatal asphyxia 401, 403, 405
Peripheral pain system 510
Periventricular intraventricular hemorrhage (PIVH) 105
- leucomalacia 105
Permissive hypercarbia 315
Personal health assessment 453
Persistent
- pulmonary hypertension 11
- - - of the newborn (PPHN) 300, 313, 322
Pharmacodynamics 409
Pharmacogenetics 373, 386
Pharmacokinetics 386
- during pregnancy 366
Phenobarbital 196
Phenytoin 197
Phosphatidylcholine (PC) 77, 93
Phosphodiesterase (PDE5) 329
Physician-patient relationship 467
Placental drug transfer 366
Platelet activating factor 178
Positive end-expiration pressure (PEEP) 284
Postnatal death 100
Postoperative heart disease 322
Prenatal exposure to indomethacin 403, 408
Pressure-volume relationship 276
Primary pulmonary hypertension (PPH) 322
PRISM score 147
Procalcitonin 230
Prophylaxis 227
Prostacyclin (PGI_2) 183, 372
Proteases 176
Protein binding 379
- kinase C (PKC) 23
Proteolytic enzymes 188
Pulmonary artery fibroblasts 27
- artery pressure 22
- artery smooth muscle cell (SMC) 11
- complications 75
- edema 271
- function 413
- - testing 439
- - tests 414
- hypertension 304
- hypoplasia 91
- oxygen toxicity 56
- vascular resistance (PVR) 102, 322
- vascular wall cells 11
Pulse oximetry 416
Pyridoxine 198
Pyrimethamine 369

Quality assessment 117
- assurance 117
- of life 104, 117, 452

Reactive oxygen species (ROS) 56
Red man syndrome 407

Renal blood flow 382
Resistance (R) 423, 440
Respiratory distress syndrome (RDS) 300, 322, 330
- failure 264, 413, 414
- mechanics 413, 419
- muscle function 432
- syncytial virus (RSV) 354
Resuscitation 48
Reticuloendothelial system (RES) 263
Retinopathy of prematurity (ROP) 36, 67, 105
Ribavirin 355
RSV-specific IVIG (RSIVIG) 359

Salbutamol 350
Score for neonatal acute physiology (SNAP) 233, 245
Scoring systems 117, 245
Seizures 193, 211
Sepsis 67, 219, 229, 231, 239, 255
- syndrome 239
Septic scoring systems 236
- shock 255, 230, 231, 243, 255, 265
Septicemia 229
Severe acute asthma 344
- sepsis 243
Severity of illness 117, 137, 147, 245
Skull fracture 207
Sodium nitroprusside 330
Spinal fluid 222
Spiramycin 369
Staphylococcus aureus 224
- epidermidis 224
Status epilepticus 193
Steroids 75
Steroid therapy 54
Stress responses 513, 528, 530
Subdural hematoma 210
Sufentanil 529
Sulfadiazine 369
Sulfur hexafluoride washout technique 443
Superoxide radical 38, 176
- dismutases (SODs) 40, 56
Supra-spinal centers 511
Surfactant 102, 271, 299, 328
- protein A (SP-A) 76
- protein B (SP-B) 77
- protein C (SP-C) 77
Systemic availability 376
- bacterial infections 264
- inflammatory response syndrome (SIRS) 3, 231, 239
- vascular resistance (SVR) 255, 325

Technology assessment 5, 456
Terbutaline 350
Theophylline 357
Therapeutic intervention scoring system (TISS) 120
Thiopentone 200
Third generation cephalosporins 400, 404
Thromboxane A_2 372
Thyroid hormone receptor (THR) 93
Thyrotropin-releasing hormone (TRH) 81
Tidal breathing flow-volume loops 419
- volumes 274, 277, 419
Tobramycin 402
Tolazoline 330
Total liquid ventilation (TLV) 305
Transcutaneous CO_2 416
Transforming growth factor βs (TGFβs) 61
Transpulmonary pressures 285
Trauma 149
Tropoelastin 12
- mRNA 18
Tumor necrosis factor (TNF) 257
Type I pneumocytes 63
Type II pneumocytes 63

Valproic acid 196
Vancomycin 400, 407
Vascular permeability 266, 332
- tone 258
Venoarterial 297
Venovenous 297
Ventilation-perfusion mismatch 328
Ventilatory flow 440
Vitamine E 42
Volume of distribution 376
- trauma 273
Volutrauma 315

Withdrawing life-sustaining treatments 480
Withholding and withdrawal of treatment 496
- of a therapy 482

Xanthines 349

MIX
Papier aus verantwortungsvollen Quellen
Paper from responsible sources
FSC® C105338

If you have any concerns about our products,
you can contact us on
ProductSafety@springernature.com

In case Publisher is established outside the EU,
the EU authorized representative is:
Springer Nature Customer Service Center GmbH
Europaplatz 3, 69115 Heidelberg, Germany

Printed by Libri Plureos GmbH
in Hamburg, Germany